Ear, Nose, and Throat Diseases

With Head and Neck Surgery

3rd edition

Founding authors:
Walter Becker, Hans Heinz Naumann, Carl Rudolf Pfaltz

Authors of the 3rd edition:

Hans Behrbohm, MD
Professor and Director
Department of Otorhinolaryngology,
Head and Neck Surgery, Facial Plastic Surgery
Park Hospital Weissensee, Berlin
Medical Faculty, Humboldt University, Berlin
Germany
In cooperation with the Institute of Medical
Development and Further Education Berlin e.V.

Tadeus Nawka, MD
Professor
Department of Audiology and Phoniatrics
Charité Hospital
Berlin, Germany

Oliver Kaschke, MD
Professor and Director
Department of Otorhinolaryngology,
Head and Neck Surgery, Facial Plastic Surgery
St. Gertrauden Hospital, Berlin
Medical Faculty, Humboldt University, Berlin
Germany

Andrew Swift, ChM, FRCS, FRCSEd
Consultant ENT Surgeon
University Hospital Aintree
Liverpool, UK

With a contribution by Thomas Verse, MD
780 illustrations
Foreword by Professor H. Stammberger

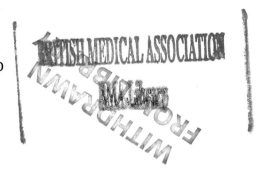
Thieme
Stuttgart · New York

Library of Congress Cataloging-in-Publication Data is available from the publisher.

1st English edition 1989
2nd English edition 1994

1st German edition 1982
2nd German edition 1983
3rd German edition 1986
1st Spanish edition 1986
1st French edition 1986
1st Italian edition 1988
4th German edition 1989
2nd Spanish edition 1992
1st Chinese edition 1995
1st Turkish edition 1996
1st Portuguese edition 1999
1st Polish edition 1999

Illustrator: Katja Dalkowski MD, Buckenhof, Germany

Contributor:
Thomas Verse, MD
Professor and Director
Department of Otorhinolaryngology,
Head and Neck Surgery
Asklepios Hospital Harburg
Hamburg, Germany

Important note: Medicine is an ever-changing science undergoing continual development. Research and clinical experience are continually expanding our knowledge, in particular our knowledge of proper treatment and drug therapy. Insofar as this book mentions any dosage or application, readers may rest assured that the authors, editors, and publishers have made every effort to ensure that such references are in accordance with **the state of knowledge at the time of production of the book.**

Nevertheless, this does not involve, imply, or express any guarantee or responsibility on the part of the publishers in respect to any dosage instructions and forms of applications stated in the book. **Every user is requested to examine carefully** the manufacturers' leaflets accompanying each drug and to check, if necessary in consultation with a physician or specialist, whether the dosage schedules mentioned therein or the contraindications stated by the manufacturers differ from the statements made in the present book. Such examination is particularly important with drugs that are either rarely used or have been newly released on the market. Every dosage schedule or every form of application used is entirely at the user's own risk and responsibility. The authors and publishers request every user to report to the publishers any discrepancies or inaccuracies noticed. If errors in this work are found after publication, errata will be posted at www.thieme.com on the product description page.

© 2009 Georg Thieme Verlag,
Rüdigerstrasse 14, 70469 Stuttgart, Germany
http://www.thieme.de
Thieme New York, 333 Seventh Avenue,
New York, NY 10001, USA
http://www.thieme.com

Cover design: Thieme Publishing Group
Typesetting by primustype Hurler GmbH, Notzingen, Germany
Printed by Gopsons Papers Limited, New Delhi, India

ISBN 978-3-13-671203-0   1 2 3 4 5 6

Foreword

After two decades of ever-increasing subspecialization, it is very encouraging and rewarding to see that otorhinolaryngology, head and neck surgery still can and should be seen as an entity. In the new edition of this marvelous textbook, Professor Hans Behrbohm and his colleagues, who have taken over authorship from Professors Walter Becker, Hans Heinz Naumann, and Carl Rudolf Pfaltz, provide all the anatomical, physiological, diagnostic, and therapeutic evidence for this, should anyone be in doubt.

This brilliantly illustrated textbook addresses advanced medical students and doctors alike, and provides a modern overview of the complexity of our fascinating specialty. As such, it may serve as both a learning and a teaching reference, summarizing our present knowledge of the different aspects of all components contributing to otorhinolaryngology, head and neck surgery.

It adds to the value and beauty of this book that not only the connections between and interdependence of various subspecialties are displayed, but the interdisciplinarity with neighboring specialties is also addressed, e.g., with neurosurgery and neurology for skull base and intracranial structures, with chest medicine specialties for tracheal and pulmonary disorders, or with gastroenterology for disorders of the upper digestive tract.

Thieme Publishers have to be congratulated for providing the plentiful and outstanding colored anatomical and schematic illustrations, in addition to the photographic images. This is a truly international textbook that will be of great benefit to all of its readers!

H. Stammberger, MD, FRCSEd(Hon),
FRCSEng(Hon), FACS(Hon)
Professor and Head
Department of General Otorhinolaryngology,
Head and Neck Surgery
Medical University of Graz
Graz, Austria

Preface

The first edition of *Ear, Nose, and Throat Diseases* was written by Professors Walter Becker (1920–1990), Hans Heinz Naumann (1919–2001), and Carl R. Pfaltz (1922–2003) and published in 1988. Since then, and over several English and German editions, this book has presented the essential knowledge of otorhinolaryngology, head and neck surgery in a concise and highly accessible format. In addition to this, it also provided advanced information to facilitate a better understanding of the diagnostic and therapeutic issues and challenges of the specialty. The scope and didactic presentation of its content made this book attractive to medical students, specialist trainees, residents, interested practitioners and specialists, both as a textbook and reference source. Because of its continuing success, a new edition of *Ear, Nose, and Throat Diseases* was very much in demand, and we are grateful to Thieme Medical Publishers for the opportunity to prepare this new volume.

We have been sensitive to the fact that the book has been important on an international scale and we have strived to maintain this status, recognizing that the range of presenting conditions and their management will vary between various countries.

As a surgical specialty, otorhinolaryngology–head and neck surgery has shown a fast-paced, progressive development with regard to diagnosis and treatment and the increased understanding of pathophysiological principles. It was therefore necessary to restructure some chapters completely and to revise and update the remaining ones in order to bring the new edition up to the present standard of scientific and technical knowledge and practice in this specialty.

As in the previous editions, basic information is presented in normal type; supplementary and advanced information is given in a smaller type.

The figures supplementing the text have received particular attention, as they are immensely important and key to understanding the text. Numerous new drawings have been prepared; all of the existing drawings have been recreated in full color as well as revised and updated where necessary. Visual findings are often the key to diagnosis for the otorhinolaryngologist, so all of the previous clinical photographs have been replaced with new images, and the number of images has been greatly increased.

Our medical illustrator, Ms Katja Dalkowski MD, has made a substantial contribution to the visual appearance of the book, and we would like to express our gratitude for her invaluable assistance and commitment to the project. Our constant contact with Mr Stephan Konnry, our editor at Thieme Medical Publishers, his thorough editorial work and clearing up of many, many details and questions made an extremely valuable and beneficial contribution to the book.

The book project was generously supported by Dr h. c. mult. Sybill Storz, to whom we are extremely grateful. We are also grateful to the patients who were willing to allow photographs of their sometimes serious diseases to be published for the purpose of medical education.

It is our hope that this new edition will continue to be a valuable practical guide to the vast range of otorhinolaryngology, head and neck surgery for its readers—the students of medicine and dental medicine, as well as physicians and surgeons who are either in training or practicing as established specialists in various disciplines within the field.

Hans Behrbohm
Oliver Kaschke
Tadeus Nawka
Andrew Swift

We would like to express our warm thanks here to our former head of department and teacher, H.-J. Gerhardt—now Professor Emeritus at the Department of Otorhinolaryngology at the Charité Hospital in Berlin (where he held the chair from 1973 to 1994)—for providing rare pictures of disease conditions from his image archive.

The *Berlin Diagnostic Workshops* have provided an important stimulus for the work on this book. We have been involved in obtaining and assessing visual and auditory organ findings for more than 10 years and have had the opportunity to discuss these discoveries with many physicians.

Hans Behrbohm
Oliver Kaschke
Tadeus Nawka

Contents

1 Ear

Applied Anatomy and Physiology

■ Embryology

Inner ear. The sensory organs for hearing and balance develop from ectoderm. The *membranous labyrinth* develops from the ectodermal otic placode. *Embryonic mesenchymal tissue* surrounding the *membranous labyrinth* is converted into cartilage and also, by a process of vacuolization, into a fine reticular network that forms the inner layer of the *perilymphatic space.* The outer layer of the cartilage forms the *labyrinthine capsule.*

Middle ear. The eustachian tube and the mucosa of the middle ear arise from a diverticulum of the first pharyngeal pouch (endoderm).

The malleus and incus develop from Meckel cartilage, which emerges from the first branchial arch and is supplied by the trigeminal nerve. The stapes develops from the second branchial arch and is supplied by the facial nerve.

Myxomatous embryonic connective tissue lies between the ectodermal and endodermal ingrowths and makes a preformed middle ear cavity. If this myxomatous tissue does not involute properly after birth, the epitympanic recess remains as a narrow cleft. This is easily occluded by inflammation and creates a predisposition for chronic ear disease to develop.

External ear. The external meatus and the tympanic membrane develop from an ectodermal diverticulum between the first and second branchial arches. Developmental disorders may therefore cause deformities of both the external and middle ears. Bilateral lesions causing severe conductive deafness or a psychologically unacceptable deformity should be corrected, for both esthetic and functional reasons (see pp. 49 and 94) (**Figs. 1.1, 1.2**).

■ Basic Anatomy

The hearing and balance systems consist of the *peripheral receptor apparatus* (i.e., the ear in the strict sense), *neurological pathways,* and *centers in the central nervous system.* Two main subdivisions can therefore be distinguished:

Peripheral part:
- The external, middle, and inner ear.
- Vestibulocochlear nerve with its two parts, the cochlear and the vestibular divisions.

Central part:
- Central auditory pathways.
- Subcortical and cortical auditory centers.
- Central balance mechanism.

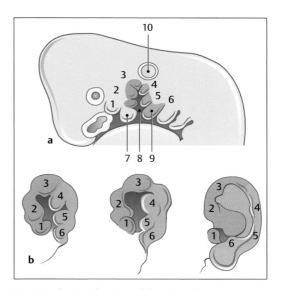

Fig. 1.1a, b Development of the external ear.
a An 11-mm embryo, lateral view.
b Development of the outer ear from six hillocks arising from the first and second branchial arches.
1, Tragus; **2**, crus helicis; **3**, helix; **4**, crus anthelicis; **5**, antihelix; **6**, antitragus; **7**, first branchial arch; **8**, branchial cleft; **9**, second branchial arch; **10**, auricular plate.

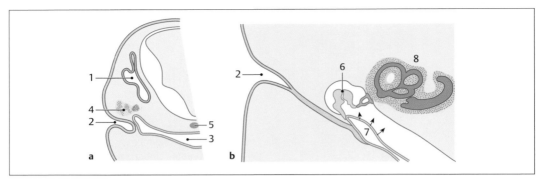

Fig. 1.2a, b Developmental stages of the external auditory canal, middle ear, and labyrinth. The epithelial auditory canal pouch with the tympanic plate opens through epithelial necrolysis (apoptosis) in the seventh month. The mesenchyme of the stapes develops from the second visceral arch; the remaining structures of the middle ear develop from the first visceral arch.

a Approx. 8th week. **1**, Otic vesicle; **2**, primary auditory canal; **3**, tubotympanic recess; **4**, mesenchymal condensation; **5**, acousticofacial ganglion.
b Approx. 7th month. **2**, Primary auditory canal; **6**, primordium of the auditory ossicles; **7** tympanic cavity; **8**, primordium for the labyrinth.

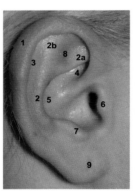

Fig. 1.3   Topography of the external ear structures. **1**, Helix; **2**, antihelix (**a**: inferior crus, **b**: superior crus); **3**, scaphoid fossa; **4**, cymba conchae; **5**, cavum conchae; **6**, tragus; **7**, antitragus; **8**, triangular fossa; **9** earlobe.

The *anatomic boundary* between the *peripheral* and *central* parts is the point of entry of the eighth cranial nerve into the brain stem (the cerebellopontine angle), at which point the peripheral part of the vestibulocochlear nerve passes into the central part, interspersed with glial cells. In functional terms, however, the peripheral neurons end in the primary centers.

■ **External Ear**

The *auricle* consists of a framework of elastic cartilage covered by skin (**Fig. 1.3**), located between the temporomandibular joint anteriorly and the mastoid process posteriorly. The skin adheres tightly to

the perichondrium on the anterior surface, but is more loosely attached posteriorly. For this reason, contusions of the anterior surface often lead to detachment of the skin–perichondrial layer and to the formation of a hematoma (see p. 55).

The *external meatus* is ≈ 3 cm long, consisting of an outer cartilaginous part and an inner bony part. The cartilaginous meatus is curved and lies at an angle to the bony part. The tympanic membrane and the middle ear lying beyond it are thus protected from direct trauma.

> **!**
> **Note:** For an otoscope to be introduced accurately, the curved cartilaginous mobile part of the external auditory meatus has to be drawn upward and posteriorly to bring it into the same axis as the bony part.

The cartilaginous part is attached firmly to the rim of the *bony meatus* by connective tissue. The bony canal is covered by a thin layer of skin that adheres to the periosteum. It contains no accessory structures, in contrast to the cartilaginous part of the meatus, which has numerous hair follicles and ceruminous glands that form wax (epidermis scale, sebaceous matter, pigment) (see p. 55).

The external meatus narrows medially. *Foreign bodies* may therefore become impacted at the junction of the cartilaginous and bony meatus. The meatal cartilage does not form a closed tube, but

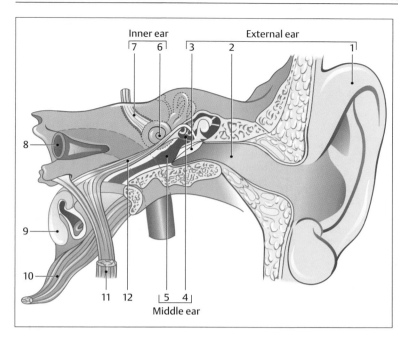

Inner ear   External ear
7   6   3   2   1

8

9

10

11   12   5   4
Middle ear

Fig. 1.4   Overview of the three sections of the ear. *External ear:* **1**, auricle; **2**, external ear canal; **3**, tympanic membrane. *Middle ear:* **4**, tympanic cavity; **5**, eustachian tube. *Inner ear:* **6** & **7**, labyrinth with internal ear canal and vestibulocochlear nerve; **8**, internal carotid artery; **9**, cartilage of eustachian tube; **10**, levator veli palatini muscle; **11**, tensor veli palati muscle; **12**, tensor tympani muscle (Toynbee muscle).

rather a channel closed superiorly by fibrous tissue. The cartilage contains several fissures (Santorini fissures), which provide a pathway for the spread of severe bacterial infection to the parotid space, the infratemporal fossa, and the base of the skull.

The auricle and the cartilaginous meatus have very rich *lymphatic drainage* to an extensive regional lymphatic network consisting of parotid, retroauricular, infra-auricular, and superior deep cervical nodes. Infections of the external meatus with regional lymphadenitis can thus cause extensive swelling in these areas.

The *sensory innervation* is supplied by the trigeminal, great auricular, and vagus nerves and the sensory fibers of the facial nerve. Irritation of the posterior meatal wall stimulates the vagus and induces the cough reflex. Hypoesthesia of the posterosuperior meatal wall occurs with facial nerve impingement from a vestibular schwannoma (see the discussion of Hitselberger sign, p. 13 and **Table 1.13**, p. 94).

Relations (**Fig. 1.4**): The cartilaginous meatus abuts anteriorly onto on the parotid gland, allowing the spread of infection or malignant tumors.

The posterosuperior wall of the bony meatus forms part of the *lateral attic wall* (the partition between the external auditory meatus and the at-

tic), the mastoid antrum, and the adjacent pneumatic system of the mastoid process. A middle ear infection can thus break through into the external auditory meatus, causing swelling of the posterosuperior wall or a fistula in acute mastoiditis. Destruction of the lateral attic wall by *cholesteatoma* may also lead to an open communication between the external auditory meatus and the attic or mastoid antrum. The anterior wall of the bony meatus forms part of the temporomandibular joint. There is therefore a risk of *fracture* resulting from a blow to the chin.

■ Middle Ear and Pneumatic System

The *middle ear cavity* consists of an extensive *pneumatic system* aerated by the eustachian tube. It has the following components:

- Eustachian tube.
- Tympanic cavity.
- Mastoid antrum.

The *eustachian tube* consists of a mobile, cartilaginous portion (two-thirds) suspended from the skull base, and a bony portion (one-third). The bony portion, together with the tensor tympani muscle, forms the musculotubal canal in the temporal bone.

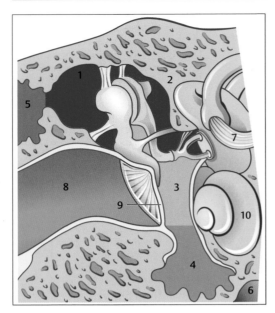

Fig. 1.5 Anatomy of the middle ear cavity. **1** & **2**, Epitympanum; **3**, mesotympanum; **4**, hypotympanum; **5**, mastoid antrum; **6**, internal jugular vein. The lower part of the attic (**2**) is markedly narrowed by the facial nerve (**7**) and the horizontal semicircular canal. **8**, External meatus; **9**, tympanic membrane; **10**, cochlea.

This canal lies adjacent to the internal carotid artery. The funnel-shaped pharyngeal ostium of the cartilaginous part (the torus tubarius) lies in the nasopharynx. The bony end opens into the middle ear.

The junction between the two parts of the tube is very narrow. This *isthmus* is the site of predilection for inflammatory stenosis of the tube. The tube serves to equalize the pressure between the middle ear and the nasopharynx, and thus to equalize the pressure on each side of the tympanic membrane (see pp. 6, 37). An increase in pressure in the tympanic cavity is usually compensated for passively via the eustachian tube to the nasopharynx, whereas a decrease in pressure usually requires active ventilation from the nasopharynx along the tube to the middle ear cavity. The tube opens and closes in response to movements of the neighboring muscles and by differences of air pressure between the nasopharynx and the middle ear cavity that tend to equalize spontaneously. The principal closing mechanism is elastic recoil of the cartilage

of the tube and the valvular action of the pharyngeal ostium of the tube. The tube opens by contraction of the tensor palati and levator palati muscles. The mechanism is partially under the control of voluntary muscle, but the reflex movements on yawning and swallowing and the muscle tone are under autonomic control. Tension opposing the opening muscles is provided by the elastic recoil of the tubal cartilage and the pressure of the peritubal tissues—i. e., the pterygoid muscles, Ostmann's fatty bodies, the venous and lymphatic plexus of the tubal mucosa, and the pterygoid venous plexus.

The *middle ear cavity* is an air-containing space lying between the external ear and the inner ear. It is divided into three parts (**Fig. 1.5**):

- Epitympanic recess or attic.
- Mesotympanum.
- Hypotympanic recess.

There are two narrow zones within the middle ear cleft. Firstly, there is an anatomic constriction between the epitympanum and mesotympanum that can lead to retention of secretions in inflammation and to deficient aeration of the attic. This is due to the considerable narrowing of this area caused by the head of the malleus, the body of the incus, numerous ligaments, nerves (the chorda tympani), and mucosal folds and pockets. This is one of the causes of chronic inflammation of the epitympanum (chronic epitympanitis), which is one of the causative factors for epitympanic cholesteatoma (see p. 68). A second narrow zone lies at the junction of the attic and the mastoid antrum (the aditus ad antrum). This may be blocked by granulation tissue in chronic inflammation, leading to deficient aeration or drainage of the mastoid cell system.

The hypotympanum is closely related to the bulb of the internal jugular vein.

The *tympanic membrane*: The lateral wall of the middle ear cavity is formed by the tympanic membrane. The tympanic membrane consists of the pars tensa and the pars flaccida. The *pars tensa* forms the stiff vibrating surface of the membrane and is attached to a fibrous ring (the *anulus fibrosus*), lying in the tympanic sulcus of the tympanic part of the temporal bone. The *pars flaccida* is the superior part of the membrane in the area of the tympanic notch (Rivinus notch) where the anulus fibrosus ends (**Fig. 1.6a,b**).

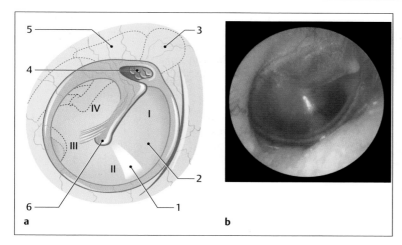

Fig. 1.6a, b **a** The macroscopic appearance of the right tympanic membrane. **1**, Light reflex; **2**, pars tensa; **3**, malleus head; **4**, pars flaccida; **5**, incus; **6**, umbo; **7**, anulus fibrosus. The visible part of the surface of the tympanic membrane is divided into four quadrants, in order of investigation: **I**, anterosuperior; **II**, anteroinferior; **III**, posteroinferior; and **IV**, posterosuperior. **b** The oto-endoscopic appearance of a normal, transparent tympanic membrane. The tympanic ring, the handle of the malleus, and the short process of the malleus are visible. The light reflex is visible in the usual position—starting from the umbo across the anterior inferior quadrant.

The microscopic cross-sectional appearance of the tympanic membrane is shown in **Fig. 1.7**. The epithelial or cuticular layer (the stratum corneum) is similar in structure to the skin of the external auditory meatus. Close to the tympanic annulus is the marginal zone of the tympanic membrane. This section shows extremely active proliferation due to papillary ingrowths into the stratum germinativum. This is another important factor in the genesis of cholesteatoma (see pp. 68–76).

The keratinizing squamous epithelium regenerates through migration of the epidermis from the center of the tympanic membrane to the periphery—in contrast to superficial desquamation, as occurs in normal skin. Migration of the outer epidermal layer forms an important part of the self-cleansing mechanism of the external meatus; this can be observed clinically in the movement of a blood clot from the tympanic membrane to the external meatus.

The *lamina propria* has an external radial layer of fibers and an internal circular layer: this is evident during myringotomy. The anulus fibrosus forms a thickening of the edge of the tympanic membrane and is formed by both layers of fiber. A lamina propria can also be seen in the pars flaccida, but it lacks the characteristic radial and circular structure described above, which provides the normal pars tensa with the necessary functional tension.

The *middle ear*, or *tympanic cavity*, is empty except for air. Only the epitympanic recess contains solid structures—the ossicular chain and the chorda tympani. The ossicular chain consists of three separate bones connecting the lateral and medial wall of the middle ear. The medial wall of the middle ear also forms the lateral wall of the labyrinthine capsule. The malleus is the most lateral of the ossicles. Its inferior portion, or handle, is incorporated into the eardrum, while the superior portion, or head, is located in the anterior portion of the attic. The incus is connected to the head of the malleus by a genuine articulation surrounded by a joint capsule. The long process of the incus ends in the lenticular process, which bends medially to articulate with the head of the stapes. The lenticular process is covered by cartilage to form the incudostapedial joint (**Figs. 1.8, 1.9**).

The *mucosa* that lines the middle ear space consists of stratified cuboidal epithelium, which changes to pseudostratified ciliated epithelium around the mouth of the eustachian tube. A few goblet cells and submucosal glands are normally present. The submucosa is very thin, so that the mucosa lies directly on the periosteum, forming a tightly bound unit called the *mucoperiosteum*. In pathologic conditions such as tubal occlusion or chronic otitis media, the structure of the mucosa changes considerably to show hyperplasia of the glands, proliferation of the goblet cells, edema of the submucosa, vascular buds, and transformation of the flattened cuboidal epithelium to columnar epithelium.

The middle ear mucosa forms several pouches and folds *(Prussak space, Tröltsch pouch)*, which narrow the junction

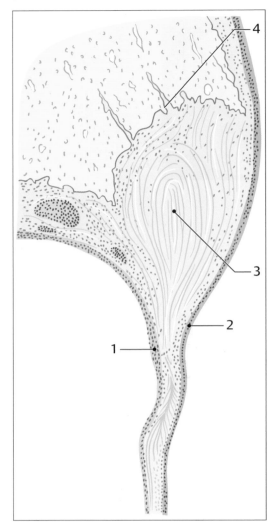

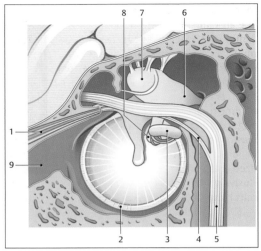

Fig. 1.8 Medial view of the middle ear, with the ossicular chain and facial nerve. **1**, Tensor tympani muscle. The pars tensa is anchored by the anulus fibrosus (**2**) in the bony niche of the tympanic ring. **3**, Stapes footplate. The handle and short process of the malleus lie lateral to the chorda tympani (**4**), as part of the facial nerve (**5**). The long process of the incus forms a joint (**8**) at its lenticular process with the head of the stapes. The body of the incus (**6**) forms the joint surface for the head of the malleus (**7**). The malleus and incus vibrate as one body in the middle part of the frequency range. The middle ear cavity is aerated via the eustachian tube (**9**).

Fig. 1.7 The microscopic appearance of a sagittal section through the posterosuperior quadrant of the tympanic membrane. **1**, Epidermis layer, similar to the meatal skin bordering the tympanic membrane; **2**, middle ear mucosa; **3**, anulus fibrosus; **4**, bony sulcus of the fibrocartilaginous ring.

favors the development of chronic *epitympanitis* and plays a considerable role in the pathogenesis of *chronic otitis media* (see p. 58–61), especially attic cholesteatoma.

The *arterial blood supply* originates from the basilar artery (the labyrinthine artery), the maxillary artery (the middle meningeal and tympanic arteries), and the stylomastoid artery. Venous drainage is via the middle meningeal veins, the venous plexus of the internal carotid artery and pharynx, and venous connections into the bulb of the internal jugular vein.

The *nerve supply* of the mucosa is provided from two sources: the tympanic branch of the glossopharyngeal nerve (cranial nerve IX) and the auriculotemporal branch of the trigeminal nerve (cranial nerve V).

between the attic and the rest of the middle ear and between the attic and the antrum. The epitympanic recess may remain as a narrow cleft with development, and if chronic hyperplastic inflammation follows an infection, the "mesenchyme" can completely obliterate the epitympanum. Ventilation and drainage of the attic is then impeded by thickened masses of inflammatory tissue, despite normal tubal function. Deficient aeration and drainage of this small space

Note: The shared sensory supply of the ear and upper respiratory tract explains why pain is referred to the ear in diseases of the teeth and the jaws, as well as of the larynx and pharynx.

Pneumatic System of the Temporal Bones

The air-containing cells of the mastoid process are continuous with the air in the middle ear. These multiple interconnecting spaces arise from the mastoid antrum, and the extent to which they are pneumatized is extremely variable. On the one hand, *pneumatization* may be well developed, extending to the temporal and occipital bones and the origin of the zygomatic arch. Acute infections of the mastoid may cause inflammatory swellings in these regions. At the other extreme, in a poorly pneumatized mastoid, the mastoid process may consist exclusively of compact bone, with the pneumatized cells lying in the immediate vicinity of the antrum.

The mastoid process begins to develop after birth as a small tuberosity, which is pneumatized synchronously with the growth of the mastoid antrum. In the first year of life it consists of cancellous bone, so that true mastoiditis cannot occur. Between the second and fifth years of life, as pneumatization proceeds, it consists of mixed cancellous and pneumatic bone. Pneumatization is complete between the sixth and twelfth years of life (**Figs. 1.10, 1.11**).

Principle of pneumatization (the concept of biological mucosal competence).
Bone is destroyed by an enzymatic lacunar osteoclastic process. The resulting bony spaces are lined by continuous ingrowth of mucoperiosteum from the antrum. A system of hollow cavities results, consisting of numerous spaces lined by mucosa and communicating with each other.

Normal tubal function is a prerequisite for biologically active, healthy middle ear mucosa, and thus for the normal process of pneumatization. The process of pneumatization can be related to the biological competence of the middle ear mucosa. The mucosa may be described as *biologically normal* or as *inferior*, depending on the degree of pneumatization. *Good pneumatization* indicates biologically competent middle ear mucosa, whereas *restricted pneumatization* indicates biological incompetence of the middle ear mucosa. Biologically incompetent middle ear mucosa may be due to two possible mechanisms—a defective enzyme system that is impairing normal pneumatization, and/or a deficient local immune system in the respiratory mucosa and middle ear mucoperiosteum that predisposes to chronic or recurrent otitis media.

Note: Characteristically, pneumatization of the temporal bone is absent or restricted in chronic otitis media.

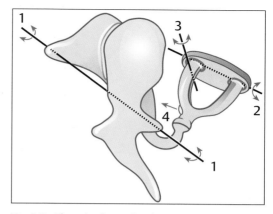

Fig. 1.9 The axis of ossicular chain movement. The malleoincudal joint can turn at a 90° angle according to the position of the footplate (**1**). The footplate itself can move from anterior to posterior (**2**) and in a lateral direction (**3**). The incudostapedial joint (**4**) moves only in a slight lateral bend.

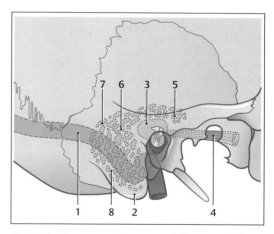

Fig. 1.10 The pneumatic system of the temporal bone. **1**, Transverse sinus; **2**, mastoid process with tip cells; **3**, mastoid antrum; **4**, eustachian tube; **5**, zygomatic cells; **6**, cells of the squamous part of the temporal bone; **7**, sinodural angle; **8**, retrosinus cells.

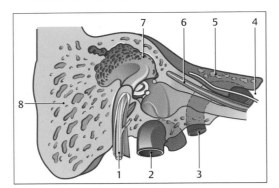

Fig. 1.11 Topographic relationships in the middle ear cavity. **1**, Facial nerve—inflammation and trauma often affect the mastoid segment; **2**, the bulb of the internal jugular vein, which is the site of predilection for extension of a glomus tumor into the middle ear cavity; **3**, the internal carotid artery—in petrositis, the inflammation can extend into the venous plexus around the carotid artery to create a cavernous sinus thrombosis; **4**, cavernous sinus; **5**, apical cells—purulent infection of the cells in petrositis (see p. 80) causes Gradenigo syndrome; **6**, the tensor tympani muscle; **7**, the tegmen tympani, which is the site of predilection for mastoiditis to penetrate into the middle cranial fossa; **8**, the pneumatic system of the mastoid process—purulent infection of the cells causes subperiosteal abscess and sigmoid sinus thrombosis.

The better pneumatized the temporal bone is, the easier it is for infection to break through the thin cortical bone. When there is poor pneumatization (known as a *dangerous mastoid process*), the inflammatory process may be concealed in the depths and lead to unexpected complications.

■ Inner Ear, Peripheral Hearing, and Balance Organs

The inner ear, or labyrinth, is embedded in the temporal bone and is divided into two functionally separate receptor mechanisms:

- The vestibule and semicircular canals (the vestibular end organ).
- The cochlea (the acoustic end organ).

The labyrinth can also be divided morphologically into *bony* and *membranous* parts.

The bony labyrinth. This is formed by the *labyrinthine capsule*, which develops by periosteal and enchondral ossification. In systemic bone diseases (e.g., Paget disease and osteodystrophy) and in localized bone disease (e.g., otosclerosis), the bony labyrinth shows characteristic histopathological and chemical abnormalities. These conditions demonstrate continuous bone remodelling.

The oval and round windows form the bony and membranous openings to the labyrinth from the middle ear cavity, and are closed by the stapes footplate and round window membrane, respectively (see p. 5).

Membranous labyrinth and inner ear fluids (Fig. 1.12a, b). The *membranous labyrinth* develops from the ectodermal otic placode. It encloses a hollow system filled with *endolymph*. This passes via the endolymphatic duct to end in a blind sac, the *endolymphatic sac,* in the posterior cranial fossa. The sac lies in the epidural space on the posterior surface of the petrous pyramid, close to the sigmoid sinus.

The *perilymphatic system* forms a hollow space consisting of the scala tympani and the scala vestibuli. The system communicates directly with the subarachnoid space in the jugular foramen via the cochlear aqueduct. Perilymph separates the membranous labyrinth from the internal layer of the labyrinthine capsule. Perilymph is the immediate substrate of the cochlear and vestibular sensory cells. The origin of perilymph is a matter of controversy; it may form from filtration of perilymphatic capillary blood and/or through diffusion of cerebrospinal fluid.

Endolymph is a filtrate of perilymph that has completely different concentrations of sodium and potassium, which are kept constant by the epithelium of the *stria vascularis* (see **Fig. 1.18a**). The electrolyte composition of the endolymph regulates the volume of the fluid circulating in the endolymphatic system. The basis of the electrolyte exchange system, which maintains a constant ion concentration, is the cellular *potassium–sodium exchange pump* found in the stria vascularis, the utricle, and the saccule. There is also passive diffusion between the endolymphatic and perilymphatic spaces, with potassium–sodium ion exchange in the endolymphatic sac. Functional disturbances of this electrolyte regulation system lead to a disorder of the middle ear known as *Ménière disease* (see p. 97).

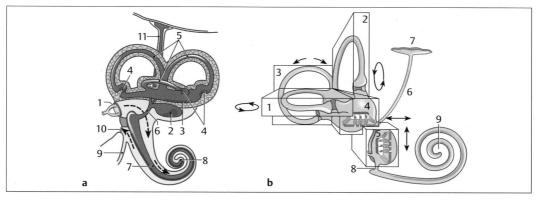

Fig. 1.12a, b **a** The inner ear. **1**, Oval window with stapes; **2**, saccule; **3**, utricle; **4**, ampulla of the semicircular canals, with cupula; **5**, membranous semicircular canals (horizontal, superior, and posterior); **6**, ductus reuniens; **7**, cochlear duct; **8**, helicotrema; **9**, the perilymphatic duct, which passes through the cochlear aqueduct; **10**, round window; **11**, endolymphatic sac on the posterior surface of the pyramid.

b The vestibular apparatus. **1**, Lateral semicircular canal; **2**, vertical semicircular canal; **3**, posterior semicircular canal; **4**, utricle; **5**, saccule; **6**, endolymphatic duct; **7**, endolymphatic sac; **8**, ductus reuniens; **9**, cochlea. Arrows mark the direction of velocity forces.

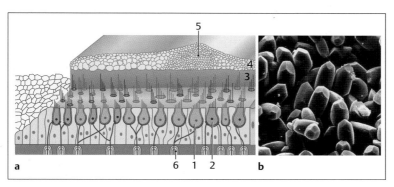

Fig. 1.13a, b **a** Static macula. A change in the polarity of the hair cells occurs below the striola. **1**, type I hair cell; **2**, type II hair cell; **3**, gelatinous layer; **4**, statolith membrane; **5**, statoliths, striola; **6**, afferent nerve fibers.

b Scanning electron-microscopic image of calcium carbonate crystals in the gelatinous layer of the utricle—otoliths.

Vestibular–Semicircular Canal System

The anatomical fine structure of the balance mechanism system is shown in **Figs. 1.13a, 1.14, 1.15**. It consists of the *utricle* and *saccule* enclosing the static *maculae* with the sensory end organs for the reception of linear acceleratory stimulation. These consist of *supporting cells* and *hair cells*, which have *cilia* embedded in a gelatinous mass consisting of sulfomucopolysaccharides. On their surface lie the *otoliths* (or statoconia), which consist of rhomboid calcium carbonate crystals (**Fig. 1.13b**). Linear acceleration changes the otolith pressure, deflecting the sensory hairs. This stimulates the sensory cell by altering the *resting potential.*

The three semicircular canals arise from the utricle and have a pear-shaped expansion at one end called the *pars ampullaris,* enclosing the sensory cells, which are stimulated by angular acceleration (**Fig. 1.16**). The sense organs consist of an *ampullary crest* (crista ampullaris), on which *sensory hair cells* are arranged in such a way that their cilia extend to the *cupula,* which reaches to the roof of the ampulla. The cupula acts as a mobile partition that closes off the pars ampullaris and is relatively impervious to endolymph (**Fig. 1.15**).

Note: The hair cells of the maculae and ampullary crests have similar structural principles. They are mechanoreceptors that respond to tangential bending of their cilia.

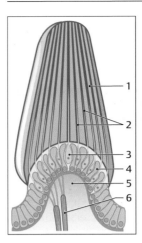

Fig. 1.14 A receptor in the semicircular canal. **1**, Cupula; **2**, cilia; **3**, sensory cells; **4**, supporting cells; **5**, crista ampullaris; **6**, afferent nerve fibers.

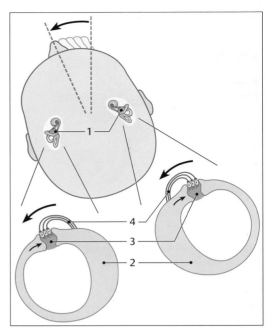

Fig. 1.16 Oscillation of the cupula. When the head is rotated (arrow), the semicircular canals rotate as well. Owing to its viscosity, the endolymph initially remains motionless and directs the cupula in the opposite direction. This causes the cilia to bend. **1**, Labyrinth; **2**, membranous canal of semicircular canal; **3**, cupula; **4**, vestibular nerve.

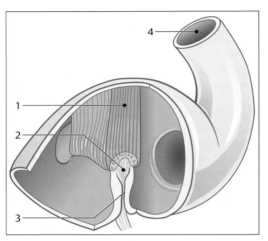

Fig. 1.15 The ampulla of a semicircular canal. **1**, Cupula; **2**, crista ampullaris; **3**, afferent nerve fibers; **4**, membranous semicircular canal.

Cochlea (Acoustic End Organ)

The macroscopic and microscopic structure of the bony and membranous cochlea are shown in **Figs. 1.17a,b, 1.18a–c**.

Functional structure of the organ of Corti. The basilar membrane supports the sensory apparatus of the organ of Corti. It stretches between the bony spiral lamina and the lateral cochlear wall and forms the border to the scala tympani. Surrounded by supporting cells, there are two types of receptor cells: one row of inner and three rows of outer hair cells, totaling ≈ 16 000 sensory cells. The hair cells have fine cilia on their free surfaces, with approximately 80 cilia per cell. So-called *tip links*, ≈ 10 μm thick, extend from the tips of the small cilia to the longer, very fine protein strings. There are ion channels where the tip links connect to the cilia, providing the basis for transduction of the sound stimulus to a receptor potential. Lying on top of the organ of Corti is the gelatinous tectorial membrane. The cilia of the outer hair cells lie below the tectorial membrane, while the cilia of the inner hairs cells do not insert into the tectorial membrane. The hair cells are secondary sensory cells and have no nerve cell processes. They receive fibers from the spiral ganglion. Approximately 90% of the nerve fibers extend to the inner hair cells, and each inner hair cell is connected to many afferent fibers, each of which undividedly connects to an individual hair cell. The remaining 10% of the nerve fibers are widely dendritic and innervate the outer hair cells. There are

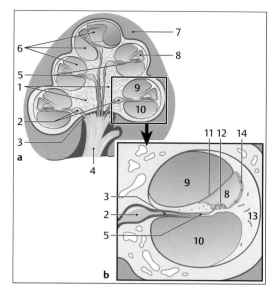

Fig. 1.17a, b Axial cross-section through the cochlea (**a**) and cochlear canal (spiral canal) (**b**). The cochlea is arranged spirally (with two and a half turns) around the central modiolus (**1**) lying horizontally. Its base lies against the lateral end of the internal acoustic meatus, and its apex is directed anterolaterally toward the medial wall of the middle ear. The spiral ganglion—i. e., the ganglion of the cochlear nerve (**2**)—is located within the modiolus, and its nerve fibers (**3**) join to form the stem of the cochlear nerve, the pars cochlearis of the vestibulocochlear nerve (**4**). The osseous spiral lamina or spiral plate (**5**) is a bony plate that runs spirally from the base to the apex (**7**). Nerve fibers pass through the channels of the spiral lamina to the spiral organ of Corti (12). The cochlear duct (scala media) (**b, 8**), filled with endolymph, lies between the scala vestibuli (**9**) above and the scala tympani (**10**) below, both of which contain perilymph (**6**). The osseous spiral lamina (**5**) and the basilar membrane form the separating wall between the scala tympani, on the one hand, and the scala vestibuli and cochlear duct on the other. The Reissner membrane (**11**) separates the scala vestibuli and the cochlear duct. The tectorial membrane (12) covers the sensory cells of the organ of Corti. The stria vascularis (**14**) forms the lateral wall of the cochlear duct and has numerous vessels. This layer of fibrous vascular tissue is the site of production of the endolymph. Laterally, it borders on the spiral ligament of the cochlea (13). The perilymphatic spaces of the cochlea, the scala tympani and scala vestibuli, communicate with each other at the apex of the cochlea (**a, 7**), at the helicotrema, (see **Fig. 1.12a, 8**) and are also connected with the perilymphatic space of the membranous labyrinth of the vestibule, containing both the utricle and the saccule (see **Fig. 1.12a, 2, 3**).

≈ 30 000–40 000 axons that lead from the spiral ganglion to form the vestibulocochlear nerve (**Fig. 1.19**).

> **Note:** The entire frequency spectrum of 18–20 000 Hz is represented in the hair cells of the organ of Corti over the entire basilar membrane. The highest frequencies are localized to the most basal segment of the cochlea and the lowest frequencies near the helicotrema in the apical turn. This arrangement forms the morphologic basis of the "tonotopic" organization of the cochlea—i. e., the point-to-point connection between the sound wave receptors and the signal-converting central neurons of the auditory system.

Central Connections of the Organ of Corti

The cochlear division of the eighth cranial nerve (pars cochlearis) is formed by the bipolar neurons of the spiral cochlear ganglion. It runs through the internal auditory meatus, unites with the vestibular division, crosses the cerebellopontine angle, and enters the brain stem at the lower border of the pons, at which point the central auditory pathway begins (**Fig. 1.20**).

The central auditory radiation incorporates the strict tonotopic arrangement, as does the *auditory cortex*. The cochlea is thus represented unrolled, as it were, from basal turn to the helicotrema. The *auditory cortex* is considerably larger than the area of Heschl's transverse striations, since these represent only the *primary auditory field* (AI) in which the auditory radiation ends. The secondary acoustic field (AII) and the posterior ectosylvian gyrus, like the visual cortex, include secondary integration areas such as the *Wernicke speech center*. Numerous commissural systems allow fibers to be exchanged between the two halves of the brain. These are very important for directional hearing.

Central Connections of the Balance Mechanism

The bipolar neurons of the vestibular ganglion send out their peripheral processes as two divided neural bundles—a superior division to the sensory cells in the macula of the utricle, the lateral and superior semicircular canals; and an inferior division to the posterior semicircular canal and the macula of the saccule (**Fig. 1.21**).

The central processes combine to form the vestibular division of the eighth cranial nerve, which

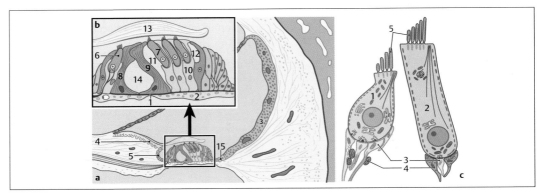

Fig. 1.18a–c **a, b** The cochlear duct (**a**) and spiral organ of Corti (**b**). The spiral organ of Corti (**b**) rests on the basilar membrane (**1, 2**) in the cochlear duct. Medially, at the free edge of the osseous spiral lamina, lies the limbus of the spiral lamina (**4**), with two labia enclosing the internal spiral sulcus (**5**). The highly vascularized stria vascularis (**3**) with intra-epithelial capillaries lies laterally. The spiral organ of Corti (**b**) consists of inner hair cells (**6**) and outer hair cells (**7**) supported by pillar cells (**8, 9**), constituting the borders of the inner tunnel (perilymph or cortilymph, **14**). Between the outer pillars (**9**) and external phalangeal cells of Deiters (**10**), which act as supporting cells for the spiral organ of Corti, lies the Nuel space, with perilymph (**11**). In the extreme lateral position, there is the outer tunnel (**12**), which borders on the external spiral sulcus (**15**) and the stria vascularis (**3**), respectively. Above the hair cells (inner and outer, **6, 7**) is the tectorial membrane (**13**), a gelatinous mass extending from the limbus of the spiral lamina (**4**). The intercellular spaces of the spiral organ (**11, 12, 14**) contain perilymph, also known as cortilymph.
c The ultrastructure of the inner and outer hair cells. **1**, Inner hair cells; **2**, outer hair cells; **3**, afferent nerve endings; **4**, efferent nerve endings; **5**, cilia.

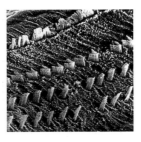

Fig. 1.19 Scanning electron-microscopic image of the spiral organ of Corti, with a view of the surface of the basilar membrane. There are three rows of outer hair cells in the lower part of the picture and one row of inner hair cells in the upper left corner of the picture.

unites in the internal auditory meatus with the cochlear division to form the vestibulocochlear nerve which has a common nerve sheath. The vestibular division sends ascending fibers to the vestibular centers after it has entered the medulla oblongata. The *secondary vestibular pathway* is connected to the spinal cord by the *vestibulospinal tract.* Its fibers end at the spinal intermediate neurons and activate the alpha and gamma motor neurons of the extensor muscles. They are therefore the antagonists of the pyramidal pathway and mainly produce flexor inhibition and activation of extensors. They form part of a phylogenetically old anti-gravity system that serves to maintain balance. In addition, there are important ascending pathways to the cerebellum, the reticular formation (a multisensory integration center), and the centers for the eye muscles (where the oculomotor muscles are coordinated), via the *medial longitudinal bundle.*

A vestibulocortical connection is provided via the thalamus. Vestibular stimulation is projected to a small area in the *ventral postcentral somatosensory region,* near the visual area. This region represents a primary vestibular cortical area.

Note: Connections between the vestibular centers, the centers for the ocular muscles, and the cervical musculature, together with the cerebellum, form the morphologic basis for the extremely precise coordination of the three functional systems. This allows objects to be visually fixed even when the head is moving. Synchronized coordination of the ocular and cervical muscles is controlled through the vestibular apparatus via the gamma neurons.

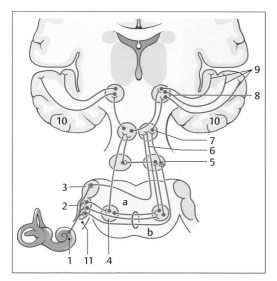

Fig. 1.20 The afferent auditory pathways. For the sake of simplicity, the pathways for only one cochlea are shown. **a**, Direct auditory pathway; **b**, indirect auditory pathway; **1**, cochlea; **2**, ventral cochlear nucleus; **3**, posterior cochlear nucleus; **4**, superior olivary nucleus; **5**, nuclei of the lateral lemniscus; **6**, lateral lemniscus; **7**, inferior colliculus; **8**, medial geniculate body; **9**, acoustic radiation; **10**, auditory cortex; **11**, vestibulocochlear nerve.

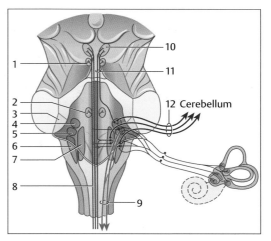

Fig. 1.21 The central vestibular connections in the brain stem. **1**, Trochlear nucleus; **2**, abducent nucleus; **3**, inferior cerebellar peduncle; **4**, superior vestibular nucleus (Bekhterev nucleus); **5**, lateral vestibular nucleus (Deiters nucleus); **6**, inferior vestibular nucleus; **7**, medial vestibular nucleus; **8**, **11**, medial longitudinal bundle; **9**, lateral vestibulospinal tract; **10**, oculomotor nucleus; **12**, vestibulocerebellar nerve fibers.

■ **Facial Nerve**

The seventh cranial nerve carries *motor fibers* for the mimetic muscles of the face, *afferent sensory taste fibers* and *visceroefferent secretory neurons* in a separate nerve bundle, the intermediate nerve. The nerve also contains the sensory fibers that supply the posterior wall of the external auditory meatus. This explains the reduced sensation of this area of skin in patients who have a vestibular schwannoma *(Hitselberger sign)* (**Fig. 1.22**).

The motor fibers originate from the facial motor nucleus in the floor of the fourth ventricle, run round the abducens nucleus (the internal "genu"), and exit at the lower border of the pons, together with the *visceroefferent fibers* of the intermediate nerve arising from the superior salivatory nucleus. The *gustatory fibers* insert into the subcortical taste centers in the nucleus of the solitary tract. All of these branches form the *nervus intermediofacialis,* which runs first in the internal auditory meatus (the meatal segment). It enters the bony canal immediately adjacent to the labyrinth (the labyrin-

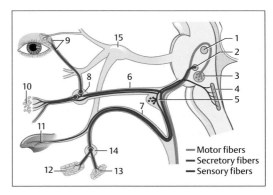

Fig. 1.22 Course of fibers in the facial nerve. **1**, Abducent nucleus; **2**, secretory nucleus of the nervus intermedius; **3**, motor nuclei of the facial nerve; **4**, nucleus of the solitary tract; **5**, geniculate ganglion; **6**, greater superficial petrosal nerve; **7**, chorda tympani; **8**, pterygopalatine ganglion with the lacrimal anastomosis; **9**, lacrimal gland with greater superficial petrosal nerve; **10**, nasal glands; **11**, taste fibers to the anterior two thirds of the tongue; **12**, sublingual gland; **13**, submandibular gland; **14**, submandibular ganglion; **15**, trigeminal ganglion.

thine segment) and runs to the hiatus in the canal for the facial nerve. At this point, the greater superficial petrosal nerve divides off from the main trunk. This branch goes to the lacrimal gland and also supplies fibers to the glands of the nasal mucosa. The first "genu" of the facial nerve lies at the level of the geniculate ganglion. The nerve then turns into the horizontal *tympanic segment* before it passes at the level of the entrance to the mastoid antrum, the second "genu," into the vertical *mastoid segment.* In this area, it branches to the stapedius muscle and the chorda tympani, which contains taste fibers for the anterior two-thirds of the tongue and carries visceroefferent fibers for the sublingual and submandibular glands. After leaving the mastoid process through the stylomastoid foramen, it divides into five extratemporal branches—the temporal, zygomatic, buccal, marginal mandibular, and cervical—to the platysma. These branches are highly variable (see **Fig. 1.114**).

The facial nerve is surrounded by a tough fibrous sheath in its course through the temporal bone. Its individual fascicles are embedded in a well-developed *epineurium* of loose connective tissue that encloses the vessels and nerves. The fiber bundles are enclosed in a *perineurium.* When injuries to the nerve are being repaired, the epineurium has to be resected from the stump, and a perineural suture has to be used so that the site of anastomosis can be adapted precisely, to prevent the formation of a scar tissue neuroma due to connective-tissue infiltration of the anastomosis (see p. 114).

!

Note: Familiarity with the details of the regional anatomy of the facial nerve is a prerequisite for understanding the neurologic diagnosis of facial paralysis (the differential diagnosis of central and peripheral paralyses and the topographic diagnosis of the lesion; see p. 47).

■ Physiology and Pathophysiology of Hearing and Balance

■ Physiology of Hearing: Middle and Internal Ear

The functions of the various parts of the ear are as follows:
- The external and middle ear transport the stimulus.
- The cochlea distributes the stimulus.
- The function of the outer hair cells is mechanoelectric transduction.
- The inner hair cells transform the stimulus.

Stimulus Transport

In the *external auditory meatus,* the resonance effect lowers the hearing threshold to between 2000 and 3000 Hz, the main range of speech frequencies.

The *tympanic membrane* is a sound pressure receptor and transformer.

The *ossicular chain* is responsible for impedance adaptation between the middle ear, in which the medium is air, and the inner ear in a fluid medium, as well as *pressure transformation.* The pressure enhancement is 1 : 17, due to the ratio between the surface of the tympanic membrane and the stapes footplate. The ratio due to the mechanical advantage of the incudomalleolar joint is 1 : 1.3. The total pressure on the stapes footplate is therefore increased 22 times (see **Fig. 1.9**).

The physical movements of molecules that we perceive as sound set the tympanic membrane in motion. The frequency of the motion is the same as that of the vibrations of the air, and its amplitude is proportional. The transmission of sound waves from the air medium to the fluid medium in the perilymphatic and endolymphatic space requires a relative increase in power, due to the increase in density—i. e., impedance adaptation through sound pressure transformation (impedance = acoustic resistance).

For normal transmission of sound to the inner ear, the tympanic membrane has to be in a normal position and have normal mobility, and the air pressure in the outer and middle ears has to be similar. Measuring the impedance at the tympanic membrane can provide information about the functioning of the sound transmission apparatus, and this method—known as *impedance audiometry*—is used for clinical investigations (see p. 36). Sound energy reaches the cochlea firstly via the sound transmission apparatus of the middle ear *(air conduction)* and secondly through the bone of the skull, which is set in motion in a sound field. The sound energy is thus transmitted directly to the cochlea via the labyrinthine capsule *(bone conduction).*

Audiometry is used to measure the hearing threshold for both air and bone conduction (see p. 27).

Stimulus Distribution

The main function of the cochlea is *mechanical frequency analysis,* which depends on its *hydrodynamics.* Periodic movements at the stapes are converted into aperiodic movements to produce a tr eling wave on the basilar membrane (**Fig. 1.23**). Since the inner ear fluids are not compressible, volume displacement at the stapes footplate leads to an equal volume displacement at the round window, and this produces a bulging of the round window membrane that is equal in extent to the depression of the stapes footplate. This volume displacement, produced by *periodic vibrations* of the stapes footplate, leads to displacement of the *cochlear duct* (scala media, Löwenberg scala; the space surrounded by the basilar membrane and Reissner membrane, between the scala vestibuli and scala tympani) (see **Fig. 1.17a,b**). This initial displacement forms a wave motion that proceeds along the partition to the helicotrema. This is an *aperiodic vibration,* or traveling wave. The wavelength becomes shorter as the wave approaches the helicotrema, but the amplitude becomes greater. The amplitude reaches a maximum at one specific point and then immediately begins to fall sharply, before dying away toward the helicotrema. The traveling wave causes a displacement between the tectorial membrane and the basilar membrane at its point of maximal amplitude, so that the cilia of the hair cells are displaced at this point, forming the sensory stimulus for these mechanoreceptors (see **Figs. 1.18c, 1.25b**).

The frequency-dependent development of the maximal amplitude on the traveling wave induces a corresponding *frequency-dependent localized stimulus* on the basilar membrane in the sensory cells of the organ of Corti that lie at the point of maximal amplitude. An initial analysis of the sound is thus achieved in accurately defined frequency stimulus patterns (Békésy's dispersion or traveling wave theory).

The maximum displacement of the traveling wave lies at a different point for each frequency: it is nearer the helicotrema for the lower frequencies and nearer the stapes footplate for the higher. The tonotopic arrangement of the cochlea means that every frequency is thus represented at a particular point on the basilar membrane (**Fig. 1.24**). Since the distribution of the maximal amplitude across the basilar membrane determines the point of excitation of the organ of Corti and thus the activity of the afferent nerve fibers in the cochlear nerve, the traveling wave hypothesis is also a "one-point" hypothesis, as suggested by Helmholtz. Each point on the basilar membrane therefore corresponds to a specific frequency.

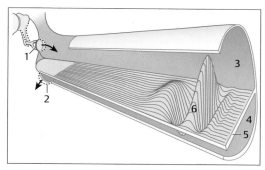

Fig. 1.23 Three-dimensional representation of the vibration of the basilar membrane. The traveling wave runs from the stapes along the basilar membrane, the tectorial membrane, and the Reissner membrane to the apex of the cochlea. The location of the maximum elongation of the basilar membrane is similar to the formation of a frequency-dependent maximum amplitude. **1**, Stapes in the oval window; **2**, round window; **3**, scala vestibuli; **4**, scala tympani; **5**, basilar membrane with spiral organ of Corti; **6**, maximum amplitude of the traveling wave.

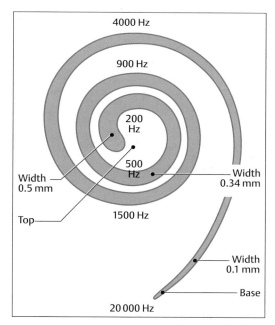

Fig. 1.24 The human basilar membrane, showing the frequency-dependent locations of sound receptors and analyzing receptors.

Mechanoelectric Stimulus Transduction

The cilia of the outer hair cells are bent to the greatest extent when the wave motion approaches the maximum range. A force pushing on the tip links

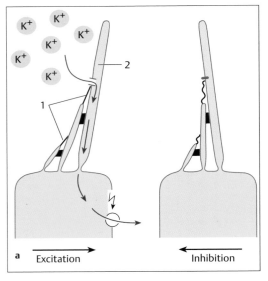

a   Excitation   Inhibition

causes the ion channels to open and changes the receptor potential. The outer hair cells carry out active, oscillating extension and thus locally intensify the travelling wave (**Fig. 1.25a**).

Stimulus Transformation

The actively intensified vibrations of the inner hair cells also cause the cilia of the inner hair cells to bend with the resulting opening of the ion channels. An influx of Ca^{2+} causes a basal discharge of glutamate as a transmitter, and the afferent nerve fibers of the vestibulocochlear nerve are consequently stimulated (**Fig. 1.25b**).

Otoacoustic Emissions

Active contractions of outer hair cells have natural modes of vibration and are subject to distortion. In this phenomenon of normal hearing, sounds emitted by the cochlea occur at certain frequencies as *spontaneous otoacoustic emissions* (SOAEs). *Evoked otoacoustic emissions* (EOAEs) can be recorded in the external auditory canal after induction by external acoustic stimuli (see p. 39).

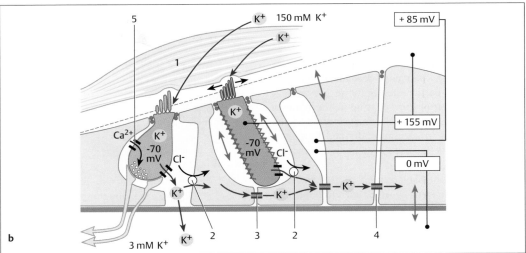

Fig. 1.25a, b   a Depolarization (excitation) of the sensory hair cells by deflection of the cilia (**2**) and opening of stretch-sensitive potassium ion channels. Stretching of the channels is induced by tension to the tip links (**1**). K^+ ions escape the hair cell at the base through stretch-sensitive channels, leading to repolarization of the cells.

b The spiral organ of Corti, showing the electromotility of the outer hair cells acting as a cochlear amplifier. The frequency-dependent length changes in the outer hair cells (blue) vibrate the spiral organ of Corti and thereby stimulate the inner hair cells (red), which are normally not in contact with the tectorial membrane (**1**). The influx of K^+ into the

hair cells is necessary for depolarization. This occurs through the high K^+ concentration of the endolymph and the endocochlear potential (+ 85 mV), which amounts to as much as 155 mV between the hair cell (resting potential –70 mV) and endolymph. Potassium ions leave the cells basolaterally by means of excitation-dependent K^+ channels (**2**) and are led through the cortilymph by means of K^+Cl^- cotransporters (**3**) and nexus channels (**4**) in the support cells into the spiral ligament. Excitation-dependent Ca^{2+} channels (**5**) regulate transmitter release during depolarization through the influx of Ca^{2+} ions.

■ Physiology of Hearing: Retrocochlear Analysis of Acoustic Information

The electrical stimulus pattern of sensory cells in the organ of Corti is converted in the peripheral cochlear neuron into the action potential pattern of the vestibulocochlear nerve. The sound stimulus—which has many parameters, such as frequency, intensity, temporal pattern, and the periodicity of the action potentials—has to be encoded to allow the information to be analyzed in the central nervous system.

Sound frequency and sound intensity coding play a very important role in the central analysis of the acoustic signal.
• *Sound intensity coding* occurs through frequency modulation. With increasing sound intensity, the number of spikes in the sensory cell discharge increases.
• In *sound frequency coding*, specific sensory cell groups in the organ of Corti are stimulated depending on the sound frequency. Tonotopicity (see below) allows these locally circumscribed stimulus patterns, produced on the basilar membrane, to be conducted by the vestibulocochlear nerve to the higher centers without distortion.

Tonotopy is a point-to-point connection between the sound receptors and the neurons analyzing the signal. Each cochlear neuron what is known as a *best frequency*—i. e., it responds only to an acoustic stimulus that has a frequency identical to the frequency assigned to it.

The acoustic system can process the duration, intensity, and frequency parameters of the acoustic signal in the following ways:
• With increasing intensity and constant frequency, the action potential rate in the nerve fibers increases, and the number of stimulated afferent neurons also increases, corresponding to the extent of the deflected area of the basilar membrane.
• At constant intensity and variable frequency, the deflected area of the basilar membrane is displaced into the appropriate segment of the organ of Corti within the cochlea, so that frequency is determined by point analysis. In addition, changes occur in the periodicity of the action potential series within the individual nerve fibers, which are analyzed by means of periodicity

analysis. This provides another means of frequency determination.

Frequency analysis by means of local pattern scanning, *intensity perception* by frequency modulation, and *time-periodicity analysis* by combined evaluation of the time and place pattern also provide information that passes to the higher auditory centers as a result of tonotopicity (**Fig. 1.26a, b**).

■ Pathophysiologic Basis of Hearing Disorders

Conductive or middle ear hearing loss is caused by lesions of the stimulus transport organ. A characteristic symptom of this type of hearing loss is that bone conduction functions better than air conduction. The depression of the hearing threshold for air conduction is associated with an increase in acoustic impedance, as seen with stapes fixation due to otosclerosis.

Sensory hearing loss is caused by lesions in the stimulus transformation organ and/or in the vestibulocochlear nerves, and is therefore better known as *sensorineural hearing loss*. Noise-induced hearing loss and *age-related hearing loss (presbyacusis)* are caused mainly by mechanical overloading of the cochlear amplifier system of the outer and inner hair cells.

Disorders of sound perception are caused by lesions in the subcortical or cortical auditory centers and by pathologic processes involving the central auditory pathway. As a result, the acoustic signals are falsely coded, stimulus patterns are wrongly analyzed, and acoustic information can no longer be integrated. The patient can then hear but not understand.

Central hearing disorders are characterized by a loss of the integrative functions of the auditory centers. Differences in level of tone, differences in loudness, and temporal differences of acoustic stimulus pattern can no longer be analyzed. Redundancy is also reduced—i. e., the information content is reduced due to loss of secondary and tertiary cochlear neurons. These disorders affect the understanding of speech (whereas hearing of pure tones may be preserved), directional hearing, and speech intelligibility.

Recruitment: In certain forms of unilateral sensorineural deafness, the loudness perception rises quickly with increasing loudness intensity, so that despite different hearing thresholds both ears hear

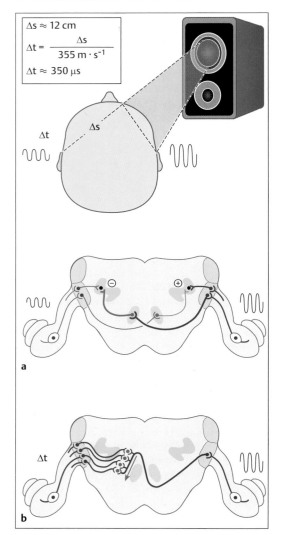

$$\Delta s \approx 12 \text{ cm}$$

$$\Delta t = \frac{\Delta s}{355 \text{ m} \cdot \text{s}^{-1}}$$

$$\Delta t \approx 350 \text{ }\mu s$$

Fig. 1.26a, b Important connections for directional hearing. When level differences are being determined to identify the sound source (**a**), the highly stimulated neurons on the lateral superior olivary nucleus are on the sound side (low inhibition, intense excitation). With the interaural time difference Δt (**b**), simultaneous maximal excitation only takes place in the neurons of the medial superior olivary nucleus on the side turned away from the sound source.

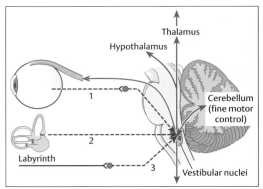

Fig. 1.27 The input and output of the vestibular nuclei. **1**, Visual information; **2**, vestibular information from the semicircular canals and otolith apparatus; **3**, kinesthetic information from the superficial and deep receptors in the skin, muscles, tendon, and joints, which react to pressure and traction forces caused by the force of gravity and inertia; **4**, vestibular nuclei.

cruitment can generally be regarded as a sign of a cochlear lesion, whereas *absent recruitment* indicates a retrocochlear lesion localized to the first or second neuron.

■ **Physiology of the Balance System**

Balance is maintained by coordination of visual kinesthetic and vestibular regulatory mechanisms. These serve for *spatial orientation, upright posture,* and *gait*. Control of all the static and motor muscle groups allows the body to counteract the influence of weight and centrifugal forces (**Fig. 1.27**).

The main functions of the vestibular system are:
- To send information to the central nervous system about the action of linear and angular acceleratory forces.
- Coordination. Movement is coordinated by continuous control of the tone of the skeletal muscles. Information from the vestibular sensory receptors is coordinated and integrated with information from the visual system. Spatial orientation is also ensured.

the tone at the same loudness once a certain threshold is reached. This phenomenon is called recruitment. The pathophysiologic basis for recruitment is loss of the cochlear amplifier mechanism, with abnormal sound processing dynamics of. *Positive re-*

The potential difference between the sensory cells and the extracellular fluid forms the physiologic basis for normal functioning of the vestibular sense organ. A constant discharge of action potentials passes along the vestibular nerve fibers, even

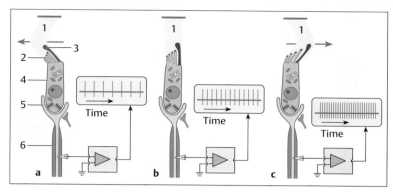

Fig. 1.28a–c The bioelectrical activity of the vestibular sensory cells at rest and in response to stimulation. Bending of the sensory hair cells away from the kinocilium (**a**) causes hyperpolarization and inhibition of the resting activity (**b**). Deflection in the opposite direction, toward the kinocilium (**c**), causes depolarization and an increase in the discharge frequency of the action potential. **1**, Gelatinous layer; **2**, cilia; **3**, kinocilium; **4**, sensory cell; **5**, synapse of the afferent nerve; **6**, afferent nerve fiber.

when the end organs are at rest *(resting activity)*. As in the cochlea, a transduction channel in the vestibular hair cells is opened by a force pushing on the tip links, allowing an influx of ions and causing the receptor potential to change. Depending on the direction of the ciliary deflection of the sensory hair cells, the resting activity is altered by an increase in the discharge frequency *(depolarization)* or by inhibition *(hyperpolarization)* (**Fig. 1.28a–c**). Modulation of resting activity thus allows the body to sense movement both in one direction and also in the opposite direction using a single receptor.

Function of the Otolith Organ: Linear Acceleration Measurement
Linear acceleration is the sensory stimulus for the horizontally orientated macula of the utricle and the vertical macula of the saccule. Shearing forces occur during linear acceleration that shift the otoliths from their base, causing shearing of the hair cells (see **Fig. 1.12b**) and providing an adequate stimulus for the sensory cells. The resulting neuronal impulses release the *maculo-ocular reflex,* producing compensatory eye movements that ensure optimal static positioning of the eyes during linear movement. The *maculospinal reflex* is also evoked, which influences the musculature of the trunk and limbs via the motor anterior horn cells in the spinal cord to ensure that the position of the body remains stable during linear movement. The otolith apparatus also has another important function: due to the continuous effect of gravity, the otoliths exert constant pressure on the underlying sensory cells, even at rest. This pressure influences the resting activity

of these mechanoreceptors. Linear acceleration— e. g., a fall, rapid lowering of the head, air travel, or fast movement in an elevator—changes this resting activity, thus guaranteeing continuous spatial orientation during vertical movement.

Function of the Semicircular Canals: Angular Acceleration Measurement
Positive or negative angular acceleration causes endolymphatic movement within the semicircular canals lying in the plane of the centrifugal force. The stimulus always affects the semicircular canals on both sides; the cupula is displaced toward the utricle on one side *(ampullopetal stimulation)* and in the opposite direction on the other side *(ampullofugal stimulation)*. As a result, resting activity increases in the semicircular canal in which the cupula is deflected in an ampullopetal direction (depolarization effect), whereas activity decreases in the contralateral canal (hyperpolarization effect). This rule applies only to the horizontal canals, since ampullofugal deflection causes depolarization in the vertical semicircular canals. This is the neurophysiologic basis for the stimulating mechanism of the vestibuloocular reflex.

The *vestibuloocular reflex* also serves for spatial orientation. It addition, it assists in stabilizing the retinal image of the visual environment and induces vestibular nystagmus. Every movement of the head causes slow, conjugated movement of the eyes in the opposite direction, to stabilize the field of vision on the retina for as long as possible during the movement. Two modifiable parameters determine the progress of the vestibuloocular reflex: the

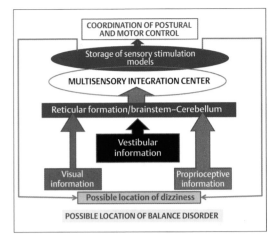

Fig. 1.29 Pathogenesis of disorders of orientation and balance. *Disorders of proprioceptive information:* loss of control over the ability to stand upright and walk straight causes a balance disorder. *Disorders of visual information:* loss of optical control of the visual field occasionally leads to *dizziness* due to a discrepancy between visual and vestibular information, causing disorientation. *Disorders of vestibular information* are due to involvement of the spatial orientation and stabilization of the gaze axis, leading to contradictory vestibular visual and kinesthetic information and *dizziness.* If central compensation of the loss of vestibular function is also absent, there is an additional balance disorder.

position of the head and the position of the eyes. The difference between these is the angle of vision (see **Fig. 1.16**).

> **Note:** The vestibuloocular reflex coordinates the speed of reflex eye movements (the slow component of nystagmus) with the speed of head movement. This ensures clear visual control of the environment during movement. Fast return of the eyes is achieved by a reflex, the fast component of nystagmus.

Conjugated eye movements due to the vestibuloocular reflex, with typical slow and fast components, are classified as vestibular nystagmus (see p. 42).

The intervertebral joints of the cervical spine and the deep muscles of the neck contain mechanoreceptors, which are connected to the reticular formation by afferent fibers and from there to the vestibular and oculomotor centers. The function of these receptors is to provide continuous information about the position and movement of the head and to allow coordination of eye movements through the *cervicoocular pathway.*

The central *vestibular system* includes the cerebellum and the reticular formation of the brain stem—i. e., it is integrated into the centers for multisensory data analysis. This allows multisensory control and coordination of posture, movement, and oculomotor functions.

■ **Pathophysiologic Basis of Functional Vestibular Disorders**

Vestibular disorders become manifest through:
- *Vertigo:* partial or complete loss of spatial orientation—e. g., apparent movement of the environment as a result of spontaneous vestibular nystagmus; and/or
- *Disturbed balance,* with an inability to maintain balance, stand upright, or walk properly (ataxia) (**Fig. 1.29**).

Vestibular disorders may be *peripheral,* caused by sudden unilateral failure of one labyrinth, or by a unilateral lesion of the vestibular nerve. They may also be *central,* caused by a lesion in the vestibular centers or their central connections to the cerebellum and reticular formation.

Every functional disturbance in a vestibular end organ causes unequal activity in the higher vestibular centers. This central imbalance initially produces a disturbance of vestibular information. The multisensory spatial orientation is therefore no longer capable of functioning, since vestibular information on the one hand and visual somatosensory information on the other hand contradict each other. This causes a disturbance of orientation, which in turn causes dizziness. If the central imbalance in the two vestibular centers influences the main neighboring coordination centers for eye movements in the reticular formation of the brain stem, spontaneous abnormal eye movements occur that have the characteristics of nystagmus (**Fig. 1.30**).

Peripheral functional failure is compensated centrally by adjustment of the difference in neuronal activity in the vestibular centers and by substitution of visual and somatosensory regulatory mechanisms for the loss of peripheral vestibular function. This process is called *central vestibular compensation.* Central vestibular disorders are only incompletely compensated by the above mechanisms (or not at all), since the multisensory connections to the vestibular centers are damaged.

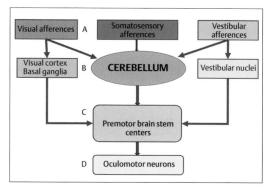

Fig. 1.30 Oculomotor system. All three sensory systems (**A**) send afferent signals via relay stations (**B**) in the premotor centers of the reticular formation of the brain stem (**C**). The motor neurons (**D**) that innervate the eye muscles begin at this point. The cerebellum is the key to coordination: visual, somatosensory, and vestibular signals are continually being compared with one another. If this structure receives contradictory information that could lead to disorientation and dizziness, the vestibular signal is modified or, if necessary, completely suppressed.

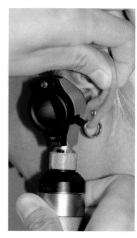

Fig. 1.31 Otoscopy with an illuminated otoscope, which consists of a disposable ear speculum, a light source, and a magnification attachment.

Methods of Investigation

- ## Inspection, Palpation, Otoscopy, Microscopy

- ### Inspection of the External Ear

The physician should look for redness, swelling, ulceration, tumors, malformations, fistula, or retroauricular scars.

Palpation

The mastoid process should be palpated with both hands to search for swelling and for sensitivity to pressure on the surface of the mastoid process and at its apex. The auricle is examined for pain when pressure is applied to the tragus or when the auricle is pulled. Finally, the regional lymph nodes in the preauricular and postauricular areas and the upper deep cervical chain are examined.

Otoscopy

The external auditory meatus and the tympanic membrane are examined, and if a perforation is present, the middle ear is also examined.

Indirect illumination with a head mirror is a difficult method of investigation for the nonspecialist, as correct adjustment of the light source and head mirror require time and practice, especially when patients are being examined in bed (see **Fig. 2.16**).

The electrical *otoscope* is more widely used, as it is easier to handle. It consists of a combination of an interchangeable *ear speculum* with a small, but strong, built-in low-voltage *light source* and a *magnification attachment* providing a magnification of 1.5–2 × (**Fig. 1.31**).

The *otomicroscope* provides a magnification of 6–12 × and is indispensable for accurate examination of the meatus, tympanic membrane, and parts of the middle ear in cases of perforation.

The *oto-endoscope* provides a wide-angled and magnified view over the tympanic membrane, allowing complete investigation of the anulus and anterior tympanomeatal angle. Rigid scopes with 0° and 30° views are used.

Technique of otoscopy. The cartilaginous part of the external meatus is stretched by pulling the auricle upward and backward. The speculum is then introduced into the long axis of the bony meatus. The instrument is held with one hand, so that the other hand remains free for handling instruments such as cotton-wool probes, hooks, an aspirator, and aural forceps (**Fig. 1.32**). The speculum has to be introduced carefully, and the end of it should not be moved abruptly, as its opening has relatively sharp edges. The wall of the bony meatus is particularly sensitive and easy to injure, and contact with it should therefore be avoided.

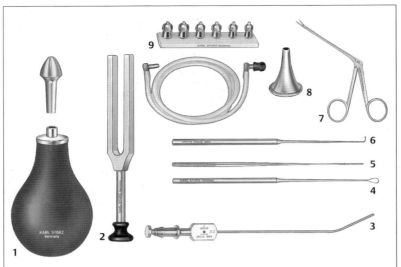

Fig. 1.32 Important ear instruments. **1**, Politzer bag with olive; **2**, tuning fork; **3**, suction tube; **4**, curette; **5**, driller for cotton pads; **6**, hook; **7**, microforceps; **8**, ear speculum; **9**, hearing tube with olives (of various sizes).

In *infants* and *young children,* the auricle is pulled downward and backward to allow the speculum to be introduced. The short cartilaginous part of the external meatus is reduced to a cleft, which can only be entered with a narrow speculum with a small lumen, making otoscopy difficult. The head has to be immobilized, either by an assistant or using a headrest on the patient's chair, to prevent unnecessary movements that can cause pain.

Wax and other material obstructing the view into the external auditory meatus has to be removed using the following methods:

- By syringing for foreign bodies, wax, and exudate.
- With the hook or curette, for hard wax.
- With the aural aspirator, for exudate or fluid wax.
- With a cotton-wool probe for exudate.

The ear is syringed with tap water at body temperature. Hard wax is softened beforehand with softening drops such as 3% hydrogen peroxide, 5% sodium bicarbonate, soft soap, olive oil, or a commercial preparation.

Note: Syringing the ear is contraindicated in:
- Dry perforations of the tympanic membrane
- Fresh injuries to the tympanic membrane and meatus
- Longitudinal and transverse fractures of the petrous pyramid, with meatal trauma

It is important to obtain a history of any previous perforation, as syringing may rupture a thin scar. In the United States, failure to take a history can result in a malpractice suit.

Mistakes to be avoided:

- A speculum that is too narrow and that penetrates too deeply into the sensitive bony meatus.
- Introducing the speculum in the wrong direction—e. g., from above downward.
- Not introducing the speculum far enough, causing its opening to be blocked by otic hairs.
- Unsatisfactory cleaning of the external meatus, so that a proper view of the tympanic membrane is not obtained.

Otomicroscopy. This is performed with a speculum under the operating microscope, with a magnification of 6–40×, in all cases in which routine otoscopic examination does not allow reliable assessment of the tympanic membrane (**Fig. 1.33**).

Oto-endoscopy. This is performed with a tele-otoscope (0° and 30° view). This allows examination of the whole tympanic membrane, meatus, and anulus, as well as assessment of perforations and pockets in the tympanic membrane, and anterior angles and open cavities after surgery (**Fig. 1.34**).

Normal Otoscopic Appearance

Characteristics of the tympanic membrane: The pars tensa is grayish-yellow. The cutis layer is often slightly injected. The surface is smooth and without any relieving features, apart from the handle of the malleus. The membrane is moderately translucent and is only transparent in scarred areas. A tympanic membrane showing the properties described above is described as *normal.* The mobility of the tympanic membrane can be assessed using a pneumatic otoscope (**Fig. 1.35**).

The tympanic membrane is moved back and forth with positive and negative pressure while it is in the field of vision. Atrophic parts flutter, and the movement of the pars tensa may be limited by scar tissue. In the presence of a perforation, the remnants of the tympanic membrane are completely immobile.

Appearance of a Pathologic Tympanic Membrane

- Injection of the vessels and inflammation are seen in otitis externa (occasionally), myringitis, and otitis media.
- Hemorrhage is red if fresh, or brownish if old. Blood vesicles are seen in influenzal otitis, and the hemotympanum is dark blue.
- Serous exudate: A fluid level can be seen, and there are air bubbles in the fluid. The tympanic membrane looks like oiled silk when there is a complete middle ear effusion. A blue tympanic membrane or "blue drum" is seen in advanced stages.
- Retraction of the tympanic membrane as a result of decreased pressure in the middle ear: The short process of the malleus protrudes externally, and there is displacement of the manubrium of the malleus posteriorly and superiorly, causing an apparent shortening of the malleus handle. The triangular light reflex is fragmented, or disappears entirely.
- Bulging due to the formation of exudate behind the tympanic membrane, at times with an irregular surface, which may be papillary, with an opaque surface.
- Atrophy of the tympanic membrane with retraction pockets results from chronic inflammation and reduced pressure. The site of predilection is the posterosuperior quadrant.
- Thickening of the tympanic membrane, as a result of degenerative changes or as the result of inflammation, produces a surface that is dark and lacking in luster.

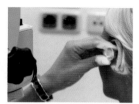

Fig. 1.33 Ear microscopy: variable magnification between 6 × and 12 ×, with a focused light supply.

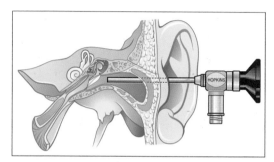

Fig. 1.34 A rigid telescope with a straight or 30° angled view and a diameter of 2.7–4.0 mm is used for oto-endoscopy. The external meatus should be stretched by pulling the auricle upward and backward, as in other otoscopy procedures.

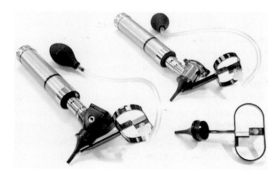

Fig. 1.35 Pneumatic otoscope with loupe (Welch Allyn, Skaneateles Falls, New York, USA).

- Scars of the tympanic membrane: These may be thickened areas, with or without calcium deposits or atrophic areas.
- Tympanic membrane perforations: These may be either central or peripheral, mesotympanic or epitympanic. Central or mesotympanic defects are the result of chronic mucosal inflammation (see p. 67), whereas peripheral or epitympanic perforations are usually associated with a cholesteatoma (p. 68).

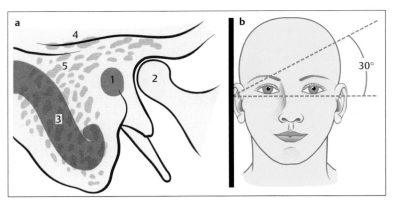

Fig. 1.36a, b Radiographs in the Schüller view. **1,** The external and internal meatus superimposed; **2,** the head of the mandible; **3,** the sigmoid sinus; **4,** the border to the middle cranial fossa; **5,** the sinodural angle.

Note: A tympanic membrane that has a surface with an opaque and dull appearance—as a result of inflammatory infiltration of the pars tensa, with hyperemia, edema, formation of bullae, desquamation of the epidermal layer, and distortion of the characteristic appearance of the handle of the malleus—is designated as abnormal or pathologic.

■ Diagnostic Imaging

The position in regional anatomy of the petrosal bone inside the skull base generates overlapping artifacts during radiographic examinations. Special radiographic images of the temporal bone, or of both sides for comparison, are therefore essential.

Conventional imaging of the petrosal bone using the Stenvers and Schüller techniques has now to a large extent been replaced by computed tomography (CT). In selected cases, however, the Schüller radiographic view is still valuable for clinical evidence.

■ Conventional Radiography

Schüller technique: This provides information about the degree of mastoid pneumatization and demonstrates the intercellular space and septal bone, the course of the sigmoid sinus, the tympanic roof (tegmen tympani), and the maxillary joint. These images are useful for diagnosing otitis media, mastoiditis, and fractures of the petrosal bone (**Fig. 1.36a, b**).

Stenvers technique: Demonstration of the inner auditory canal, and the width of the canal in particular. The horizontal and superior arches of the equilibrium/vestibular organ, as well as the petrosal apex, are also well displayed. These images are useful in cases of acoustic neuroma, destructive processes in the internal ear, and transverse fractures of the petrosal bone (**Fig. 1.37a–c**).

■ Computed Tomography

High-resolution CT images of the petrosal bone in axial and coronal views, with slice thicknesses of 1 and 2 mm, have largely replaced conventional radiographic imaging in image-guided diagnosis. In addition to clear depiction of anatomical structures, CT images precisely show inflammatory changes such as soft-tissue enlargement (mucosal swelling, cholesteatoma, or tumor masses) and fluid retention, as well as osseous destruction or fractures (**Fig. 1.38a, b**). A new CT technique known as *multislice spiral CT* also allows three-dimensional interpretation of the middle and inner ear structures.

■ Angiography

The following supplementary *neuroradiologic investigations* are indicated for suspected vascular neoplasms or space-occupying lesions in the middle or posterior cranial fossa and cerebellopontine angle (CPA):
• Carotid angiography.
• Vertebral angiography.

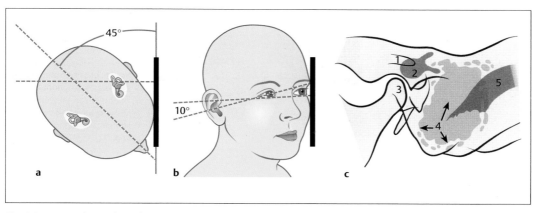

Fig. 1.37a–c Radiographs in the Stenver view. **1,** Internal auditory meatus; **2,** vestibule, with the superior and horizontal semicircular canals; **3,** mandibular condyle; **4,** pneumatic system; **5,** sigmoid sinus.

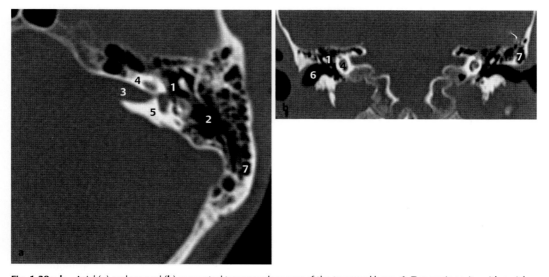

Fig. 1.38a, b Axial (**a**) and coronal (**b**) computed tomography scans of the temporal bone. **1,** Tympanic cavity with ossicles; **2,** antrum; **3,** internal acoustic canal; **4,** cochlea; **5,** labyrinth; **6,** external acoustic canal; **7,** pneumatized mastoid cells.

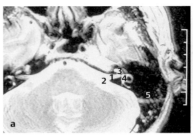 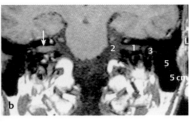

Fig. 1.39a, b Axial (**a**) and coronal (**b**) magnetic resonance images of the temporal bone area. **1**, vestibulocochlear nerve in the internal acoustic canal; **2** cerebellopontine angle (CPA); **3**, cochlea; **4**, labyrinth; **5**, pneumatized mastoid. The arrow in **b** shows an intrameatal vestibular schwannoma (see p. 92).

■ Magnetic Resonance Imaging

Magnetic resonance imaging (MRI) is an optimal method for detecting inflammatory, traumatic, or neoplastic pathology in the temporal bone and skull base. It is routinely used with T1-weighted and T2-weighted spin-echo sequences, producing thin-slice images, sometimes with contrast administration (gadolinium diethylenetriamine pentaacetic acid, Gd-DTPA). Very small vestibular neuromas in particular (acoustic neuromas) can be optimally visualized (**Fig. 1.39a, b**). The enhanced soft-tissue display is very helpful for assessing the extent of any neoplasms, complementing CT images.

Using high-resolution T2-weighted sequences such as the *constructive interference in steady state* (CISS) sequence—a three-dimensional magnetic resonance sequence that displays cerebrospinal fluid spaces—even details of the membranous labyrinth and neuronal structures of the inner ear canal and cerebellopontine angle become visible. The *volume-rendering* technique can even produce three-dimensional images of the entire inner ear, as well as of the topological relationships in the entire temporal bone. In addition, it provides virtual endoscopic visualization of the inner ear region.

Views can be taken in all three planes without secondary reconstruction using a computer and without the need for special positioning of the patient. Pathologic formations (e. g., tumors, ischemic lesions) can be differentiated from normal structures using contrast administration (Gd-DTPA). Other specific MRI techniques include *functional MRI* (f-MRI), which makes localized perfusion changes in the brain visible, and *magnetic resonance angiography*, which can reveal intracranial tumors (glomus tumors) and vascular structures.

■ **Functional Assessment of the Eustachian Tube**

Tests of tubal function are always necessary in all patients with middle ear hearing loss, particularly before an operation to improve hearing.

■ Qualitative Assessment of Tubal Function

Valsalva test. This test is used to demonstrate normal tubal patency without the need for any external aids. Failure of the test does not prove pathologic occlusion of the tube, but further functional tests may be required.

After taking a deep breath, the patient pinches his nose and closes his mouth in an attempt to blow air into his ears.

Otoscopy shows bulging of the tympanic membrane, and auscultation reveals crackling.

> **Note:** In patients with infection of the nose and nasopharynx, inflation of air involves a risk of transmitting infected secretions into the middle ear, causing tubogenic otitis media. In patients with an atrophic scar of the pars tensa, rupture of the tympanic membrane is also possible, especially during air insufflation or catheterization of the tube.

Toynbee test. This test is used to confirm normal tubal air patency with a simple and safe method. During swallowing, pressure in the middle ear falls if the nose is closed off. This can be seen on otoscopy as a drawing-in of the tympanic membrane.

Hearing Investigations

Testing Hearing without an Audiometer

Hearing Threshold for Whispered Voice and Conversational Speech

Two-syllable words are articulated at a decreasing distance from the patient until the test words can be correctly repeated. The distance is recorded in meters. Alternatively, the examiner can say numbers or words at a fixed distance with decreasing loudness. When severe unilateral deafness is being assessed, and also when the hearing distance for conversational speech is being measured, it is necessary to mask the contralateral ear. Each ear is tested separately, with the better ear being tested first. The contralateral ear canal is closed with a finger.

Requirements:
- A sufficiently large, quiet room (6 m long).
- Good acoustic properties (no smooth walls with distorting echoes).

Tuning Fork Tests

A C^1 fork with a frequency of 512 Hz is used.

Weber test. This test is based on binaural comparison of bone conduction. The tuning fork is placed in the center of the skull at the hairline. A patient with normal hearing or with symmetrical hearing loss localizes the tone either in the center of the head or equally in both ears. A patient with unilateral conductive hearing loss (middle ear) localizes the tone in the affected ear, whereas a patient with unilateral inner ear deafness localizes the sound in the healthy ear.

Theoretical explanations:
- In middle ear disorders, the mobility of the ossicular chain is reduced and it thus transmits less sound energy than it does in normal physiologic conditions (Mach's sound wastage theory).
- Pathologic processes in the middle ear cause an increase in the mass of the sound conduction apparatus, so that increased forces are exerted at the oval window, due to inertia. This leads to greater stimulation of the inner ear (inertia theory) (**Fig. 1.40a–c**).

Rinne test. This test is based on monaural comparison of air conduction with bone conduction. If air conduction is better than bone conduction, Rinne's test is *positive.* This is the finding in normal hearing or sensorineural hearing loss (inner ear). If bone conduction is better than air conduction, Rinne's test is *negative.* This is found in conductive or middle ear hearing loss.

The patient is asked whether the tuning fork placed in front of the ear is heard better than when it is placed behind the ear, on the mastoid process, without striking it again. If the patient cannot decide with certainty, the decay period of the tuning fork should be determined precisely for both air and bone conduction separately (**Fig. 1.41a–c**).

Gellé test. This can be used to test the mobility of the ossicular chain in cases of otosclerosis (see p. 81) and fixation of the incus. The test has now been replaced by impedance audiometry (see p. 36) (**Fig. 1.42a, b**).

> **Note:** Assessment of the hearing distance for whispered and conversational speech, along with tuning fork tests, provides valuable information about the site of a hearing disorder. These tests are still the basic diagnostic methods in otologic examinations (**Table 1.1**).

Audiometry: Fundamental Physical and Acoustic Concepts

See **Tables 1.2, 1.3, 1.4, 1.5, 1.6, 1.7.**

Pure-tone Audiometry

An *audiometer* is an electric tone generator used to determine the hearing threshold for pure tones—i.e., tones free of harmonics within a frequency range from 125 to 12 000 Hz.

The *hearing threshold* is measured for both air and bone conduction in decibel steps. The *normal hearing threshold is* indicated by a straight line at 0 dB. Hearing loss is measured in decibels relative to this threshold for all frequencies and is recorded on an audiogram (**Fig. 1.43**).

The decibel (dB) is a relative value that compares one sound pressure to another. The reference point in audiometry is the human hearing threshold of 1000 Hz. The sound pressure necessary to produce the subjective impression of hearing at a threshold of 1000 Hz is 20 µPa (2×10^{-4} µbar) (see **Table 1.3**). This is the average value for young individuals with normal hearing and is the reference point for the physical or absolute measurement of the hearing threshold

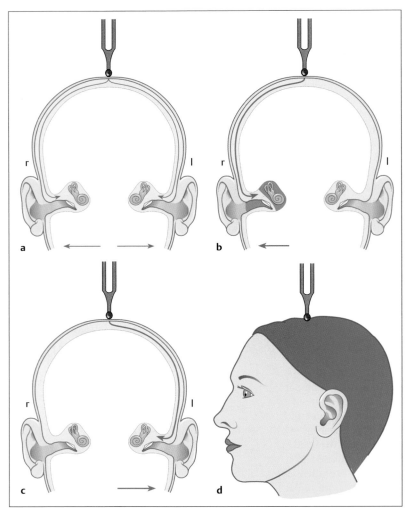

Fig. 1.40a–d The Weber test. A vibrating tuning fork is placed on the midline of the skull.
a Equal loudness perceived in both ears means symmetrical hearing.
b Lateralization of sound to the affected ear (right) is present in cases of conductive hearing loss.
c In cases of sensorineural hearing loss, the sound is lateralized to the better ear (left).
d Correct orientation of the tuning fork.

in decibels (sound pressure level, SPL). The *relative hearing threshold* for pure tones is a simpler method of demonstrating and describing the hearing threshold. The reference point is no longer the absolute sound pressure, but the just-audible threshold of hearing, measured in dB (hearing level, HL). This makes it possible to use a coordinate system with a horizontal zero line. The *absolute hearing threshold* is curved in comparison with the relative hearing threshold. The reason for this is that greater sound pressure is needed at high and low tones to produce a similar sensation of sound near the threshold than for the central part of the frequency range around 1000 Hz (see **Fig. 1.44**).

A disorder of sound conduction can be identified by assessing the difference between the hearing threshold for air and bone conduction, in the same way as with tuning fork tests.

Relationship between Air Conduction and Bone Conduction

Normal conduction of sound to the inner ear via the sound-conducting apparatus is defined as *air conduction* (conduction via earphones). Sound is also conducted via the bones of the skull to the inner ear, either via the middle ear (*osteotympanic* or *craniotympanic bone conduction*) or by direct transmission via the labyrinthine capsule (*osteal* or *cranial bone conduction*) (conduction via a vibrator).

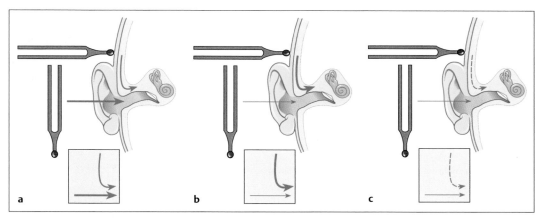

Fig. 1.41a–c The Rinne test. Air and bone conduction are compared in the same ear.
a Rinne positive, normally hearing ear. Air conduction is perceived louder or longer than bone conduction in the test ear.

b Rinne negative, conductive hearing loss. Bone conduction is perceived louder or longer than air conduction.
c Rinne positive, sensorineural hearing loss. Air conduction is perceived louder or longer than bone conduction, but the duration is shorter than in normal hearing.

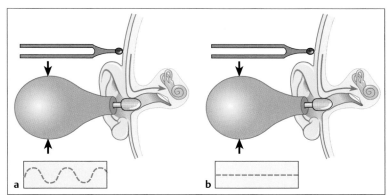

Fig. 1.42a, b The Gellé test. A fixed ossicular chain causes conductive hearing loss.
a Compression of the Politzer bag induces fluctuations of loudness in the normal ear.
b The fluctuations are absent when the ossicular chain is immobile.

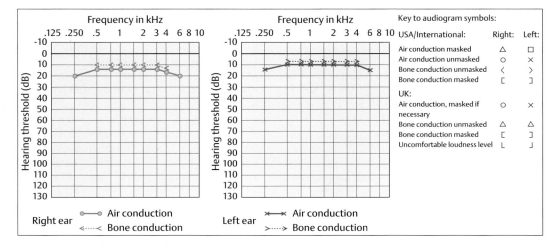

Fig. 1.43 A normal pure-tone audiogram.

Table 1.1   Evaluating the results of clinical hearing tests

	Discrepancy between hearing distance for whispered and conversational speech	Weber test	Rinne test
Normal individual	None	Midline	Positive
Conductive hearing loss	Usually small	Lateralized to the poorer-hearing ear in unilateral hearing loss	Negative or equivocal
Sensorineural hearing loss	Usually large	Lateralized to the better-hearing ear in unilateral hearing loss	Positive
Degree of hearing loss	Distance for hearing conversational speech: Slight (> 4 m) Medium (< 4 m, > 1 m) Severe (< 1–25 cm) Total deafness < 25 cm		

Table 1.2   Properties of sound

Sound	A molecular vibration of an elastic medium propagated as a waveform (in air, water, bone, and all other media)
Speed of sound	340 m/s in air, 1400 m/s in water
Sound pressure (Pa)	This is the predominant change of pressure in a sound field. It is a function of time at any particular point and is expressed in pascal units
Mass unit	The old-fashioned unit was the microbar (µb), dynes/cm^2. The SI unit for absolute sound pressure is the pascal (Pa), equivalent to newtons per m^2 (1 Pa = 1 N/m^2 = 10 µb)

Table 1.3   Hearing or dynamic range and sound pressure level

Hearing range (0 dB)	The lower limit—i. e., the hearing threshold at 1000 Hz—is 20 µPa
(120 dB)	The upper limit or pain threshold is 20 Pa
Sound pressure level (SPL)	The unit is the decibel, a logarithmic unit calculated as follows: Lp = 20log$_{10}$(p/p_0) dB, where p ist sound pressure being measured and p$_0$ ist reference pressure, defined as 20 µPa.

Table 1.4   Hearing range and decibel (dB) scale

Sound source	Intensity ratio	dB
Jet engine	1 : 10^{13}	130
Riveting hammer	1 : 10^{12}	120
Drilling machine	1 : 10^{11}	110
Printing machine	1 : 10^{10}	100
Weaving machine	1 : 10^9	90
Machine workshop	1 : 10^8	80
Street traffic	1 : 10^7	70
Normal speech	1 : 10^6	60
Soft radio music	1 : 10^5	50
Soft speech	1 : 10^4	40
Whispering	1 : 10^3	30
Quiet living room	1 : 10^2	20
Rustling of leaves	1 : 10	10
Hearing threshold	1 : 10^0	0

Table 1.5 Sound intensity, sound volume, and loudness

Scale of sound intensity	This is a physically defined decibel scale based on the square amplitude value of tones, rather than on a subjective assessment of the loudness of the tone
Volume of loudness level	Measured in phons, a logarithmic unit. The tone is compared subjectively with a reference sound of 1000 Hz. The sound pressure level (SPL) of the reference tone is adjusted so that the test tone and reference tone sound equally loud. The result in decibels SPL is expressed in phons. A sound with a loudness level of 50 phon produces the same sensation of loudness as a reference tone at 1000 Hz at an SPL of 50 dB
Loudness	The unit is the sone, which is a linear scale depending on subjective comparison with a measured value. The loudness of a test tone is compared with that of a reference tone of 1000 Hz and 40 dB SPL
Isophon curves	See **Fig. 1.40**. Consist of curves of the same loudness level measured in phons, but at different frequencies (in Hz) and SPL (dB)
Hearing range	Between the hearing threshold at 4 phons and the threshold of pain at 130 phons (see **Fig. 1.40**)

Table 1.6 Tone, timbre, noise

Tone	A pure sinusoidal vibration in the audible range characterized by frequency
Frequency	Vibrations per second in hertz
Timbre	A sound contains overtones in addition to the basic tone, which determine the subjective color of the sound
Noise	Sound whose pressure in the sound field is not a periodic function of time
White noise	Consists of equal components of all the audible frequencies from 18 to 20 000 Hz
Loud noise	May be distressing or cause actual damage

Table 1.7 Impedance

Acoustic impedance	Resistance to the flow of sound pressure waves through a medium, proportional to:
	The mass of the vibrating system
	Its resistance
	Its elasticity
Resistance	The frictional resistance in the joints, ligaments, and muscles of the sound-conducting apparatus
Reactance	An imaginary component determined by the stiffness and mass of the system
Compliance	The flexibility of the tympanic membrane

! Note: The audiometric characteristic of conductive or middle ear hearing loss is that the threshold for air conduction is poorer than that for bone conduction, producing an air–bone gap.

Conductive hearing loss results from an increase in impedance (**Fig. 1.45a–d**). If the elastic recoil due to air in the middle ear and mastoid process increases, mobility in the middle and low tones decreases at constant mass and tension. The resonance point of the middle ear is displaced to the upper frequencies. Conductive hearing loss is characterized by greater loss of hearing for air conduction in the lower frequencies—as seen, for example, in ossification of the stapes annulus in *otosclerosis* (**Fig. 1.45c**; see also **Fig. 1.101**). The conduction system is increasingly damped by the increase in mass and tension, and the resonance point of the middle ear is thus displaced into the lower tones. The hearing loss that results that is greater for air conduction in the middle and higher tones—e. g., as occurs with glue ear exudate in the middle ear (**Fig. 1.45b**) and impacted wax.

Conductive hearing loss independent of frequency is caused by simultaneous elastic stiffening and dampening of the sound conduction apparatus. This may occur in advanced *otosclerosis*, in *middle ear cholesteatoma* with destruction of the ossicular chain, in *tympanosclerosis*, and in *congenital anomalies*. A flat air conduction curve is found in such cases.

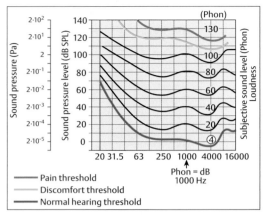

Fig. 1.44 Human auditory field. The sound pressure (in Pa), the sound pressure level (in dB), and the loudness (in phon) are shown together in a coordinate system with the spectrum of human hearing in hertz. The abscissa shows frequencies, the ordinate decibels and phon. Isophons are curves of equal loudness. The curves for decibels and phon coincide only at 1000 Hz and deviate from each other above and below this frequency.

> **Note:** The bone conduction threshold curve is an expression of the function of the inner ear and, to a limited extent, of its central connections.

This rule applies with a few unimportant exceptions—e. g., bony closure of one or both windows.

The audiometric characteristic of all forms of sensorineural hearing loss (inner ear and retrocochlear hearing loss) is that the thresholds for air and bone conduction coincide (**Fig. 1.46a–d**). Supplementary *suprathreshold tests* have to be performed to differentiate inner ear hearing loss from retrocochlear hearing loss.

Demonstration of Recruitment

Patients with *inner ear hearing loss* showing *recruitment* often have difficulty in hearing relatively soft tones. In contrast, they hear loud conversational speech as well as individuals with normal hearing. They find excessive loudness upsetting due to distortion and painful sensations, as the *threshold of discomfort* is exceeded. In inner ear deafness, recruitment occurs in the frequency range of the damaged hair cells, which require a considerably higher sound pressure in comparison with the nor-

mal hair cells to produce a response. The resulting reduction of the dynamic hearing range has extremely deleterious effects as far as hearing of speech is concerned (see **Fig. 1.44** and pp. 108–110).

The following tests are used:

Fowler test. *Principle:* This test is based on a subjective comparison of loudness between the right and left ears. A tone of the same frequency and loudness is presented alternately. A recruitment phenomenon is present if a difference in the hearing threshold between the two sides disappears as the loudness of the test tone increases (**Fig. 1.47**).

> **Note:** Demonstration of the recruitment phenomenon is currently accepted as indicating an inner ear or hair cell lesion, whereas this phenomenon is usually absent in retrocochlear neural hearing loss due to vestibular schwannoma, for example.

Tone intensity difference threshold (Lüscher test).
Principle: The threshold of intensity difference in decibels at the same distance above the hearing threshold is smaller in an ear affected with recruitment than in the normal ear.

Short increment sensitivity index (SISI) test. *Principle:* A test tone is produced 20 dB above the patient's threshold and is increased by 1 dB every 5 seconds with a duration of 0.2 s. Negative results are obtained in retrocochlear lesions with pathologic fatigue. The score is greater than 80 % in patients with cochlear hearing loss showing recruitment.

Demonstration of Pathologic Fatigue

Pathologic auditory fatigue is a sign of a retrocochlear hearing loss. It can be demonstrated using the technically simple *tone decay test* and the *Békésy test.* These two methods have now been largely replaced by measurement of auditory evoked potentials (AEPs; see p. 37), which allows objective testing of auditory functions and considerably more accurate diagnosis of retrocochlear hearing disorders.

■ Speech Audiometry

Speech audiometry is an integral part of audiometric methods of investigation. The ability to hear and understand speech is more important in human communication than the ability to hear pure tones. Speech audiometry therefore has both diagnostic and therapeutic significance. To understand the re-

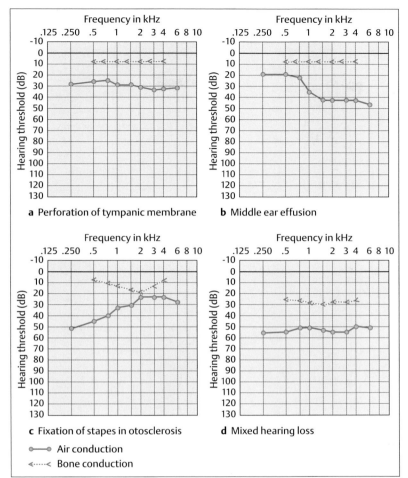

Fig. 1.45a–d Audiograms showing conductive hearing loss (right ear).

a Perforation of tympanic membrane

b Middle ear effusion

c Fixation of stapes in otosclerosis

d Mixed hearing loss

○—○ Air conduction

◁·····◁ Bone conduction

sults of speech audiometry, it is necessary to know the frequencies contained in speech. The fundamental vocal frequencies for men (125 Hz) and women (250 Hz) are shown in a tone threshold audiogram in **Fig. 1.48**.

The loudness of speech is perceived as an acoustic image, the frequencies of which extend from 100 to 8000 Hz. *Hearing loss for speech* is assessed using two-syllable test words, and maximum discrimination is also measured using one-syllable test words (**Fig. 1.49a**).

Speech audiometry is not performed in the same way as testing of the vocal speech (see p. 127)—i.e., with an increasing distance between the patient and the sound source—but rather by varying the loudness as measured in decibels, i.e., with a speech sound level above 20 µPa (see p. 30, **Table 1.2**).

The speech or test material is recorded on a disk and is presented to the patient either using earphones or in a free field using a loudspeaker with varying loudness levels. The percentage of numbers, words, or sentences understood correctly at each loudness level is then assessed.

The dependence of speech comprehension on the loudness level is tested using speech audiometry. In the standardized test (e.g., the *Freiburg speech test*), multisyllable numbers are first used. This can provide a rapid rough estimate of the extent of hearing loss.

An individual with normal hearing understands 50% of numbers presented at 18.5 dB. This normal value forms the basis for assessing hearing loss for numbers. The patient's ability to comprehend monosyllabic words is also tested.

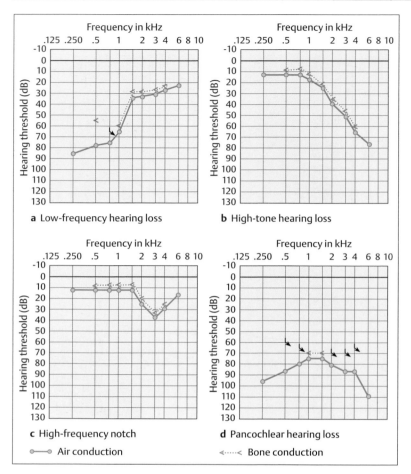

Fig. 1.46a–d Audiograms showing sensorineural hearing loss.

↳ = no response

a Low-frequency hearing loss

b High-tone hearing loss

c High-frequency notch

d Pancochlear hearing loss

●——○ Air conduction   ◄·····◄ Bone conduction

These words are considerably more difficult to understand than multisyllabic numbers. The purpose of the monosyllable test is to assess percentage comprehension and ultimately to achieve 100% comprehension values, if possible, by increasing the loudness level. Normal individuals hear 100% of monosyllables at 65 dB, and in favorable conditions at 50 dB, whereas 100% speech comprehension cannot be achieved even in normal individuals at a sound pressure level of less than 50 dB.

Speech audiometry allows quantitative measurement of hearing. The speech audiogram indicates the percentage of syllables, words, or sentences that the individual has heard correctly in each test series. The result of a speech audiogram depends not only on hearing, but also on higher cognitive functions such as memory, language comprehension, and motor speech. Other factors that influence the results include whether the patient's mother tongue is being used and the patient's vocabulary range.

Comparison of pure-tone and speech audiograms. Discrepancies between the results of pure-tone and speech audiometry are mainly found in retrocochlear hearing disorders. In such cases, hearing for speech is considerably worse than hearing for pure tones. The pathophysiologic basis for this is described on p. 17.

Diagnosis of *central hearing disorders* is based on tests of the central understanding of speech. The classic methods of testing hearing fail in such cases due to the phenomenon of *redundancy*. This is the safety margin within the auditory pathways, which can transmit and analyze billions of information units, whereas only 100 are necessary for recognizing and decoding acoustic information. A disorder of the central summation and integration capacity can only be demonstrated with difficulty—e. g., by distorting speech by filtering out high frequencies and inserting periodic interruptions of the speech signal, or with binaural application of garbled test words, reducing the information content of normal speech to a minimum (Feldmann dichotic speech test).

Note: Speech audiometry is indispensable for:
- Assessing residual hearing for speech. This makes it possible to predict the probable benefit to be expected from a hearing aid. The loss of discrimination and the threshold of discomfort can be measured.
- Assessing the need for hearing aids and surgery to improve hearing.
- Investigating central hearing loss. This allows assessment of the integrative performance of the auditory centers.
- Assessment, for insurance purposes, of a loss of hearing for speech leading to a loss of earning capacity.

■ Objective Hearing Tests

Behavioral, pure-tone audiometry is based on a subjective response from the patient. In contrast, objective audiometry makes it possible to carry out testing without eliciting a patient response. This method uses tests based on involuntary physiologic reactions and "objective" parameters. These objective responses support the interpretation of pure-tone audiometry and are very important for audiometric diagnosis in infants, small children, and patients with mental and cognitive impairment.

Three main methods are used in objective audiometry:
- Measurement of changes in the acoustic impedance of the tympanic membrane: *impedance audiometry.*
- Measurement of acoustically evoked bioelectric responses of the cochlea, vestibulocochlear nerve and tract, or cerebral cortex: *auditory evoked potentials (AEPs).*
- Measurement of spontaneous or acoustically evoked vibrations of the cochlea: *otoacoustic emissions (OAEs).*

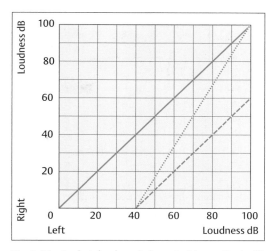

Fig. 1.47 Fowler's loudness balance test in a patient with unilateral left-sided sensorineural hearing loss, with a 40-dB loss at 1 kHz.

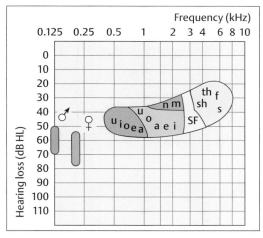

Fig. 1.48 The speech field. The fundamental voice frequency is 125 Hz in men and 250 Hz in women. Vowels are formed between 500 Hz and 4000 Hz and are spoken ≈ 10–20 dB louder than consonants in normal conversational speech. Several consonants lie in a higher frequency range (s, t) and therefore cannot be perceived by patients with high-frequency deafness; "e" as in "bed," "a" as in "bar." Dark green area = region of the first formant; medium green area = region of the second formant; light green area = region of the speaker's formant (SF); red area = resonance of the nasal tract.

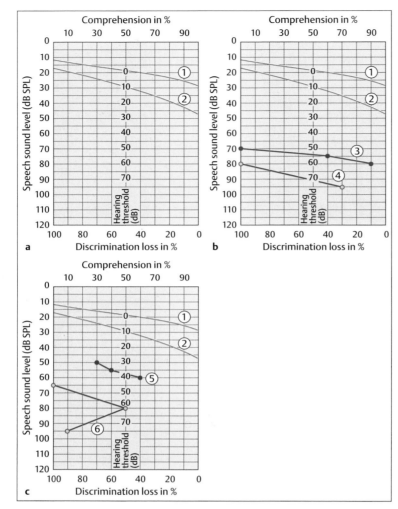

Fig. 1.49a–c Speech audiometry is carried out using uniform test content consisting of multisyllabic numbers and monosyllabic words.

a An individual with normal hearing understands 50 % of numbers heard at 18.5 dB and 100 % of those heard at 30 dB (**1**). For monosyllabic test words (**2**), intelligibility is 50 % at 30 dB and 100 % at 50 dB.

b In patients with conductive hearing loss, a parallel shift toward higher sound levels occurs in the performance–intensity function (**3**), but nearly 100 % comprehension can still be achieved at sufficiently high levels (**4**).

c Sensorineural hearing loss leads to a flattening of the performance–intensity function for monosyllabic words (**5**). Loss of intelligibility and a decline in speech recognition at higher sound levels are signs of abnormal speech processing, such as that caused by cochlear damage or neural disturbances (**6**).

Impedance Audiometry

This technique is part of the functional diagnosis of the sound conduction apparatus. It includes the following two investigation methods:

- *Tympanometry:* This involves recording the impedance (see p. 14) or indirect measurement of pressure in the middle ear, when the tympanic membrane is intact, by means of pressure in the external meatus. This is an indirect test of tubal function.
- *Measurement of the acoustic reflex:* The change in impedance caused by the acoustic stapedial reflex is measured.

Technique

The external auditory meatus is closed by an airtight plug, through which three tubes pass. One tube carries the test tone; the second is connected to the pressure regulator, which allows positive or negative pressure (± 400 mmH₂O) to be produced in the external auditory meatus. A microphone is connected to the third tube, allowing measurement of the sound pressure of the test tone reflected from the tympanic membrane as the impedance changes (**Fig. 1.50**).

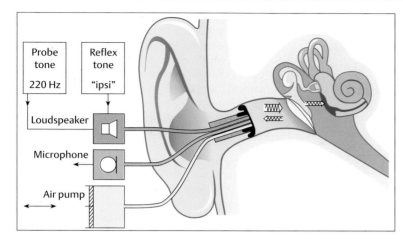

Fig. 1.50 Tympanometry. Tubes passing through an airtight plug transmit the test tone and the reflected tone. The flexibility of the tympanic membrane, compliance, is calculated from the measured sound level. Pressure-dependent displacement of the tympanic membrane is regulated by an air pump.

Tympanometry. Normally, there is no pressure differential between the two sides of the tympanic membrane, so that the acoustic resistance of the tympanic membrane is minimal. Recording the impedance of the tympanic membrane during a change in pressure in the external auditory meatus allows the pressure difference on the two sides of the tympanic membrane to be determined by measuring its compliance. The greater the pressure differential, the greater is the impedance of the tympanic membrane. Recording the impedance at pressures from -300 mmH$_2$O to $+300$ mmH$_2$O produces a curve with a peak at zero for a normally mobile tympanic membrane. This represents the maximum flexibility—i. e., compliance—of the tympanic membrane, and thus minimal impedance. The apex of this curve is lower if the tympanic membrane is stiffened by scar tissue or damped by exudate in the middle ear. It becomes higher with increasing compliance due to atrophic scars of the pars tensa (**Fig. 1.51a–d**).

Stapedial reflex. The *principle* of this test is that a sound stimulus greater than 70 dB above the threshold induces a reflex contraction of the stapedius muscle. This causes a change of impedance at the tympanic membrane, which can be recorded graphically. The effect is absent when the tympanic membrane is immobile, when the ossicular chain is disrupted, and when the stapes is fixed in the oval window by otosclerosis. In simulated deafness, this reflex is activated by loudness approaching the norm. In this case, simulation can be assumed.

The stapedial reflex is an acousticofacial reflex. The afferent limb is the vestibulocochlear nerve and parts of the central auditory pathway up to the auditory centers. The efferent limb is formed by the connections between the auditory centers and the facial nucleus, and finally by the facial nerve. Measurement of the stapedial reflex is therefore very useful in topical diagnosis of facial paralysis.

Testing the threshold for the stapedial reflex is of considerable diagnostic importance for assessing the following hearing disorders: otosclerosis, recruitment (Metz recruitment is reduction of the difference between an elevated hearing threshold and the threshold for the stapedial reflex, with increasing hearing loss for high tones), retrocochlear deafness, and brain stem lesions.

The stapedial reflex is absent in:

- Retrocochlear sensorineural deafness as a result of auditory fatigue—i. e., in vestibular schwannoma.
- Otosclerosis and other middle ear diseases.
- Facial nerve damage proximal to the point at which the stapedius muscle is innervated.
- Brain stem lesions with damage to the central reflex arc.

Auditory Evoked Potentials (AEPs)

The patient is repeatedly exposed to an acoustic stimulus, either regularly or irregularly, and an electroencephalogram (EEG) is used to assess whether there is any change in brain activity. The AEPs are recorded from the scalp using needle or surface electrodes. As the amplitudes of the AEPs

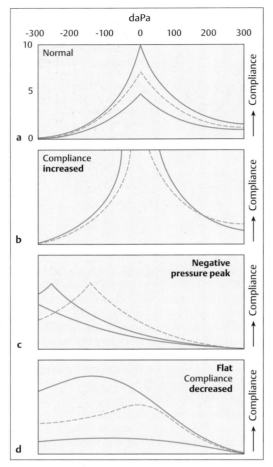

Fig. 1.51a–d Summary of the four most important results of a tympanogram. The curve shows the compliance of the tympanic membrane to changes in pressure in the external canal.

a Normal: the apex of the curve (daPa) lies close to 0 on the pressure scale when the pressures in the meatus and in the middle ear are equal.

b Increased compliance: the apex of the curve will be abnormally high if the tympanic membrane is extremely mobile. This situation may occur with atrophic scars of the pars tensa or interruption of the ossicular chain.

c Negative peak pressure: the apex of the curve is displaced below 100 daPa due to reduced pressure in the middle ear.

d Flat tympanogram with no compliance peak. This is seen when the tympanic membrane is dampened due to the middle ear effusion. This type of curve also occurs if the tympanic membrane is perforated, but the equivalent (or ear) canal volume (ECV) will then be high.

are very small relative to the total activity of the brain, averaging the potentials is necessary (see **Fig. 1.49**). Averaging means that the individual response, which is concealed on the EEG by the "noise" of brain activity, can be distinguished by mathematical analysis of numerous evoked individual potentials. The intermittent acoustic stimulus produces a uniform potential during a time interval that always occurs at the same time and can be amplified by repetitive summation of the EEG segment.

The properties and shape of AEPs depend partly on the time at which they occur after presentation of the acoustic stimulus, or their latency (in milliseconds). Several types of AEP can be distinguished on the basis of different sites of origin and latency.

Classification

Electrocochleography (ECochG). This measures the potentials arising in the cochlea and vestibulocochlear nerve. These potentials occur ≈ 1–3 ms after the stimulus is presented. The two most useful diagnostic parameters are *cochlear microphonics* (CM) and the *action potential* of the vestibulocochlear nerve (PI).

Auditory brain stem response (ABR) audiometry (brain stem evoked response audiometry, BERA). This measures the potentials arising in the vestibulocochlear nerve and brain stem structures, with a latency of up to ≈ 10 ms. The latency of individual potentials, particularly between potential peaks I and V, is very important for recognizing retrocochlear hearing disorders (**Fig. 1.52**).

Auditory middle latency potential (AMLP) audiometry. This measures potentials with a latency of 10–100 ms that originate in the thalamus and primary auditory cortex.

Cortical evoked potentials (CEPs). This measures potentials with a latency of 100–1000 ms, which express generalized higher-order cortical function.

Measurement of the auditory brain stem response (ABR) and electrocochleography (ECochG) are two of the most important diagnostic methods for accurate differentiation between cochlear and retrocochlear deafness. The latter is due to space-occupying formations in the CPA (e. g., vestibular schwannoma), a tumor of the posterior cranial fossa, or multiple sclerosis. AEP is also very useful for investigating deafness in infants and young children. It can also be used to assess residual function of the central nervous system in patients with severe head injuries, coma, or other conditions marked by a complete loss of consciousness. It does not, however, replace pure-tone audiometry or tympanometry (including the stapedial reflex), which still form the basis for audiometric evaluations. ABR is also tested intraoperatively in order to monitor hearing.

Otoacoustic Emissions (OAEs)

Otoacoustic emissions are sound signals emitted from the inner ear in response to acoustic stimulation. The signals are vibrations produced by the biomechanical cochlear amplifier (see p. 16). They occur spontaneously or in response to an acoustic stimulus and are transmitted in retrograde fashion across the ossicles to the tympanic membrane. The membrane acts like a loudspeaker membrane, so that emitted vibrations can be measured as sound waves in the external ear canal. These active cochlear vibrations can be detected by a sensitive microphone.

Otoacoustic emissions are clinically important, as they reflect the functional integrity of the cochlea. OAE detection depends on normal middle ear function for good transmission to the tympanic membrane.

Classification

Spontaneous OAEs (SOAEs). Vibrations can arise spontaneously in the cochlea without any external stimulus. They are detectable as low-level, continuous tones in ≈ 50 % of individuals with normal hearing.

Transient evoked otoacoustic emissions (TEOAEs). Emissions are detected in response to an acoustic stimulus (click) in individuals with normal cochlear function. An averaging technique is used (as in ABR; see p. 38). This measurement is used as an objective audiometric testing method (**Fig. 1.53a**). TEOAEs occur in normal hearing and confirm cochlear integrity; they are absent in patients with middle ear disease or cochlear hearing loss with a threshold increase of ≈ 30 dB. The amplitude in infants with normal hearing is usually higher than in adults.

Distortion product otoacoustic emissions (DPOAEs). Acoustic distortions in the cochlear amplifier can be detected by stimulation with two

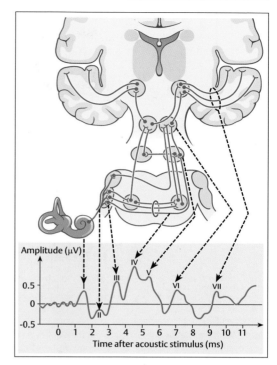

Fig. 1.52   Auditory brain stem response (ABR). The typical waveform consists of five or seven waves (I–VII), which reflect the acoustically induced activity of the anatomical structures of the auditory system (see **Fig. 1.20**).

continuous tones that have different, but adjacent, frequencies. DPOAEs are intimately linked to outer hair-cell function. This is another frequently used objective audiometric testing method (**Fig. 1.53b**).

The most important application of otoacoustic emissions is for screening cochlear function in newborns, infants and small children. DPOAEs can be used to detect early discrete lesions of the outer hair cells, and they provide an important noninvasive screening method for cochlear impairment that can even be used without sedation or general anesthesia. OAEs can also be used to investigate nonorganic hearing loss, to objectify audiometric findings in adults, and to assess cochlear function in risk groups (ototoxic medication).

!

Note: In the absence of OAEs, additional audiologic tests such as auditory evoked potentials and pure-tone audiometry should be used.

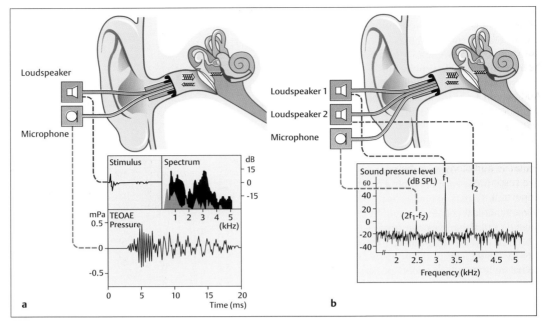

Fig. 1.53a, b   **a** The system for measuring transient evoked otoacoustic emissions (TEOAE). A measuring probe with a microphone and loudspeaker is placed in the external ear canal. A click impulse is induced by the loudspeaker, and evoked emissions from the cochlea are recorded by the miniature microphone.

b The system for measuring distortion products of otoacoustic emissions (DPOAE). The cochlea is stimulated with two tones (f_1 and f_2). The sound pressure changes as a response in the external ear canal are recorded by the microphone along with the primary tones. The curve represents the frequency spectrum of the microphone signal.

■ Hearing Tests in Infants and Young Children

> **Note:** Every child who does not respond normally to sound stimuli soon after birth—and at the latest after the first 6 months—must undergo otologic examination.

Since even a completely deaf child passes through a period of crying and babbling, serious hearing loss only begins to be suspected when speech does not develop. Most children with hearing disorders are therefore presented to the general practitioner or otologist between the first and third years of life. As hearing is not an obvious condition in the newborn, it needs to be detected using screening, which is indicated in particular in the following cases:

- Necessary treatment for more than 48 hours in an intensive-care unit.
- Positive family history of hearing impairment.
- Manifest craniofacial anomalies.

Universal screening: Every newborn should be screened on the second or third day after birth during the second routine examination. Eighty percent of all hearing problems can be detected using this method. The organization required for this method of screening depends on the local health-care system.

Additional screening should be performed at routine pediatric visits or in a preschool medical examination.

Tests

Otoacoustic emissions (OAEs). If OAEs are present, the peripheral hearing is satisfactory, but this does not exclude a hearing disorder. The degree of any hearing loss cannot be determined.

Auditory brain stem response (ABR). If an ABR is not elicited, severe hearing loss is present. The hearing threshold can be determined when auditory evoked potentials are measurable.

Pediatric audiology with behavioral tests. Subjective responses in pediatric audiometric testing are important methods and can be performed at virtually any age, but should be age-appropriate. The reliability of the test results is variable.

Test Methods

Reflex audiometry. Nonspecific responses to auditory stimuli, such as sucking responses, motor responses (Moro reflex, acousticopalpebral reflex) or breathing responses, can be elicited in normal infants from birth on. The reflexes can be stimulated only by a loud noise (nearly 80 dB).

Response audiometry. By the second half of the first year of life, acoustic stimuli evoke typical response patterns. A normally hearing infant turns his or her head toward the sound source that is out of the range of vision.

Distraction test. A tester attracts the child's attention with a toy, and the examiner presents an acoustic stimulus invisible to the child and observes the reaction.

Visual reinforcement audiometry (VRA): An acoustic stimulus is combined with the activation of a moving toy. After conditioning, the child moves toward the toy when it hears the acoustic stimulus.

Play audiometry. As a variation of pure-tone audiometry, tasks and responses to tone testing are incorporated into a play setting (e. g., while playing, the child has to react when an acoustic stimulus is presented).

Pediatric speech audiometry. Children aged 3–4 years can be examined using audiometric speech tests specially designed for children (e. g., the Pediatric Speech Intelligibility Test).

Table 1.8 Checklist for suspected congenital or early acquired hearing loss

Family history	Hearing and speech disorders, psychiatric and neurologic diseases, congenital anomalies
History of pregnancy	Virus infection with rubella, measles, influenza, herpes zoster, coxsackievirus, or *Toxoplasma;* drugs such as thalidomide or aminoglycosides; diseases such as diabetes or neuropathy; or vaccination
Perinatal history	Forceps or other mechanical damage, asphyxia, prematurity, kernicterus
Postnatal history	Infectious disease, vaccination reaction, diseases of the central nervous system, trauma to the skull, intoxication, and drugs
Hearing	Reaction to noise and speech, directional hearing, the time when the hearing disorder began, and the progress of the symptoms
Speech	Age at which the first sounds, words, and sentences were uttered

Note: The sense of hearing is a vitally important factor for acquiring speech. It is therefore essential for hearing loss in a child to be recognized and treated. The earlier the treatment is instituted, the more successful it is. Treatment should be started in the second half of the first year (**Table 1.8**; see also **Table 1.25**).

■ Vestibular Function Tests

Investigations of the vestibular system comprise:
1. Case history and analysis of symptoms.
2. Testing of the vestibulospinal reflexes.
3. Testing for spontaneous and provoked nystagmus.
4. Experimental testing of the vestibular and optokinetic systems.

■ Case History

The subjective feeling of dizziness is generally regarded as being an expression of a disturbed neuronal discharge pattern in the cortical projection

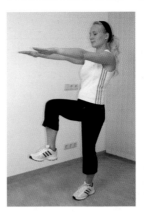

Fig. 1.54 The Unterberger stepping test. The patient is asked to walk on the spot with the eyes closed.

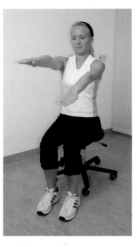

Fig. 1.55 The patient's position for static positional tests. A spontaneous deviation reaction and spontaneous tone reaction in the arm are observed while the patient is sitting on a chair.

areas. A thorough case history is required in order to achieve a structured analysis, allowing differential-diagnostic classification of:

- Peripheral vestibular dizziness.
- Central vestibular dizziness.
- Nonvestibular dizziness.

The case history should include questions about previous illnesses, medications, and noxae. Questions regarding the type of subjectively perceived dizziness, as well as its duration and intensity, are important. Dizziness-causing factors and secondary symptoms are also important details to clarify.

■ Vestibulospinal Reflexes

In peripheral vestibular lesions, the body's center of gravity is usually displaced to the side on which the labyrinthine lesion is located. In central disturbances of balance, the pattern of unsteadiness of gait and the direction of falling are irregular. Body sways can also be registered on an electronic scale (posturography).

Romberg test. The patient is asked to stand with the feet together (touching each other) and to close the eyes. A check is made to see whether there is then any unsteadiness or a tendency to fall.

Blindfold gait and walking a straight line. Only gross abnormalities of gait are diagnostically important. The patient deviates to the same side as in the Romberg test.

Unterberger stepping test (Fig. 1.54). *Stepping on the spot with the eyes closed:* patients with peripheral disorders show rotation of the body axis to the side of the labyrinthine lesion; in central disorders, the deviation is irregular. Only deviations of more than 40° are of diagnostic significance.

Static positional tests
(see also p. 45)

Spontaneous deviation reaction, past pointing. Parallel displacement of *both* arms (with arms in the supine position) occurs in accordance with the vestibulospinal reflexes.

Spontaneous tone reaction in the arms. The arm on the side of the cerebellar lesion sinks as a result of loss of tone of the muscles (**Fig. 1.55**).

Finger–nose pointing test. The index finger of the outstretched arm is brought to the tip of the nose with the eyes closed. Ataxia and disorders of coordination (overshooting) indicate an ipsilateral cerebellar lesion or a disorder of positional sense and deep sensation.

■ Spontaneous and Provoked Nystagmus

Nystagmus. This is a conjugated, coordinated eye movement around a specific axis; the movement consists of rhythmically alternating slow- and fast-beating phases. The direction of the fast component of the nystagmus determines the laterality of the nystagmus.

Tests

Observation with and without Frenzel's glasses.

This is used for the diagnosis of a *spontaneous nystagmus*. The patient is examined in a darkened room with +15-diopter lenses that almost completely suppress optical fixation, so that the visual fixation suppression of the vestibular nystagmus is eliminated (**Fig. 1.56**).

Direct gaze, with and without fixation, is used to recognize *fixation nystagmus*. Lateral gaze and gaze upward and downward are used to confirm *gaze-directional* or *gaze-paretic* nystagmus.

The direction (←), frequency (≫—), and amplitude (=) of the eye movements observed are recorded on a Frenzel's chart (**Figs. 1.57**).

Electronystagmography (ENG).

The eye is a dipole in which the cornea is electropositive and the retina electronegative. The periocular electrical field therefore changes when the eyes move. This change in the corneoretinal potential is proportional to the amplitude, frequency, and speed of the nystagmus. It can be picked up and recorded by electrodes and analyzed. The direction of the eye movements is demonstrated by a positive or negative corneoretinal potential (**Fig. 1.58a–c**).

Video nystagmography (VNG).

The eye movements are recorded by a touchless video camera. The position of the dark pupil of the eye can be recorded by a processor that analyzes the eye's horizontal and vertical rotation.

Spontaneous Nystagmus

This term includes all eye movements that have the character of nystagmus and are not induced by external stimulation of the vestibular and visual systems (**Fig. 1.59**). The fast component usually beats toward the side of the functionally dominant vestibular center.

Three main forms of spontaneous nystagmus can be distinguished:

Spontaneous vestibular nystagmus.

This disorder may be due either to a peripheral vestibular disorder, in which case the fast component of the nystagmus always beats toward the dominant labyrinth; or it may be caused by a central vestibular disorder. The inhibitory impulses on the vestibular center are suppressed (see p. 20). The nystagmus beats on the side of the lesion.

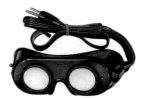

Fig. 1.56 Frenzel's glasses with magnifying lenses allow assessment of nystagmus.

Recovery nystagmus may be due either to a central compensatory process after a peripheral lesion, or to the recovery of peripheral function. In both cases, it is directed toward the side of the dominant vestibular center—i. e., in this case toward the affected ear.

Gaze-evoked and gaze-paretic nystagmus.

This form of nystagmus is always induced by a central lesion. Often it beats to both sides and in both the horizontal and vertical planes. It only appears after deviation of the globe by more than 30° for at least 30 s.

An exceptional form of toxic gaze-evoked nystagmus may occur after barbiturate or alcohol poisoning, due to release of the central inhibitory effect.

This form of nystagmus is due to a lesion affecting voluntary motor control of gaze, which in serious cases is accompanied by paralysis of gaze. Transitions from gaze-evoked to gaze-paretic nystagmus are fluid. The latter is characterized by a nystagmus to the side of the gaze paresis.

This is due to a congenital or acquired disorder (such as multiple sclerosis) of the gaze centers of the reticular formation of the pons (the center for horizontal gaze movement) and of the tegmentum of the midbrain (the center for vertical gaze movements). These centers are involved in central voluntary motor control of gaze (integration of voluntary gaze impulses and visual and vestibular afferents), binocular coordination via the medial longitudinal bundle (see **Fig. 1.21**), and the rhythm of nystagmus. Lesions in this area of the brain stem therefore lead to serious abnormalities of gaze movements and nystagmus—such as changes in the rhythm and form of beat, dissociation of movements of the right and left eyes, extinction of the fast phase of nystagmus, unilateral or bilateral enhancement of optokinetic nystagmus, gaze-evoked and gaze-paretic nystagmus, and internuclear ophthalmoplegia.

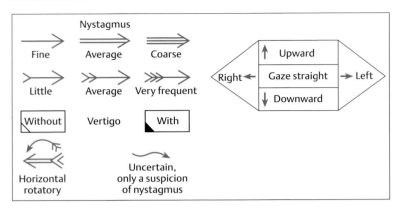

Fig. 1.57 Symbols for recording nystagmus and vertigo (left). The direction is recorded on a Frenzel's chart (right).
→ = direction,
≡ = amplitude,
≫― = frequency.

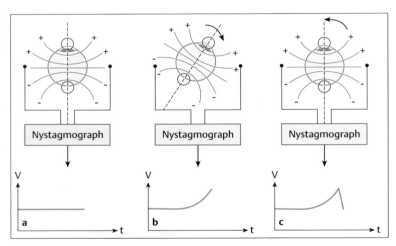

Fig. 1.58a–c The principle of nystagmography.
a Gaze straight ahead. The nasal and temporal electrodes are positive, and the isoelectric baseline is horizontal.
b The eyeball is turned slowly to the right (slow phase). The nasal electrode is positive, the temporal electrode is negative, and the baseline is displaced superiorly.
c The eyeball returns quickly (fast phase), the baseline returns to the neutral position, and both electrodes are positive.

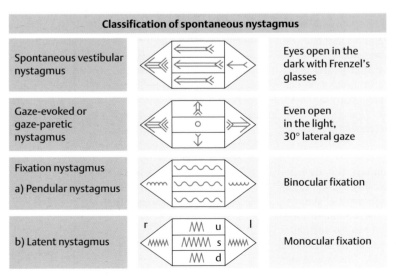

Fig. 1.59 Classification of spontaneous nystagmus (u = upward, s = straight, d = downward).

Fixation nystagmus. This form of nystagmus does not have any typical fast or slow components, but rather a pendular movement. It almost always occurs with binocular fixation, but may rarely be seen with monocular fixation. It is often congenital and may even be hereditary. Synonyms for it include *congenital* or *hereditary pendular nystagmus.*

The three main forms of spontaneous nystagmus should not be confused with the following:

- *Endpoint nystagmus,* a short-lived, nonpathologic, rapidly decaying beat at the extremes of gaze—i. e., more than 50° deviation.
- *Fatigue nystagmus,* which occurs during prolonged lateral gaze due to fatigue of the lateral rectus muscle, similar to tremor in skeletal muscles. This is also nonpathologic.
- *Adjustment nystagmus,* which is due to adjustment of movements of a nystagmoid character when fixing on an object in the visual field. There is a rapid beat that fatigues quickly. This, too, is nonpathologic.

Provoked Nystagmus

Unlike spontaneous nystagmus, this is exclusively a vestibular-induced nystagmus that only appears after specific stimuli, such as changes in the position of the body or of the head.

Frenzel's glasses are used to investigate this condition. The same criteria are used for assessing provoked nystagmus as for spontaneous nystagmus; however, the duration of eye movements is also taken into account. One of the following patterns of nystagmus may be seen:

- *Transitory* nystagmus, which lasts less than 60 s.
- Continually beating *persistent* nystagmus.
- *Head-shaking nystagmus*—i. e., "release" spontaneous nystagmus of peripheral or central origin. This may be transitory or persistent.

Provocation Measures

Head-shaking. Spontaneous nystagmus can be provoked by gentle, passive, horizontal shaking of the patient's head.

Positional testing (static). The nystagmus is induced by adopting various body positions in slow motion (supine, lateral decubitus, head-hanging). The vestibular apparatus and the otolithic organs in particular are exposed to various gravitational stimuli in the different positions (**Fig. 1.60a**).

Positional testing (dynamic). This involves a unilateral quick movement of the patient back to a head-hanging position for 60 s. The test is repeated on the opposite side (*Dix–Hallpike maneuver*) (**Fig. 1.60b**).

It is a useful test for diagnosing *benign paroxysmal positional vertigo* (BPPV, see p. 100). The classic finding includes, after a short latent period of 5–10 s, a horizontal or rotatory downward-beating nystagmus toward the underlying ear, with an increase in intensity. Later, after 15–30 s, it decreases and a marked subjective feeling of vertigo arises. Occasionally, a transitory nystagmus beating in the opposite direction occurs when the patient sits up. In addition to this *paroxysmal positional nystagmus,* persistent or transitory direction-determined nystagmus, regular direction changing, and irregular positional nystagmus may be observed. The latter is always of central origin.

■ Experimental Tests of the Vestibular System

These tests and analysis of them should be performed by a specialist.

Turning test. The rotatory or turning test uses *angular acceleration* as the stimulus for investigating the sensitivity of the horizontal semicircular canals. Rotation around an axis passing through the head stimulates one or more semicircular canals on each side, depending on the head position. The left and right sides are stimulated in an opposing fashion. Rotation of the head in one direction (e. g., to the right) induces nystagmus toward the same side (rotatory nystagmus). When the rotation ceases, the nystagmus reverses to the opposite direction (postrotatory nystagmus). The test is carried out in a darkened room using a rotating chair.

Using the rotatory test, it can be determined whether the vestibular apparatus is functioning properly or whether there are signs of a functional or regulatory disorder (imbalance to one side, swinging).

Caloric labyrinthine testing. The principle involved in these tests is illustrated in **Fig. 1.61a–c**. The horizontal semicircular canal is brought into a vertical position in the supine patient. Cooling or warming the labyrinthine capsule by irrigation with water at 30°C or 44°C for 30–40 s induces convection currents and a slight change in the volume of the endolymph. This produces move-

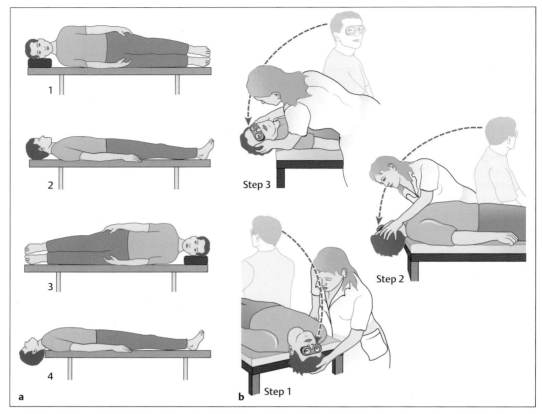

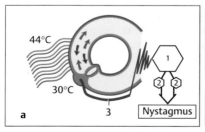
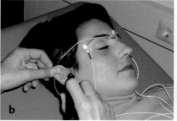
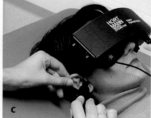

Fig. 1.60a, b **a** Positional testing (static). Beginning with a supine position on the examining table, the patient rolls onto the right side and then rolls back to the supine position and continues rolling onto the left side. After that, the patient adopts a head-hanging position.

b Positioning test (dynamic). A dynamic provocation is carried out. Starting in the sitting position, the patient adopts a head-hanging position, and the upper body is then swiftly brought back to the sagittal plane (step 1). The head is then turned to the left (or right) and the patient adopts the head-hanging position for each side (steps 2 and 3).

Fig. 1.61a–c Principle of caloric labyrinthine tests.
a Temperature changes at the lateral labyrinthine capsule cause a change in the density of the perilymph, leading either to an influx away from the ampulla (cold stimulus) or to an influx toward the ampulla (warm stimulus). The oscillation of the cupula produces a neural stimulus that is transmitted by the vestibular nerve (**3**) to the vestibular nucleus (**1**) and ocular muscle nucleus (**2**).
b Examination with electrode deflection.
c Examination with video nystagmography.

ment of the endolymph, which deflects the cupula. This process has exactly the same electrophysiologic effect as deflection of the cupula by angular acceleration (see **Fig. 1.28a–c**)—i. e., it induces nystagmus via the vestibuloocular reflex.

The *extent of the caloric response* (the nystagmus and the subjective feeling of dizziness) gives some indication of the function of the stimulated labyrinth. *Reduced excitability* indicates partial functional loss, and *lack of response indicates subtotal or complete loss of function.* The advantage of caloric tests is that the labyrinth on each side can be investigated separately.

Fistula test. In the presence of a fistula in the horizontal semicircular canal or elsewhere in the labyrinthine capsule (see p. 8), caused by an inflammatory osteolytic process such as cholesteatoma, a sudden increase in pressure in the external auditory meatus produces a subjective feeling of dizziness, objective nystagmus, and lateropulsion (**Fig. 1.62**). The same phenomenon can also occur when there are adhesions between the membranous labyrinth and the stapes footplate (fistula symptom without a labyrinthine fistula, see p. 81).

Technique: A Politzer balloon with a perforated olive is introduced into the meatus. Compression induces nystagmus toward the affected ear and aspiration to the other side.

Pseudofistula symptom: Inflation or aspiration of air in a patient with a large defect in the tympanic membrane produces cooling of the horizontal semicircular canal, which induces a caloric labyrinthine reaction and thus nystagmus. However, this always beats toward the sound ear for both compression and aspiration.

> *!*
> **Note:** The fistula symptom always has to be tested in chronic otitis media with marginal perforation of the tympanic membrane, especially when there is a suspicion of cholesteatoma of the middle ear.

Optokinetic Function and Pursuit Tracking

The optokinetic and eye-tracking tests are among the most sensitive methods available for detecting central oculomotor lesions. They are indispensable for distinguishing peripheral from central disorders of balance, as the two systems are functionally very closely linked.

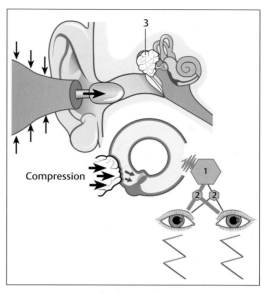

Fig. 1.62 A positive fistula test due to erosion of the right lateral semicircular canal by cholesteatoma. **1**, Vestibular nucleus; **2**, oculomotor nerve nuclei; **3**, cholesteatoma.

Principle: Observation of an object moving within a stationary visual field (foveal stimulation) or observation of the displacement of the entire visual field (foveoretinal stimulation). Only the latter induces the optokinetic reflex—a conjugated reflex eye movement that shows a slow movement in the direction of the displacement of the moving object or visual field (gaze following movement) and a fast phase (the central correction movement) in the opposite direction. This is described as *optokinetic nystagmus.*

Brain stem lesions, especially of the pons and cerebellum, produce the changes involved in optokinetic nystagmus, such as unilateral directional preponderance, disintegration of coordinated movement of the left and right eye, and complete unilateral or bidirectional disintegration of coordinated movement. Gaze-evoked or gaze-paretic nystagmus and simultaneous abnormalities of optokinetic nystagmus are characteristic early symptoms of multiple sclerosis.

■ Investigation of the Facial Nerve

The first and most important investigation serves to differentiate central from peripheral paralysis:
- In *central paralysis,* the function of the branches to the forehead is preserved.

- In *peripheral paralysis,* all three branches are affected. The secretion of tears and sensitivity for taste are affected, and hyperacusis may occur due to disruption of the stapedial reflex.

The *topographic diagnosis* of peripheral lesions of the facial nerve is shown in **Fig. 1.22**.

Taste. The anterior two-thirds of the tongue is innervated by the chorda tympani. The test stimulus is 20% sugar, 10% saline, or 5% citric acid solution (see **Fig. 3.2 c**).

Gustometry. The peripheral taste fibers are stimulated electrically, and the threshold is measured in milliamperes (see p. 242).

Schirmer test. The Schirmer test uses paper strips inserted into the eye for several minutes to measure the production of tears. The eyes are closed for 5 min. The paper is then removed and the amount of moisture is measured. Sometimes a topical anesthetic is administered to the eye before the filter paper, to prevent tear production due to irritation from the paper. The use of the anesthetic ensures that only basal tear secretion is measured. The reduction in the secretion of tears due to interruption of the lacrimal anastomosis in the greater superficial petrosal nerve is measured on the paralyzed side (see **Fig. 1.22**).

The *stapedial reflex* is measured using impedance audiometry (see p. 37).

Electrical and Magnetic Excitability Tests

The severity and prognosis of a paralysis can only be determined by *electrodiagnosis.*

Note: Every facial paralysis, of whatever cause, has to be investigated as early as possible using electrodiagnostic methods.

Three stages of a lesion can be distinguished:
- *Neurapraxia:* There is complete absence of function, but without interruption of the axon. This stage is reversible.
- *Axonotmesis:* There is disruption of the axon with preservation of the connective-tissue framework of the nerve (endoneurium, perineurium, and epineurium). These lesions usually do not recover completely.

- *Neurotmesis:* There is disruption of the axon and of the supporting tissues. This is irreversible without surgical intervention.

Electromyography (EMG). Muscle action potentials are picked up by a needle electrode on voluntary contraction of the facial musculature. The EMG is of relatively little value in the acute phase of facial paralysis, since denervation potentials only appear 12 days after the start of the paralysis.

Electroneuronography (ENoG). The sums of the action potentials of the facial musculature induced by contraction in response to maximal percutaneous faradic stimulation are measured. The proportion of degenerated fibers can be assessed approximately by comparing the summation potential between the healthy and the paralyzed side.

Nerve excitability test (NET). The strength of current in milliamperes that is sufficient to induce a muscle twitch at a constant duration of impulse of 0.3 ms is assessed. The threshold for the two facial nerves varies to an insignificant extent (0.4 mA) in the same individual. A difference in threshold between the two sides that is greater than or equal to 3.5 mA is abnormal. An increase in the threshold indicates progressive degeneration of the nerve fibers or progressive axonotmesis.

Transcranial magnetic stimulation (TCMS). The stimulation is administered by applying a quickly changing magnetic field above the motor cortex and the facial nerve. The summation potential is diverted by the mimetic muscles. This makes it possible to measure the motor transmission speed and the location of the nerve lesion.

In the acute phase of paralysis, the results of NET and ENoG (rheobase and chronaxy) provide important information about the extent and progression of degenerative processes in the nerve and are decisive in determining the choice of treatment.

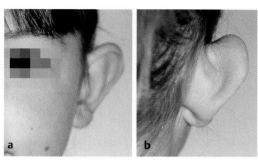

Fig. 1.63a, b   Bat ears are characterized by hypertrophy of the conchal cartilage or failure of the auricle to fold.

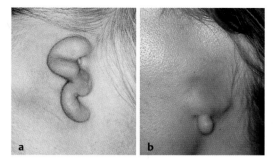

Fig. 1.64a, b   Dysplasia of the auricle: type II microtia (**a**) and anotia, absence of the auricle (**b**).

Clinical Aspects of Diseases of the External Ear

■ Congenital Anomalies

In addition to wide variation in the position, size, and shape of the auricle, there are also numerous disfiguring anomalies. Classifying auricular deformities provides an overview of these congenital dysplasias, at increasing degrees of severity:

- *First-degree dysplasia*: minor deformities (e. g., prominent ear, macrotia, scaphoid deformity, lobular deformities, cup ear deformities types 1 and 2).
- *Second-degree dysplasia*: some characteristics of a normal auricular structure are present (e. g., first- and second-degree microtia, cup ear type 3).
- *Third-degree dysplasia*: absence of a normal auricular structure (e. g., third-degree microtia, anotia).

Lop ear (bat ear). This is one of the most common disfiguring anomalies (**Fig. 1.63a, b**). It is often caused by hypertrophy or excess curvature of the conchal cartilage, or by failure of the auricle to fold due to underdevelopment or absence of the antihelix.

Treatment: The deep conchal cavity is corrected, and an antihelixplasty is performed. The angle between the auricle and the head is reduced to the ideal value of 30° and the scaphoconchal angle to 90°. The operation should be performed during preschool years.

Microtia, anotia. *Microtia* (abnormal smallness of the auricle of the ear, **Fig. 1.64a**) and *anotia* (absence of the auricle or the ear, **Fig. 1.64b**) are often associated with auditory canal stenosis or atresia and with middle ear deformities. Deformities of the external ear and the middle ear can also occur in connection with other facial deformities (e. g., Franceschetti syndrome (**Fig. 1.65**), mandibulofacial dysostosis, Treacher–Collins syndrome).

Congenital aural fistulas and auricular appendages. These are usually located in front of the auricle. They are due to incomplete closure of the first branchial cleft or incomplete fusion of the auricular hillocks. Three groups can be distinguished on the basis of the embryologic association and site:

1. Preauricular fistulas, between the angle of the mouth and the tragus.
2. Fistulas that begin in front of the ascending helix and lead toward the meatus, or open externally inferior to the angle of the jaw as a hyomandibular fistula (**Fig. 1.66**).
3. A small fistula or pitted depression affecting any part of the auricle.

Treatment: Treatment is excision, with careful consideration of the danger of damaging the parotid gland or facial nerve (see pp. 112 and 435).

■ Reconstructive Operations on the Auricle

Reconstructive procedures on the auricle vary in difficulty. Correcting an anomaly of the auricle's shape (remodeling the auricular cartilage) can be relatively simple in the hands of a skilled surgeon

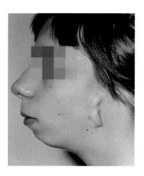

Fig. 1.65 Franceschetti Syndrome: deformity of the auricle and middle ear, with facial deformities.

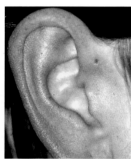

Fig. 1.66 Preauricular fistula.

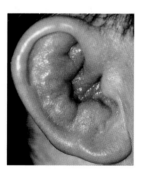

Fig. 1.67 Perichondritis of the auricle.

and can lead to very satisfactory results. However, reconstruction of the entire auricle is one of the most difficult tasks in plastic surgery in this area.

Thorough familiarity with skin and cartilage transplantation techniques is a prerequisite for the success of this reconstruction procedure. Costal cartilage is an ideal source for graft, and specialist instruments are required for modeling the graft. Staged surgery is necessary. Revision surgery may be required. Providing skin to create the new auricle is not easy and requires the construction of rotation and sliding flaps from the neck and from the region of the hairline. Prostheses should be considered as an alternative in difficult cases.

Reconstruction of the external auditory meatus and the sound-conducting apparatus is discussed in the section on anomalies of the middle ear (see p. 94).

■ Inflammations of the External Ear

■ Nonspecific Inflammation

Classification. Bacterial or fungal inflammation of the skin of the external auditory canal, with or without inflammation of the tympanic membrane (myringitis).

Clinical Features. *Acute exudative inflammatory phase:*

- Swelling of the skin of the auditory canal with lubricious, often fetid secretion.
- The tympanic membrane is often not visible, due to shifting of the auditory canal.
- There is an accumulation of detritus in the auditory canal.
- The cartilaginous part of the meatus is painful.
- Painful limitation of motion of the adjacent temporomandibular joint.
- The regional retroauricular lymph nodes may be so enlarged and tender to pressure in serious cases that the condition bears a strong resemblance to *pseudo-mastoiditis.*

Chronic inflammatory phase:

- The meatus is wide, the epithelial lining is atrophic, and dry scales of epidermis accumulate.
- There is intense itching, which causes scratching by the patient. This promotes the development of *superinfection* with acute dermatitis, with or without perichondritis (**Fig. 1.67**).

Pathogenesis

- Maceration of the meatal skin by exogenous and endogenous factors, such as fluid, mechanical and chemical damage, allergy, and diabetes.
- Reduction of the elasticity of the meatal skin and atrophy of the ceruminous and sebaceous glands.
- Loss of the protective film of secretion, with drying of the meatal skin, disturbance of its chemical balance, and increased susceptibility to infection by bacteria and fungi.
- Disturbance of the pH balance of the meatal skin, leading to the growth of anaerobic bacteria.

Factors that encourage the elimination of pathogens in the meatal skin include:

- Low pH values.
- Fatty acids in the secretions of the sebaceous glands.
- Normal lysozyme content of the secretions of the ceruminous glands.
- A normal self-cleaning mechanism, with external migration of the meatal epithelium.

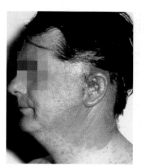

Fig. 1.68 Erysipelas of the skin.

Disturbance of protective factors—as may occur in allergy, with displacement of the pH to alkaline values, reduction of the protective film, and changes in the composition of the secretions due to mechanical stimulation or recurrent inflammation—can cause chronic or recurrent otitis externa.

Diagnosis and differential diagnosis
- The inflammation is localized to the auricle, external auditory meatus, and regional lymph nodes.
- Inflammation is often associated with etiological skin conditions such as eczema or psoriasis.
- Extension to the outer and middle layers of the tympanic membrane (myringitis) is only an exceptional occurrence.
- The middle ear and mastoid are not affected by the disease.
- Conductive deafness due to obstruction of the external auditory meatus is unusual and mild in nature.
- It is important to exclude acute otitis media, mastoiditis, and the acute phase of a chronic middle ear inflammation with cholesteatoma.
- Pain when pressure is applied to the tragus strongly suggests otitis externa.

Investigations. These include otoscopy, a specimen of pus for bacteriology, possibly irrigation of the ear, hearing and tuning-fork tests, audiography, and imaging. If there is any clinical suspicion of mastoiditis or other infective complications, a CT scan should be done.

Treatment. The external auditory meatus is cleaned manually under vision, ideally with a microscope, or by irrigation with water at 37°C. The external auditory meatus is dried, and eardrops consisting of locally active broad-spectrum antibiotics and a corticosteroid are instilled several times a day during the moist phase. In severe cases, sys-

temic antibiotics are given. Once the acute inflammatory phase subsides, local applications of ointments based on a combination of an antibiotic and a steroid are used. However, certain antibiotics, notably neomycin, can themselves cause an allergic skin reaction. In these cases, the local use of 70–80% pure alcohol is indicated, and in the acute inflammatory phase, a fine gauze wick should be introduced into the ear. This is moistened repeatedly with alcohol, which opens the external auditory meatus and reduces the swelling of the meatal skin by absorbing moisture.

■ **Specific Forms of Inflammation of the External Ear**

Bacterial and Viral Diffuse Otitis Externa
A characteristic form of *erysipelas* occurs in streptococcal infection. In *swimmer's otitis,* due to maceration of the skin by halogen-containing swimming-pool water and deep penetration of virulent organisms, there is usually a deep-seated cellulitic inflammation (**Fig. 1.68**), with *perichondritis.* In addition to swimmer's otitis externa, confined to the external ear, a tubal form of swimmer's otitis media may also occur.

Clinical Features. These include fever, generalized illness, regional lymphadenitis, and pain when the auricle is pulled or pressure is applied to the tragus. A cellulitic form can extend to surrounding tissues and organs, such as the parotid gland, mastoid, and skull base, and in exceptional cases can cause osteomyelitis of the temporal bone and septicemia (*necrotizing otitis externa;* see p. 53). In severe cases of otitis externa, especially in infants and young children, there is complete obstruction of the ex-

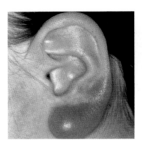

Fig. 1.69 Edematous swelling of the lobule of the auricle is a pathognomonic sign in patients with Lyme disease.

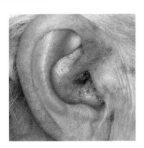

Fig. 1.70 Herpes zoster oticus.

ternal auditory meatus, with an accompanying retroauricular lymphadenitis. The ear is displaced laterally, and the patient may appear to have mastoiditis.

Treatment. Systemic antibiotics; local reduction of the swelling of the skin of the external auditory meatus with 70–95% alcohol, chloramine in a 1 : 1000 irrigation, or local application of topical antibiotics with or without a steroid.

Furuncle of the Ear (Otitis Externa Circumscripta)

The patient is in good general condition, but has local pain in the ear. A characteristic finding is a circumscribed, exquisitely painful swelling in the cartilaginous part of the external auditory meatus (hair follicles), modest regional lymphadenitis, and pain when pressure is applied to the tragus or the auricle is pulled.

Treatment. Gauze wicks soaked with alcohol (70–95%) are used until the furuncle points and bursts spontaneously. Incision and systemic antibiotics are only exceptionally indicated in patients with severe pain, a protracted course, or marked swelling.

Note: The glucose content of the urine and blood should be checked in patients with recurrent furunculosis of the external meatus.

Lyme Disease (Lyme Borreliosis)

Lyme disease is a multisystemic bacterial infection caused by species of bacteria belonging to the genus *Borrelia*. It is transmitted to humans by the bite of an infected hard tick.

The early infection often starts with flu-like symptoms such as headache, stiff neck, fever, muscle aches, and fatigue. An enlarging rash, known as erythema migrans (EM), develops days to weeks later at the site of the bite (**Fig. 1.69**). Neurological problems such as severe headaches, meningitis, or cranial nerve involvement can occur at a later stage. Changes in smell or taste, vocal cord and facial nerve paralysis, vertigo with nystagmus, and hearing and swallowing disorders are typical otolaryngological symptoms. Progression of the infection is characterized by central nervous symptoms such as cognitive changes (memory problems, difficulty in finding words, confusion, decreased concentration, problems with numbers) and behavioral changes (depression, personality changes).

Herpes Zoster Oticus

This disease is characterized by multiple herpetic vesicles arranged in groups on the auricle, the external auditory meatus, and occasionally the tympanic membrane (**Fig. 1.70**). In severe cases, disorders of hearing and balance and facial paralysis may occur (see **Table 1.16**, p. 99, and p. 111).

Bullous Myringitis

This disease usually occurs in association with an influenzal infection. It is occasionally combined with otitis media, in which case the patient has conductive deafness. Initially there is a moist, bluish-livid bullous inflammation, which can extend to the tympanic membrane. After a few days, the hemorrhagic vesicles dry out and heal without complications. The patient usually reports extremely severe pain.

!

> **Note:** If the middle ear is involved, systemic antibiotics must be administered immediately due to the danger of superinfection.

In most cases, treatment is limited to simple cleansing of the external meatus and otoscopic control. Antibiotics are only given for protection against secondary infection.

Necrotizing Otitis Externa
Severe necrotizing inflammation can develop from commonplace otitis externa, especially in patients with diabetes, whether latent or manifest. The infection is generally caused by optionally anaerobic Gram-negative organisms, usually *Pseudomonas aeruginosa*. The infection spreads through the tissue clefts of the cartilaginous meatus and extends into the depths of the retromandibular fossa and along the base of the skull as far as the jugular foramen, and it leads to insidious osteomyelitis of the temporal bone.

Diagnosis. The hallmark of this condition is pain in and around the ear. In addition to examining the auditory canal and carrying out a hearing test, it is necessary to examine the neighboring cranial nerves (examination with Frenzel glasses for spontaneous nystagmus; examination of the facial nerve, trigeminal nerve, and abducent nerve), ultrasound examination of the parotid and neck, microbiological culture and sensitivity tests, CT/MRI of the base of the skull, blood sugar profile, C-reactive protein (CRP), erythrocyte sedimentation rate (ESR), hemoglobin, and full blood count.

Treatment. Treatment of diabetes and intensive anti-inflammatory therapy with broad-spectrum antibiotics (e. g., ciprofloxacin) is fundamental. Local treatment of the external acoustic meatus promotes the drainage of infective secretions. In severe cases, generous drainage of the retromandibular space, infratemporal fossa, and pterygopalatine fossa together with debridement of necrotic tissue from the external meatus may become necessary. Ligation or resection of the internal jugular vein may also be indicated if it is involved.

Prognosis. Even with massive antibiotics and extensive surgery, the prognosis is poor, due to septicemia and sinus thrombosis.

■ **Chronic Inflammation**

Tuberculosis and *syphilis* (stage 2) cause local, circumscribed lesions of the external ear and auditory meatus. The therapy is focused on local dermatological treatment and specific high-dose antibiotic treatment.

■ **Otomycosis and Eczema**

Otomycosis
Clinical Features. The infection is caused by a fungus and is limited to the external auditory meatus. There may be a recent history of antibiotic drops being used to treat bacterial infection. Typically, a fine, easily removable coating that is loose and fluffy, varying in color from whitish-yellow to greenish-black, is visible. The patient reports itching, but rarely describes pain.

Diagnosis. Culture and sensitivity tests demonstrate fungal mycelium.

Treatment. The mainstay of treatment is manual cleaning, but irrigation should be avoided if possible to prevent the formation of a "moist chamber," which promotes the growth of the fungus.

Antimycotic agents, such as 1 % clotrimazole or clioquinol, can be applied locally unless contraindicated by perforation of the tympanic membrane. Antibiotics should not be used. Daily painting of the meatus with thiomersal or 2 % acetic acid spray helps. In severe cases, systemic antimycotics such as fluconazole can be used.

Course. The course is chronic and recurrent.

Eczema of the Ear
Clinical Features. The disease follows an episodic course, with intermittent acute exacerbations. The entry of fluid such as sweat or water during washing, or the presence of a moist exudate, promote colonization by pathogenic bacteria or fungi in the relatively enclosed external meatus.

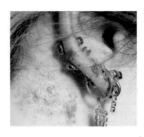

Fig. 1.71 Contact dermatitis caused by jewelry containing nickel.

In the acute stage, there is deep-red inflammatory swelling with moist vesicles and pustules. Later, crusts accumulate. Rhagades form around the meatal introitus, and fetid debris collects. The usual picture is one of nonspecific acute otitis externa, but occasionally the appearance may progress to chronic myringitis with superficial granulations.

In the chronic stage, the skin is atrophic, dry, scaly, and may be partly lichenified. The patient reports chronic irritation. Occasionally, stenosis may occur.

Diagnosis and differential diagnosis. *Contact eczema* may be due to cosmetic solutions, hair sprays, glasses frames made of metal or plastic, cement or flour dust, or medications—e. g., antibiotics. Skin tests have to be performed in order to identify the antigen (**Fig. 1.71**).

Microbial eczema is mainly due to infection with staphylococci or to oral mycosis. A swab should be taken for culture and sensitivity tests.

Seborrheic eczema is the most common form. It is often combined with acne.

Endogenous eczema is a localized manifestation of a generalized eczema.

Treatment. Elimination of the allergen and local treatment, as detailed above.

■ Trauma

Sharp or Blunt Trauma to the External Ear
Any injury to the auricle and cartilaginous part of the external auditory meatus can damage the perichondrium, causing cartilaginous necrosis. A distinction is made between auricle lacerations and avulsions either of the whole auricle or parts of it.

Treatment. For lacerations, primary closure of the wound with monofilament suture material (6–0 or 7–0) is recommended, and the duration of antibi-

otic treatment depends on the degree of contamination. In comprehensive lacerations with cartilaginous involvement and extensive skin damage, it is recommended—following wound debridement if necessary—to close the wound, starting on the posterior aspect of the auricle, with monofilament suture material.

The cartilage should be repaired with 5–0 absorbable suture material, and the skin of the anterior surface with monofilament 6–0 suture material. Replantation of the avulsed part of the auricle in the acute situation is also the treatment of choice for partial avulsion injuries; ischemia periods of up to 8 hours are tolerable and still allow the graft to take. If the graft does not take, plastic reconstruction is necessary in the interval.

Prognosis. Bacterial infection can cause perichondritis, with partial or complete destruction of the cartilaginous framework, leading to cauliflower ear (see **Fig. 1.73**) or atresia of the meatus.

Hematoma of the Auricle
This arises from closed blunt injury, with dissection of the skin and perichondrial layer from the cartilage and the formation of a subperichondrial hematoma (**Fig. 1.72**).

Treatment. The aim of treatment is to remove the seroma or hematoma and to achieve long-term adaptation of the perichondrium to the cartilage in order prevent leakage into the seroma cavity.

In general, drainage from the anterior surface can be carried out, with the incision being made in the fossa of the helix (scapha). Following curettage and readaptation of the skin with monofilament suture material, light compression for 3–5 days with a dental roll, secured with through-and-through sutures, is recommended. For drainage from the posterior surface of the auricle, an incision has to be made in the cartilage to reach a seroma/hematoma on the anterior surface, and a cartilage window may be necessary to achieve adherence of the perichondrium layers. Antibiotic treatment is recommended in order to prevent perichondritis.

Note: Repeated aspiration may cause a seroma or superinfection, leading to perichondritis.

If a hematoma is not treated, connective-tissue organization, secondary calcification, and deformity of the auricle occur, leading to cauliflower ear (**Fig. 1.73**).

Frostbite

Grade 1: Cyanosis of the skin due to vascular spasm.
Grade 2: Ischemia with formation of vesicles.
Grade 3: Deep necrosis of tissue.

Treatment. Sterile dressings, antibiotics, intravenous vasodilators, and possibly stellate ganglion block are used, depending on the severity of the injury. The area has to be kept dry.

Burns require the same treatment as burns to the skin; particular attention needs be given to the close relationship between the skin and the cartilage.

Late complications include necrosis of the auricle and atresia or stenosis of the external auditory meatus.

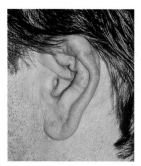

Fig. 1.72 Auricular hematoma (othematoma).

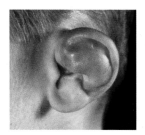

Fig. 1.73 Untreated hematoma or infection can lead to a deformity of the auricle—cauliflower ear.

■ Wax and Foreign Bodies

Wax

!

> **Note:** Collections of wax and cell debris are unusual if the self-cleaning mechanism of the external auditory meatus is undisturbed. The present widespread habit of cleaning the external ear daily with ready-made cotton swabs is inappropriate and can sooner or later lead to the development of chronic otitis externa.

Wax is a yellowish-brown mass consisting of secretions of the sebaceous and ceruminous glands, desquamated epithelium, hair, and particles of dirt.

Plug of wax. The normal symptom is deafness when the external auditory meatus is completely closed, but occasional complaints include a roaring noise in the head and a feeling of dizziness.

Differential diagnosis. A plug of epidermis, foreign body, dried blood, purulent exudate, and cholesteatoma of the meatus or of the middle ear.

A *plug of epidermis* is a compact white mass consisting of desquamated epithelial crusts, which usually adhere firmly to the skin of the meatus.

Treatment. The ear is irrigated with water at 37°C. Manual syringes are now rarely used, and electrically controlled water jets with controlled pressure are used instead. It should be ensured that a perforation of the tympanic membrane is not hidden

behind the plug of wax. This should be excluded by taking a careful history. If the patient does have such a perforation, the wax should be removed manually by a specialist. Hard wax should be first softened with soft soap drops, 5 % sodium bicarbonate, olive oil drops, or 3 % hydrogen peroxide for up to 1 week before syringing. The moist external auditory meatus should be mopped out with cotton applicators. Local steroid or antibiotic creams or eardrops should be prescribed for patients with inflammation of the meatus. For medicolegal reasons, the patient's hearing should be tested after this procedure.

Foreign Bodies

Foreign bodies are diagnosed using careful otoscopy. The findings vary depending on the object and the length of time it has been in the ear. In children, a careful history should be taken to establish the nature of the foreign body. Depending on their age, children may be able to indicate that they have a foreign body in the ear, or they may present with symptoms of ear pain or discharge. Insects can cause injury to the canal or tympanic membrane as a result of scratching or stinging.

Physical pain or bleeding may occur with objects that abrade the ear canal or rupture the tympanic membrane, or as a result of the patient's attempts to

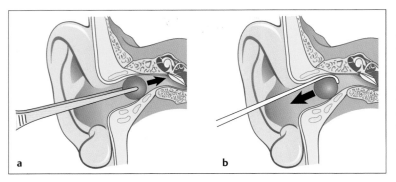

Fig. 1.74a, b Attempts to remove a foreign body with simple forceps (**a**) may displace the foreign body more deeply, and it may perforate the tympanic membrane, causing dislocation of the ossicles and injury to the facial canal. The foreign body can be removed easily without danger to the patient using a hook, under otoscopic or microscopic guidance (**b**).

remove the object. Hearing loss may be observed. If the presentation is delayed, erythema and swelling of the canal and a foul-smelling discharge may be present.

> **Note:** Foreign bodies that cannot be removed by syringing should be removed manually, with general anesthesia being administered in small children.
> If a perforation of the tympanic membrane is known of or suspected, the ear should not be syringed.
> Blind attempts to extract foreign bodies without otoscopic control, or attempts to extract them under vision with unsuitable instruments and inadequate anesthesia, should be avoided. Instrumental removal of foreign bodies from the meatus should therefore only be carried out by a specialist, except for the simplest cases.
> **Figure 1.74a,b** shows correct and incorrect methods of extracting a foreign body from the meatus.

■ Tumors

■ Benign Tumors

These include retroauricular atheroma, cicatricial keloid, hemangioma and lymphangioma, dermoid tumors, fibroma, papilloma, keratoma, lipoma, and nevi.

Treatment. The treatment consists of tumor resection.

Meatal tumors include *hyperostosis,* caused by periosteal stimulation and resulting in appositional bone growth with progressive narrowing of the lumen of the meatus; and *exostosis,* a true bony tumor arising from the ossification centers in the anulus tympanicus. This tumor should only be removed if it is causing stenosis. *Chondrodermatitis nodularis*

circumscripta helicis causes painful nodes on the ear that should be distinguished from a premalignant lesion by the marked pain that occurs when pressure is applied.

■ Precancerous and Malignant Tumors

The classification, symptoms, diagnosis, and differential diagnosis are shown in **Table 1.9**.

Precancerous Lesions
Premalignant lesions often progress to true carcinoma, and they should therefore always be treated with radical surgery, in the same way as true tumors. Biopsy excision is not advisable, and any tumor of the external ear suspected of being malignant should be excised with a wide margin. The mainstay of treatment is surgery; radiotherapy or cryosurgery are second-best options.

Precancerous lesions such as senile keratosis (**Fig. 1.75a**) or Bowen disease are excised with a healthy margin. Periodic follow-up is necessary.

Malignant Tumors
Basal cell carcinoma. Surgical excision of basal cell carcinoma in an otherwise healthy patient is decisive for the prognosis (**Fig. 1.75b**). A two-step surgical procedure is the method of choice. The first step involves temporary wound coverage of the defect after resection of the tumor. After histological confirmation that the wound margins are tumor-free, the defect can be covered in a second operation, which may require reconstruction of the auricle. For very small tumors, a one-step procedure is possible, with primary wound closure after intraoperative histological control of the wound margins using frozen-section histology.

Table 1.9   Precancerous and malignant tumors of the external ear

	Form	Color	Skin surface	Cartilage invasion	Regional lymph-node metastases
Cutaneous horn	A sharply limited warty growth of the epidermis	Inconspicuous	Slightly nodular, intact	None	None
Senile keratosis	Smooth mass with indistinct borders	Yellowish-brown	Rough, intact, occasionally covered by crusts	None	None
Bowen disease	Smooth round lump	Intensive brownish-red	Smooth but intact	None	None
Basal cell carcinoma	Sharply demarcated smooth, slowly growing mass	Hyperemic, sometimes much more pigmented than the surrounding skin (special form: pigmented basal cell carcinoma)	Often superficially ulcerated, crusted, raised edges with an atrophic center (or central ulcer)	Perichondrium sometimes infiltrated, tumor relatively immobile at its base	Rarely
Squamous cell carcinoma	Exophytic tumor of relatively rapid growth with indistinct margins	Often hyperemic	Ulcerated, raised edges, superficially nodular, firm	Always The tumor is not movable; occasionally perichondritis	20 %
Malignant melanoma	A round mass, sometimes verrucous, rapidly growing	Dark-brown to black, occasionally weakly pigmented, the amelanotic melanoma	Smooth to slightly nodular, occasionally ulcerated or bleeds easily to touch	Perichondrium often infiltrated and the tumor is relatively immobile at its base	Frequent Also early distant metastases, especially to the lung

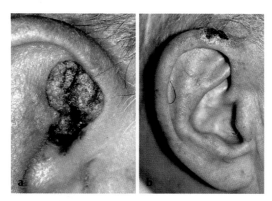

Fig. 1.75a, b   **a** Senile keratosis of the auricle. **b** Basal cell carcinoma.

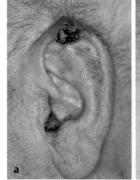 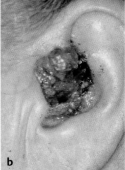

Fig. 1.76a, b   Squamous cell carcinoma. **a** A small erosive carcinoma invading the helix. **b** Carcinoma growing out of the external meatus.

Keratinizing squamous cell carcinomas. These are infiltrating, often ulcerated carcinomas (**Fig. 1.76a, b**). In 20 % of patients, the lesions have early metastases to the regional lymph nodes. The treatment of choice is *radical surgery,* with no regard for the cosmetic result. Radiotherapy is only successful for tumors less than 1 cm in diameter that are not ulcerated, have not infiltrated the perichondrium, and have not metastasized to the regional lymph nodes. In all other cases, *partial or complete excision of the auricle* is the method of choice. Neck dissection is performed when there are regional lymph-node metastases.

Carcinoma of the external auditory meatus. This represents ≈ 5 % of all aural carcinomas. In comparison with tumors of the auricle, the prognosis is unfavorable due to late diagnosis and because the tumor penetrates early into the parotid space or the middle ear. The treatment of choice is extensive resection of the tumor with radical neck dissection and, if necessary, parotidectomy.

Pigmented nevus and suspected malignant melanoma. These should be treated with primary excision of the tumor, without previous biopsy. Depending on the histological results, it may be necessary to carry out a secondary surgical excision, dictated by the extent and depth of the tumor (see p. 405), with regional neck dissection or radical neck dissection and, if necessary, parotidectomy. Postoperative radiotherapy, chemotherapy, or immunotherapy may also be necessary. Surgery should only be considered when distant metastases have been ruled out.

Clinical Aspects of Diseases of the Middle and Internal Ear

■ Disorders of Ventilation and Drainage of the Middle Ear Spaces

Pathophysiology. Most chronic middle ear diseases are based largely on two functional disturbances: *impaired middle ear ventilation* and *inflammation.* Impairment of ventilation due to eustachian tube dysfunction is based on a mucosal inflammation in the nasopharynx, leading to inflammation of the middle ear mucosa.

Pathogenesis. The eustachian tube does not open regularly on swallowing, due to one of the following factors:

- A dysfunctional tensor veli palatini muscle.
- Swelling of the tubal mucosa caused by chronic inflammation of neighboring structures, such as the sinuses or tonsils or by allergy.
- Obstruction of the ostium of the tube by hypertrophic adenoids, in a child or adult.
- Infiltration of the tube by a malignant tumor of the nasopharynx.

The middle ear is thus no longer aerated, and the remaining air is resorbed, producing a decrease in pressure that acts as an irritant to the middle ear mucosa.

In *short-term tubal occlusion* or persistent, reduced pressure in the middle ear, the following changes may occur:

- Edema of the mucosa.
- Middle ear fluid, due to transudation of the constituent parts of the serum.
- Stiffening of the ossicular chain, with retraction of the tympanic membrane.

Note: Ventilation and drainage disorders of the middle ear are usually caused by a dysfunctional opening mechanism of the tube, but mechanical obstruction of the tube by a lesion in the nasopharynx may also occur.

In *long-standing tubal occlusion* and reduced pressure in the middle ear, the following changes may occur:

- Metaplasia of the middle ear mucosa from the flat epithelial cells of the mucoperiosteum to form columnar, ciliated, mucus-producing goblet cells.
- Increase in secretory activity of the goblet cells and mixing of the mucus with the transudate already present in the middle ear, causing a *seromucinous exudate.*
- Formation of cholesterin-containing mucosal cysts (cholesterol granuloma).

The seromucinous exudate and mucosal changes substantially reduce the aeration of the middle ear, thus causing a vicious circle.

The metaplasia of the middle ear mucosa also affects the submucosa, causing firstly a proliferation of the connective tissue and secondly maturation of a local immunologically active cellular defense mechanism. The active secreting goblet cells produce a mucus blanket, which serves to transport newly formed immunoglobulins to the mucosal surface. The previously inactive mucoperiosteum of the middle ear is thus converted into a secreting hyperplastic respiratory mucosa, characterized by its newly acquired property of responding to every new stimulus (mechanical, chemical, bacterial, enzymatic, allergic, or autoimmune) with a completely mature defense mechanism. This consists of the following:

- Mucociliary elements, which form the transport medium for the superficially active mucus blanket.
- Enzymatic elements, which consist in particular of bactericidal lysozymes and protease inhibitors.
- Locally produced immunoglobulins.

The result of this increased activity in the local and mucosal immune system is that each bacterial stimulus causes hyperplasia or metaplasia of the superficial epithelium and induces mucosal edema with a cellular infiltrate. The resulting increase in the volume of the middle ear mucosa thus starts a vicious circle of deteriorating ventilation and drainage.

This hyperactivity of the middle ear mucosa continues after cessation of the external stimulus and ultimately leads to *tympanosclerosis*. Enzymes and the pathologic concentration of metabolic products and mediators of inflammation (lipoids, mucopolysaccharides) cause progressive metaplasia of the middle ear mucosa, resulting in fibrosis and sclerosis of the middle ear and formation of cholesterol granulomas. These changes lead to an irreversible tympanosclerotic condition.

Basically, two main forms of disorders of ventilation and drainage can be distinguished: the first occurs acutely and is reversible, while the second follows a chronic course that is only partially reversible.

Acute Tubal Occlusion (Serotympanum)

Clinical Features. A feeling of pressure in the ear occurs during a head cold (rhinopharyngitis), often accompanied by stabbing pain, deafness, and a crackling noise when swallowing.

Diagnosis. Otoscopy shows a retracted tympanic membrane (**Fig. 1.77a, b**) and hyperemia of the handle of the malleus and of the vessels of the tympanic membrane. If a transudate occurs, there is an amber discoloration of the pars tensa and occasionally a fluid level and air bubbles in the

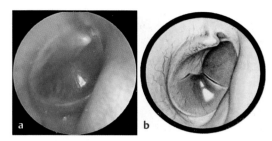

Fig. 1.77a, b Serous otitis media. The tympanic membrane is slightly retracted and transudate is visible in the tympanic cavity. The malleus handle is perceptibly shortened, the light reflex is widened.

middle ear. The patient also has mild to moderate conductive hearing loss.

Differential diagnosis. Acute otitis media has to be ruled out.

Treatment. This is initially directed at the underlying disease. Rhinopharyngitis is treated with decongestant nose drops, vasoconstrictors, and antihistamines to reduce hyperemia and edema in the tube. Antibiotics are given if there are dangerous signs of progression to otitis media or of acute nasal pharyngitis. Hypertrophic adenoids are removed later if necessary, and sinusitis is treated.

Note: Oral analgesics, rather than analgesic ear drops, should be used to treat pain in the ear. Ear drops obliterate the otoscopic appearance of the tympanic membrane by macerating the superficial epithelium and can make it difficult to recognize otitis media.

Course and prognosis. The symptoms usually resolve rapidly, but occasionally the disease progresses to chronic seromucinous otitis media.

Note: The Valsalva maneuver or air insufflation should not be performed when there is acute inflammation in the nasopharynx, due to the danger of transmitting infectious microorganisms to the middle ear and causing tubal otitis media.

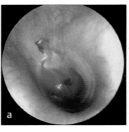
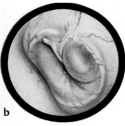

Fig. 1.78a, b Chronic seromucinous otitis media. The pars tensa of the tympanic membrane is protracted, while the pars flaccida is retracted. A bulb filled with yellow-brown liquid expands the tympanic membrane.

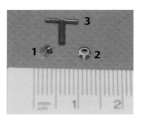

Fig. 1.79 Different types of ear ventilation tube. **1, 2,** Silver ear tubes coated with gold, sizes I and II; **3,** Silastic tube for long-term placement.

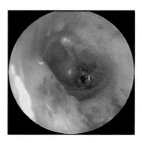

Fig. 1.80 Middle ear drainage is achieved by inserting a metal tube ("grommet").

Chronic Seromucinous Otitis Media

Clinical Features. There is a feeling of pressure and fullness in the ear, often following an infection of the upper airway, and there is a considerable decrease in hearing on one or both sides. Noises are heard in the ear when yawning, swallowing, and sneezing. Pain is absent.

Pathogenesis. Tubal obstruction and the resulting reduction in tympanic pressure predominate. Obstructive processes in the nasopharynx and disorders of tubal kinetics, particularly incompetence of the muscles opening the tube in cleft palate, and viral infections are the most common underlying mechanisms.

Diagnosis. Otoscopy shows a markedly retracted tympanic membrane with localized protrusion, an exudate in the middle ear, and dark discoloration behind the tympanic membrane (the so-called "blue drum"), with a blackish fluid level or air bubbles. There is conductive deafness for the entire frequency range up to 50 dB. A typical flat curve is found. A search for the primary cause shows enlargement of the adenoids, sinusitis, allergy, or tumor (**Fig. 1.78a, b**).

Differential diagnosis. This includes *hemotympanum* (the dark-brown exudate behind the tympanic membrane on occasion lends this a bluish tinge) and *chronic otitis media,* evidenced by perforation, cholesteatoma flakes, and purulent exudate. Adhesions may occur after recurrent otitis, shown by a markedly retracted tympanic membrane with thick scars, tympanosclerotic deposits, and abnormal tubal function. In adult patients with unilateral symptoms, biopsy from the nasopharynx should be considered to exclude tumor; some tumors are submucosal and not clearly apparent.

Treatment. If necessary, surgical restoration of tubal patency by adenoidectomy or revision adenoidectomy under direct vision, and elimination of any sinus infections.

Selective insertion of a ventilation tube after paracentesis and drainage of the middle ear (see **Fig. 1.84**), when clinically indicated by symptoms, is the treatment of choice.

An incision is made in the anteroinferior quadrant of the tympanic membrane, under general anesthesia in children and under local anesthesia in some compliant adults. The middle ear effusion is aspirated, and long-term drainage is provided for at least 6 months using a ventilation tube (or "grommet"; **Figs. 1.79, 1.80**). Alternatively, watchful waiting can make it possible to avoid surgery, as the disease resolves in many cases. Adjuvant treatment consists of steroids with antibiotic cover and mucolytic drugs. Other alternatives—such as local aerosol treatment (intranasal or tubotympanic application), α-chymotrypsin (tubotympanic, transtympanic, or systemic administration), hyaluronidase, and corticosteroids (intratympanic application)—are not generally used, but have been investigated in research studies. Antiallergic treatment includes antihistamines and intranasal steroids if there is positive evidence of allergy. Acute otitis media is often present even if the immunological findings are normal. Mastoiditis has to be ruled out, otherwise mastoidectomy should be considered.

Course and prognosis. Long-term healing is only achieved in a proportion of patients. In others, there is a progressive, chronic course leading to adhesive processes as a result of connective-tissue organization of the seromucinous exudate and development of cholesterol granuloma and tympanosclerosis. Hyaline degeneration of the mucoperiosteum may also occur, with the formation of sclerotic submucosal plaques as a result of local metabolic disturbances (**Fig. 1.81a, b**).

Syndrome of the Patulous Eustachian Tube

Clinical Features. These include *autophony,* which is a rumbling reverberation of the patient's own voice, and a noise in the ears synchronous with breathing, due to movements of the tympanic membrane and resonance in the nasopharynx.

Pathogenesis. The symptoms represent a masking effect of the lower and middle tones, evoked by resonance and respiratory noise. The primary cause is insufficiency of the closing mechanism of the tube (see p. 3). The secondary cause is disappearance of the fat bolster around the opening of the tube, a gaping ostium caused by hormonal disturbances, and possibly also by use of the contraceptive pill.

Diagnosis. The diagnosis is made by impedance audiometry and tubal function tests.

Treatment. If possible, the basic cause is dealt with. The patient also needs to have the cause of the symptoms explained.

■ Nonspecific Inflammation of the Middle Ear and Mastoid

> **Note:** Inflammatory diseases of the middle ear are important because of their frequency and the life-threatening complications associated with them due to the close relationship between the middle ear and the cranial cavity.

Acute Otitis Media

Clinical Features. In the first phase of *exudative inflammation,* lasting for 1–2 days, there is an increase in temperature to 39–40°C, and in severe

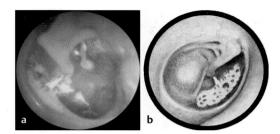

Fig. 1.81a, b Tympanosclerosis.
a Hyaline degeneration of the mucoperiosteum occurs with the formation of sclerotic submucosal plaques.
b The posterior half of the tympanic membrane shows atrophic scarring, and plaque has formed on the anterior half.

cases, rigors, and occasionally meningism in children. The patient has a severe pulsating pain, which is worse at night than during the day. There is a muffled noise in the ear synchronous with the pulse, deafness, and sensitivity of the mastoid process to pressure. In older patients, there is often no fever.

The second phase, involving *resistance and demarcation,* lasts 3–8 days. The pus and middle ear exudate usually discharge spontaneously, after which the pain and fever subside. This phase can be considerably shortened by administering topical therapy (meatal cleansing, application of an astringent solution). Early antibiotic administration does not alter the clinical course of the disease significantly, and it does not prevent spontaneous perforation of the tympanic membrane.

In the third, *healing* phase, lasting 2–4 weeks, the aural discharge dries up and hearing returns to normal.

> **Note:** Acute middle ear inflammation may have a serious course, even if the tympanic membrane does not perforate.

Pathogenesis. *Routes of infection:* The tubal route is the most common. Hematogenous infection is unusual and occurs in measles, scarlet fever, typhus, and septicemia. Exogenous infection requires rupture of the tympanic membrane or previous perforation, allowing bathwater or dirt to penetrate during irrigation of the ear. Incorrect methods of re-

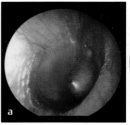
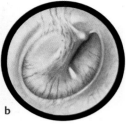

Fig. 1.82a, b Acute otitis media.
a The tympanic membrane is erythematous and bulging, and the handle of the malleus shows hyperemia.
b The tympanic membrane also has radiating hyperemia.

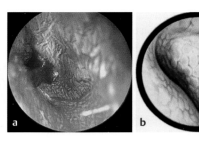

Fig. 1.83a, b Acute otitis media (desquamative phase). The tympanic membrane is severely bulging and a livid red, partially blue-gray appearance with scales, as a result of severe desquamation.

moving a foreign body from the external meatus are also another cause.

> **Note:** In healthy individuals, the middle ear is sterile if the tympanic membrane is intact.

Type of organism: the infection is monomicrobial. In decreasing order of frequency, the infecting organisms are: streptococci in adults, pneumococci in children, *Haemophilus influenzae, Moraxella catarrhalis,* and various staphylococci. A viral infection may prepare the way for secondary bacterial infection (herpes simplex and zoster, flu viruses). The inflammation usually affects not only the mucosa of the middle ear, but also that of the entire respiratory system.

> **Note:** Every attack of acute otitis media is accompanied by mastoiditis.

Diagnosis. In the first phase, otoscopy shows hyperemia, then moist infiltration and opacity of the surface of the tympanic membrane. The contours of the handle of the malleus and its short process disappear (**Fig. 1.82a, b**). The patient has conductive deafness. At the height of the exudative phase, the tympanic membrane bulges, particularly its posterosuperior quadrant. Pulsation is also seen. The inflammation may extend to the external meatus, obliterating the boundary between the meatus and the tympanic membrane (**Fig. 1.83a, b**). The accompanying mastoiditis makes the mastoid pro-

cess tender to pressure. In influenzal otitis, hemorrhagic bullae form on the external auditory meatus and the tympanic membrane.

In the second phase of acute otitis media, immediately before spontaneous rupture, a pinhole-sized fistula forms, usually in the posterosuperior quadrant. This discharges a pulsating, thin, fluid, odorless pus. Radiography with the Schüller view or preferably CT scanning shows clouding of the cell system without osteolysis—i.e., the bony septa appear sharp. Imaging is indicated only if there are severe clinical symptoms (facial palsy, dizziness, vertigo, severe sensorineural hearing loss).

In the third phase of acute otitis media, the inflammation and thickening of the tympanic membrane resolve, the pulsations disappear, and the discharge becomes mucoid and finally ceases. The perforation closes spontaneously, leaving a fine scar. Hearing returns to normal. CT scans show gradual clearing of the cell system.

Differential diagnosis. *Otitis externa* needs to be considered. In otitis externa, there is pain when pressure is applied to the tragus, and the exudate does not pulsate, is usually fetid, and is never mucoid. There is little or no deafness, and the cell system appears normal on radiographs.

Treatment
1. Systemic antibiotics at high dosages are given if condition worsens after 48 h. Hospital admission and intravenous application of amoxicillin and other broad-spectrum penicillins are indicated. Culture and sensitivity tests are carried

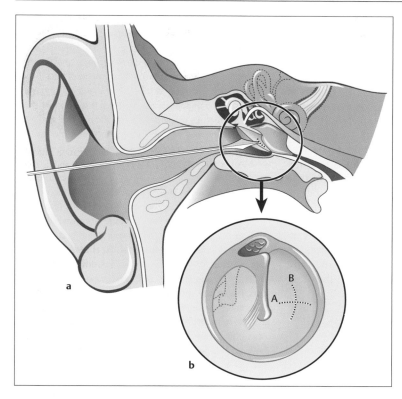

Fig. 1.84a, b   The principle of paracentesis.
a The position of the myringotomy knife relative to the external meatus and tympanic membrane.
b Incision into the anterior lower quadrant of the pars tensa. **A**, Correct incision; **B**, alternative incision.

out and appropriate antibiotics are administered if the tympanic membrane perforates.

2. Nasal drops are given to decongest the nasopharyngeal mucosa around the opening of the tube.
3. Analgesics (liquid paracetamol is recommended for children) and mucolytic drugs can be given.

Paracentesis (**Fig. 1.84a, b**), performed using a myringotomy with placement of a tympanostomy tube, is indicated in the following circumstances:

- Marked bulging of the tympanic membrane.
- Persistent high fever and severe pain.
- Unsatisfactory spontaneous perforation, with incomplete differentiation of the tympanic membrane.

If *symptoms of early mastoiditis* occur, with discrete facial palsy, acute meningitis, or labyrinthitis, and if the appearance of the tympanic membrane is inconclusive, surgery is indicated.

!

Note: Drops containing cortisone and antibiotic solution should not be used locally for aural discharge. They are ineffective, and also carry a risk of resistance to antibiotics developing. However, regular meatal cleansing should be performed for acute otitis media after the tympanic membrane perforates. The meatus can be irrigated with water at body temperature. The external meatus is then dried. Closing the meatus with cotton wool or gauze strips provides an ideal moist environment for inoculation with Gram-negative bacteria or fungi, and the meatus therefore has to be kept open.

Course and prognosis. In the first, acute phase, there is a danger of early otogenic complications, depending on the virulence and resistance of the organism, until the patient's own resistance develops and the bacterial infection is controlled with antibiotics.

During the second phase, complications occur very rarely. However, latent otitis media and the resulting occult mastoiditis may develop during this period due to insufficient antibiotic dosage, increased resistance of the organism, or inadequate resistance on the part of the patient. The general findings at otoscopy then do not correlate with the severity of the pathologic changes taking place in the middle ear and mastoid process. The paucity of symptoms leads to a false assumption that the otitis media has healed rapidly and completely. After an apparently symptom-free interval, late otogenic complications can occur in the third phase (see pp. 65 and 76). This course resembles that of the previously described, dreaded pneumococcal-type III mastoiditis.

In the third phase, most cases of acute otitis media and its concurrent mastoiditis heal completely. However, if latent otitis media and mastoiditis become established in the second phase, late otogenic complications may develop in the third period—i. e., 2–3 weeks after the start of the otitis. The symptoms include:

- Reappearance of fever.
- Recurrence of aural pain and discharge.
- Headaches.
- Worsening of the patient's general condition.
- Elevated erythrocyte sedimentation rate (ESR).

■ Specific Types of Inflammation of the Middle Ear and Mastoid

Acute Otitis Media in Infants and Children

Severe forms are unusual nowadays, thanks to effective diagnosis and treatment with antibiotics. However, they can occur in patients with immune deficiency or after inappropriate therapy. They are characterized by:

- Severe general symptoms, with high fever, meningeal and cerebral irritation, vomiting, loss of appetite, and disturbance of sleep.
- Immediate improvement of the child's condition after spontaneous perforation or paracentesis.
- A protracted course with numerous recurrences or exacerbations, with combined otitis media and bronchopneumonia, digestive and feeding upsets, and pyelonephritis.

Note: The younger the child, the more severe the generalized symptoms are and the more discrete the local signs are. The gastrointestinal symptoms are sometimes the most pressing.

Infants and young children have a predisposition to tubal middle ear infection because the tube is short, straight, and wide; because of the uniform character of the mucosa of the middle ear and the upper respiratory tract; and due to a higher frequency of infections of the respiratory tract, hyperplasia of the lymphoid tissue of the Waldeyer ring, poor aeration of the middle ear cavity, which is still partially filled with myxomatous tissue or hyperplastic mucosa, and a difference in the way in which the general and mucosal immune system react, caused in part by the genotype and in part by the phenotype.

Local symptoms. These include pressure in the ear, tugging on the affected ear, and painful reactions to pressure and traction. The tympanic membrane is grayish-red in color and bulges only slightly. Spontaneous perforation is not common; its site of predilection is the anteroinferior quadrant. Discharge is uncommon, as pus drains through the short, wide, and straight eustachian tube. If discharge occurs, it is stringy and pulsating. Mucosal polyps may form in the middle ear; regional retroauricular lymphadenitis causes a swelling behind the ear. If the petrosquamosal fissure is open, the pus may penetrate directly from the middle ear beneath the periosteum, causing marked swelling behind the ear.

Treatment. Treatment consists of oral antibiotics. If the infection is severe, intravenous antibiotics are given. Decongestant nose drops and analgesics can also be administered. The ear is irrigated with physiologic saline solution at body temperature.

Paracentesis (see **Fig. 1.84a, b**) should be carried out with the patient under general anesthesia early if the tympanic membrane does not perforate spontaneously.

If indicated on clinical grounds, *cortical mastoidectomy* should be performed early, even if radiographs are normal. *Cortical mastoidectomy* is carried out under general anesthesia in infants and young children in whom the mastoid process is incompletely pneumatized or not pneumatized at all. The infected part of the mastoid process is cleared via a retroauricular access route, with wide opening and drainage of the mastoid antrum (**Fig. 1.85**).

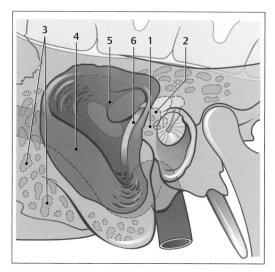

Fig. 1.85 The principle of cortical mastoidectomy. The posterior meatal wall (1) and attic wall (2) remain intact, while the cell system of the mastoid process (3) is cleared via a retroauricular approach. The anatomy of the external auditory meatus is not altered by this operation. 4, Sigmoid sinus; 5, mastoid cavity; 6, facial nerve (mastoid segment).

Course. The course is usually protracted, with intermittent exacerbations. There is often quick improvement and healing after surgical treatment of the affected ear. The prognosis is good with the correct treatment, but there is otherwise a danger of periantral osteomyelitis developing (infantile occult antritis), with vomiting and generalized toxic symptoms. In this case, immediate antrotomy is indicated.

Specific forms. *Influenzal otitis*: This is a hemorrhagic, bullous, acute middle ear inflammation. Primary infection with influenza A virus, combined with secondary bacterial infection *(Streptococcus pneumoniae)*, can take a fulminating course with complications (facial paralysis, labyrinthine irritation, meningitis).

Measles otitis: Hematogenous viral otitis media with subsequent tubal secondary infection, often leading to purulent mastoiditis.

Scarlatinal otitis: Acute necrotizing inflammation, with subtotal perforation of the tympanic membrane, necrosis of the ossicular chain, and osteomyelitis of the temporal bone.

Mastoiditis

The most frequent complication of middle ear inflammation is *mastoiditis,* an extension of the infection from the middle ear cavity to the pneumatic system of the temporal bone. In contrast to the mucosal inflammation, which always accompanies otitis media (see p. 61), the infection extends to, and causes dissolution of, bone. An unusually well-pneumatized bone infection can extend to the petrous pyramid (petrositis) and more rarely to the diploë of the temporal bone, causing osteomyelitis.

Clinical Features. Mastoiditis becomes manifest when there is a change in progress during resolution of acute otitis media.

General: Worsening of the general condition, rise in temperature, leukocytosis, and markedly increased ESR.

Local: Increasing pain in the ear, synchronous with the pulse and radiating to the temporal bone and the occiput; reappearance or increase in the aural discharge, which is creamy, odorless, and purulent. The patient also has hearing loss.

Pathogenesis. Acute otitis media with concomitant mastoiditis usually resolves without complications. The development of complications depends on:

- The anatomic relationships between the respiratory system and middle ear space. Because of the narrow connection between the antrum and the mastoid cells, there is poor aeration from the eustachian tube.
- The virulence and resistance of the organism.
- The local immune resistance of the mucosa.
- The patient's general immune resistance.
- The patient's general condition. Generalized diseases such as diabetes, immunodeficiency, allergy, and disorders of the liver and kidneys are important.

Diagnosis

- Aural discharge.
- Tenderness to pressure over the mastoid.
- Retroauricular swelling, with a protruding ear.

This classic triad of symptoms is now seldom seen, as otitis media is treated with antibiotics. This is especially true of the critical period that used to occur in the third week, during the preantibiotic era. The symptoms of mastoiditis are now more discrete and its course more insidious than they

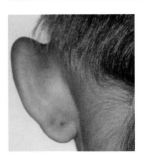

Fig. 1.86 Subperiosteal abscess, due to acute otitis media with mastoiditis.

used to be, so that this complication is easily overlooked. For this reason, the following otoscopic findings, which are also present during antibiotic treatment, need to be treated with caution:

- A pale but still thickened tympanic membrane.
- Circumscribed inflammation and thickening of the tympanic membrane in the posterosuperior quadrant.
- Thickened opaque tympanic membrane.
- Formation of a nipple on the tympanic membrane, with a fine pinpoint fistulous opening.
- Prolapse of the posterior meatal wall, which occurs relatively often in small children (see p. 2).

Local findings over the mastoid process and in the surrounding area:

- *Subperiosteal abscess*: Soggy swelling of the skin is caused by edema due to spread of the infection. Reddening and a taut, elastic, fluctuating swelling of the skin over the mastoid process (**Fig. 1.86**).
- *Zygomatic bone inflammation*: There is swelling of the zygomatic process, with extension to the cheek and eyelids in an extensively pneumatized bone. This is relatively common in children.
- *Bezold mastoiditis*: Visible and palpable tender swelling of the lateral triangle of the neck, with torticollis. This is due to an abscess tracking from the mastoid apex in the fascial spaces of the digastric, sternocleidomastoid, splenius, and longissimus capitis muscles.
- *Radiographic signs* in the Schüller view and/or CT of the temporal bone show a decrease in radiolucency due to a reduction in the air content in the respiratory system, haziness and opacity of the mastoid cells, haziness of the fine bony structures as a result of decalcification and liquefaction of the bony septa between the cells, bone

destruction with foci of liquefaction, and erosion of neighboring structures.

Differential diagnosis (pseudomastoiditis) (see p. 51). Furuncle of the external ear canal, parotitis, or cervical lymphadenitis.

Treatment

> **Note:** Mastoiditis in which the inflammation is no longer confined to the mucosa but has extended to the bone should be treated surgically.

It is incorrect to assume that inflammation of the pneumatic system of the temporal bone can be cured by antibiotics once it has invaded the bony structures. The poor vascularization of the mucosa and bone makes it impossible to maintain a satisfactory concentration of antibiotic in the tissues. The poorly aerated cells, filled with hyperplastic mucosa and granulations, are an ideal culture medium for bacteria, particularly anaerobes.

Indications for mastoidectomy: The operation is indicated if bone infection is thought to be present at any stage of otitis media:

- Symptoms of otogenic intracranial complications.
- Signs of a subperiosteal collection.
- A focus of liquefaction of mastoid cells on CT scans of the temporal bone.
- Facial paralysis.

In the healing phase—i. e., in the critical third week of otitis media—the operation is also indicated when there is:

- Recurrence of aural discharge, pain, and subfebrile temperature.
- Worsening of the general condition and an increase in CRP.
- Aural discharge persisting for 4–5 weeks and resisting treatment, in the presence of good pneumatization of the temporal bone, with reduced air content on radiographs, and without serious generalized symptoms.

Principle of mastoidectomy: The diseased tissue in the cell system of the mastoid process is excised via a retroauricular skin incision under general anesthesia. A wide connection is created between the mastoid antrum and the mastoid cavity, and from the latter to the middle ear cavity (see **Fig. 1.85**).

Course and prognosis. Two forms of true mastoiditis with bone destruction can develop from the mastoiditis accompanying otitis media, even during antibiotic treatment:

- *Acute mastoiditis:* This is marked by purulent liquefaction of the bony septa of the pneumatic system, with external rupture to form a subperiosteal or retroauricular abscess. The course is rapid and the symptoms marked. Paralysis of the facial nerve is possible.
- *Chronic mastoiditis:* This is partly a productive inflammation, with obliteration of the spaces of the pneumatic system by inflammatory granulation tissue; and partly a continuous inflammatory breakdown of bone. The course is therefore insidious, and the symptoms are initially mild.

The prognosis is good with correct treatment, but otherwise there is a danger of late otogenic complications (see p. 76).

Chronic Otitis Media

Chronic Mucosal Inflammation (Chronic Mesotympanic Otitis)

Clinical Features. *There is a chronic discharge of mucoid, purulent, odorless exudate.* The otitis is associated with periods of complete freedom from symptoms, alternating with acute exacerbations. The exudate may be creamy and purulent in the acute phase and then becomes mucoid and stringy as the infection resolves. However, it is always odorless.

Hearing: The patient has conductive hearing loss. Pain is absent, and the general condition is good.

Pathogenesis. The disease is not one that has a single cause, but rather it is the end result of several different primary disease processes. The inflammation remains confined to the mucosa, but in certain patients it can lead in time to rarefying osteitis—i. e., chronic inflammatory destruction of the ossicles, such as the long process of the incus. In contrast to cholesteatoma, this destructive bone process is unusual and less likely to extend and progress. Vascular obliteration can occur due to heavy scar tissue deposits in the vascular subepithelial connective-tissue layer, leading secondarily to nutritional disturbances of the neighboring bony tissue (aseptic bone necrosis).

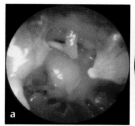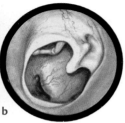

Fig. 1.87a, b Chronic otitis media (mesotympanic). There is a large central perforation in the tympanic membrane, with only a thin edge left. The promontory is visible through the perforation. The long process of the incus, the stapes tendon, and the round window niche are visible.

Pathogenetic factors:
- Constitutionally reduced mucosal (immunological) competence (see p. 7).
- Type, pathogenicity, virulence, and resistance of the bacterial organisms.
- Anatomic conditions in the middle ear, such as pneumatization, and connections between the attic, antrum, middle ear cavity, and eustachian tube.
- Disordered function of the eustachian tube— e. g., in patients with cleft palate.
- Generalized diseases such as allergy, immune defects, cachexia, and diabetes.

Diagnosis. The *history* shows a chronic recurrent aural discharge with reduced hearing. The *otoscopic findings* include a central defect of the tympanic membrane (**Fig. 1.87a, b**), scarring of the pars tensa, and occasionally aural polyps due to mucosal hyperplasia in acute exacerbations.

CT scanning (as well plain Schüller radiographs) show either reduced pneumatization or opacity of the cell system, if it is well pneumatized; occasionally, signs of bony destruction and formation of new bone (sclerosis) are seen. These are regarded as signs of chronic mastoiditis.

The *audiogram* shows conductive hearing loss.

Differential diagnosis. *Cholesteatoma* is associated with a marginal defect in the tympanic membrane and a fetid discharge.

Aural tuberculosis shows several central perforations of the tympanic membrane, with marked hearing loss.

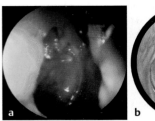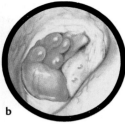

Fig. 1.88a, b   Chronic otitis media (epitympanic). The marginal defect in the tympanic membrane in the posterosuperior pars tensa and in the pars flaccida is causing osteitis in the bony lateral wall of the epitympanum. Granulations or polyps are typical signs.

Middle ear carcinoma causes a marginal defect with exuberant tissue extending into the meatus, and bone destruction in the attic and the meatal wall.

Treatment. *Conservative measures for drying the middle ear:* The external meatus is cleaned periodically. It can be irrigated with physiologic saline at body temperature. In the acute phase, pus is taken for culture and sensitivity tests, and appropriate systemic and local antibiotics are given, with care being taken not to use ototoxic drugs.

Aural polyps are removed with a wire snare or microforceps. Chronic infection of the nasopharynx and paranasal sinuses must be looked for.

Surgery: Mastoidectomy can be carried out to eliminate foci of infection in the temporal bone and middle ear cavity. Tympanoplasty can be performed to reconstruct the sound-conducting apparatus—i. e., the tympanic membrane and ossicular chain.

Course and prognosis. The course is episodic, with exacerbations caused by exogenous infection—e. g., from bathwater—and tubal infection. Complications are very rare. Progression to cholesteatoma is exceptional, and hearing loss is usually progressive. The prognosis is good in relation to survival, but poor with regard to function. An early tympanoplasty should therefore be carried out after intensive preparation (see **Figs. 1.95, 1.96**).

Age in itself is not a contraindication to surgical treatment. The key objective of the operation is to close the perforation, to avoid recurrent infection of the middle ear

mucosa via the external ear canal. Improvement of hearing can only be achieved in a small proportion of the children, and this should be taken into account and discussed during the process of obtaining consent for the operation.

Every patient presenting with active mucosal inflammation with frequent infections that do not settle with conservative medical management should be treated as early as possible using *tympanoplasty*, since the extent of the destruction of the sound-conducting apparatus increases with every inflammatory episode. If a hearing aid is necessary, tympanoplasty is also indicated, since chronic otorrhea makes it impossible to wear an earpiece.

> **Note:** Chronic mucosal inflammation is a form of chronic otitis media in which the inflammation is mainly confined to the mucosa. It does not usually cause progressive bone destruction and is therefore free of complications, but it has a protracted course.

Chronic Bone Suppuration (Chronic Epitympanic Otitis Media)

As a result of a marginal defect of the tympanic membrane in the posterior superior pars tensa or in the pars flaccida, inflammation spreads to parts of the bony lateral wall of the epitympanum. Granulations or polyps are typical signs of granulating ostitis (**Fig. 1.88a, b**).

Acquired Cholesteatoma of the Middle Ear

A cholesteatoma is a skin growth that occurs in the middle ear. It is usually due to repeated infection, which causes ingrowth of the skin of the eardrum. Progressive inflammation develops on the basis of a marginal tympanic membrane perforation, with osteitis on the lateral epitympanic wall. Cholesteatomas often take the form of a cyst or pouch that sheds layers of old skin, which builds up inside the middle ear.

Clinical Features

- Fetid otorrhea that is sometimes minimal or completely absent; when present, it is always purulent, and never mucoid.
- Progressive hearing loss, possibly dizziness.
- Otalgia and fever in acute exacerbations.
- Dull headaches or a feeling of pressure in the head.

Pathogenesis

!
> **Note:** An acquired middle ear cholesteatoma is not a tumor, but rather a chronic inflammation which, unlike chronic mucosal inflammation, causes progressive destruction of the bony cells and structures.

Promoting factors:
- Disordered ventilation and drainage of the middle ear (chronic reduction of pressure) with hypopneumatization.
- Displaced squamous epithelium as a result of increased capacity for growth of the meatal skin in the upper part of the anulus tympanicus (the papillary ingrowths form the later *matrix,* either as a result of invagination of the pars flaccida or by formation of a retention pocket in the pars tensa).
- An increased proliferative tendency in the stratum germinativum (see **Fig. 1.7**), caused by the stimulus of inflammation.
- Incompletely resolved embryonic hyperplastic mesenchymal remnants in the submucosa of the middle ear, which later form the *perimatrix.*

Histopathogenesis: A cholesteatoma may form a compact sac of desquamated lamellae, arranged like the layers of an onion and connected with a fairly thick pedicle to its site of origin in the tympanic membrane (the pars flaccida or tensa). Alternatively, it may consist of a widely fanned-out cholesteatoma matrix lining the antrum and mastoid cavity and sending off shoots into the furthest bony niches of the bony process. The latter type of cholesteatoma therefore has a reticular or dendritic, branched structure. The latter occurs more commonly in a tensa cholesteatoma than in a flaccida cholesteatoma. Bone destruction is caused firstly by enzymes (e. g., collagenase) formed in the perimatrix, and secondly by osteoclastic destruction of bony tissue—i. e., chronic osteomyelitis.

!
> **Note:** A prerequisite for the development of a cholesteatoma is direct contact between the keratinizing squamous epithelium in the external meatus and mucoperiosteum of the middle ear that has been damaged by inflammation.

This can happen as a result of:
- A *marginal perforation* with a destruction of the protective barrier of the anulus fibrosus.

- *Papillary ingrowths*—e. g., in the region of the pars flaccida or of the destroyed anulus fibrosus.
- Formation of a *retraction pocket* in the pars tensa.
- *Traumatic displacement* of keratinizing squamous epithelium after longitudinal pyramidal fractures or ruptures of the tympanic membrane, with the development of posttraumatic otitis media.

The same pathogenetic factors (see p. 67) are involved in the genesis of cholesteatoma as to that of chronic mucosal inflammation.

Diagnosis. An inflammatory middle ear cholesteatoma can be classified from several different points of view (primary, secondary, or topographic anatomy). The method using the site of origin appears to be the most sensible from the diagnostic point of view and clearer than the other classifications. Cholesteatoma can thus be classified as follows:
- *Tensa cholesteatoma* (synonym: secondary middle-ear cholesteatoma).
- *Flaccida cholesteatoma* (synonyms: primary or genuine attic or epitympanic cholesteatoma).
- *Occult cholesteatoma* (synonyms: cholesteatoma behind an intact tympanic membrane, or congenital cholesteatoma).

The *tensa cholesteatoma* (**Fig. 1.89a, b**) develops from a retraction pocket caused by chronic inflammation, usually in the posterosuperior quadrant of the pars tensa. It is characterized by a posterosuperior marginal perforation. Inflammatory granulations, fetid exudate with flakes of cholesteatoma, and circumscribed destruction of the surrounding posterosuperior meatal wall are often found in the region of the edge of the perforation. Conductive hearing loss is also present, due to destruction of the ossicular chain. The site of predilection is the incudostapedial joint.

The *flaccida cholesteatoma* (**Fig. 1.89c, d; Fig. 1.90a–c; Fig. 1.91a, b**) arises from papillary ingrowth of the keratinizing squamous epithelium in the region of the Shrapnell membrane, in the presence of simultaneous chronic epitympanitis. The stimulus of inflammation induces increased proliferation of the squamous epithelium. Circumscribed perforation of the pars flaccida, often covered by a crust and usually also accompanied by destruction of the lateral attic wall, is therefore

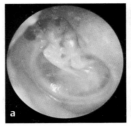 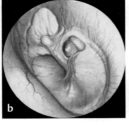 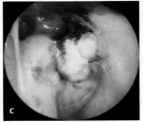 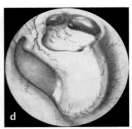

Fig. 1.89a–d   Chronic otitis media with cholesteatoma.
a, b A marginal tympanic membrane defect in the anterior upper quadrants.

c, d A large marginal perforation in upper posterior quadrant. The chronic inflammation has destroyed the postero-superior auditory wall.

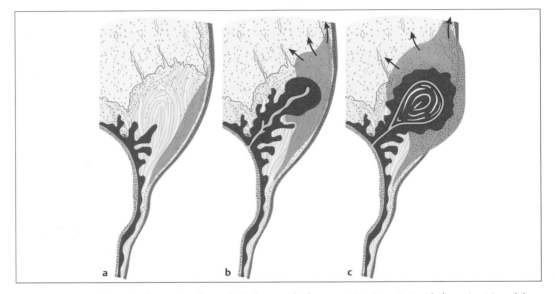

Fig. 1.90a–c   Histological pathogenesis of an attic cholesteatoma.
a Papillary growth of the stratum corneum (the future matrix) of the pars flaccida down toward the attic. The connective tissue is loose, and the submucosa (the future perimatrix) is hyperplastic and chronically inflamed.
b Invagination of the pars flaccida into the attic as a result of hypoventilation and reduced pressure in the epitympanum.

The future matrix is in contact with the perimatrix and there is early bone destruction.
c Activation of the basal cell layer of the matrix by chronic inflammation. Proliferation of keratinizing squamous epithelium and destruction and undermining of the mucosa in the middle ear, with replacement by the "foreign" squamous epithelium from the invaginated pars flaccida and formation of a cholesteatoma sac.

characteristic of this type of cholesteatoma. Medial to this lie inflammatory granulation tissue and fetid exudate with flakes of cholesteatoma. The patient has conductive hearing loss and also, in the advanced stages, involvement of the inner ear.

Occult cholesteatoma develops gradually and remains asymptomatic for a long time behind an intact tympanic membrane with no demonstrable perforation. In most cases, this involves a flaccida cholesteatoma that develops without a perforation by papillary ingrowth into the epitympanum, extending from there to the neighboring middle-ear space (**Fig. 1.92**). The pneumatization and the mucosal folds determine the pathways of spread of the cholesteatoma. In rare cases, it may be a congenital cholesteatoma.

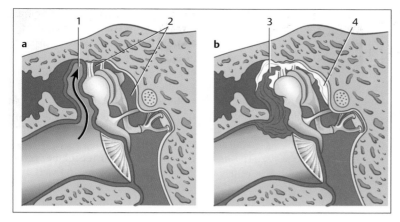

Fig. 1.91a, b Development of an attic cholesteatoma.
a Retraction and invagination of the pars flaccida into the epitympanum occurs as a result of persistently reduced pressure in the middle ear. The keratinized squamous epithelium is thus displaced into the middle ear. **1**, Invaginated pars flaccida; **2**, attic.
b Chronic inflammation causes hyperplasia of the mucosa of the attic and thus prevents adequate aeration of the region. **3**, Cholesteatoma sac; **4**, hyperplastic mucosa and "mesenchymal cushion" of the attic.

Common diagnostic characteristics. *Radiology: Axial and coronal high-resolution CT* of the temporal bone is the most useful and versatile procedure for demonstrating bone destruction in the petrous pyramid, soft-tissue abnormalities in the middle ear, and extension of the cholesteatoma into the cranial cavity. Schüller and Stenver views can partly show the grade of pneumatization, but have limitations for demonstrating destructive processes.

Audiometry: The audiogram shows conductive hearing loss, possibly combined with sensorineural deafness. Extension into the labyrinth causes progressive sensorineural deafness.

Vestibular tests: If the labyrinthine capsule is intact, spontaneous and provoked vestibular nystagmus do not occur. Erosion of the lateral semicircular canal causes a positive fistula test sign (see p. 47).

Facial nerve function: Erosion of the bony canal of the facial nerve and its mastoid or tympanic segment, or extension into the internal meatus, first cause neurapraxia and later progressive axonotmesis.

Differential diagnosis

- *Inactive chronic mucosal inflammation* with adhesions between the promontory and an atrophic pars tensa.
- *Carcinoma of the middle ear or external meatus.*
- *Tuberculosis of the middle ear.*

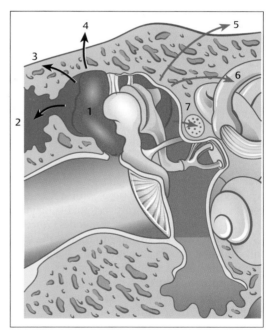

Fig. 1.92 Pathways of cholesteatoma extension: from the epitympanum into the attic (**1**); posteriorly, toward the mastoid and the sigmoid sinus (**2**) and the posterior (**3**) and middle cranial fossa (**4**); or medially, toward the internal meatus (**5**); and anteriorly toward the labyrinth (**6**) or the facial canal (**7**). **1**, attic (see also **Fig. 1.4.**).

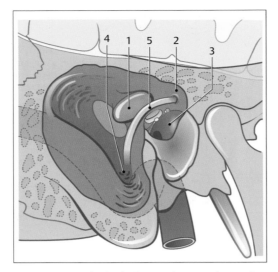

Fig. 1.93 Principle of radical mastoidectomy. There is eburnation of the mastoid, and the antrum (**1**), attic (**2**), middle ear cavity (**3**), and small mastoid cavity (**4**) are opened widely. Dissection of the bony facial canal as far as the second knee (tympanic segment) (**5**). These structures are united in a common cavity opening into the external meatus. If a tympanoplasty is to be performed, then a modified radical operation is carried out: the middle ear cavity is closed off from the mastoid cavity, and the sound-conducting apparatus is reconstructed.

Treatment. *Conservative treatment* with antibiotics, irrigation of the ear (also with a drainage tube), and antibiotic and corticosteroid-containing eardrops are ineffective, since antibiotics (whether systemic or local) are not able to control the local inflammation or the displacement of squamous epithelium into the middle ear space.

Surgical treatment: Surgical treatment of chronic otitis media with cholesteatoma involves a curative procedure, with radical removal of the inflammation, and a reconstructive procedure, with reconstructive surgery of the middle ear.

> **Note:** There are two goals in surgery for cholesteatoma:
>
> 1. Radically eliminating inflammation by removing the matrix, perimatrix, and invaded bone
> 2. Maintaining and reconstructing the sound-conducting apparatus

Mastoidectomy: In the curative part, the attic, middle ear cavity, antrum, and infected pneumatic spaces of the mastoid process are exposed using a retroauricular or endaural approach. The mastoid and antrum cells are exposed and resected. Two mastoidectomy principles are used here, depending on the extension of the cholesteatoma:

1. The *closed* or *intact canal wall* technique. The bony posterior meatal wall and lateral attic wall are preserved (see **Fig. 1.85**).
2. The *open* or *canal wall–down* technique: After removal of the posterior bony meatal wall, the mastoid, attic, epitympanum and middle ear cavity are brought into continuity with the external meatus (**Fig. 1.93**).

Subtotal petrosectomy: After a mastoid cavity has been created using the canal wall–down technique, additional portions of the temporal bone are resected. The surgical cavity is obliterated with abdominal fat, and the eustachian tube and external ear canal are permanently closed.

Radical removal of the cholesteatoma matrix and perimatrix is carried out under microscopic control. The radical cavity heals within a matter of weeks, developing an epidermal layer (**Fig. 1.94a,b**). The disadvantage of this operation is that the sound-conducting chain is not reconstructed, so that the functional result is generally poor. In addition, there is an open connection between the middle ear, the mastoid cavity, and the external auditory meatus, so that chronic otorrhea is common due to tubal or exogenous infection.

Tympanoplasty: The purpose of this part is to reconstruct sound pressure protection of the round window and sound pressure transformation between the tympanic membrane and the oval window, by:

- Closing the perforation of the tympanic membrane with fascia or perichondrium.
- Reconstructing the direct connection between the tympanic membrane and stapes footplate if the ossicular chain is defective (ossiculoplasty).
- Separating the middle ear cavity from the external meatus by reconstructing the posterior meatal and lateral attic walls with a bony or cartilaginous graft or preserving the intact bony meatal wall.

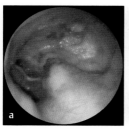 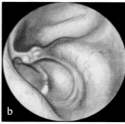

Fig. 1.94a, b View into an open cavity following a radical mastoidectomy. The cavity is completely epithelialized.

Radical elimination of the infection and reconstruction of the sound-conducting apparatus are usually performed in a one-stage procedure, but a radical mastoidectomy is still occasionally performed in preference to a tympanoplasty for the following indications:

1. Cholesteatoma with intracranial complications.
2. Cholesteatoma with facial nerve paralysis.
3. Extensive reticular–dendritic cholesteatoma in a well-pneumatized temporal bone.

The main goal of radical mastoidectomy is to control the disease. This therapeutic approach can be expanded by performing a tympanoplasty, which is done as a secondary procedure after complete healing of the infection; the aim is to achieve ossicular reconstruction. This expanded approach is not practised in all countries, however, as the theories underlying the treatment vary.

Principles of tympanoplasty: In 1952, Wullstein introduced a scheme of five basic types of operation for reconstructing the middle ear (**Fig. 1.95a–e**). Only type I and type III are of practical importance nowadays, as fenestrations of the semicircular canal are no longer performed and the importance of the lever mechanism of the ossicles was overestimated. Closure of the perforation of the tympanic membrane using fascia or perichondrium is the type I operation and is called *myringoplasty*. Type III involves reconstruction of the ossicular chain (ossiculoplasty), the aim being to restore the sound-pressure transformation from the tympanic membrane to the footplate in the oval window. The condition of the stapes is particularly important for this procedure. Three primary situations are encountered (**Figs. 1.95a–e, 1.96a–f**):

1. *Stapes intact*: The reconstructive procedure establishes a bridge between the tympanic membrane and/or the malleus handle and the head of the stapes. The connection is provided by an alloplastic (synthetic) prosthesis, known as a *partial ossicular replacement prosthesis* (PORP) (**Figs. 1.96 d, 1.97a**).
2. *Stapes crura absent, footplate mobile*: An alloplastic prosthesis, known as a *total ossicular replacement prosthesis* (TORP), is placed between the footplate and the tympanic membrane (**Figs. 1.96 f, 1.97b**).
3. *Footplate absent or fixed*: An opening is made in the oval window and subsequently closed with autologous tissue (type V tympanoplasty; **Fig. 1.95e**).

Ossiculoplasty can be carried out using different materials, mainly consisting of alloplastic implants (gold, titanium, plastic, ceramic). Remnants of true ossicles are used whenever possible.

Course and prognosis. Untreated cholesteatoma is the most dangerous form of chronic middle ear inflammation (see **Fig. 1.92**). At any time, healthy patients can develop the following life-threatening intracranial complications:

- Labyrinthitis and meningitis.
- Sinus thrombosis and septicemia.
- Epidural or subdural abscess, with meningitis.
- Temporal lobe or cerebellar abscess.

> **!**
> **Note:** Conservative treatment almost never achieves healing of a cholesteatoma. Surgery is therefore always indicated, due to the danger of intracranial complications.

Congenital Cholesteatoma of the Temporal Bone
This is a rare form of cholesteatoma, with no obvious connection with the external meatus or tympanic membrane. It is usually an occult lesion behind an intact tympanic membrane and only exceptionally develops from an embryonic ectodermal remnant within the temporal bone. It is also known as true or primary cholesteatoma.

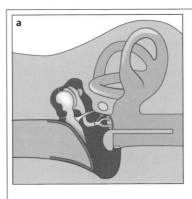

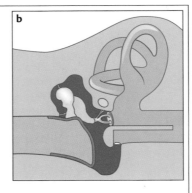

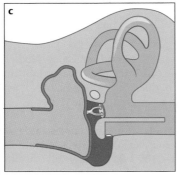

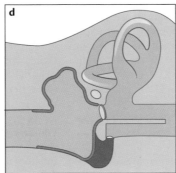

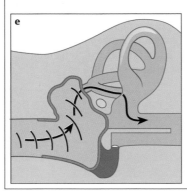

Fig. 1.95a–e The five classical types of tympanoplasty as defined by Wullstein.
a Type I: simple myringoplasty. The perforation of the tympanic membrane is closed with fascia or perichondrium.
b Type II: reconstruction of the defective ossicular chain by bridging the defect with autologous bone or cartilage grafts.
c Type III: direct transmission of sound waves from the tympanic membrane to the stapes by the columella effect. A shallow tympanum is created.
d Type IV: the ossicular chain is absent; sound is transmitted directly to the oval window, and sound protection is provided for the round window. A small tympanum is formed.
e Type V. In this case, the oval window is completely closed by bony fixation of the footplate. A window is made in the horizontal semicircular canal so that sound is transmitted directly to this fenestration, as in the similar operation for otosclerosis. Types IV and V have both now been abandoned in favor of interposition of an artificial columella (type IV) or—instead of type V—by removing the footplate and interposing a bony, cartilaginous, or synthetic prosthesis, as in stapedectomy for otosclerosis (see **Fig. 1.102**).

Course of Specific Forms of Cholesteatoma

Cholesteatoma is rare in infants and young children, but increases in frequency after the age of 6 years.

Cholesteatoma is relatively rare in old age. It is then usually due to reactivation of an old inflammatory process, which proceeds insidiously and may become manifest initially through the development of complications such as:

- Dizziness.
- Rapidly progressive hearing loss.
- Facial paralysis.
- Meningitis.

Petrositis due to progressive bone destruction, formation of sequestra, and invasion of the labyrinth, facial canal, and cranial cavity, with an epidural or subdural abscess, may develop insidiously. One pathogenetic factor is diabetes, due to the reduction in general resistance and local tissue metabolic disorders. The postoperative healing process is often prolonged, and the prognosis on the whole is poor.

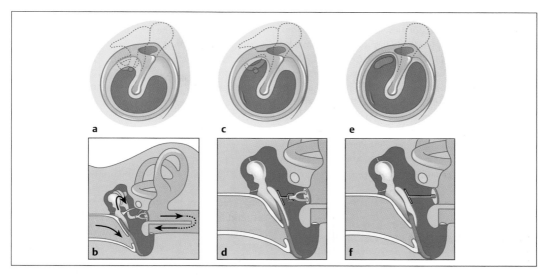

Fig. 1.96a–f Principles of tympanoplasty.

a Simple perforation of the tympanic membrane; the ossicular chain is intact.

b Closure of the defect in the pars tensa with underlay graft (fascia or perichondrium, *red*) and reconstruction of the sound pressure protection and transformation mechanism.

c Tympanic membrane perforation with a defect of the long process of the incus.

d Closure of the perforation. Reconstruction of the sound-conducting apparatus by interposing an alloplastic prosthe-

sis (partial ossicular replacement prosthesis, PORP) between the malleus and the stapes—the columella effect. There is a slice of cartilage (*blue*) between the prosthesis and tympanic membrane.

e Defect of the incus and stapes with retention of the long process of the malleus and the footplate of the stapes, in a subtotal perforation of the tympanic membrane.

f Bridging of the defect of the ossicular chain by interposing an alloplastic prosthesis (total ossicular replacement prosthesis, TORP).

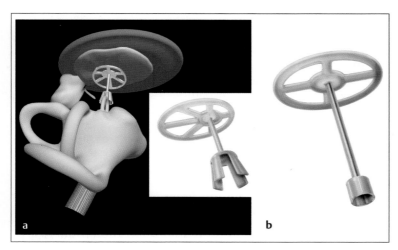

Fig. 1.97a, b **a** Positioning of an alloplastic PORP prosthesis, which is placed on the head of the stapes.

b TORP prosthesis. The oval plate is connected to the tympanic membrane; the small end is placed on the stapes footplate.

Meatal cholesteatoma can arise either from the pathologic proliferative tendency of the meatal epidermal lining in the bony part, or it may be the result of a rupture of a middle ear cholesteatoma from the antrum into the part of the meatus immediately lateral to the tympanic membrane.

Posttraumatic cholesteatoma arises as a result of a longitudinal pyramidal fracture extending into the external meatus. This allows meatal epidermis or a part of the tympanic membrane to be displaced into the middle ear space. The displaced keratinizing squamous epithelium initially forms an innocent epidermal cyst; a bone-destroying cholesteatoma with a matrix and perimatrix arises later, after the cyst has become infected.

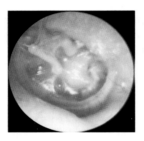

Fig. 1.98 Adhesive otitis. The tympanic membrane is retracted, scarred, and thickened, but intact.

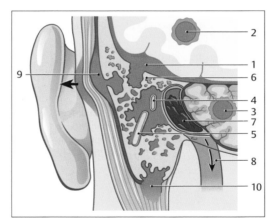

Fig. 1.99 Pathogenesis and pathways of spread of otogenic complications. **1**, Extension into the middle cranial fossa, causing a subdural abscess; **2**, meningitis or temporal lobe abscess; **3**, extension into the posterior cranial fossa, causing meningitis or cerebellar abscess. Intratemporal complications: **4**, labyrinthitis; **5**, otogenic facial paralysis; **6**, petrositis; **7**, sinus thrombosis with thrombophlebitis; and **8**, sepsis. Extratemporal complications: **9**, external rupture of mastoiditis to form a subperiosteal abscess; **10**, rupture of the mastoid apex to form an infratemporal Bezold abscess.

Adhesive Otitis (Middle Ear Fibrosis)

Clinical Features. The tympanic membrane is retracted, scarred, and thickened, but intact. The patient has severe conductive hearing loss (**Fig. 1.98**).

Pathogenesis. The condition is caused by recurrent otitis with cicatricial fibrosis of the poorly aerated middle ear, formation of cholesterol granuloma, and fixation of the ossicular chain.

■ Otogenic Infective Complications

Otogenic complications (**Fig. 1.99**) are otologic emergencies that should be investigated and treated by a specialist without delay. Evaluation using audiometric and neurovestibular examinations, as well as CT scanning, should be carried out as soon as possible. Indications for surgery have high priority.

Labyrinthitis

Clinical Features. Dizziness, nausea, vomiting, whistling noises in the ears, and deafness develop within a short period. The patient has no fever and no pain.

Pathogenesis. In *acute otitis media,* toxins diffuse through the labyrinthine windows and the infection extends along the vessels (see p. 77).

In *chronic otitis media* with cholesteatoma, a fistula forms in the labyrinth and the infection extends directly into the perilymphatic space. After a transverse fracture of the temporal bone or operative trauma, there is direct damage to the membranous labyrinth, with secondary infection (see **Fig. 1.62**).

Diagnosis. The patient has the cochlear and vestibular symptoms of rapidly progressive inner ear failure.

Differential diagnosis. Ménière disease, sudden deafness, and acute vestibulopathy.

Treatment. Intravenous antibiotics are administered in high doses by continuous infusion. The middle ear should be drained, and a mastoidectomy may have to be performed. Mastoidectomy using the canal wall–down technique or subtotal petrosectomy is performed for cholesteatoma. An additional labyrinthectomy has to be performed in cases of purulent labyrinthitis with meningitis. After trauma with temporal bone fractures, surgery is only undertaken if there is simultaneous cerebrospinal fluid (CSF) otorrhea, facial nerve paralysis, or meningitis.

Course and prognosis. Because of the varying pathologic anatomy, several different clinical forms of labyrinthitis are possible: serous in posttraumatic or viral cases; purulent due to bacterial invasion of the perilymphatic space; circumscribed due to a labyrinthine fistula in cholesteatoma; and generalized with involvement of the entire labyrinth due to extension of infection or generalized infection. In the latter form, the course is fulminant, with irreversible total loss of function. The infection is capable of extending to the meninges.

Epidural Empyema

Clinical Features. Dull pulsating pain in the head, otorrhea, and subfebrile temperature occur. There is no completely characteristic pattern of symptoms.

Pathogenesis. Acute or chronic infection extends from the mastoid process into the epidural space, due to destruction of the inner table by infection. The infection may also spread via preformed pathways along the perforating vessels in the bone, which remains intact.

Diagnosis. Characteristically, the condition has very few symptoms. It is usually an incidental finding at mastoidectomy, but it can be demonstrated using neuroradiographic techniques, including angiography, CT, and MRI.

Treatment. Immediate mastoidectomy with wide exposure of the dura, drainage, and antibiotics are indicated.

Course and prognosis. The prognosis is good if the disease is recognized early. Otherwise, there is a danger of pachymeningitis developing, with extension to the leptomeninges.

Subdural empyemas are rare and only occur during the course of diffuse meningitis.

Otogenic Meningitis

Clinical Features. These include headaches, stiffness of the neck, scaphoid abdomen, increasing loss of consciousness, photophobia, restlessness, tonic–clonic convulsions, and facial paralysis. Otorrhea, otalgia, and even deafness may be absent or occult. Typically, there is a bounding pulse, irregular breathing, and a fever of 39–40°C. The patient may have an oculomotor or abducens paralysis and abnormal optic fundi.

Pathogenesis. The cause is the spread of an acute or chronic bacterial infection, usually due to pneumococci, into the subarachnoid space:

- By *direct continuity,* due to inflammatory destruction of the bony walls.
- *Along preformed pathways,* via the perforating vessels and nerves in the bone—e. g., via the caroticotympanic nerves.
- By a thrombophlebitis extending along the diploic veins.
- *Via the labyrinth* and as a result of spread into the internal auditory meatus (rare).

Diagnosis. In addition to the typical clinical symptoms of acute meningitis, including CSF abnormalities, there are signs of acute, subacute, or chronic middle ear inflammation of varying degrees of severity. If the hearing is more or less normal and the otoscopic findings are equivocal, the signs of inflammation of the pneumatic system on radiographs of the temporal bone (in CT scan, Schüller or Stenver views) can be decisive in making the diagnosis and establishing the indication for surgery.

The CSF shows pleocytosis, a marked increase of protein, and a reduced sugar and chloride content. The pressure is greater than 200 mmHg. In the acute phase, bacteria—usually pneumococci—can be found in the fluid.

Differential diagnosis. This includes viral or epidemic meningococcal meningitis and tuberculous meningitis.

Treatment. High dosages of antibiotics are administered intravenously on the basis of an antibiogram—e. g., penicillin 40–60 million U/24 h for a pneumococcal infection. Repeated lumbar punctures are carried out to assess the CSF.

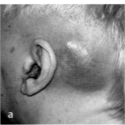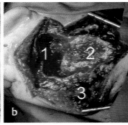

Fig. 1.100a, b Otogenic sinus thrombosis.
a Painful swelling of the mastoid.
b The intraoperative situation after drainage of the thrombophlebitis. **1**, Opened mastoid cavity; **2**, ligated sigmoid sinus with infected thrombus; **3**, severely inflamed tissue on the mastoid.

The *blood–brain barrier* for antibiotics varies greatly, depending on the severity of the meningitis. Some of the antibiotic is inactivated by binding to the CSF protein. Third-generation cephalosporins such as ceftazidime (an antipseudomonal cephalosporin and therefore useful for otogenic meningitis due to chronic otitis media), cefotaxime, and ceftriaxone penetrate the blood–brain barrier very well. Intrathecal antibiotics are only used in exceptional cases. Immediate drainage of the middle ear cavity by mastoidectomy is required, with wide exposure of the dura.

Course and prognosis. The disease ends fatally if it is untreated or not treated correctly. The prospects of recovery are ≈ 90 %, provided that the otitis media is recognized as causing the meningitis at an early stage and provided that energetic treatment is started.

> **Note:** Any unexplained attack of meningitis must be suspected of having a nasal or otologic origin.

In doubtful cases with obscure otoscopic and radiographic findings, the risk of an exploratory operation is less than that of an expectant policy if the middle ear space is infected. Intensive antibiotic treatment does not lead to resolution unless the primary focus of infection has been eliminated by surgery.

Otogenic Sinus Thrombosis

Clinical Features. A perisinus abscess, periphlebitis, and incipient sinus thrombosis lead to the same diagnostic difficulties as an epidural empyema. The release of emboli of infective thrombi alone causes the characteristic signs of *septicemia*. These include:

- Chills.
- A spiking temperature chart, with several peaks on the same day.
- Increased pulse rate.
- Headaches.
- Vomiting.
- Somnolence.
- Neck stiffness (accompanying meningitis).
- Dyspnea due to septic lung metastases or pneumonia.
- Jaundice due to septic metastases in the liver or to nonspecific reactive hepatitis.

Pathogenesis. Infection due to mastoiditis or cholesteatoma destroys bone in continuity, so that it can rupture into the perisinus space. A perisinus abscess forms, with periphlebitis of the sigmoid sinus, followed by sinus phlebitis. The thrombus is initially mural, but later it occludes the lumen and extends superiorly to involve the transverse and sagittal sinuses and the mastoid emissary vein, and inferiorly toward the internal jugular vein.

The thrombus undergoes thrombolysis due to bacterial infiltration, and septic metastases are caused by blood-borne infected emboli.

Diagnosis. The following symptoms during acute otitis media or chronic otitis media with cholesteatoma suggest sinus thrombosis (**Fig. 1.100a, b**):
- High fever above 40°C.
- Spiking temperature with chills.
- Swelling and sensitivity to pressure over the mastoid emissary foramen at the posterior border of the mastoid process (Griesinger sign).
- Induration and tenderness of the internal jugular vein and of the anterior border of the sternocleidomastoid muscle.
- Petechiae in septic coagulopathy.
- Splenomegaly.

Laboratory investigations: Blood culture is strongly positive. Urinalysis shows hematuria due to septic interstitial focal nephritis, albuminuria, and cylindruria.

Radiology: CT scans show bone destruction in the area of the sinus. Angiography shows narrowing or occlusion of the sigmoid sinus in the venous phase of carotid angiography.

Differential diagnosis. This includes miliary tuberculosis, typhus, malaria, brucellosis, viral pneumonia, and cystopyelitis.

Treatment. Immediate surgical excision of the primary inflammatory focus in the mastoid and sigmoid sinus by mastoidectomy for cholesteatoma is performed (**Fig. 1.93 b**; see also p. 72). The sigmoid sinus has to be widely exposed; an incision is performed or the sinus wall is incised, and thrombectomy is performed. The internal jugular vein is ligated and divided, with a margin of healthy tissue. Parenteral antibiotics are given in high dosages for a long period, as well as anticoagulants, if possible determined by the results of culture and sensitivity tests.

Course and prognosis. The patient should be monitored with serial CT scans to check the changes in the surrounding tissue. The disease is fatal if it is not treated correctly, or if the basic cause and its secondary consequences are not recognized promptly. Eighty percent of patients are cured when adequate treatment is started early.

> **Note:** Every unexplained case of septicemia requires rigorous investigation of the ear, including radiographic diagnosis, since the otitis media that is primarily responsible may go unrecognized due to a lack of other typical clinical signs.

Otitic Hydrocephalus

This disease is caused by increased intracranial pressure due to obstruction of CSF drainage caused by a sterile otogenic sinus thrombosis.

Clinical Features

- Failing vision.
- Vomiting.
- Double vision.
- Jacksonian epilepsy.
- Pareses and disorders of sensation.

Pathogenesis. A relatively asymptomatic chronic mastoiditis follows an acute otitis media, leading to sterile erosion of perisinus bone and sigmoid sinus phlebitis with formation of a mural thrombus, extending to the confluence of the sinuses and the superior sagittal sinus. This causes occlusion of the pacchionian granulations, which interferes with resorption of CSF, leading to increased CSF pressure.

Diagnosis

- Abducens paralysis without Gradenigo syndrome (see p. 80).
- Increased CSF pressure without pleocytosis.
- Free CSF circulation without CSF obstruction.
- Congested optic fundi with failing vision.
- Opacity and osteolytic perisinus lesions in temporal bone CT scans.
- A history of acute otitis media 3–5 weeks previously.

Differential diagnosis

- Petrositis (see p. 80) with arachnoiditis in the cerebellopontine angle.
- Carotid aneurysm at the petrous apex.

Treatment. Treatment includes mastoidectomy, exposure of the sinus, thrombectomy, and neurosurgical decompression to allow drainage of the CSF.

Course and prognosis. These are good if the disease is recognized and treated early. Otherwise, the disease progresses to blindness and the development of Jacksonian epilepsy.

Otogenic Brain Abscess

This is one of the most serious late complications of chronic inflammatory middle ear cholesteatoma.

Clinical Features. See **Table 1.10**.

Pathogenesis. The disease can spread by *direct continuity* via one of the following pathways:

1. Through the tegmen tympani, to form a temporal lobe abscess.
2. Through the sigmoid sinus to the posterior cranial fossa, to form a cerebellar abscess.
3. From the labyrinth to the endolymphatic sac, to form a cerebellar abscess (see **Fig. 1.99**).

Another pathway is via vessels (the diploic veins, advancing septic thromboangiitis of the cerebral veins), or via the internal auditory meatus in cases of labyrinthitis.

Clinical Features of temporal lobe abscess

- Speech disturbances, revealed by a history of aphasia and difficulty in understanding words. (This disorder of speech is exclusively sensory and is never motor.)
- Central hearing disorders, which are mostly discrete.
- Acoustic hallucinations.
- Disorders of smell, which are usually discrete.
- Visual disturbances such as quadrant hemianopsia and gaze paresis.

Table 1.10 Clinical Features of otogenic brain abscess

1. Initial stage	Meningism, nausea, headache, psychological changes, fever
2. Latent stage	Epileptiform attacks, neurologic signs
3. Manifest stage	Vomiting and bradycardia, psychological changes, focal signs of aphasia, alexia, agraphia, hemiplegia, epileptic attacks, and ataxia in cerebellar abscess. Symptoms due to spread to neighboring organs include cranial nerve paralyses, visual field defects, disorders of the oculomotor system and of posture
4. Terminal stage	Stupor, coma, conjugated deviation to the side of the lesion, bradycardia, and Cheyne–Stokes respiration

- Neuropathies of cranial nerves III–VII.
- Crossed lesions of the pyramidal tracts.

Differential diagnosis of a temporal lobe abscess.
Intracerebral tumor.

Clinical Features of a cerebellar abscess
- Disorders of the oculomotor and postural system.
- Nystagmus: coarse spontaneous nystagmus to the side of the lesion, vestibular provocation nystagmus with irregular positional nystagmus, gaze-directional nystagmus due to secondary damage to the pons, gaze-paretic nystagmus to the side of the lesion.
- Ataxia, intention tremor, dysmetria, adiadochokinesia, hypotonia, and symptoms due to spread to neighboring organs such as paralysis of cranial nerves III, V, VI, VII, IX, and X.

Differential diagnosis of a cerebellar abscess. Labyrinthitis, acute vestibulopathy, multiple sclerosis, cerebellar tumor, and cerebellopontine angle syndrome need to be considered.

Investigations. In addition to otologic examination, these include:
- Neurotologic investigations: AEP, ENG, and electrodiagnostic methods for the facial nerve.
- Neuro-ophthalmologic investigation of the optic fundi, visual field, and ocular motor nerves.
- Neurologic and neuroradiologic investigations, including CT, MRI, EEG, brain scan, and possibly angiography, echoencephalography, and investigations of the CSF.

Treatment. The primary focus is removed by an otologist, using mastoidectomy. Intracranial drainage can be performed during the same operation. Primary removal of the brain abscess can be achieved by craniotomy in a neurosurgical procedure. Isolated aspiration of the abscess has now been abandoned, except in a few exceptional circumstances. It is more effective to eliminate the focus of infection radically by surgery along the pathway of infection. In addition to surgery, appropriate, intense antibiotic therapy is administered.

Course and prognosis. Despite intensive surgical treatment, the mortality is still 5–8 %. The defect often heals, but there may be neurologic deficits after neurosurgical excision of the abscess.

Petrositis (Petrous Apex Syndrome)
Pathogenesis. Good pneumatization of the entire petrous pyramid is a prerequisite for the development of petrositis. As a result of extension of inflammation from the middle ear to the perilabyrinthine cells, purulent liquefaction in the cells of the petrous apex results, often accompanied by osteomyelitis. The classic Gradenigo triad is due to the close relationship of the pyramidal apex to the trigeminal nerve and abducens nerve. The symptoms of this triad include otorrhea, ipsilateral irritation of the trigeminal nerve, and abducens paralysis. The facial, vagus, and glossopharyngeal nerves are also often paralyzed. In addition, the patient may have signs of labyrinthitis due to extension of the inflammatory process. The symptoms of primary otitis media may be hidden due to antibiotic treatment. Predisposing factors include advanced age and diabetes.

Diagnosis. The main symptoms are:
- Trigeminal neuralgia.
- Abducens paralysis with double vision.
- Dizziness and deafness.
- Deep, throbbing headache.
- Abnormal CT scans of the temporal bone.

Differential diagnosis. Brain abscess and sinus phlebitis.

Treatment. A combination of administering high-dose and prolonged parenteral antibiotics and surgery. Mastoidectomy is performed, with translabyrinthine clearance and drainage of the apical cells, ensuring that the facial nerve is protected.

Prognosis. If the disease is recognized early and treated effectively, the prognosis is relatively good. However, the prognosis is poor in patients of advanced age and those with diabetes (development of circumscribed meningitis at the base of the brain, with subsequent multifocal microinfarction of the pons).

■ Specific Diseases of the Middle Ear and Mastoid Process

Wegener Granulomatosis

The disease is characterized by a combination of necrotizing granuloma formation and vasculitis. It can become manifest in adult patients as chronic bilateral serous otitis media. It can cause facial nerve paralysis and conductive hearing loss, as well as sensorineural hearing loss secondary to vasculitis of the stria vascularis. The inflammation damages renal and pulmonary structures. In consultation with a rheumatologist, treatment with cyclophosphamide and steroids is recommended. Inserting tympanic ventilation tubes may help alleviate the hearing loss.

Tuberculosis

Tuberculosis of the middle ear may be due either to a miliary process or to tubal extension of a localized infection from the nasopharynx. Multiple and persistent perforations of the tympanic membrane, severe loss of hearing, facial paralysis, and otorrhea are suspicious signs, but the diagnosis can be difficult to confirm. Confirmation is based on a positive tuberculin skin test and demonstration of acid-fast bacilli in the otorrhea or on tissue staining. The first-line treatment is medical, with antituberculous antibiotics. Surgical therapy may be necessary in order to debride bony sequestra.

Syphilis

Syphilis of the middle ear is extremely rare in comparison with syphilis of the internal ear and vestibulocochlear nerve. It becomes manifest in the secondary and tertiary stages and also as metasyphilitic or congenital disease.

Clinical Features. These include dizziness, tinnitus, rapidly progressive nonfluctuant hearing loss, and headaches due to chronic syphilitic meningitis.

Pathogenesis. The disease is due to a specific labyrinthitis and neuritis of the vestibulocochlear nerve, the latter arising during the course of a meningovascular syphilitic meningitis. In the tertiary stage and also in congenital and metasyphilitic disease, the nervous apparatus degenerates and atrophies due to meningovascular or parenchymatous syphilis, with progressive demyelinization of the vestibulocochlear nerve.

Diagnosis. The diagnosis is established by serum specimens that test positive on the *Treponema pallidum* hemagglutination (TPHA) or fluorescent treponemal antibody absorbed (FTA-abs) tests.

Differential diagnosis

- Ménière disease with a fluctuating course.
- A cerebellopontine angle tumor, which has typical neuroradiologic findings.
- Vertebrobasilar insufficiency, which occurs in the elderly, with discrete neurologic findings.

Treatment. Long-term penicillin is given in high doses.

Course and prognosis. Early diagnosis and correct treatment can stop progression, but the outlook for function being restored is poor.

■ Noninflammatory Diseases of the Labyrinthine Capsule

Otosclerosis

Otosclerosis is a localized disease of the bony labyrinthine capsule, the cause of which has not yet been identified. Spongy bone hardens around the base of the stapes. This condition fixes the stapes to the opening of the inner ear, so that the stapes no longer vibrates properly. Otosclerosis can also affect the malleus, incus, and the bone that surrounds the inner ear, resulting in disruption of sound transmission to the inner ear. Untreated otosclerosis eventually results in total deafness, usually in both ears. The exact diagnosis is made by histology, but only 10 % of patients with histologic evidence of the disease have clinical otosclerosis: 8–10 % of whites, 1 % of Japanese, and fewer than 1 % of blacks have histologic diseases.

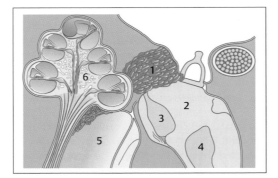

Fig. 1.101 Pathology of otosclerosis. **1**, Focus of otosclerosis; **2**, vestibule; **3**, utricle; **4**, saccule; **5**, internal acoustic
canal, **6**, cochlea.

Clinical Features. Depending on the site of the
otosclerotic focus, the symptoms include:

- Conductive hearing loss of the middle ear type,
  in ≈ 80 % of patients.
- Mixed conductive and sensorineural hearing
  loss, in ≈ 15 % of patients.
- Pure sensorineural hearing loss, in ≈ 5 % of patients.

The disease becomes manifest *subjectively* through:

- Slowly progressive hearing loss, which usually
  affects one ear initially, but later affects both ears
  in most patients.
- Constant, progressive tinnitus.

The disease never causes otalgia, otorrhea, dizziness, or disorders of balance.

Pathogenesis. This disease appears to have multifactorial causes, with the following being the most
important:

Heredity: In 50–60 % of patients, there is a familial disposition with dominant inheritance, possibly due to a hereditary enzyme defect. As clinical otosclerosis only occurs in
10 % of patients with histologic disease, the pattern of inheritance appears to be recessive. The chance of inheriting
the disease from a parent with clinically manifest disease is
≈ 20 %, and ≈ 10 % from a parent with histologic disease.

Disorders of hormone and bone metabolism: Pregnancy
coincides with a period of progression of clinically manifest
otosclerosis in half of female patients with the disease.
Abnormal lysosome formation of and increased enzyme
activity of the histiocytes and osteocytes in the labyrinthine

capsule, as well as enzymatic collagenolysis and bony remodeling have been demonstrated. The newly re-formed bone
fixes the stapes footplate in the oval window (**Fig. 1.101**).

Local infection with measles virus: As elevated levels of
measles virus–specific immunoglobulins, acting as antigens,
have been found in the perilymph in otosclerotic patients, it
is thought that infection with measles virus may be an
etiological factor. Measles-like structures have also been
found in otosclerotic foci using transmission electron microscopy.

Autoimmunity: Some immunological findings have suggested that autoimmune reactions play a role in the pathogenesis of otosclerosis.

> **Note:** Otosclerosis is due to an extremely localized dis-
> order of mineral or bone metabolism, with an abnormal
> increase of enzyme activity in the mesenchymal cells of
> the labyrinthine capsule, mainly determined by genetic
> factors but also by hormonal disturbances.

Diagnosis.

- Positive family history.
- Otoscopy occasionally shows hyperemia of the
  promontory as it shines through the tympanic
  membrane (Schwartze sign).
- Functional symptoms: Pure-tone audiography
  usually shows pure middle-ear hearing loss, occasionally mixed hearing loss, and rarely pure
  sensorineural deafness with positive recruitment. There is often a characteristic notch in
  the bone conduction curve at 2000 Hz (the
  Carhart notch). Impedance audiometry usually
  shows a normal curve at normal pressures. However, the stapedial reflex is often suppressed due
  to otosclerotic fixation of the footplate.
- Radiography usually shows very good pneumatization of the temporal bone.

Differential diagnosis.

- Congenital anomalies of the middle ear.
- Posttraumatic dislocation or fracture of the os-
  sicles.
- Postinflammatory fixation of the ossicles (mal-
  leus head).
- Adhesive processes.
- Tympanosclerosis.

Treatment. *Surgery* is indicated when there is sufficient inner ear function and the contralateral ear is not deaf. Three major components need to be taken into account when recommending surgery for otosclerosis: overall hearing loss, the extent of the air–bone gap, and the degree of handicap experienced by the patient. Although these three components are interrelated, it is not possible to predict the extent of one on the basis of the others. They have to be assessed independently.

In some countries, a trial of a hearing aid is recommended initially before surgical options are used, as hearing aids are usually very effective early in the course of the disease.

Two surgical techniques are used in otosclerosis:

Stapedectomy: The principle of this operation is to open the middle ear and expose the stapes footplate in the oval window niche. The fixed stapes is removed. The oval window is then closed with connective tissue, and the stapes is replaced with an alloplastic or wire prosthesis, or with an autologous cartilage graft. Complete removal of the footplate is no longer recommended.

Stapedotomy: After exposure of the oval niche, the footplate is perforated and a tiny, piston-like prosthesis is inserted and fixed to the long process of the incus (**Fig. 1.102**).

In cases of far-advanced otosclerosis with high-grade sensorineural hearing loss and no benefit from hearing aids, bilateral cochlear implantation can optimize performance.

The alternative treatment in sensorineural hearing loss is fitting a hearing aid. Other less successful forms of treatment include fluoride administration, which theoretically becomes incorporated into bone and inhibits progression of the otosclerosis. This treatment is not able to reverse conductive hearing loss, but may slow the progression of both the conductive and sensorineural components of the disease process.

Course and prognosis. Bilateral manifestations of the disease occur in 70 % of cases. Both ears can be operated on with stapedotomy, with an interval of at least 6 months between the procedures. If one ear has severe sensorineural hearing loss, surgery on the better-hearing ear is not indicated.

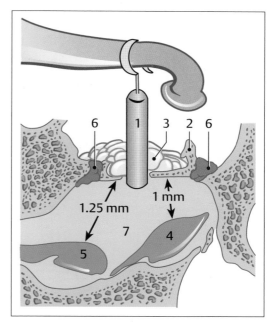

Fig. 1.102   The principle of stapedectomy, with reconstruction of the sound-pressure transformation mechanism. A suitable piston (**1**) is placed in the opening in the footplate (**2**) and its wire loop is fixed to the crura of the incus. Loose connective and fat tissue (**3**) is placed around the piston and the footplate to close off the perforation. The small distances between the stapedial footplate and the saccule (**4**) and utricle (**5**) are surgically important. **6**, Otosclerotic focus on the footplate; (**7**) vestibule.

Note: The earlier in life otosclerosis becomes manifest, the more rapid and unfavorable is its course.

In the vast majority of cases, the prognosis with surgical treatment is excellent. The rate of hearing deterioration over time after stapedotomy has not been found to exceed that due to presbyacusis. Patients with otosclerosis very seldom develop total deafness, and they continue to be able to hear with a hearing aid. The older the patient, the less the tendency for further hearing loss to occur due to the process of otosclerosis.

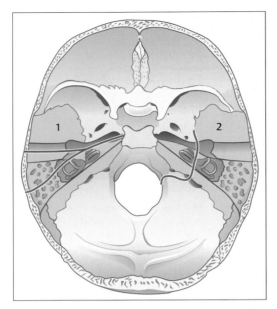

Fig. 1.103   Temporal bone fractures. **1**, Longitudinal fractures; **2**, transverse fracture.

Otologic Manifestations of Generalized Skeletal Disorders

The temporal bone, and the labyrinthine capsule in particular, can be affected by other generalized skeletal disorders:

- Osteogenesis imperfecta.
- Paget disease.
- Localized fibrous dysplasia.
- Osteogenesis imperfecta tarda with blue sclera (Lobstein type).

■ Trauma of the Middle and Inner Ear

Thorough familiarity with injuries to the ear and their consequences is essential for every practicing doctor. These lesions are usually caused by accidents, and the patients are therefore first seen by doctors working in accident and emergency departments or by general practitioners.

Frequency. Although injuries to the ear only make up 2–3 % of all injuries, 45 % of fractures of the base of the skull extend to the temporal bone, affecting the middle and inner ear.

Note: The ear and nasal sinuses should be examined as early as possible after every head injury. It is incumbent on the doctor who first sees the patient to investigate the following:

- Fresh bleeding or CSF leakage from the ear or nose.
- Evidence of blood or brain tissue in the external auditory meatus or the nose.
- Facial paralysis.
- Hemotympanum, rupture of the tympanic membrane, or a break in the outline of the anulus tympanicus and the external meatal wall.
- Hearing loss.
- Dizziness, disorders of balance, and nystagmus.
- Bleeding from the nasopharynx.

Temporal Bone Fracture

Pathogenesis. *Direct fractures* are caused by the effect of external force concentrated on a small surface—e. g., by gunshot wounds. The result is a penetrating, perforating fracture with brain damage.

Indirect fractures are due to diffuse external forces. The course of the fracture can run either:

- Along the pyramidal axis (i. e., *a longitudinal fracture*), extending into the middle ear.
- Across the pyramidal axis (i. e., *transverse fracture*), extending into the bony labyrinth and internal auditory meatus.

In both cases (**Fig. 1.103**), the dura may be torn, producing an open connection between the pneumatic system of the temporal bone and the subarachnoid space of the cranial fossae. The patient is then in danger of latent infection ascending via the eustachian tube to the meninges.

Clinical Features of longitudinal pyramidal fractures (mainly affecting the middle ear)

- Hemotympanum or CSF in the middle ear cleft (**Fig. 1.104**).
- Tearing of the tympanic membrane (**Fig. 1.105**).
- Bleeding from the external auditory meatus.
- A break in the contour of the tympanic ring.
- Step formation in the external auditory meatus, which should be differentiated from a posteriorly displaced fracture of the mandibular condyle.
- Middle ear deafness.
- Facial paralysis in ≈ 20 % of patients—usually neurapraxia or partial axonotmesis.
- Occasionally, CSF otorrhea.

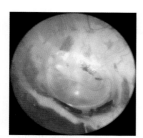

Fig. 1.104 Cerebrospinal fluid (CSF) in the tympanic cavity after a temporal bone fracture.

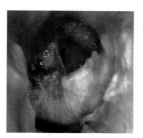

Fig. 1.105 Traumatic perforation of the tympanic membrane.

!

Caution: Syringing or manipulations must not be performed within the external auditory meatus.

Diagnosis. This is based on otoscopic findings and high-resolution CT scans.

Clinical Features of transverse pyramidal fractures (mainly affecting the inner ear)

- Intact external auditory meatus.
- Intact tympanic membrane, possibly with hemotympanum or CSF in the middle ear cleft (see **Fig. 1.104**).
- Hearing loss.
- Vertigo.
- Spontaneous nystagmus beating to the healthy ear.
- Facial paralysis in ≈50% of patients, usually showing axonotmesis or neurotmesis.
- Cerebrospinal fluid leak via the eustachian tube to the nasopharynx.

Diagnosis. This is based on otoscopic and functional findings and high-resolution CT scans. Additional investigations include EMG and neuronography, and the Schirmer test and gustometry for facial nerve paralysis (see p. 47).

Treatment of longitudinal and transverse pyramidal fractures. The treatment is dictated by the ever-present risk of otogenic meningitis. Prophylactic antibiotics are therefore administered in the form of high-dose, long-term parenteral broad-spectrum agents.

The temporal bone has to be explored if early or late complications occur (**Table 1.11**).

Emergency surgery definitely needs to be performed for the indications detailed above, as soon as the general condition of the patient permits. As the

Table 1.11 Pyramidal fracture

Indications for early otologic intervention

- Early meningitis, treated by mastoidectomy
- Bleeding from the sigmoid sinus, treated by opening of the mastoid and packing or ligature of the sinus
- Persistent CSF otorrhea, treated by repair of the dura and possible obliteration of the mastoid cavity.
- Facial paralysis with signs of progressive axonotmesis, treated by decompression if there is more than 90% denervation shown by neuronography
- Depressed fracture of the external auditory meatus, treated by reconstruction of the meatus because of the danger of secondary atresia
- Gunshot wounds of the temporal bone, treated by debridement of the fragmented area

Indications for late otologic intervention

- Antibiotic-resistant traumatic otitis media
- Chronic mastoiditis, treated by mastoidectomy
- Late facial nerve paralysis with symptoms of denervation, treated by facial nerve decompression
- Posttraumatic hearing loss, treated by tympanoplasty and ossiculoplasty
- Posttraumatic cholesteatoma, treated by mastoidectomy and tympanoplasty

CSF, cerebrospinal fluid.

patient has usually suffered multiple injuries, the various disciplines have to be prioritized as follows:
1. Traumatology.
2. Neurosurgery.
3. Otology.
4. Maxillofacial surgery.
5. Ophthalmology.

Course and prognosis. The following complications are possible, particularly as a result of unsatisfactory treatment or missed diagnoses:

Early complications:
- Acute otitis media with mastoiditis.
- Extension of the infection to the subarachnoid space, causing early meningitis or an infected labyrinthitis extending to the meninges.

Late complications:
- Chronic otitis media with mastoiditis.
- Late otogenic meningitis.
- Epidural abscess.
- Otogenic brain abscess.
- Posttraumatic cholesteatoma.

Labyrinthine Concussion
Posttraumatic disorders of inner ear function (deafness and dizziness) in the presence of normal otoscopic and radiographic findings are summed up under the heading of labyrinthine concussion.

Clinical Features. These include tinnitus, unilateral or bilateral sensorineural hearing loss with positive recruitment and high-tone loss or a notch at 4000 Hz; dizziness particularly after changing position or after rapid movements of the head; and disorders of balance.

Pathogenesis. The condition is usually due to organic mechanical damage to the membranous labyrinth, similar to acute acoustic trauma (see p. 88). Microfractures of the labyrinthine capsule accompanied by bleeding into the perilymphatic and endolymphatic space, and mechanical disturbances of the microcirculation causing degeneration of the cochleovestibular sensory cells, may also occur.

Diagnosis
- Normal otoscopic findings.
- Normal radiographs (Schüller and Stenver views; CT scan).
- A pure-tone audiogram showing a sensorineural hearing loss with a notch at 4000 Hz or high-tone loss with recruitment.
- Vestibular provocation nystagmus in the presence of vertigo, and more rarely spontaneous nystagmus; possibly reduced sensitivity to caloric stimulation.

Differential diagnosis
- Acute acoustic trauma in which vestibular symptoms are absent.

- Posttraumatic psychogenic hearing loss in which the findings are inconsistent and vestibular symptoms absent.

Treatment
- Intravenous low-molecular-weight dextran infusion (if there is no general contraindication—e. g., hypertension, heart rhythm disturbance, or allergy).
- Corticosteroids intravenously (if there is no contraindication—e. g., diabetes, hypertension).
- Antivertigo drugs are administered for dizziness.

Course and prognosis. In young patients and patients with normal circulation, recovery is rapid. Cochlear symptoms often only resolve incompletely. Irreversible vestibular defects are compensated centrally (see p. 20). Cochleovestibular symptoms, especially dizziness, often progress in elderly patients.

Direct Injuries to the Tympanic Membrane and Middle and Internal Ear
Clinical Features. *Injury to the tympanic membrane:* This is accompanied by momentary pain, slight bleeding from the ear, and slight hearing loss.
  Middle ear injuries: There is profuse bleeding, pain and hearing loss, a pulsating sound in the ear, and occasionally facial paralysis.
  Inner ear injuries: There is immediate tinnitus, hearing loss, dizziness, nausea, and vomiting.

Pathogenesis. Damage to the tympanic membrane and to the middle and internal ear can be caused by slapping injury or by the introduction of pointed objects such as matchsticks, toothpicks, knitting needles, hairpins, and twigs into the ear; and by careless removal of foreign bodies, by occupational injuries (hot cinders, welding sparks), acid burns, or gunshot wounds.

Diagnosis. Otoscopic findings include a tympanic membrane perforation with jagged, frayed, blood-streaked, and occasionally rolled-in edges (see **Fig. 1.105**). Blood is found in the external auditory meatus, mixed with perilymph, in injuries to the inner ear. *Conductive deafness* is found in middle ear injuries, *sensorineural deafness,* or mixed deafness if the inner ear is involved, and in severe lesions there is *complete deafness* and spontaneous nystagmus.

Immediate total peripheral *facial nerve paralysis* is found in fractures involving the bony tympanic segment of the facial nerve canal (see **Fig. 1.22**). CT can reveal a retained bullet or a bullet track.

Treatment. In simple tympanic membrane rupture, the fragments of the membrane are repositioned and splinted aseptically using a thin Silastic or plaster sheet under the operating microscope. Systemic prophylactic antibiotics are administered.

> **Caution:** Nonsterile instruments should not be used in the ear, and the ear should not be syringed.

In *combined injuries* of the tympanic membrane, middle ear, and inner ear, immediate exploration of the middle ear cavity and labyrinthine capsule is carried out with the operating microscope (tympanoplasty). Any perilymph leakage—e.g., from the round window—is stopped by closing the labyrinthine fistula. Prophylactic antibiotics are administered. Simultaneous facial nerve paralysis is treated by surgical decompression of the facial nerve if a disruption of the bony facial nerve canal is detectable. Otherwise, steroids and expectant management are recommended (see p. 112 and **Fig. 1.115**).

Course and prognosis. Simple injuries to the tympanic membrane and middle ear usually heal smoothly and without functional deficit if they are treated correctly by an otologist. Involvement of the labyrinth is usually followed by irreversible cochleovestibular failure. The prognosis for the facial paralysis is very good if continuity of the nerve has been preserved, but after neurotmesis there is irreversible paralysis if surgery is not undertaken.

Barotrauma

Clinical Features. Acute pain, pulsating tinnitus, hearing loss, occasionally vertigo and disturbance of balance.

Pathogenesis. Sudden changes in air pressure, producing an absolute or relative reduction of pressure in the middle ear, cause bleeding into the middle ear mucosa and into the tympanic membrane, and on occasion even rupture of the tympanic membrane and of the round window membrane. This may occur after rapid decompression or recompression from a low-pressure or high-pressure chamber, a rapid dive from a great height in a non-pressurized aircraft, or after surfacing too quickly from deep-sea diving.

The condition is caused by a sudden closure of the tube, which is compressed by the rapid rise in atmospheric pressure or by the associated increase in tissue pressure. After ≈ 2 h of closure of the tube, the Valsalva maneuver and politzerization are ineffective, as mucosal edema and serous–hemorrhagic exudate in the middle ear cavity have occurred due to the reduced pressure in the middle ear. The disorder is called *aerotitis* or *barotitis*.

Diagnosis. This is based on the history. The otoscopic findings show retraction of the tympanic membrane, occasionally subepithelial hemorrhage in the pars tensa, transudate behind the tympanic membrane, or a hemotympanum. Audiological tests show conductive hearing loss.

Treatment. This includes decongestant nose drops, possibly paracentesis, analgesics, and oral anti-inflammatory agents. Prophylaxis is important, and the patient should avoid flying or diving during inflammation of the nasopharynx, nose, and paranasal sinuses. Anatomic deformities in the nose and nasopharynx obstructing nasal respiration and favoring the development of inflammatory diseases of the eustachian tube should be dealt with. These diseases include septal deformity, hypertrophy of the turbinates, and adenoidal hypertrophy. Immediate tympanotomy should be performed for barotrauma with severe sensorineural hearing loss, to allow assessment of the round window so that a possible perilymph fistula due to rupture of the round window membrane can be closed.

Caisson Disease and Diving Accidents

These accidents occur in people who work underwater at depths where the pressure is several times that of atmospheric pressure. They can also occur in amateur sports divers who surface too quickly from too great a depth.

Clinical Features
- Dizziness, vomiting, headache.
- Severe tinnitus and rapidly progressive hearing loss.
- The above symptoms have a latent period of minutes to hours.
- Disorders of vision, ataxia, and clouding of consciousness in severe cases.

Pathogenesis. When working at several times atmospheric pressure, either in a caisson or when diving to depths greater than 10 m, a considerable quantity of air, including relatively insoluble nitrogen, is taken into solution. Gaseous nitrogen is released into the blood if the patient decompresses too quickly from the caisson or surfaces too rapidly from depths greater than 10 m. This can lead to the formation of small gas emboli within the cerebral end arteries. These cause deficits in the area of supply of the cerebral vessels, including that of the inner ear. This explains the symptoms described above.

Diagnosis. Previous history of an accident. Sensorineural hearing loss, spontaneous and provocation vestibular nystagmus, and in serious cases ataxia and neurologic deficits.

Treatment. Hyperbaric oxygen is given.

Course and prognosis. This depends on the degree of severity of the gas emboli and on the time taken to institute treatment. In serious cases, the patient may become blind or deaf, suffer from balance disorders, may be paralyzed, or may even die.

Acute Acoustic Trauma

!

Note: There is an important basic difference between explosion and gunfire injuries. The physical-acoustic properties of an explosion are qualitatively identical to those of gunfire, but are completely different quantitatively. In an explosion, there is a high-pressure wave, but the shock wave lasts more than 1.5 ms, whereas with gunfire the peak of the pressure wave lasts less than 1.5 ms.

Clinical Features. *Blast trauma:* There is marked, persistent earache, occasionally with bleeding from the affected ear, deafness, and tinnitus.

Gunshot trauma: There is a short stabbing pain in the ear, marked continuous tinnitus, and deafness.

Pathogenesis. In both explosion and gunshot trauma, the causes are partly direct and mechanical, due to bleeding, and partly indirect, with a metabolic effect on the microcirculation causing partially reversible damage to the sensory cells of the organ of Corti. The severity and site of the lesion in the cochlea directly depend on the sound pressure level of the acoustic energy and its maximum frequency. In explosion trauma, ruptures of the tympanic membrane and other middle ear lesions often occur.

Diagnosis. Only *explosion injury* causes abnormal otoscopic findings; in addition, the audiogram shows sensorineural or mixed hearing loss. In *gunshot trauma,* there is a notch at 4000 Hz, or a high-tone loss, and positive recruitment.

Treatment. Intravenous infusion of low-molecular-weight dextran and a vasodilator such as pentoxifylline within 24 h of the trauma if possible. Tympanoplasty has to be performed in cases of visible middle ear injuries such as tympanic membrane perforation and defects in the ossicular chain.

Course and prognosis. Traumatic *middle ear lesions* usually heal without complications after surgical repair. The prognosis is good.

Inner ear lesions are partially reversible, but in some patients there is continuing degeneration of sensory cells and secondary increased degeneration of the peripheral neurons.

Chronic Noise Trauma

In contrast to acute acoustic trauma, this condition is the result of damage to the inner ear caused by weaker, but more prolonged, noise. Chronic noise-induced hearing loss is now a considerable hazard in the younger population, as they are exposed to loud music and other noises associated with leisure activities. The severity of the lesion therefore depends not only on the sound pressure peaks of the noise (noise level), but also on the exposure time and on the individual patient's sensitivity to the effect of noise. Exposure to levels below 85 dB (A) for 8 h/day is considered safe. Emotional factors also play an important role and produce autonomic symptoms that have deleterious effects on the entire body.

Clinical Features. *Subjectively,* there is a sense of pressure in the ears and in the head, a feeling of hearing loss, generalized tiredness and lack of concentration, and often tinnitus. The subjective symptoms are often reversible, since the patient becomes used to the noise. Few patients are aware of the developing deafness in the early phases.

Objectively, a pure-tone audiogram of chronic noise trauma initially shows a notch at 4000 Hz, typically in both ears. Later, the threshold for the lower frequencies rises, and finally the deafness spreads to the speech frequencies. Further loss of hearing follows as a result of the physiologic aging process. In the early phases of its development, chronic noise deafness shows a certain tendency toward recovery when the patient is no longer exposed, but with increasing exposure this tendency declines.

Pathogenesis. Depending on the intensity and duration of exposure, the ear may react to sounds in one of the following ways:
1. A physiologic *adaptation of threshold* may develop.
2. After more prolonged exposure, the ear may react with *fatigue* or with the appearance of a temporary threshold shift (TTS), which can be related directly to acoustic damage that is proportional to the exposure time and has a linear relationship with the sound intensity. The "physiologic" TTS usually recovers within minutes and at the most 2 h after the end of exposure to the noise.
3. A *permanent threshold shift* (PTS) may develop, which is an expression of pathologic fatigue and irreversible damage to the hearing organ. This is caused by metabolic decompensation of the sensory cells due to a disturbance of the balance between supply and demand in energy metabolism. This is caused by increased oxygen consumption or by decreased supply during permanent intensive acoustic exposure. The outer hair cells degenerate first, and the inner cells last. Not all individuals are affected equally. Some highly susceptible people lose their hearing ability faster than others. Intracellular conditions presumably have an influence on this—e. g., the adenosine triphosphate (ATP) level. In a person who is constantly exposed to noise, it is not possible to determine whether or not any hearing loss is due to the noise.

Diagnosis. The hearing loss is of long standing, and a social history reveals occupational exposure or lifelong social habits that are responsible. A pure-tone speech audiogram is important.

Differential diagnosis
- Endogenous heredodegenerative sensorineural deafness in which there is a positive family history.
- Infective and toxic damage to the inner ear and vestibulocochlear nerve, particularly by ototoxic antibiotics.
- Progressive sensorineural deafness in severe generalized diseases such as diabetes, chronic nephritis, and hypertension.

!

Note: The limits of noise causing damage to the ear are as follows:
- Equivalent continuous sound pressure (Leq) in the range of 85–90 ± 2.5 dB and higher must be regarded as damaging to the ear.
- Single sound impulses exceeding a peak of 135 dB also damage the ear.

Treatment. No active methods of treatment for dealing with the cause are available. If hearing in social situations becomes inadequate, a hearing aid should be prescribed. Prophylaxis, including the provision of hearing protectors, is very important. *Protection of hearing:*
- Elimination or reduction of noise through technical improvements to machinery.
- Protection of personnel from noise using ear protectors.
- Limitation of the time of exposure to noise and frequent rest periods.
- Medical prophylaxis against damage to hearing, prescribed by occupational medical health staff.

!

Note: A cotton wool plug does not protect against noise trauma to the ear.

Course and prognosis. The disease progresses to advanced hearing loss and tinnitus, which may decompensate.

■ Tumors of the Middle and Internal Ear, Vestibulocochlear Nerve, and Facial Nerve

Nonchromaffin Paraganglioma (Glomus Tumor)
This is the most frequent true tumor of the middle ear. It develops from neuroectoderm. The structure

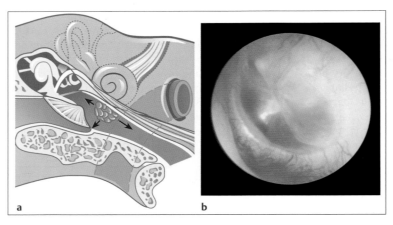

Fig. 1.106a, b Glomus tympanicum tumor.
a The arrows mark the possible direction of tumor growth.
b A small red tumor becomes visible.

of the tumor is similar to that of the chemoreceptor tissue of the carotid body. It is characterized by extensive vascularity. Because of its structural and functional relationship to the carotid body, this tumor is also considered in the section on chemodectomas (see p. 397).

Clinical Features. These are very variable, depending on the site of origin and extent of the tumor, and include:

- Unilateral tinnitus, synchronous with the pulse.
- Unilateral hearing loss and feeling of pressure in the ear.
- Disorders of balance.
- Lesions of the lower cranial nerves causing facial paralysis, paralysis of the soft palate, hoarseness, disorders of swallowing, and paralysis of the tongue in the late stage.

Pathogenesis. The tumor develops from nests of epithelial cells surrounded by a high vascular stroma. The sites of predilection are the bulb of the internal jugular vein, the tympanic plexus, and the lesser superficial petrosal nerve. They can be grouped by site and extent as follows:

1. Glomus tympanicum tumors limited to the middle ear cavity (**Fig. 1.106a**).
2. Glomus jugulare tumors limited to the middle ear cavity and the bulb of the jugular vein, without destruction of bone (**Fig. 1.106b**).
3. Glomus jugulare tumors destroying bone and invading the whole of the mastoid as far as the petrous apex.
4. Glomus jugulare tumors with intracranial extension.

Diagnosis. Otoscopy shows the tumor shining through the tympanic membrane. The tumor is often red. If the tumor breaks through into the external meatus, a polyp that bleeds easily can be seen (**Fig. 1.107a, b**).

The hearing loss is conductive in the early stage, but later becomes sensorineural, and finally the patient may be completely deaf if the tumor erodes into the labyrinth.

The hypoglossal, glossopharyngeal, or vagus nerves may be paralyzed in tumors arising primarily from the bulb of the jugular vein (the jugular foramen syndrome).

Intracranial extension is accompanied by pontine and cerebellar syndromes, in addition to facial paralysis, trigeminal hypoesthesia, deafness, and vestibular symptoms.

Supplementary investigations include CT scans with contrast enhancement, to allow three-dimensional comparison of the two temporal bones and the jugular foramen and jugular bulb area. The tumor extension is best evaluated using MRI, magnetic resonance angiography, and subtraction angiography (which allows embolization of the main afferent vessels in selected patients during the same session).

Treatment. Tumors in groups 1 and 2 (see above) can be removed easily and radically with otologic surgery. Tumors in group 3 require a combined cervicotemporal approach, and those in group 4 a two-phase neurotologic procedure designed to remove the tumor completely while preserving the facial nerve.

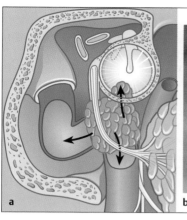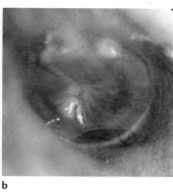

Fig. 1.107a, b Glomus jugulare tumor.
a The arrows mark the possible direction of tumor growth into the epitympanum, the hypotympanum, and through the tympanic membrane.
b There is a blue-colored tumor shining through the tympanic membrane.

Preoperative angiographic embolization of the larger and tumor-feeding vessels reduces intraoperative blood loss. In group 4 tumors, tumor control using radiotherapy has been proposed as an alternative form of treatment.

Course and prognosis. The tumor grows slowly. In advanced stages with extensive intracranial invasion, life-threatening situations occur due to compression of the brain stem or thrombosis of the carotid artery.

Middle Ear Carcinoma

In most patients, this involves a keratinizing squamous cell carcinoma, arising at the junction between the external auditory meatus and the tympanic membrane, which has penetrated into the middle ear.

Adenocarcinomas and adenoid cystic carcinomas arising primarily from the middle ear mucosa are very rare, as are sarcomas.

Clinical Features

- Neuralgic pain around the ear.
- Blood-stained otorrhea, which is very fetid.
- Progressive hearing loss.
- Occasionally, dizziness, disorders of balance, facial nerve paralysis, and intense headache if the tumor is infiltrating into the dura.

Diagnosis

- Otoscopy shows a readily bleeding aural polyp (**Fig. 1.108**).
- Destruction of the tympanic membrane by hemorrhagic granulations.
- Destruction of the posterior meatal wall.

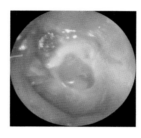

Fig. 1.108 Middle ear carcinoma.

- Peripheral facial paralysis, enlargement of the regional lymph nodes, conductive hearing loss, combined conductive and sensorineural hearing loss or even deafness, spontaneous vestibular nystagmus to the healthy side, depending on the extent of the tumor.
- Tumor expansion into the parotid gland and regional lymph-node metastases.
- CT scans show extensive destruction of the temporal bone arising from the middle ear cavity and the external auditory meatus.

Differential diagnosis

- Chronic otitis media with cholesteatoma.
- Necrotizing otitis externa.

Treatment

- Radical expansive operation with subtotal petrosectomy, parotidectomy, neck dissection, and reconstruction of the facial nerve.
- Postoperative radiotherapy.

Course and prognosis. Despite combined surgery and radiotherapy, the prognosis is poor due to early expansion and the lesion's tendency to metastasize.

Table 1.12 Subjective symptoms of vestibular schwannoma

Focal symptoms

- Tinnitus (incidence 70 %)
- Unilateral progressive deafness (45 %)
- Sudden hearing loss (40 %)
- Fluctuating deafness (10 %)
- Dizziness (30 %)

Associated symptoms

- Unilateral facial nerve spasm or paralysis
- Double vision
- Ataxia
- Clumsiness on moving the arms
- Unilateral disturbances of sensation of the face

Symptoms of increased cranial pressure

- Occipital headache
- Projectile vomiting
- Decrease in vision and papilledema
- Personality changes

Vestibular Schwannoma (Acoustic Neuroma)
Clinical Features. See **Table 1.12**.

Pathogenesis. This is a histologically benign tumor arising from the Schwann cells of the neurilemma. It usually arises in the transitional zone between the neuroglia and the neurilemma of the pars superior of the vestibular nerve. The tumor is a generally slow-growing one and may also grow inside the labyrinth or arise from the cochlear nerve, but only in rare cases.

Depending on their site of origin, these tumors may be divided into:

- *Lateral vestibular schwannomas,* which lie in the internal auditory meatus and exclusively cause localized symptoms; and *mediolateral vestibular schwannomas* in the region of the porus, lying partly in the internal meatus and partly in the cerebellopontine angle and causing both localized symptoms and symptoms due to impairment of neighboring organs.
- *Medial vestibular schwannomas,* which arise in the cerebellopontine angle and cause slight symptoms in cranial nerve VIII, but marked symptoms due to involvement of the adjacent cranial nerves, brain stem, and cerebellum, and finally the symptoms of increased intracranial pressure.

Three stages can be distinguished, depending on the size of the tumor (**Fig. 1.109a-c**):

1. Small intrameatal tumors with a diameter of 1–8 mm, which cause focal symptoms.
2. Medium-sized tumors with a diameter of up to 2.5 cm, with intrameatal and intracranial extension, which cause focal symptoms and slight symptoms caused by involvement of neighboring neural structures.
3. Large tumors more than 2.5 cm in diameter, causing focal symptoms, symptoms due to involvement of neighboring neural structures, and symptoms of increased intracranial pressure, depending on their size.

Diagnosis. See **Table 1.13**. Diagnostic investigations include:

- Pure-tone and speech audiometry, stapedial reflex.
- Auditory evoked potentials.
- Vestibular tests with nystagmography.
- MRI with Gd-DTPA enhancement.

Differential diagnosis

- Ménière disease (see p. 97).
- Sudden sensorineural hearing loss (see p. 101).
- Primary congenital cholesteatoma of the cerebellopontine angle.
- Vascular compression syndrome.
- Secondary acquired occult middle ear cholesteatoma with perilabyrinthine extension and rupture into the internal auditory meatus (see p. 68).
- Meningioma and facial nerve neuroma.
- Congenital syphilis causing vascular cochleovestibular symptoms (see p. 81).

Treatment. Intrameatal tumors (stage 1) can be removed using an extradural transtemporal approach through the middle cranial fossa (**Fig. 1.110a**). In asymptomatic patients with good hearing, a "wait-and-scan" approach with regular follow-ups can be considered. Stereotactic radiosurgery (with the gamma knife) is a possible treatment. The indication depends on the quality of hearing and the patient's age and wishes.

Medium-sized tumors (stage 2) are removed via a translabyrinthine (**Fig. 1.110b**) or retrosigmoid route (**Fig. 1.110c**). The mortality is zero, but 85 % of patients become totally deaf. Facial nerve function, however, can be preserved in 85 % of patients. Large tumors (stage 3) are treated using a retrosigmoid or suboccipital neurosurgical approach.

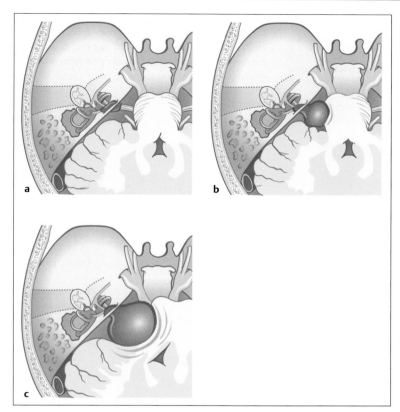

Fig. 1.109a–c The three stages of a vestibular schwannoma.
a Intrameatal tumor.
b Intrameatal and extrameatal tumor.
c A mainly extrameatal medial tumor compressing the brain stem and the cerebellum.

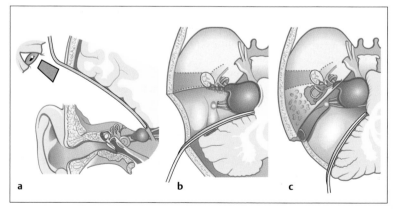

Fig 1.110a–c Otologic and neurosurgical routes of access to the internal meatus.
a The transtemporal approach through the middle cranial fossa.
b, c The translabyrinthine and retrosigmoid approaches.

Table 1.13 Objective symptoms of vestibular schwannoma

Focal symptoms

- Retrocochlear sensorineural hearing loss, with negative recruitment, pathologic hearing fatigue: abnormal SISI test, abnormal decay on Békésy audiogram, and discrepancy between pure-tone and speech audiogram. Stapedial reflex absent. Pathologic ABR and electrocochleography
- Vestibular symptoms include spontaneous nystagmus to the healthy ear and loss of caloric labyrinthine responses

Associated symptoms

- Peripheral, usually slight, facial paralysis, neurodiagnostic axonotmesis and positive Hitselberger sign
- Abducens paralysis
- Loss of the corneal reflex
- Hypoesthesia of the trigeminal nerve
- Occasionally, palatal paralysis

Symptoms due to brain stem compression

Disorders of oculomotor nerves. In stage III tumors, pontine compression causes the following:

- Gaze-evoked nystagmus to the side of the tumor
- Direction-changing irregular positional nystagmus
- Abnormal or absent optokinetic nystagmus

Cerebellar symptoms

In stage III, often include dysdiadochokinesia and ataxia

Symptoms of increased intracranial pressure

Papilledema and projectile vomiting

ABR, auditory brain stem response; SISI, short increment sensitivity index.

!

Note: The possibility of a vestibular schwannoma must always be suspected in all patients with unilateral progressive sensorineural hearing loss or unilateral recurrent loss of hearing, and a thorough neuro-otologic examination and neuroradiologic examination (including MRI and evoked response audiometry) must be performed.

!

Note: In patients with von Recklinghausen neurofibromatosis (NF2), one or more neuromas of the auditory or facial nerve may be suspected.

Facial Nerve Neuroma

Clinical Features. The tumor causes slowly progressive facial paralysis or hemifacial spasm. Depending on its site, the tumor may cause symptoms similar to those of acoustic neuroma (vestibular schwannoma).

Bony Tumors

These rare tumors include:

- Osteoma.
- Giant cell tumor.
- Solitary plasmacytoma.
- Histiocytosis (reticuloendotheliosis; Letterer–Siwe disease, Hand–Schüller–Christian disease, eosinophilic granuloma).

■ Congenital Anomalies of the Middle and Internal Ear

Simultaneous congenital anomalies of the middle and internal ear are rare, but those affecting the middle and external ear together are common, occurring in one in 10 000 normal births.

Combined Anomalies of the External and Middle Ear

Clinical Features

- Dysplasia.
- Microtia.
- Meatal atresia.
- Facial deformities.
- Deafness.

Pathogenesis. The following factors may be responsible for these anomalies:

- Genetic factors, chromosomal abnormalities, or mutation of genes.
- Exogenous factors, including hypoxia, radiation, ultrasound, and thalidomide.
- Combined exogenous and genetic factors, causing polygenic multifactorial anomalies.

The developmental process (described on p. 1) is restricted or disturbed by these factors.

Diagnosis

- Inspection.
- High-resolution CT scan.
- Auditory evoked potentials.
- Vestibular tests.

Treatment. Surgery is performed or a hearing aid is prescribed.

Purpose of treatment:

1. Construction of an esthetically satisfactory auricle using rib cartilage, followed by creation of an external meatus in a second procedure.
2. Improvement of hearing, either by reconstructing the sound conducting apparatus with tympanoplasty (see **Fig. 1.96 d**, **f**) or by prescribing a hearing aid.

Timing of the operation:

A patient with bilateral meatal atresia with a conductive hearing loss of 50 dB should undergo surgery on one ear in the third to fourth year of life. However, it is preferable to reconstruct the external auditory meatus and to carry out a tympanoplasty after pneumatization is complete and when the auricle has reached its final size—i. e., after the eighth year of life. Otoplasty is performed after the fifth year of life.

A bone conduction hearing aid is prescribed for patients with bilateral atresia as early as possible—i. e., in the second half of the first year of life—to allow speech to develop normally.

Congenital Anomalies of the Internal Ear

These are rare and are summarized in **Table 1.14**.

Table 1.14 Congenital anomalies of the internal ear

Mondini syndrome	Isolated dysplasia of the cochlea
Congenital CSF otorrhea	Due to a fistula of the oval window with a patent cochlear aqueduct (gusher syndrome)
Thalidomide embryopathy	A labyrinthine dysplasia with aplasia of the petrous pyramid
Rubella embryopathy	Labyrinthine anomalies with dysplasia of the middle ear

CSF, cerebrospinal fluid.

Clinical Aspects of Cochleovestibular Disorders

■ Toxic Damage to the Hearing and Balance Apparatus

Exogenous ototoxins include drugs such as aminoglycosides, cytostatics and diuretics, as well as industrial products, tobacco, and alcohol.

Endogenous ototoxins include bacterial toxins and the toxic metabolites that arise in metabolic disorders such as diabetes and renal disease.

Clinical Features

- Tinnitus is usually the first symptom.
- Progressive bilateral sensorineural hearing loss, initially for high tones, but later from high to middle and lower frequencies.
- Positional vertigo with nausea.
- Balance disorders with persistent vertigo and unsteadiness of gait.
- Oscillopsia—i. e., a weakness of fixation

■ Ototoxic Drugs

Aminoglycoside Antibiotics

Pathogenesis. Aminoglycoside antibiotics are retained for a longer period and in higher concentrations in inner ear fluids than in other body tissues and fluids. Ototoxic aminoglycosides destroy both cochlear and vestibular sensory cells; streptomycin is mainly vestibulotoxic, whereas dihydrostreptomycin is ototoxic. Neomycin and kanamycin are strongly ototoxic, and gentamicin is both ototoxic and vestibulotoxic.

> **Note:** The development of inner ear damage depends on the dose and the half-life of the ototoxic antibiotic and on the patient's renal function.

Treatment

- Immediate cessation of aminoglycoside administration.
- Intravenous infusion of low-molecular-weight dextran solutions.
- Intravenous infusion of a vasodilator and systemic corticosteroids.

Course. The disease usually progresses for up to 6 months after the antibiotics are stopped; the prognosis therefore has to be guarded, as the inner ear damage is largely irreversible.

Cytostatics

Cisplatin and cyclophosphamide produce a direct toxic effect on the hair cells of the cochlea, while cisplatin also has neurotoxic effects. Other platinum-based cytostatic drugs, such as carboplatin, appear to be less ototoxic, but hearing loss may still occur.

Note: Any patient being treated with aminoglycosides or cytostatic drugs must have the following investigations: renal function tests and an audiogram once or twice a week during the course of treatment.

Diuretics

Diuretics, including furosemide and ethacrynic acid, can also damage the inner ear. The extent of the lesion varies, and it affects mainly the outer hair cells, due to disturbance of the regulation of ion concentration caused by a lesion in the stria vascularis. These lesions are reversible in ≈ 90 % of patients.

Other Ototoxic Antibiotics

Metabolic damage to the cochlear hair cells can be caused by quinine and salicylate. The initially reversible effect can become irreversible in overdosed, long-term treatment.

■ Ototoxic Occupational Toxins

- Arsenic compounds.
- Mercury salts.
- Lead salts.
- Organic phosphate compounds.
- Sulfur and tetrachlorocarbon compounds.
- Carbon monoxide.
- Benzol, nitrobenzol, and aniline.

■ Inflammatory Lesions of the Hearing and Balance Apparatus

Herpes Zoster Oticus (Ramsay Hunt Syndrome)

The most common site of zoster infection in the head and neck, after herpes zoster ophthalmicus, is that affecting the ear. Herpes zoster oticus can occur at any age, but it mainly does so between 40 and 60 years of age.

Clinical Features

- Reduced general condition and/or subfebrile temperature.
- Erythema and vesicles on the auricle and the external meatus (see **Fig. 1.70**).
- Regional lymphadenitis (discrete).
- Severe neuralgic pain.
- Peripheral facial paralysis in 60–90 % of patients.
- Severe sensorineural (retrocochlear) hearing loss in 40 % of patients.
- Vertigo and balance disorders in 40 % of patients, with release nystagmus to the healthy side.

Pathogenesis. This disorder is due to a viral infection. The portal of entry is unknown. The virus may spread via the bloodstream to the CSF and meninges, causing encephalomyelomeningitis with neuritis of the spiral or vestibular ganglion.

Diagnosis

- Inspection of the auricle and otoscopy.
- Audiogram and impedance test.
- Vestibular tests.
- Tests of facial nerve function.
- Schirmer test.
- Testing of glossopharyngeal and vagus nerve function.
- Viral serology.
- Lumbar puncture with CSF examination (for diagnosis of serous meningitis).

Differential diagnosis

- Myringitis bullosa.
- Idiopathic facial paralysis.

Treatment

- Antiviral treatment with aciclovir or famciclovir (antiviral agents that inhibit DNA synthesis of type I and II herpes simplex virus, as well as varicella-zoster virus).
- Gammaglobulin.
- Antibiotics (to avoid superinfection).
- Local dermal treatment with lotions or ointment.

Course and prognosis. Complete recovery is possible within 4 weeks, but recovery is often only partial in cases of facial nerve paralysis. The cochleovestibular loss is usually irreversible.

Other Viral Infections
Influenza, measles, adenovirus, chickenpox, coxsackievirus, and mumps viruses often cause a vestibular neuritis, with corresponding symptoms.

The virus of *epidemic parotitis* (mumps) has a particular affinity for the cochlea and usually causes unilateral serous labyrinthitis, destruction of the hair cells, or degeneration of the organ of Corti. Neurolabyrinthitis with destruction of the spiral ganglion may occur. The vestibular part of the labyrinth is almost never attacked by the mumps virus.

!
> Note: Infection with the mumps virus is the most frequent cause of unilateral complete deafness in young children.

Course. The course is usually mild or abortive with respect to the primary disease.

Prognosis. This is poor, with irreversible damage.

Serous Labyrinthitis
This condition is a toxic or virally determined abacterial serous inflammation of the perilymphatic and endolymphatic spaces, with partial or total destruction of cochlear and vestibular sensory cells. The loss of cochlear and vestibular function is usually irreversible.

■ Immunologic Diseases of the Inner Ear

Recognized autoimmune syndromes can lead to inner ear disease. Rapid bilateral and often asymmetrical cochlear hearing loss, occasionally with a fluctuating course, is typical. There may be accompanying vestibular symptoms.
- Cogan syndrome.
- Wegener granulomatosis.
- Recurrent polychondritis.
- Primary autoimmune disease.

■ Trauma

(See pp. 84–89).

■ Vestibular Disorders

Ménière Disease
Clinical Features. The classic triad originally described by Ménière in 1861 consists of attacks of:
- Tinnitus—continuous low frequency with varying intensity (**Table 1.15**).
- Fluctuating hearing loss and dysacusis.
- Attacks of rotatory vertigo.

The typical attack begins acutely and consists of the three symptoms listed above, followed by nausea, vomiting, and other autonomic symptoms. Patients feel sensations of aural fullness. The tinnitus and hearing loss may change before and during the attack. Characteristically, the tinnitus improves, while hearing becomes poorer. Mostly, hearing improves again following the attack. A marked improvement in hearing during the attack itself is called *Lermoyez phenomenon.*

The symptoms are usually unilateral. In the disease-free intervals, hearing often returns to normal and the tinnitus disappears, at least in the early phases of the disease. In the later stages, there is

Table 1.15 Classification of tinnitus

Subjective tinnitus	
Conductive tinnitus	Obstruction of the ear canal
	Middle ear disease
Sensorineural tinnitus	Cochlear damage
	Cochlear nerve disturbance
Central tinnitus	Damage to the central auditory pathway
Objective tinnitus	
Vascular tinnitus	Vascular malformations
	Arteriovenous fistulas
	Paragangliomas
Myogenic tinnitus	Velopharyngeal myoclonus
	Middle ear myoclonus

fluctuating hearing loss for low tones. In the end stage, hearing loss is unilateral, severe, and pancochlear. The patient also reports persistent tinnitus. Initially, the cochlear symptoms predominate.

There is no predisposing factor, apart from psychological stress.

Pathogenesis. The disease is caused by a disturbance of the *quantitative* relation between the volume of the perilymph and endolymph. In addition, a disorder of the *qualitative* electrolyte composition of the two fluids causes abnormal osmotic pressure regulation within the membranous labyrinth. This causes endolymphatic hydrops.

The primary cause of this increase of pressure within the endolymphatic space is a disorder of resorption of the potassium-rich endolymph. This leads to an increase in osmotic pressure. When this exceeds a certain level, the Reissner membrane lying between the endolymphatic and perilymphatic spaces ruptures, allowing the endolymph and perilymph to mix. Sites of predilection for the rupture are the helicotrema, the basal turn of the cochlea and the utricle, and part of the saccule lying opposite the ampulla of the semicircular canals. This explains the genesis of the cochleovestibular symptoms in the classic Ménière attack.

Rupture of the hydropic labyrinth and the resulting mixing of the potassium-rich endolymph with perilymph, which is normally low in potassium, leads to a considerable increase in potassium content in the intercellular spaces of the perilymphatic network, in which the afferent neurons of the acoustic and vestibular nerves run. These are paralyzed by depolarization due to the increase in potassium, thus causing the symptoms of cochleovestibular failure. The process may last from a few minutes to several hours and is reversible in the early phases of the disease—which explains the clinical recovery, especially the fluctuating hearing loss.

Psychological factors such as stress can act as a trigger mechanism for an attack, but are not primarily responsible for the development of the disease.

Diagnosis. See **Table 1.16**.

Treatment. *During an attack:*
- Bed rest.
- Intravenous infusion of fluid and electrolytes for prolonged vomiting.
- Intravenous antivertigo and antiemetic drugs.
- Low-molecular-weight dextran and systemic vasodilator infusions to improve the labyrin-

thine circulation and to increase the flow of perilymph and endolymph.
- Psychotropic drugs should not be given during an attack because of the danger of central disinhibition of the vestibular system, causing worsening of the symptoms.

In the symptom-free interval:
- Antivertigo antihistamine (betahistine).
- Thiazide diuretics.
- Psychological support, if necessary psychotropic drugs.

When there is a protracted course, with repeated attacks that disable the patient:
- Destruction of the vestibular end organ while retaining social hearing: intratympanic application of gentamicin to the round window, which selectively destroys the sensory cells of the vestibular end organ.
- Neurectomy of the vestibular nerve via a transtemporal approach to the internal meatus.
- Surgical exposure and drainage of the endolymphatic sac (saccotomy; the operation is based on the hypothesis of hydrops decompression).

In patients with poor hearing and marked tinnitus:
- *Labyrinthectomy*: Surgical ablation of the severely damaged inner ear using transtympanic or translabyrinthine exposure of the internal meatus, with resection of the intrameatal portion of the vestibulocochlear nerve. This operation produces complete deafness and is only indicated in selected cases when other alternatives are not adequate.

Course. One of the characteristics of Ménière disease is that its course is unpredictable. At one end of the spectrum, there are *abortive forms,* which heal after a few attacks without permanent deafness. At the other end, the disease may progress episodically over several years with symptom-free intervals of varying duration. However, over the course of time, the fluctuating hearing loss becomes irreversible. In addition, there is also an *acute form,* in which several attacks lead rapidly to almost complete deafness and to severe disability due to the disturbance of balance. In these cases, elimination of the diseased vestibular part of the inner ear by transtympanic application of gentamicin, or by one of the surgical routes described above, is indicated.

Table 1.16 Synopsis of the most important disorders of balance and hearing

Diagnosis	Subjective symptoms	Audiogram	Vestibular symptoms	Associated neurologic signs	Other clinical signs
Acute unilateral vestibular paralysis	Acute rotatory dizziness and prolonged dizziness, possibly positional. Nausea, vomiting, no loss of consciousness, normal hearing and no tinnitus	Normal	Spontaneous nystagmus to the sound side, possibly positional nystagmus, no response to caloric stimulation, ataxia. Galvanic tests are usually abnormal, with an increased threshold	None	Often diabetes, acute infection by viruses or toxoplasmosis, or hypertension or hypotension, immune disorder
Ménière disease	Episodic vertigo, unilateral tinnitus, unilateral hearing loss, and fluctuating hearing loss	Unilateral fluctuating sensorineural hearing loss with positive recruitment, and often a flat or low tone curve	Spontaneous nystagmus to the healthy side after the attack, reduced caloric response	None	None
Vestibular schwannoma	Progressive unilateral hearing loss, progressive disorder of balance, occipital headache, occasionally also recurrent hearing loss with partial remission, tinnitus	Unilateral retrocochlear sensorineural hearing loss, at first for high tones. Stapedial reflex lost. Absent recruitment and marked loss of discrimination for speech and with a discrepancy between the pure-tone and speech audiograms, and pathological ABR	Spontaneous nystagmus to the healthy side, possibly gaze-evoked nystagmus to the diseased side, positional nystagmus, abnormal caloric responses, possibly abnormal optokinetic responses in the presence of compression of the brain stem and cerebellum	Associated symptoms, absent corneal reflex, abnormal glabellar tap, facial weakness, and positive Hitselberger sign, papilledema, and abducens paralysis in large tumors	None

ABR, auditory brain stem response.

Bilateral disease is relatively uncommon, occurring in only 10% of patients.

Acute Vestibular Loss (Vestibular Neuronitis, Vestibular Neuritis)
Clinical Features. See **Table 1.17**.

Pathogenesis. The site of the pathophysiological lesion (labyrinth or vestibular nerve) is not known. The cause may be a disturbance of the microcirculation due to an infection (e. g., neurotropic virus or other agents such as *Rickettsia,* or protozoa such as *Toxoplasma gondii*), an autoimmune disease, or a metabolic disorder.

This disorder has some similarities with sudden sensorineural hearing loss in its course, unilateral involvement, and acute onset.

Diagnosis. See **Table 1.16**.

Differential diagnosis. See **Tables 1.16, 1.17**.

Treatment. *Early acute phase:*
- Bed rest.
- Symptomatic treatment with antivertigo drugs and sedatives.
- Intravenous rheological drugs.
- Antibiotics, when there is objective evidence of bacterial infection.
- Corticosteroids for suspected autoimmune disease.

Table 1.17   Clinical Features of acute vestibular paralysis (vestibular neuronitis)

A previously healthy patient suffers from:

- Rotatory dizziness
- Nausea and vomiting
- Dizziness persisting for days or weeks
- Ataxia

Typically, the following are absent:

- Tinnitus
- Hearing loss
- Loss of consciousness
- Double vision or visual field defects

Soon after the acute phase:

- Active physiotherapy, including exercises to train balance.
- No psychotropic drugs!

Course and prognosis. The symptoms subside within a few days, with spontaneous recovery of equilibrium (vestibular compensation). Younger patients tend to recover more quickly than older patients. Despite a persistent caloric hypoexcitability of the affected labyrinth, vestibular function recovers. Latent disequilibrium with a tendency to fall may persist in older patients.

Benign Paroxysmal Positional Vertigo (BPPV) (Cupulolithiasis)

Clinical Features. The characteristic symptoms are sudden frequent attacks of severe rotatory vertigo provoked by certain movements. Symptoms sometimes occur at night during movement while asleep.

Pathogenesis. Benign paroxysmal positional vertigo is a peripheral lesion of the end organ. The theory is that vertigo is incited by particles floating in the endolymph of a semicircular canal (canal lithiasis). The particles are usually otoconia separated from the macula. During certain movements, the increased mass of the otoconia causes a nonphysiologic deflection of the cupula and subsequently the typical symptoms.

Diagnosis. The Dix–Hallpike maneuver is used to test for BPPV (see p. 46).

Treatment. Initial treatment consists of therapeutic maneuvers designed to displace and reposition the canaliths (canalith repositioning procedure or Epley maneuver).

Neural and Central Vestibular Disorders

Clinical Features. The following symptoms indicate that a balance disorder has a central cause:

- Sudden attacks of dizziness of short duration (1–2 s).
- Fluctuating dizziness with loss of consciousness.
- Dizziness with "drop attacks," which are brief attacks of muscle-tone loss in which the patient sinks to the ground but does not become unconscious.
- Dizziness with double vision and other disturbances of vision such as hemianopsia, scotoma, etc.
- Dizziness with dysarthria and change of personality.

Pathogenesis. Central vestibular disorders are usually the result of *multifocal lesions* of the brain stem. They are therefore usually accompanied by symptoms of disorders of the visual oculomotor and somatosensory system (**Tables 1.18, 1.19**).

The investigation and treatment of this group of vestibular disorders fall within the specialty of neurology. The most frequent cause is vascular insufficiency in the brain stem region, which can lead to ischemic lesions or hemorrhages.

Bilateral Vestibular Loss

This balance disorder is caused by severe, bilateral hypofunction or complete loss of the peripheral vestibular apparatus. Systematic causes are possible, as well as bilateral diseases of the vestibular apparatus.

Systemic causes

- Ototoxicity (drugs, industrial toxins).
- Endogenous lesions (renal disturbances).

Local disturbances

- Labyrinthitis (bacterial, viral, autoimmune).
- Acquired labyrinthine disorders (anomalies, acute loss).
- Vestibular nerve disease (polyneuropathy, NF2).

Clinical Features
- No nystagmus, but oscillopsias.
- Balance disturbance.
- Bilateral sensorineural hearing loss.

Different Causes of Peripheral Vestibular Disorders

Cervical syndrome includes cervicobrachial neuralgia and brief attacks of dizziness dictated by the position and changes in position of the head, occasionally associated with tinnitus and pain in the nape of the neck, which may radiate to the occiput and the forehead area. Objective findings include neck-torsion nystagmus. The cause is a lesion in the joints of the cervical spine and in the muscles on the back of the neck (see p. 375). An acute onset of deafness with vestibular failure in this condition may also be due to embolism of the labyrinthine artery. In the majority of cases, the symptoms develop independently. The prognosis for functional recovery is unfavorable.

Posttraumatic cervical syndrome is mostly due to whiplash injury and causes almost the same symptoms after a symptom-free interval of several weeks, but the objective vestibular signs such as positional nystagmus are more pronounced. In addition, sensorineural hearing loss can occur and may persist for weeks and months. Other causes of posttraumatic vestibular disorders are blunt head trauma with labyrinthine contusion and concussion, temporal bone trauma with fractures, and postsurgical conditions (ear and temporal bone surgery).

Motion sickness is a sensory conflict, or mismatch, between the visual and vestibular systems that produces symptoms of malaise, fatigue, yawning, hypersalivation, nausea, and vomiting. Prevention relies on anticipating and visually perceiving the motion with as much of the visual field as possible. Training can induce the development of central patterns to reduce susceptibility. Medical treatment with antivertigo drugs (scopolamine, dimenhydrinate) is possible.

Perilymphatic fistula: A connection—either congenital or induced by trauma (e.g., barotrauma, acoustic trauma)—between the perilymphatic space and middle ear, usually through the round or oval window, can lead to vestibular or acoustic impairment. The fistula can be inspected and repaired by covering the window niches with fat

Table 1.18 Pathogenesis of central vestibular disorders

Inflammation
- Meningitis
- Meningoencephalitis
- Cerebellar abscess

Trauma
- Cerebral concussion and contusion

Space-occupying processes
- Infratentorial tumors
- Cerebellopontine angle tumors
- Glomus tumors
- Arachnoid cysts

Vascular processes
- Vertebrobasilar insufficiency
- Basilar artery migraine
- Arteriovenous anomalies

Intoxication
- Barbiturates
- Alcohol

Degenerative diseases of the central nervous system
- Multiple sclerosis
- Syringobulbia
- Cerebellar degeneration

tissue under local anesthesia, and this should be considered immediately.

Tullio phenomenon is a vestibular symptom that is induced by acoustic stimulation, usually with the sound at high levels on high and low frequencies. Possible causes are a hypermobile stapes footplate, adhesions between the footplate and saccule, or perilymphatic fistula.

■ Hearing Disorders

Sudden Sensorineural Hearing Loss

Clinical Features. Initially, there is a feeling of pressure in the ear, followed by tinnitus, which is usually marked, followed by severe hearing loss beginning within minutes and occasionally leading immediately to complete deafness.

Table 1.19 Synopsis of central balance disorders

	Neurotologic signs	Neuroophthalmologic signs	Neurologic sign
Encephalitis	Spontaneous nystagmus, often disassociated; positional nystagmus (irregular); gaze-evoked nystagmus; pathologic optokinetic reflexes	Papilledema	Meningism, somnolence, restlessness, cerebellar symptoms, focal neurologic symptoms, abnormal spinal fluid chemistry
Cerebral concussion	Positional (provocation) nystagmus, pathologic vestibulospinal reflexes	–	Headaches, memory defects, poor mental concentration
Infratentorial tumor with brain stem compression	Spontaneous nystagmus, positional nystagmus (irregular) gaze-evoked and gaze-paretic nystagmus, pathologic optokinetic nystagmus, pathologic vestibulospinal reflexes with ataxia, pathologic caloric responses	Eye muscle paresis, papilledema, horizontal and vertical gaze paresis	Focal neurologic symptoms of cranial nerves V, VII, IX, and X, dysphagia, pyramidal signs, extremity paresis, dissociated sensation, headache, vomiting
Vertebrobasilar insufficiency with involvement of pons and medulla	Vestibular spontaneous nystagmus, vestibular provoked nystagmus, pathologic vestibulospinal reflexes, pathologic optokinetic reflexes	Horner syndrome	Cerebellar ataxia, motor hemiparesis, disturbed sensation, involvement of cranial nerves V, VII, IX, and X
Multiple sclerosis	Vestibular spontaneous nystagmus, irregular positional nystagmus (irregular), gaze-evoked and gaze-paretic nystagmus, abnormal caloric responses, abnormal optokinetic reflexes, pathologic vestibulospinal reflexes, ataxia	Dissociated (disconjugate) nystagmus horizontal and vertical gaze paralysis, bilateral internuclear ophthalmoplegia, retrobulbar neuritis	Multiple attacks of multilocular demyelinating disorders of the central nervous system with spastic paralysis, urinary incontinence, intention tremor, dysdiadochokinesis, and paresthesia and dysesthesia
Barbiturate intoxication	Vestibular spontaneous nystagmus, irregular positional nystagmus (irregular), gaze-evoked nystagmus, abnormal vestibular ocular and optokinetic reflexes	Oculomotor disorders	Cerebellar ataxia, dysarthria, somnolence

Pathogenesis. *Idiopathic sudden hearing loss:*
- Viral infection.
- Disturbance of microcirculation of the inner ear.
- Autoimmune reaction.

The types of disorder are shown in **Table 1.20**.

Diagnosis. The symptoms are usually unilateral. Audiography shows sensorineural hearing loss restricted to the higher and middle frequencies, with recruitment or complete deafness. Causes of symptomatic sudden hearing loss should be excluded by a test diagnostic battery including: impedance audiometry, otoacoustic emissions, and vestibular tests. Additional tests focus on arterial hypertension, hyperlipidemia, infections (e. g., neurotropic viruses, syphilis, borreliosis, toxoplasmosis). After a period of recovery, cerebellopontine angle tumors are ruled out by ABR testing and MRI (but caution is needed with the latter, as there is a danger of acoustic stress during the test procedure).

Treatment. *Idiopathic sudden hearing loss:*
    The aim is to improve the microcirculation and oxygenation of the cochlea as soon as possible through:
- Intravenous low-molecular-weight dextran infusions and/or a systemic vasodilator.
- Corticosteroids.

Symptomatic sudden hearing loss:
    Therapy is initiated immediately to treat the above-mentioned causes.

Course and prognosis. If treatment is instituted within 24 h, there is often partial or complete recovery within several days. Spontaneous remission also often occurs. The prognosis is poor for patients with diabetes, arterial hypertension, or established irreversible vascular disease.

Chronic Progressive Idiopathic Sensorineural Hearing Loss

This disease is defined as having an onset before the age of 50, usually starting between 30 and 50 years of age. The cause is unknown; intrinsic or extrinsic pathophysiological factors are not evident. A recessive genetic defect may be involved.

Clinical Features. Bilateral involvement, with a variable course of hearing loss, is characteristic. There is a sudden onset and gradual progression of hearing loss, frequently accompanied by tinnitus. Severe hearing loss or complete deafness can develop over a period of years or decades.

Diagnosis
- Progressive bilateral sensorineural hearing loss.
- Exclusion of etiologic factors (metabolic, genetic, autoimmune, infectious, toxic, etc.).
- Exclusion of retrocochlear, psychogenic, and central hearing loss.

Treatment and prognosis
- Hearing rehabilitation (hearing aid, lip-reading training).
- Cochlear implant.

Presbyacusis
This type of symmetrical sensorineural hearing loss is an age-related disease affecting persons over 50 years of age. Approximately one-third of persons over the age of 65 have significant hearing loss, averaging 35 dB or more on pure-tone audiometry.

Clinical Features. These include bilateral hearing loss, initially for high tones and later for middle frequencies. A "social deafness" is gradually established, i. e., the patient can no longer take part in conversation with several people at the same time. Hearing for speech is affected by loud noise, and loud sounds cause discomfort due to positive recruitment. Pure-tone hearing is often better than the hearing for speech, and hearing for syllables often better than that for sentences (*schizacusis*). Other symptoms include noises in the ears and psychological disturbances, which increasingly isolate the elderly deaf patient from his environment, causing depression, mistrust, and delusions of persecution.

Pathogenesis. *Physiologic presbyacusis.* This is a degenerative process in the inner ear and central nervous system (CNS), without exogenous damage. The degenerative process is caused by a disorder of DNA synthesis, deposition of pigment (lipofuscin), extracellular deposition of cholesterin and lipids, conversion and breakdown of collagen substances, and loss of intercellular fluid.

Pathologic presbyacusis. Supplementary inner ear and CNS lesions are caused by exogenous factors, such as environmental noise, and by lifestyle factors such as diet, smoking, alcohol, physical and psychological stress, hypertension, and maturity-onset diabetes. In summary, this is a multifactorial disease of the peripheral and central auditory systems that starts earlier than physiologic presbyacusis.

Four types of presbyacusis can be distinguished on the basis of morphologic degenerative lesions:
1. *Sensory presbyacusis* due to hair cell degeneration. The audiogram shows high tone loss.
2. *Neural presbyacusis:* A large proportion of the population of cochlear neurons is lost, so that the predominant symptom is loss of discrimination for speech.
3. *Strial presbyacusis,* due to degeneration of the stria vascularis. This causes abnormalities in endolymph production and secretion, with repercussions on the energy metabolism of the hair cells. Audiography shows a flat curve of pancochlear hearing loss with retained discrimination for speech.
4. *Conductive cochlear presbyacusis:* An age-related degenerative process in the cochlear duct causes lesions in the structure of the basilar membrane. This affects stimulus transport in the cochlea (see p. 14) and is demonstrated on audiography by bilateral symmetrical sensorineural deafness causing a characteristic sloping curve, with a linear increase in hearing loss above 1000 Hz.

Diagnosis. The patient has bilateral (usually symmetrical) sensorineural deafness. The audiometric curve depends on the type.

Differential diagnosis. Marked unilateral sensorineural deafness has to be distinguished from vestibular schwannoma or a cerebellopontine angle tumor. Marked unilateral or bilateral tinnitus, synchronous with the pulse, has to be differentiated from an intracranial aneurysm of the posterior cranial fossa or a glomus tumor. Other causes, ototoxic or metabolic, should be taken into consideration.

!

Note: Elderly patients with hearing loss require early rehabilitation of communication to the same extent as young patients with hearing loss, provided that their mental powers are not severely limited.

Treatment
- Auditory rehabilitation (hearing aid, auditory training, lip-reading course).
- Psychosocial rehabilitation (family, social programs for integration of hearing-disabled people).

Course and prognosis. The degree and time course of the hearing loss is highly variable. Its progression cannot be predicted.

Clinical Aspects of Central Hearing Disorders

See **Table 1.20.**

Acoustic Agnosia
Synonyms for this condition include sensory aphasia, psychogenic or word deafness, sensory deaf-mutism, and central deafness.

Clinical Features. The main symptoms include acoustic inattention due to an absence of the acoustic ability to differentiate, disturbances of perception, slurred articulation, animated gestures, and miming. Directional hearing is lost, and the patient suffers paramusia, amusia, and loss of musicality.

Pathogenesis. The causes may be cerebral or skull trauma, encephalitis, or prenatal, perinatal, or postnatal damage to the central nervous system.

Diagnosis. A clinical diagnosis of acoustic agnosia can only be made using neuropsychological tests. Investigations also include electroencephalography, CT and MRI, and evoked response audiometry.

Treatment. Long-term treatment includes acoustic differentiation exercises, articulation training, and prescription of a hearing aid for objectively confirmed sensorineural deafness. A hearing aid is of no use for true sensory agnosia. Rhythmic exercises, music therapy, and exploitation of visual observations can improve the patient's comprehension (e. g., through lip-reading).

Table 1.20 Synopsis of hearing disorders and their treatment

Anatomic substrate	Function	Type of disorder	Effect on hearing	Treatment	Prognosis for auditory reha-bilitation
Conductive hearing loss (middle ear)					
Middle ear	Conduction	Discontinuity due to infection of the ossicular chain, ventilation disorders of the middle ear, or stiffening of the ossicular chain and the tympanic membrane with increasing acoustic resistance—i. e., increased impedance	Quantitative hearing loss due to mechanical loss of sound energy	Surgery or a hearing aid	Good
Sensorineural hearing loss (inner ear)					
Inner ear	Mechanical frequency analysis, stimulus transformation of a mechanical into a bioelectrical stimulus, and possibly coding	Destruction of the sensory cells in the inner ear due to traumatic, vascular, metabolic, toxic, or inflammatory damage	Quantitative hearing loss combined with a qualitative worsening of speech intelligibility, due to loss of frequency analysis and stimulus transformation coding; distortion effect due to recruitment	Hearing aid, hearing training, and lip reading. Trial of medical treatment	Relatively good. Depends on the degree of hearing loss
Peripheral neuron	Coding, transmission of nerve impulses; lateral inhibition and interneural inhibition ensure acoustic selectivity	Degeneration of the peripheral neuron due to inflammatory, vascular, traumatic, or metabolic injury	Quantitative and qualitative deterioration of hearing for speech due to abnormal coding, loss of neurons, unsatisfactory selectivity, and inability to discriminate	Hearing aid, hearing training, and lip reading	Doubtful
Auditory perception (central)					
Central auditory pathways and centers	Integration—i. e., assembly of individual nervous impulses in a functional modulated activity; storage of auditory memory; decoding of acoustic information	Degeneration of the central pathways and the ganglion cells in the primary and secondary hearing centers due to inflammatory, vascular, traumatic or metabolic lesions	Mainly complete loss of the information content due to unsatisfactory integration and decoding of the acoustic signal. Partial loss of the auditory memory. The final phase is complete central deafness	Hearing aid useless. In selected cases, hearing training or lip reading	Poor

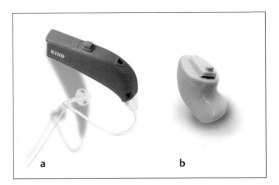

Fig   1.111a, b Different types of hearing aid.
a A behind-the-ear device.
b An in-the-ear device with an earmold fitted.

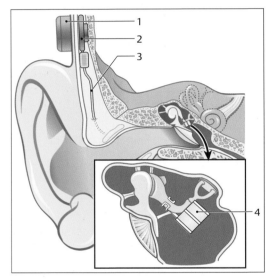

Fig. 1.112   The principle of an implantable hearing aid. An externally worn microphone and speech processor (**1**) transmits sound through the skin to an implanted receiver (**2**). A cable (**3**) connected to a tiny transducer (**4**) directly vibrates the ossicles by mimicking the natural motion of the ossicular chain, sending an enhanced signal to the cochlea.

Rehabilitation of Hearing Disorders with Hearing Aids

Note: The assessment of hearing disorders in relation to the potential for social rehabilitation should be based not only on the degree of severity and site of the hearing loss, but also on the patient's age and physical, mental, and speech development. The aim of auditory rehabilitation is to restore or improve auditory communication, which is crucial for social functioning and the patient's well-being.

A variety of rehabilitative options are available, depending on the nature and degree of the hearing loss and the degree of handicap it involves.

Surgery. This is an option for patients with conductive hearing loss due to functional disturbances of the middle ear (see p. 73, **Fig. 1.96 a–f**).

Hearing aids. These selectively amplify auditory signals. The acoustic signal is received by a microphone, amplified and processed, and then delivered to the ear through a loudspeaker. Hearing aids can be worn behind the auricle or inside the ear canal (**Fig. 1.111a, b**). The fitting of a hearing aid is an important procedure involving several steps: establishing the indication in an audiological examination; selecting and trying out hearing aids; final selection of the hearing aid and provision of follow-up care.

Bone-anchored hearing apparatus (BAHA). Devices with an acoustic amplifier and a transducer are connected to the cranial bone via a bone-anchored system. Mechanical vibrations are transduced directly to the cranial bone to improve sound transmission. BAHA systems are mainly used in patients with untreatable diseases of the external meatus or with severe hearing loss.

Active middle ear implants. An amplifier implanted under the skin transforms sound waves into electrical impulses, which are converted into mechanical vibrations in a transducer. The vibrations are transmitted directly to the ossicles or cranial bone (**Fig. 1.112**).

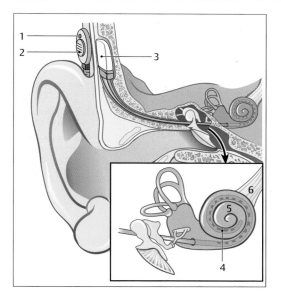

Fig. 1.113 The principle of a cochlear implant. The acoustic signal is received by a microphone (**1**) worn behind the ear and is processed by an external speech processor (**2**). An electronic receiver (**3**) is implanted into the temporal bone under the skin. It is connected to an electrode array (**4**) inserted into the cochlea (**5**). The electrodes directly stimulate the vestibulocochlear nerve (**6**).

Cochlear implant (CI). A subcutaneously implanted device can transform sound waves into electrical impulses that directly stimulate the vestibulocochlear nerve with intracochlear electrodes. Patients with almost complete deafness due to an absence of cochlear function are candidates for implantation (**Fig. 1.113**). In children, best results are obtained when the CI procedure is done before the age of 1 year because of the early brain plasticity in the growing child. Before implantation, the responsiveness of the vestibulocochlear nerve has to be tested using the promontory test with a transtympanic electrode. Subjective hearing impressions can be recorded in adults, whereas electrical brain stem responses are used for recordings in children. The surgical procedure is standardized and safe. Modern trends in CI procedures include bilateral implants and implants in children with a low auditory threshold. Children with sensorineural hearing loss more than 60 dB are also provided with CI because they can benefit from better acoustic information arriving at the auditory cortex. The success of the implantation depends on further rehabilitation being provided by speech and language therapists and teachers for hearing-impaired people. Speech recognition is also supported by teaching the patients to lip-read. Over 90 % of patients derive definite benefit from a CI and more than 50 % can achieve open speech. Patients who have only had hearing loss for a short period benefit most from implantation.

Vibrotactile aids. Acoustic signals are picked up by a microphone and converted into vibrations that are transmitted to the wrist or fingers.

Assistive devices. Devices include optical or vibrating wake-up alarms, light flashers, telephone amplifiers, text telephones, television headphones, and digital communication devices such as fax machines, text messaging, and the Internet.

Training. Hearing-impaired patients can be trained in selective listening, using listening tactics or auditory training. Using hearing aids and other assistive devices, as well as learning how to lip-read and how to improve their own speech are also important training exercises for patients.

Pediatric Hearing Disorders (Pediatric Audiology)

Significant hearing impairment is present at birth in 0.8–2.3 per 1000 newborns in Europe. During the first year of life, permanent hearing loss occurs in one in 1000–2000 children. Causes of pediatric hearing disorders, which can be classified into genetic and acquired forms, are listed in the **Tables 1.21, 1.22, 1.23, 1.24**.

The presence of hearing loss profoundly affects the subsequent development of speech and has specific consequences for rehabilitation and personality development in these children. If there is the slightest sign of hearing impairment in an infant or young child, an audiologic evaluation should be performed. Parents and special services for infants and children should be informed about the time course of speech development in children (**Table 1.25**).

Table 1.21 Genetic forms of deafness and hearing loss

Sporadic recessive deafness

Progressive morphologic lesion present at birth, usually with total degeneration of the cochlea and the peripheral cochlear neuron

Types:	Hypoplasia or aplasia of the labyrinth with almost complete loss of function of the cochlea and the vestibule
• Michel	
• Mondini	
• Scheibe	

Dominant hereditary degenerative hearing loss

Progressive disorder with an irregular course. First becomes manifests at or after puberty. Often combined with other inherited symptoms to form a circumscribed syndrome such as those detailed below

Waardenburg syndrome	Congenital anomalies of the facial skeleton, dystopia canthorum; blepharophimosis; disorders of pigmentation of the eyes, hair and skin (albinism); degenerative atrophy of the cochlea and the ganglion cells
Usher syndrome	Hereditary progressive sensorineural hearing loss with retinitis pigmentosa. Degeneration of the cochlea and the spiral ganglion
Refsum syndrome	The same symptoms are found as in Usher syndrome, with the addition of polyneuropathy and ataxia. Often, this condition first becomes manifests between the ages of 10 and 20
Alport syndrome	Progressive inner ear hearing loss, bilateral, but often asymmetrical, beginning in the second decade of life, associated with a nonspecific chronic glomerulonephritis and interstitial nephritis. The frequency is one per 200,000 births. The renal disorder is inherited, and the inner ear lesion may be a secondary nephrogenic effect
Pendred syndrome	Perceptive hearing loss with labyrinthine dysplasia associated with thyroid gland disorders

Chromosomal anomalies

Anomalies of the external and middle ear associated with numerous other organ anomalies and developmental disorders of the inner ear

Trisomy 13	Labyrinthine hypoplasia with aplasia of the spiral organ of Corti and the stria vascularis
Trisomy 18	Similar changes, with atresia of the vestibulocochlear nerve
Cri-du-chat syndrome	Similar malformations associated with laryngeal anomalies

Audimutism

This term is inaccurate, as it does not adequately characterize delayed development of speech. The child is mute despite being able to hear. The term "audimutism" in the strictest sense should be confined to children who, after the third year of life, can only make themselves understood by gestures and are unable to speak any words, but are not mentally defective and demonstrate normal hearing. There is a connection between audimutism and brain damage in early childhood. The term "deaf-mutism" has therefore been replaced by "absent or delayed speech development."

Classification and Effects of Hearing Disorders Depending on the Degree of Severity

Normal hearing. The hearing threshold of the pure-tone audiogram does not exceed 20 dB for any frequency.

Slight hearing loss. On the pure-tone audiogram, there is hearing loss of > 20 dB or at most 40 dB over the entire frequency range. Hearing loss of this extent does not usually cause delay in the development of speech in a child of normal intelligence.

Conductive hearing loss can usually be treated medically. Sensorineural hearing loss has to be treated individually with a hearing aid, supplemented by language training by a hearing therapist. Individual schooling and hearing training are not indicated.

Moderate hearing loss. In this case, the average hearing loss in the main speech frequencies of 250–4000 Hz is between 40 and 60 dB. This causes considerable difficulty in understanding speech, so that speech development is delayed. Prescription of a hearing aid is absolutely indicated, and children require early hearing and speech education. Initially, the children should attend a special school for the deaf, but they can usually attend a normal school later, provided they have a hearing aid and normal intellectual development.

Severe hearing loss. The average hearing loss in the main speech frequencies is greater than 60 dB, and tones above 1000 Hz are most severely affected. Provided that the child has normal intellectual development, a hearing aid is certainly indicated, since good speech communication can be developed with even the least residual hearing using electroacoustic methods and early speech and hearing training. These children should attend special schools for the deaf. They should have several years' training in lip-reading to encourage visual compensation for the loss of auditory function.

Bilateral complete deafness. This form is fortunately very rare. Even patients with almost total deafness often have residual hearing, which can be demonstrated using electroacoustic methods and exploited using high-performance hearing aids. The child should be educated in a separate school for the deaf. In these schools, sign language is currently being replaced by the use of real speech: practice in articulated speech is provided using the sense of vibration and training in lip-reading, partly directly and partly with a video recorder. In selected cases, both children and adults can be considered for a *cochlear implant*, which involves the implantation of a multichannel cochlear prosthesis.

Multiple handicap. A special group of deaf children also have intellectual retardation, behavioral disturbances, extensive organic brain damage, or delay in motor development causing failure to speak. A demanding therapeutic program needs to be estab-

Table 1.22 Prenatally acquired (exogenous) deafness and hearing loss

Intrauterine infection	
Rubella embryopathy	Developmental disorders of the middle and inner ear, severe bilateral sensorineural hearing loss
Congenital syphilis	Progressive degeneration of the inner ear and the peripheral neuron associated with interstitial keratitis and dental defects (Hutchinson triad)
Toxoplasmosis	Inflammatory damage to the inner ear
Viral infections	Mumps, herpes zoster, poliomyelitis, influenza, cytomegalovirus
Toxic damage due to:	Quinine, aminoglycosides, and thalidomide which causes multiple anomalies
Further exogenous damage due to:	Diabetes mellitus in the mother, fetal hypoxia, irradiation

Table 1.23 Perinatally acquired (exogenous) deafness and hearing loss

Perinatal hypoxia	Injury to the cochlea and its centers in the brain stem
Premature birth	Hemorrhage into the cochlea
Kernicterus (perinatal hyperbilirubinemia)	Rh-incompatibility, massive deposits of bilirubin in the cochlear centers and occasionally in the cochlea itself with corresponding cochleoneural deafness

lished for this group with a team including an otologist, phoniatrist, neurologist, child psychiatrist, psychologist, and speech pathologist.

Voice and speech disorders due to deafness. Deafness mainly affects the ability to communicate in children, but it can also affect adults. Physiologic auditory verbal communication requires both a normal voice and speech apparatus and also normal feedback through the ear.

Altered speech in those born without hearing or in those who become deaf or partially deaf in later life, is known as otogenic dyslalia.

Table 1.24 Postnatally acquired (exogenous) deafness and hearing loss

Infective diseases	
Meningitis and meningo-encephalitis	Labyrinthitis and cochleovestibular neuritis with damage to the sensory cells and peripheral neurons; central lesions
Mumps	Cochlear and neural lesions (see pp. 96 and 421)
Measles	Degeneration of the cochlea and its peripheral neurons due to infective damage, serous labyrinthitis
Otitis media	Recurrent otitis, infective toxic damage to inner ear associated with sensorineural deafness

Table 1.25 Timetable of speech development

Up to the 7th week	Crying
6 weeks–6 months	First babbling period, beginning of auditory feedback
6–9 months	Second babbling period, hearing predominant
8–9 months	Echolalia, imitation and first understanding of speech
9–12 months	Beginning of deliberate speech
13–15 months	Early precise use of significant words, symbolic function of speech
12–18 months	One-word sentences, developmental stammering
18–24 months	Two-word sentences; unformed sentences of several words, first age of questioning
End of 2nd year of life	Nongrammatical sentences, establishment of consciousness of symbols
From 3 years onward	Formed sentences of several words, adoption of first grammatical principles
From 4th year of life	Second questioning age, first establishment of logical and emotional relationships, maturation of the thinking–speaking process

The Completely Deaf Child

In a child with no hearing or only residual islands of hearing, there is no auditory feedback, and the child develops a typical, monotonous form of speech, which distinguishes the totally deaf child from a child with normal hearing or partial hearing loss. The best rehabilitation results are achieved through:

- Early diagnosis and treatment.
- Early prescription of a hearing aid.
- Prolonged auditory training and early voice and speech training in special preschools and schools for the deaf to develop the missing sound components of speech and speech content.
- Cochlear implant in selected cases.

Cochlear Implantation

Indications
- Bilateral cochlear deafness.
- Residual hearing that is not usable for speech understanding or speech development despite the use of hearing aids.
- Intact acoustic nerve and central hearing tract.
- Postlingual deafness. Acquired deafness after definitive speech development.
- Prelingual deafness. Acquired deafness before speech development, or congenital deafness.

Procedure

Preoperative examination and evaluation. After the cause of deafness has been determined and the functional integrity of the vestibulocochlear nerve and central hearing tract has been tested, the child's psychosocial environment also has to be assessed. This involves assessing the child's general development and language development level, as well as the general communication situation.

Surgical procedure. A subcutaneous device is implanted after complete mastoidectomy. An electrode is inserted into the scala tympani via an opening in the basal turn of the cochlea (cochleostomy).

Postoperative fitting of the speech processor. After complete wound healing, the implanted speech processor is adapted to optimize the hearing result. Lifelong technical checking and adjustment are necessary.

Hearing and speech training. Postlingually deaf patients are able to compare auditory impressions conveyed by the implant with their stored auditory impressions. They learn how to understand these new impressions within a few months. By contrast, prelingually deaf children experience hearing as a new sense modality and learn and develop language in the same way that a normally hearing child does. This process usually takes several years, and it requires special rehabilitation centers for the children.

Clinical Aspects of Disorders of the Facial Nerve

The symptoms and differential diagnosis of central and a peripheral lesions of the facial nerve are discussed above (see pp. 13 and 47). Only the effects of peripheral lesions of the facial nerve and their causes, characteristics, and treatment are therefore discussed here.

Inflammatory or Otogenic Facial Paralysis
A form of peripheral facial paralysis that is at least partly reversible may be caused by neurotropic viruses such as herpes zoster (see pp. 52 and 96), coxsackievirus, or poliomyelitis virus, and by neuroallergic polyradiculitis, Guillain–Barré disease, or sarcoidosis. The latter is also known as Heerfordt–Mylius syndrome, with uveitis and parotitis in addition to facial paralysis (see p. 417). However, the most important and most common form for the otologist is *otogenic facial paralysis*, which occurs as:
- A complication of acute otitis media or mastoiditis, which is treated with antibiotics and immediate mastoidectomy; the lesion is usually a neurapraxia. The prognosis is always good, provided the patient is not affected by diabetes or immunodeficiency.
- A complication of middle ear cholesteatoma invading the bony facial canal. Extension of the inflammation to the nerve sheath and endoneurium causes axonal degeneration and demyelinization of the mastoid, tympanic, and labyrinthine segments. The condition is treated with mastoidectomy and decompression of the nerve. The prognosis is occasionally poor, despite intensive antibiotics and decompression of the facial nerve, as the nerve is usually only partially reinnervated and does not fully heal.

Idiopathic Facial Paralysis (Bell's Palsy)
As the term "idiopathic" indicates, the cause of this is unknown. It may be a disturbance of microcirculation leading to serous inflammation, with edema developing. The bony canal is rigid, and the resulting compression of the nerve leads to ischemia and venous congestion, so that a vicious circle starts. The annual incidence of Bell's palsy is ≈ 20–30 per 100,000 population. The condition occurs most often in the 15–45-year-old age group and it is much less common in children under the age of 10.

More recent evidence now suggests that the condition may be caused by herpesvirus—specifically, herpes simplex virus type 1.

Diagnosis. Topographic diagnosis of the facial nerve is carried out (see p. 47) and causes involving inflammation, trauma, or tumor are excluded.

In ≈ 80 % of patients, electrodiagnosis shows neurapraxia, with a good prognosis. In 20 % of patients, there is partial axonotmesis. In ≈ 5–10 % of patients with idiopathic facial paralysis, the axon degeneration progresses between days 4 and 10 despite treatment with corticosteroids. If neuronography shows that more than 90 % of neurons have degenerated, decompression is indicated.

Treatment
- Intravenous infusion of low-molecular-weight dextran.
- Corticosteroids. Schedule for prednisone in the treatment of idiopathic facial paralysis: 60 mg for 4 days, reducing by 5 mg daily to 5 mg on the 15th day, followed by intermittent dosage of 5 mg for 10 days.
- Antiviral drugs (aciclovir). The evidence for using aciclovir is inconclusive, but the agent is generally recommended, as undetected slow virus infections are suspected.
- It has been recommended that surgical decompression needs to be performed within 2 weeks of the onset of total paralysis in order for it to be effective. This is a rather controversial area, and there is a lack of consensus regarding the value of facial nerve decompression in this setting.

During the first 2 weeks of the paralysis, electromyography does not provide prognostically valid information. During this period, therefore, electrodiagnostic and neuronographic investigations should be carried out every 2 days to identify patients who require decompression treatment.

Melkersson–Rosenthal syndrome is an unusual form of idiopathic facial paralysis. Symptoms include recurrent facial paralysis, furrowed tongue and cheilitis, and facial edema. The cause is unknown, treatment with steroids is unsatisfactory, and the prognosis is uncertain.

Traumatic Facial Paralysis

Causes. The second most common cause of facial paralysis is trauma, which includes blunt, penetrating, and iatrogenic forms. Most commonly, traumatic injuries to the facial nerve are caused by temporal bone fractures.

Frequency. Less than 5% of temporal bone fractures involve the otic capsule; of these, half are associated with facial nerve injury. Facial paralysis occurs in 10–20% of all longitudinal pyramidal fractures and in 50% of all transverse fractures. Seventy-five percent of all paralyses develop completely within 24 h of the trauma and 90% of late-onset paralyses resolve spontaneously.

Prognosis. The two most important prognostic factors for recovery from facial nerve paralysis are the severity of the condition and the time of onset. Nearly 40% of patients with immediate-onset complete paralysis have a poor recovery. The severity of a pyramidal fracture is determined by the type of the lesion, such as depression of the canal, damage to the nerve by a splinter of bone, shearing of the nerve without fracture of the bony canal, or a nerve sheath hematoma leading to edema. Electrodiagnosis is the only reliable method of determining which patients will develop rapid degeneration of the axons and will therefore not recover fully without decompression.

Treatment. The functional goals in facial nerve surgery are to protect the eye, restore the nasal airway, and reestablish oral competence. Cosmetic goals include improved balance and symmetry of the face at rest and coordinated movement of the facial musculature. In the acute setting, the best functional results are obtained with direct facial nerve anastomosis and interpositional nerve grafts. If transection of the nerve occurs in cases of traumatic injury, end-to-end anastomosis is recommended. If part of a facial nerve is sacrificed and reananstomsis

leads to unwanted tension, interpositional grafting can be as good as direct reanastomosis. Conservative treatment is limited to steroids and is indicated when any suspicion of direct nerve injury has been excluded. The expected rate of peripheral axonal nerve regeneration is ≈ 1 mm per day, but it varies widely. Adequate facial tone can recover within 6 months, and motion can progressively improve over a further 1–3 months.

Reconstructive Surgery after Facial Paralysis

Facial paralyses are due to various lesions of the facial nerve. Their severity depends on the extent to which the continuity of the nerve has been preserved and which segment of the nerve is affected (**Fig. 1.114**).

In cases of crushing and constricting injury, depression of the bony canal, and direct injury to the nerve by bone splinters, exposure of the nerve along its intratemporal course in the region of the bone damage is sufficient for decompressing the nerve. Occasionally, slitting of the nerve sheath is also required in order to release a hematoma. Lesions of the facial nerve in the facial region due to skull fractures, knife and stab wounds, and surgical trauma are relatively unusual. A lesion of all nerve branches is caused solely by damage to the main trunk of the nerve (see **Figs. 1.21, 1.114**); peripheral injuries usually only affect individual branches.

Principles of treatment. A search should be made for the site of injury to the nerve, if possible within 48 h. The nerve should be resutured using microsurgery, if necessary with a nerve graft from the great auricular or sural nerve. An old injury should be managed by attempting to reconstruct the nerve in the region of the lesion, and if this is not possible, by anastomosing the branches of the facial nerve to the opposite side in the form of a "crossover," using sural nerve grafts.

Loss of continuity may be due either to a clean division of the nerve or to an extensive defect. requiring one of the following procedures:
1. End-to-end suture is indicated after division of the nerve if the proximal and distal stumps can be approximated without tension. The epineurium is resected from the nerve stumps. Suturing is performed by passing the needle through the connective-tissue sheath surrounding the fascicular bundles (**Fig. 1.115**).

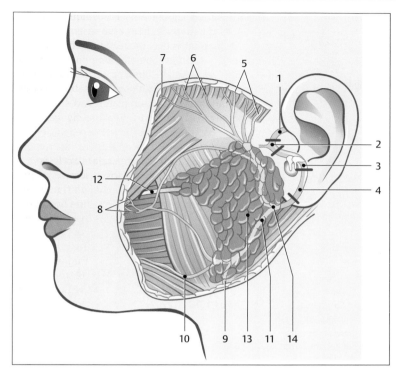

Fig. 1.114 Anatomy of the course of the facial nerve relative to exposure of the nerve. *Intratemporal section:* **1**, meatal segment; **2**, labyrinthine segment; **3**, tympanic segment; **4**, mastoid segment. *Extratemporal section:* **5**, temporal rami; **6**, zygomatic rami; **7**, temporofacial portion; **8**, buccal rami; **9**, cervical rami; **10**, marginal mandibular ramus; **11**, cervical part; **14**, extratemporal part. *Other structures:* **12**, parotid duct; **13**, parotid gland.

2. *Rerouting* consists of exposing the damaged nerve over a wide area and shortening its route by lifting the nerve out of the bony canal. This allows tension-free repair with end-to-end suture, even for extensive defects (**Fig. 1.116**).
3. *Autogenous nerve grafts* (cable nerve grafting), with free grafting from the great auricular nerve, sural nerve, or medial and lateral antebrachial nerves, are used for large defects if the freshened nerve stumps cannot be apposed without tension.

In most cases of irreversible facial nerve damage, satisfactory recovery of function can be achieved by one of these surgical techniques. When there is extensive damage of the nerve and its immediate surroundings, and especially when there are defects in the cerebellopontine angle, reinnervation of the muscles of facial expression can only be achieved using nerve replacement techniques.

The peripheral stump can be anastomosed to a cranial nerve such as the ipsilateral hypoglossal or accessory nerve. Individual branches of the still-functioning healthy side can be anastomosed with free autologous nerve grafts to the facial nerve using a cross-face (or faciofacial) anastomosis.

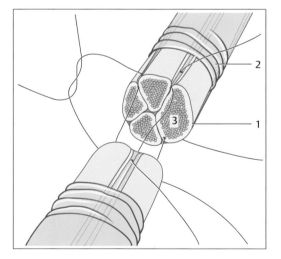

Fig. 1.115 Perineural–fascicular nerve suture. Perineural reconstruction starts with the central fascicle, followed by suture of the epineurium. **1**, Perineurium; **2**, epineurium; **3**, fascicle.

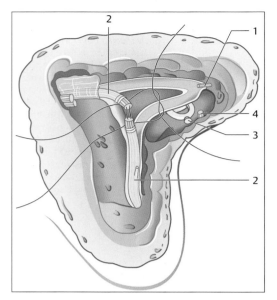

Fig. 1.116 Facial nerve decompression and reconstruction. Decompression and reconstruction in the internal auditory canal can be performed using the translabyrinthine approach. The greater petrosal nerve (**1**) is cut and the facial nerve (**2**) is rerouted and anastomosed in the mastoid. **3**, Stapes; **4**, malleus handle.

The best results are achieved with *hypoglossal–facial anastomosis,* which has to include resection of the epineurium.

In cases of facial nerve defects in the area of the cerebellopontine angle after tumor resection, end-to-end anastomosis with fibrin adhesive or nerve transplantation is performed (Dott's operation).

Facial function should not be expected to return earlier than 6 months after nerve repair or grafting, and 12–18 months may be needed before maximal recovery is seen. In long-standing paralyses, irreversible changes develop over an interval of more than 18 months. These involve fibrosis of the nerve, degeneration of motor end plates, and disuse atrophy of the muscle fibers. Irreversible changes of this type may preclude successful nerve repair or grafting. Reconstruction procedures using regional muscle transfer, such as temporalis muscle or masseter muscle, or free tissue transfer with reinnervation, can be used. Static sling techniques, additional ancillary lid procedures, and brow lifts can also be performed.

Synopsis of Ear Symptoms

See **Tables 1.26, 1.27**.

Table 1.26 Local symptoms and signs of ear disease

Pressure sensation	*Unilateral or bilateral, constant or intermittent:* cerumen, tubal problem, Ménière disease, glomus tumor
Pain (otalgia)	*Dull, penetrating sensation:* early otitis media or parotitis
	Pulsating: caused by acute otitis media or furuncle in the external canal
	Stabbing or intermittent: otalgia secondary to radiation therapy; bad teeth; temporomandibular joint syndrome; parotitis; tumor of the base of the tongue, tonsil, hypopharynx, or larynx
Aural discharge (otorrhea)	*Smell:* fetid in otitis externa and cholesteatoma
	Color: yellow with cerumen and pus; hemorrhage in influenzal otitis
	Consistency: watery in cerebrospinal otorrhea, mucoid in chronic secretory otitis, greasy in external otitis and cholesteatomas
	Pulsating: otitis media with perforation
	Nonpulsating: external otitis

Table 1.27 Functional ear symptoms

Tinnitus	*Type:* whistling, buzzing, ringing, hissing; crackling are often due to tubal problems
	Occurrence: constant, intermittent, may occur in attacks, as in Ménière disease
	Character: synchronous with pulse in hypertonia, cranial aneurysm, or glomus tumor
Hearing loss	High-tone loss caused by acoustic trauma or presbyacusis
	Low-tone loss caused by Ménière disease, otitis media, otosclerosis
	Decreased speech intelligibility, due to a loss of discrimination (inner ear or cranial nerve VIII lesion)
	Fluctuating, episodic, as in Ménière disease and sudden hearing loss
	Improvement in noisy environment, reported to be typical of conductive hearing loss
	Unilateral in Ménière disease, cranial nerve VIII tumors
	Bilateral in age-induced and noise-induced losses
Vertigo	Turning vertigo in Ménière disease and acute vestibular paralysis (vestibular neuronitis)
	Elevator and swing vertigo due to inner ear involvement
	Blackout spells due to extravestibular or orthostatic cause
	Episodic in Ménière disease
	Continuous vertigo occurs in vestibular paralysis
	Spontaneous and episodic in Ménière disease
	Provoked by head movement and position change of the body, caused by the inner ear, the cervical syndrome, vertebrobasilar insufficiency
	Unsteadiness in gait and standing is caused by central vestibular disturbance and multiple sclerosis
	Otologic disorders with vertigo: • Nausea, vomiting—occurs in acute vestibular paralysis and Ménière disease • Double vision—indicates a brain stem lesion • Loss of consciousness—is due to a brain stem or a space-occupying intracranial lesion

2 Nose, Nasal Sinuses, and Face

Applied Anatomy and Physiology

■ Basic Anatomy

■ External Nose

The supporting structure of the nose consists of bone, cartilage, and connective tissue. **Figure 2.1** shows the most important elements. The *bony* superior part of the nasal pyramid is often broken in typical fractures of the nasal bones, but it may also be fractured in injuries to the central part of the face. The *cartilaginous* inferior portion is less at risk, at least in mild blunt trauma, because of its elastic structure, but it is endangered in stab wounds, lacerations, and gunshot injuries. The shape, position, and properties of the bone and cartilage of the nose have a considerable influence on the shape and esthetic harmony of the face (see p. 212) and on the function of the nasal cavity.

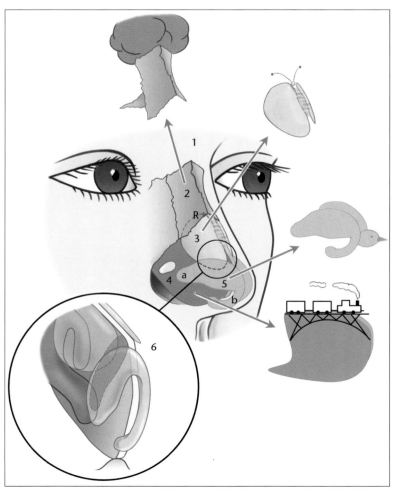

Fig. 2.1 The nasal skeleton. **1**, Glabella; **2**, nasal bone; **3**, lateral nasal cartilage; **4**, cartilaginous nasal septum; **5**, alar cartilage with lateral (**a**) and medial crus (**b**); **6**, nasal valve between the cranial alar and caudal lateral cartilages. **R**, Rhinion. The bony portion of the nose is completely rigid. The flexible cartilaginous portion begins at the rhinion. The distal caudal lateral cartilages can move like the wings of a butterfly, whereas the alar cartilages move more like the wings of a bird. The nasal septum is the center of stability.

The following *blood vessels* in the external nose are of practical importance:

- Facial artery and its branches.
- Dorsal nasal artery, arising from the ophthalmic artery.

Profuse hemorrhage can arise from these vessels when the central part of the face is injured.

The angular vein is also clinically important. Thrombophlebitis arising from a furuncle of the upper lip or the nose can spread via the ophthalmic vein to the cavernous sinus, causing a cavernous sinus thrombosis (see p. 189 and **Fig. 2.2**).

The external nose derives its *sensory nerve supply* from the first and second branches of the trigeminal nerve (see **Fig. 2.15a, b**). The muscles derive their *motor nerve supply* from the facial nerve.

■ Nasal Cavity

The interior of the nose is divided by the nasal septum into two cavities, which are usually unequal in size. Each side may be divided into the *nasal vestibule* and the *nasal cavity* proper (**Fig. 2.3a, b**). The nasal vestibule is covered by epidermis containing hairs (vibrissae) and sebaceous glands. The latter are the site of origin of a nasal furuncle, which can thus only develop in the nasal cavity in the vestibule.

The medial wall of the nasal vestibule encloses the supporting structure of the anterior part of the cartilaginous septum and the membranous septum—i. e., the *columella*. The roof of the vestibule is formed by the bird wing–shaped

lower lateral or alar cartilage, the medial crus of which extends into the columella and the lateral crus of which supports the external wall of the vestibule (**Figs. 2.1, 2.3a, b**). The alar cartilage determines the shape of the nasal tip and the nasal apertures. Correcting this area is often an important part of rhinoplasty.

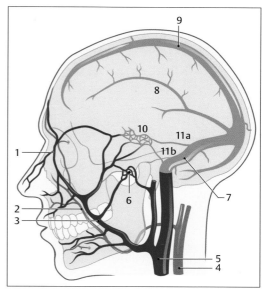

Fig. 2.2 Important vascular relationships in the face. **1**, Site for ligation of the angular vein; **2**, facial artery; **3**, facial vein; **4**, common carotid artery; **5**, internal jugular vein; **6**, pterygoid plexus; **7**, sigmoid sinus; **8**, inferior sagittal sinus; **9**, superior sagittal sinus; **10**, cavernous sinus; **11a**, superior petrosal sinus; **11b**, inferior petrosal sinus.

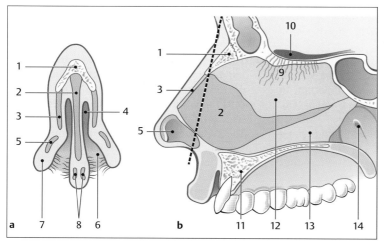

Fig. 2.3a, b   a Section through the anterior nose, showing the vestibule and the limen nasi. The dashed line in **b** shows the sectional plane of **a**. The limen nasi is located at the junction of the pink and red areas.

b Medial nasal wall. **1**, Bony nasal bridge; **2**, nasal septum; **3**, upper lateral nasal cartilage; **4**, nasal cavity; **5**, alar cartilage; **6**, nasal vestibule; **7**, nasal ala; **8**, nasal columella with medial crus of the cartilaginous ala; **9**, filaments of the olfactory nerve; **10**, olfactory bulb; **11**, palatine bone; **12**, perpendicular plate of the ethmoid; **13**, vomer; **14**, pharyngeal eustachian tube ostium.

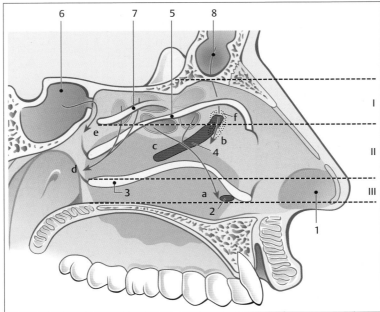

Fig. 2.4   Lateral nasal wall. I, Superior meatus; II, middle meatus; III, inferior meatus. **1**, Nasal vestibule; **2**, opening of the nasolacrimal duct; **3**, origin of the inferior turbinate; **4**, semilunar hiatus; **5**, insertion of the middle turbinate; **6**, sphenoid sinus; **7**, insertion of the superior turbinate; **8**, frontal sinus. **a,** Drainage of the antral cavity; **b,** drainage of the frontal sinus; **c,** drainage of the anterior ethmoid cells; **d,** drainage of the posterior ethmoid cells; **e,** drainage of the sphenoid sinus; **f,** area of infundibulum (dotted area).

The *internal nasal valve* or limen nasi is a very important structure from the physiologic point of view. It lies at the junction of the vestibule and the nasal cavity. It is formed by a prominence of the anterior edge of the upper lateral or triangular cartilage on the lateral wall of the nose (**Fig. 2.3a**). The internal nasal valve is normally the narrowest point in the entire cross-section of the nasal cavity, making it an important factor in nasal respiration (see p. 135).

The *nasal cavity* extends from the internal nasal valve to the choana. The structure of the floor and roof of the nose, the medial wall, and the *nasal septum* is shown in **Fig. 2.3a, b**.

The outline of the lateral wall of the nasal cavity is more complex than that of the medial wall. It contains several structures that are important in the functioning of the nose and nasal cavity (**Fig. 2.4**):

- Three nasal turbinates (superior, middle, and inferior)
- Drainage of the paranasal sinuses (frontal sinus and maxillary sinus through the hiatus semilunaris in the middle meatus, located between the inferior and middle turbinate; the sphenoid sinus has an ostium of its own in the sphenoethmoidal recess)
- Opening of the nasolacrimal duct into the inferior meatus

The superior, middle, and inferior meatus are located inferior to the three turbinates (**Fig. 2.4**); the paranasal sinuses and the nasolacrimal duct open into them. These openings are of diagnostic and therapeutic importance.

- The inferior meatus, located between the floor of the nose and the insertion of the lower turbinate, lacks a sinus ostium, but contains the opening of the nasolacrimal duct ≈ 3 cm posterior to the external nasal opening and 3 mm posterior to the head of the inferior turbinate (**Fig. 2.4**).
- The middle meatus, between the inferior and middle turbinate, is of clinical importance because the frontal recess, the anterior ethmoid cells, and the maxillary antrum open into it (**Fig. 2.4**).
- The superior meatus, between the middle and superior turbinate, contains the opening for the posterior ethmoid cells. The sphenoid ostium is located on the anterior wall of the sphenoid sinus, at the level of the superior meatus (**Fig. 2.4**).

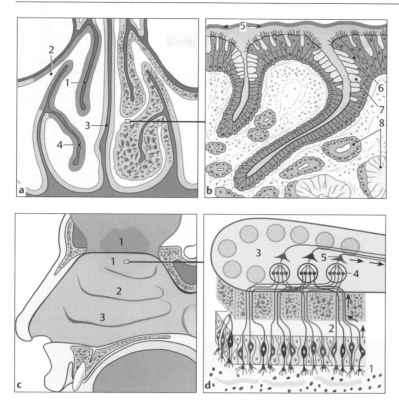

Fig. 2.5a–d **a** Frontal section through the nasal cavity. The nasal mucosa is constricted on the left side and normal on the right.
b Respiratory mucosa. **1**, Middle turbinate; **2**, antrum with ostium; **3**, nasal septum; **4**, inferior turbinate; **5**, layer of mucus; **6**, respiratory epithelium with cilia; **7**, goblet cells; **8**, mucosal glands.
c Sagittal section through the nose with the septum reflected superiorly. **1**, Olfactory region; **2**, middle turbinate; **3**, inferior turbinate.
d **1**, Scent molecules dock onto receptors; **2**, bipolar nerve cells; **3**, olfactory bulb with **4**, glomerulus (microcenter) and **5**, mitral cells.

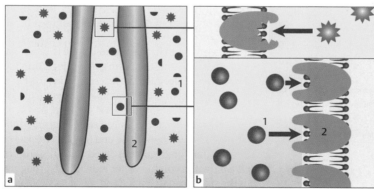

Fig. 2.6a, b **a** **1**, Scent molecules, **2**, scent receptors. Each olfactory cell bears only a single type of receptor. There are 350 types of receptor in humans. A receptor can recognize up to 100 structurally similar molecules in a scent category.
b Scent molecules only fit one specific receptor. They trigger a biochemical reaction and a subsequent electrical signal, which is transmitted to the olfactory center in the brain.

The nasal cavity is lined by two types of epithelium: respiratory and olfactory (**Figs. 2.5a–d, 2.6a, b**). *Respiratory epithelium* coats the entire airway and its projections and extensions (e. g., the paranasal sinuses and the middle ear), from the nasal introitus to the bronchi. It shows morphologic variation in different parts of the respiratory tract. **Figure 2.5c, d** shows the structure of the respiratory epithelium of the nasal cavity. The epithelium is columnar-ciliated with goblet cells and a layer of mixed glands, a fairly well demarcated lymphoid cell zone and well developed venous cavernous spaces in the turbinates and around the ostia (**Fig. 2.5a**).

The *olfactory mucosa*, innervated by fibers of the olfactory nerve, covers the area of the olfactory cleft, the cribri-

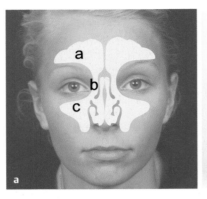

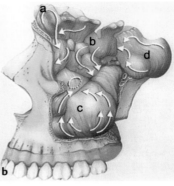

Fig. 2.7a, b The paranasal sinuses.
a Arrangement of the paranasal sinuses in the facial skeleton.
b The mucosal surface of the paranasal sinuses is substantially larger than that of the nose. The arrows indicate the mucociliary transportation of secretions out of the sinuses to the nose.
a, Frontal sinus; **b**, ethmoid cell system; **c**, maxillary sinus; **d**, sphenoid sinus.

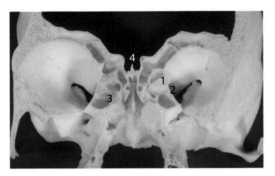

Fig. 2.8 Anatomy of the ethmoid bone. **1**, Labyrinth; **2**, perpendicular lamina; **3**, ethmoidal bulla; **4**, crista galli.

form plate, part of the superior turbinate, and the part of the septum lying opposite it. The structure is shown in **Fig. 2.5 d**, and its topographic extent in **Fig. 2.5c**. Bowman glands occur specifically in this area. They produce a lipo-lipid secretion that covers the olfactory region and aids in olfactory perception due to the enzymes it contains. It is entirely dissimilar to the secretion of the glands of the respiratory epithelium.

■ **Paranasal Sinuses**

The paranasal sinuses are pneumatized cavities in the bone adjacent to the nose (**Fig. 2.7a, b**).

Ostiomeatal Complex
The ostiomeatal complex is a functional entity in the anterior ethmoid complex that represents the final common pathway for drainage and ventilation of the frontal, maxillary, and anterior ethmoid cells (see **Fig. 2.9**). Any or all cells, clefts, and ostia, as well

as their dependent sinuses, can become diseased, contributing to the symptoms and pathophysiology of sinusitis.

Ethmoidal Labyrinth
The central structure in this system of pneumatized cavities is the ethmoid bone. The *anterior ethmoid* is the morphologic connection and secretion channel between the nose and the frontal and maxillary sinuses. The tight spaces and clefts normally ensure ventilation and drainage of the sinus mucosa. The anterior ethmoid is central to the pathogenesis of acute, recurrent, and chronic inflammations of the frontal and maxillary sinuses, since ≈ 90 % of all diseases of the frontal and maxillary sinuses begin here.

The central part of the ethmoid bone is T-shaped. In the median plane, the *crista galli* projects into the anterior fossa (**Fig. 2.8**). The *falx cerebri* inserts here. The *perpendicular plate* (lamina perpendicularis) abuts anteriorly onto the septal *cartilage* and dorsally onto the *vomer*. The paired *ethmoidal labyrinth* is situated between the nose and orbit. It consists of 10 to 15 pneumatized cells lined with *respiratory epithelium*. The volume varies individually; roughly, it is the size of a matchbox standing on its short side.

The *lamina cribrosa* passes into the *ethmoidal notch* (incisura ethmoidalis) of the frontal bone. The *olfactory nerves* extend from the olfactory rim to the olfactory bulb.

The ethmoid air cells are differentiated into anterior and posterior groups. They are derived from an embryonic paired anlage that coalesces in the first year of life to form a single ethmoid cell. There are communications between all of the ethmoid cells on one side. There are often also common ostia for the anterior ethmoid complex in the middle meatus and for the posterior ethmoid complex in the superior meatus (see **Fig. 2.4**). Unlike all the other nasal sinuses, the ethmoid labyrinth is fully formed at birth.

Superiorly, it is related to the anterior part of the base of the skull and is an avenue of spread for rhinogenous intracranial infections. The cranial closure of the ethmoidal labyrinth is formed by frontal bone.

Laterally, the lamina papyracea separates the ethmoid cells from the orbital cavity and is a pathway of spread for orbital complications. It is very thin in children.

Posteriorly, the ethmoid labyrinth is related to the sphenoid sinus. The posterior closure of the ethmoid labyrinth is formed by the sphenoid bone. The optic nerve often runs very close to the posterior ethmoid cells, or even within them. This may explain some cases of retrobulbar neuritis.

Medially, the ethmoid labyrinth is related to the middle and superior turbinates.

Maxillary Sinus

The *maxillary sinus* is the largest sinus, with an average volume of 15 mL. The paired sinuses often develop asymmetrically, and the resulting differences in the thickness of the bony wall may give rise to incorrect radiologic diagnoses. The sinus usually consists of a single chamber, but it may have recesses and may even contain separate loculi. This can give rise to difficulties in diagnosis and treatment.

The ostium of the maxillary sinus occupies the superior part of the medial wall of the sinus; it opens not directly into the nose, but sagittally into a three-dimensional space, the *ethmoidal infundibulum.* The infundibulum opens into the nose in the *hiatus semilunaris* in the middle meatus (**Fig. 2.9**).

The *superior* or *orbital wall* of the maxillary sinus also forms the floor of the orbit. The infraorbital nerve passes through it.

The *medial wall* is also the lateral wall of the nasal cavity. The *anterior wall* contains the infraorbital foramen.

The *posterior wall* separates the sinus from the pterygopalatine fossa. The maxillary artery, the pterygopalatine ganglion, and branches of the trigeminal nerve and autonomic nervous system lie within the pterygomaxillary fossa (see **Fig. 2.12**).

The *floor* of the maxillary sinus is related to the dental roots in the alveolus, particularly those of the second premolar and the first molar. Odontogenic sinusitis can originate from this site.

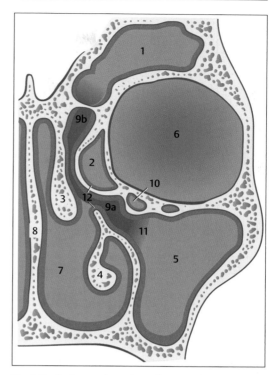

Fig. 2.9 Ostiomeatal unit (green). **1**, Frontal sinus; **2**, ethmoid sinus; **3**, middle turbinate; **4**, inferior turbinate; **5**, maxillary sinus; **6**, orbit; **7**, nasal cavity; **8**, nasal septum; **9a**, ethmoidal infundibulum; **9b**, frontal recess; **10**, orbital ethmoidal cell; **11**, natural ostium; **12**, semilunar hiatus.

Before the second dentition erupts—i.e., until about the seventh year of life—the maxillary sinuses are usually very small, since the maxilla contains the tooth buds of the second dentition. The maxillary sinus does not develop its final form and size until after the second dentition appears.

Frontal Sinus

The *frontal sinus* varies in shape and extent more than the maxillary sinus. The average frontal sinus has a capacity of 4–7 mL. There is often a considerable difference in size between the right and left cavities in the same person. The frontal sinuses may be completely absent on one or both sides in 3–5 % of individuals, but they may also be very extensive and contain loculi. The latter favor the development of inflammatory complications. In the drainage system of the frontal sinus, the frontal infundibulum

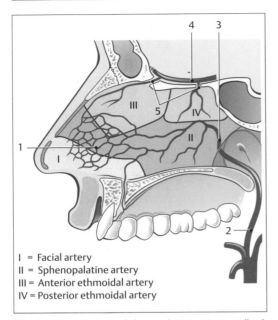

I   = Facial artery
II = Sphenopalatine artery
III = Anterior ethmoidal artery
IV = Posterior ethmoidal artery

Fig. 2.10 Vasculature of the nasal cavity. **1**, Kisselbach area; **2**, internal maxillary artery; **3**, sphenopalatine artery; **4**, ophthalmic artery; **5**, anterior and posterior ethmoid arteries. I–IV: areas supplied by arteries to the nose.

merges into the frontal recess (ethmoidal bone) at the hiatus semilunaris in the middle meatus.

The frontal sinuses form after birth and are not completely developed until the second decade of life. A bony septum separates the two sinuses. The floor of the frontal sinus forms part of the roof of the orbit and is a pathway for the spread of inflammatory orbital complications. The canal of the supraorbital nerve traverses the floor of the frontal sinus.

The posterior wall of the frontal sinus forms part of the bony anterior cranial fossa, making it a typical pathway for the spread of rhinogenous intracranial complications due, either to frontonasal injury or as a complication of sinusitis (see p. 188).

Sphenoid Sinus

The sphenoid sinus does not begin to develop until the age of 5 years.

The *sphenoid* is the most posterior of the sinuses. It occupies the skull base at the junction of the anterior and middle cranial fossae in the body of the sphenoid bone. There are marked individual variations in shape and size, and the capacity of

the sinus is 0.5–3.0 mL. The sphenoid sinus may be entirely absent in 3–5% of individuals. The ostium of the sphenoid sinus lies on the anterior wall of the body of the sphenoid bone in the sphenoethmoidal recess, behind and somewhat above the superior turbinate (see **Fig. 2.4**).

The *superior wall* of the sphenoid sinus is related to the anterior and middle cranial fossae and is a pathway of spread for rhinogenous intracranial complications. The optic chiasm and optic foramen are closely related. The sella turcica and pituitary gland lie on the roof of the sphenoid sinus, which can therefore be used for surgical access to the pituitary.

On the *lateral wall* of the sphenoid sinus lie the cavernous sinus, the internal carotid artery, and the second, third, fourth, fifth, and sixth cranial nerves. The optic canal may lie freely in the lateral wall of the sphenoid sinus, as may the internal carotid artery and the third and sixth cranial nerves.

The *floor* of the sphenoid sinus is related to the roof of the nasopharynx and the choana (see **Fig. 2.4**).

Mucosa of the Paranasal Sinuses

The *mucosa* of the paranasal sinuses (see **Fig. 2.13**) consists of *respiratory epithelium. Goblet cells* and *seromucous glands* produce a secretion forming a two-layered film on the mucosa surface.

The lining of the paranasal sinuses is simpler than that of the nasal cavity. Cavernous erectile tissue may be found in the mucosa around the ostia, and this can affect the patency of the ostia (see p. 119). This variability in the opening of the ostia is supplemented by simultaneous variations in the volume of the neighboring turbinates (see **Fig. 2.5a**). Functionally, they form the *ostiomeatal unit.*

Blood Supply

The *blood supply* to the nasal cavity and nasal sinuses is provided by both the internal and external carotid arteries and their accompanying veins. **Figure 2.10** shows the blood supply of the *medial* nasal wall, and **Fig. 2.93** shows the supply of the *lateral* nasal wall.

The *external* carotid artery supplies the nose internally via the internal maxillary artery and externally via the facial artery. The sphenopalatine artery is an important branch of the internal maxillary artery.

The *internal* carotid artery gives rise to the ophthalmic artery, and from there to the anterior and posterior ethmoidal arteries.

There is a particularly rich and relatively superficial plexus of small vessels (the *Kiesselbach plexus*) located on the anterior part of the nasal septum (**Fig. 2.9**). It is supplied ultimately by both the internal and external carotid arteries.

Venous drainage is provided by the ophthalmic and facial veins and the pterygoid and pharyngeal plexuses. It is therefore located both partially intracranial to the cavernous, coronary, and transverse sinuses, and partially extracranial (see **Fig. 2.2**).

The *cavernous spaces* within the mucosa of the nasal turbinates are very important clinically, as are those on the nasal septum and around the ostia of the nasal sinuses. The filling of these spaces with venous blood is highly variable and is under autonomic control. By regulating the thickness of the mucosa, the cavernous spaces of the turbinates can change the cross-sectional areas of the nasal cavity and of the ostia of the nasal sinuses, thus controlling respiration, ventilation, and drainage (see **Fig. 2.5a**).

Lymphatic Drainage

The lymphatic drainage consists of two parts: an *anterior system*, which collects the lymph from the nasal pyramid and drains to the submandibular superficial cervical lymph nodes; and a *posterior system*, which drains the posterior part of the nasal cavity and the nasopharynx to the retropharyngeal lymph nodes and jugular nodes.

Nerve Supply

The nasal cavity and nasal sinuses have a sensory and autonomic (secretory and vasomotor) nerve supply. In addition, they include the special sensory function of the olfactory nerve.

The *sensory nerve supply* is provided by the first and second branches of the trigeminal nerve. The complex autonomic innervation for secretion and vasomotor supply is shown in **Fig. 2.11**.

Autonomic innervation: The *sympathetic fibers* for vasoconstriction arise from the first to the fifth thoracic segments of the spinal cord, and synapse in the superior cervical ganglion. The postganglionic fibers follow the blood vessels to the mucosa of the nose and nasal sinuses. Some fibers run through the pterygopalatine ganglion without synapsing.

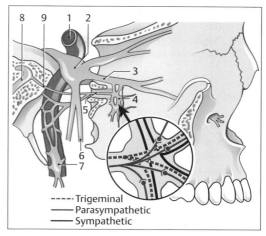

Fig. 2.11 Nerve supply of the nasal mucosa. **1**, Internal carotid artery with sympathetic plexus; **2**, Gasserian ganglion; **3**, maxillary nerve; **4**, pterygopalatine ganglion; **5**, nerve of the pterygoid canal; **6**, mandibular nerve; **7**, superior cervical ganglion; **8**, facial nerve with intermediate nerve; **9**, greater petrosal nerve. The inset shows the course of fibers in the pterygopalatine ganglion: the black lines indicate sympathetic fibers, the solid red lines indicate parasympathetic fibers, and the dotted red line indicates the trigeminal nerve.

The pathway for the *parasympathetic fibers* for vasodilation is from the lacrimomuconasal nucleus along the intermediate nerve to the geniculate ganglion and then along the facial nerve, the greater superficial petrosal nerve, and the nerve of the pterygoid canal to the pterygopalatine ganglion.

The preganglionic parasympathetic fibers synapse in the pterygopalatine ganglion. From there, they supply the mucosa of the nose and nasal sinuses with secretory and vasodilator fibers.

The *pterygopalatine* or *sphenopalatine ganglion* plays a key role in the functioning of the nose and nasal sinuses. It is the main site of its autonomic innervation and has three roots:

1. Parasympathetic fibers, which supplement secretory and vasodilator functions.
2. Sympathetic fibers for vasoconstriction and inhibition of secretion.
3. Sensory fibers from the trigeminal nerve, which arise in the trigeminal ganglion and run in the maxillary nerve.

The nose and maxillary sinus are closely related both anatomically and functionally to the *maxilla*. This bone forms the upper half of the masticatory system and also forms the main part of the middle third of the facial skeleton. The upper jaw is important in diseases of the nose, due to its immediate relationship to the nose and nasal sinuses.

■ Basic Physiology and Pathophysiology

The nose is both a *sensory organ* and a *respiratory organ*. In addition, the nose performs an important function for the entire body by providing both physical and immunologic protection from the environment. Finally, it is also involved in the formation of speech sounds. The nose is also a major esthetic unit in the center of the face. It balances and unites the other esthetic units, paired and unpaired, such as brows, cheeks, forehead, and lips.

■ The Nose as an Olfactory Organ

The human sense of smell is poorly developed in comparison with that of most mammals and insects. Nevertheless, it is still very sensitive and almost indispensable for the individual. For example, taste is only partly a function of the taste buds, which can only recognize the qualities of sweet, sour, salty, and bitter. All other sensory impressions caused by food, such as aroma, bouquet, are mediated by olfaction. This *gustatory olfaction* is due to the fact that the olfactory substances of food or drink pass through the olfactory cleft during expiration while eating or drinking. The sense of smell can stimulate appetite but can also depress it. It also provides a warning against spoiled or poisonous foods and toxic substances—e. g., gas. The sense of smell is particularly important in the field of psychology; marked affects may be induced or inhibited by smells. It should also be remembered that a good sense of smell is essential for people in certain occupations—e. g., cooks and confectioners; wine, coffee, and tea merchants; perfumers; tobacco blenders; and chemists. Finally, physicians need a "clinical nose" for making diagnoses.

The *olfactory area* of the nose is relatively small, at ≈ 2–5 cm^2. The cell bodies of the olfactory cells are located in the olfactory epithelium covering the superior nasal passage, the cranial nasal septum, and the middle turbinate (see **Fig. 2.5c**). The olfactory cells are primary sensory cells that project directly into the olfactory bulb. Their axons are bundled into the olfactory filaments, which pass through the cribriform plate to the olfactory bulb. Between a hundred and a thousand axons together reach each mitral cell. Glutamate is the neurotransmitter between the sensory cells and mitral cells and the messenger of the mitral cells. Other neurotransmitters are γ-aminobutyric acid and dopamine. Important ganglia for further processing within the central nervous system are located in the hippocampus and amygdala, which are responsible for processing emotions and memory content. Finally, conscious olfactory perception occurs at the level of the cortex (superior temporal gyrus, orbitofrontal cortex, insula region).

The olfactory epithelium can regenerate within 100 days, which is unique for sensory organs.

During olfaction, scents first dock onto the olfactory binding protein in the olfactory region. In this way, they reach the scent receptors located on the bipolar olfactory receptor neurons. The receptors are located within the membrane, where they bind to a specific olfactory G protein (second messenger; cyclic adenosine monophosphate).

Richard Axel and Linda Buck were the first to examine the sense of smell at the molecular level. They discovered that every olfactory cell is specialized for only a single class of scent and is equipped with only one type of receptor. Human beings have 350 types of receptor. One receptor can recognize up to a hundred molecules with structural similarities. Scent molecules have to fit into a receptor like a key into a lock. Docking of a molecule activates a chemical cascade. The scent is transformed into a electrical signal, which is transmitted to a scent center in the brain. The two scientists were awarded the Nobel Prize in 2005 for this discovery.

Only volatile substances can be smelled by humans. These substances have to be soluble in water and lipids. Only a few molecules can be sufficient to stimulate the sense of smell. On average, 10^{-15} molecules per milliliter of air are enough to exceed the stimulation threshold.

It is said that there are ≈ 30 000 different olfactory substances in the atmosphere; of these, humans can perceive ≈ 10 000 and are able to identify ≈ 200.

The sense of smell, like other senses, demonstrates the phenomenon of *adaptation*. The sensitivity of the olfactory organ is also dependent on hunger. A very hungry individual can perceive several olfactory stimuli better than one who has just eaten, and this is a useful physiologic regulating mechanism.

Olfactory Disorders (Table 2.1)

Sinonasal olfactory disorders. These are the most common disorders encountered in otolaryngology. Inflammatory or noninflammatory changes impede the transportation of scents to the olfactory cleft or damage the olfactory epithelium directly.

- Infectious causes: chronic recurrent rhinosinusitis
- Noninfectious causes: allergies, polyposis, hyperplastic rhinosinusitis, postirritative and toxic, postinfectious, rhinitis sicca
- Noninflammatory causes: anatomic (malignant and benign tumors, stenoses, choanal atresia, adhesions, septum deviations) or nasal congestion, nerve reflexes, idiopathic rhinitis (formerly called nasal hyperreactivity), side effects of drugs

!

Note: Esthesioneuroblastoma is a highly malignant lesion, the most serious tumor that can affect the olfactory epithelium. It needs to be considered in every patient with an olfactory disorder.

Nonsinonasal olfactory disorders. Viral infections can lead to primary damage to the olfactory cells. Typically, patients experience a subjective loss of the sense of smell immediately after an infectious disease. Neurologic, congenital, toxic, and psychiatric conditions may involve olfactory disorders, as well as head injuries. Dysosmias may be an initial symptom of Alzheimer disease, preceding loss of cognition and abnormal behavior. In Parkinson disease, olfactory disorders often occur before motoric disorders. Noxious substances such as carbon dioxide, formaldehyde, or tobacco smoke can directly damage the olfactory cells. Congenital dysosmias (e. g., Kallmann syndrome) are rare.

A large body of clinical evidence suggests that olfactory disorders are associated with certain neurological and psychiatric diseases (**Table 2.2**), and as such may be associated with pronounced emotional changes. One of the most common findings is temporal lobe epilepsy, which is associated with an olfactory aura. Olfactory hallucinations are usually unpleasant and lead to corresponding emotional effects, frequently with feelings of "déjà vu," which in turn elicit motor and sensory phenomena.

An olfactory disorder is regarded as idiopathic if all other causes have been ruled out.

Table 2.1 Disorders of olfaction—dysosmias

Quantitative disorders	Hyperosmia—oversensitivity
	Normosmia—normal sensitivity
	Hyposmia—reduced sensitivity
	Anosmia—complete inability to perceive scents
Qualitative disorders	Parosmia—altered perception of scents in the presence of a stimulus
	Phantosmia—perception of scent in the absence of a stimulus
	Anosmia—inability to identify perceived scents

Table 2.2 Dysosmia associated with neurological or psychiatric disorders

Abnormal recollection of smells (déjà vu, jamais vu)
Illusions/hallucinations
Schizophrenia
Alcoholism
Senile dementia
Depression

The Vomeronasal Organ

Adolf Butenandt (1903–1995), a Nobel prizewinner from Munich, coined the term *pheromones* for molecules that are produced by a species and evoke certain reactions in animals of the same species. The vomeronasal organ (Jacobson organ) is essential for social and mating behavior in all mammals. With the exception of some of the higher primates, mammals mate only when the female is fertile. Information on the timing of ovulation is conveyed to males by means of pheromones. Numerous observations and studies indicate that pheromones also convey signals in humans.

The vomeronasal organ consists of tiny, paired, blindly terminating channels located in the anterior nasal septum. Its morphology suggests that the organ is a functioning sensory epithelium. Further studies are needed to identify its central connections with the hypothalamus and elucidate its functional significance.

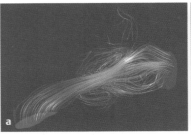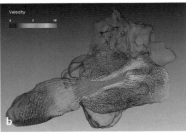

Fig. 2.12a, b   Flow patterns in the nose. Images courtesy of T. Hildebrandt, Birkenwerder, Germany.

■ The Nose as a Respiratory Organ

In humans, the only physiologic respiratory pathway is via the nose. Mouth breathing is abnormal and is activated only as an emergency supplement to nasal respiration. The physiology of the air stream through the normal nose during inspiration and expiration can be summarized as follows. Average ventilation through a normal nose during normal breathing is 6 L/min, and 50–70 L/min during maximum ventilation. The internal nasal valve or limen nasi is the narrowest point in the normal nose. It acts as a nozzle, and the speed of the airstream is very high at this point (**Fig. 2.12a, b**)

The nasal cavity between the valve and the head of the turbinates acts as a diffuser—i. e., it slows the air current and increases turbulence. The central part of the nasal cavity, with its turbinates and meatus, is the most important part for nasal respiration. The column of air consists of a laminar and a turbulent stream. The ratio of laminar to turbulent flow considerably influences the functioning and condition of the nasal mucosa.

The airstream passes in the reverse direction through the nasal cavities during expiration. The expiratory airstream shows much less turbulence in the central part of the nose, reducing the exchange of heat and products of metabolism between the airstream and the nasal wall in comparison with inspiration and enabling the nasal mucosa to recover during the expiratory phase. Inspiration through the nose followed by expiration through the mouth causes the nasal mucosa to dry out rapidly.

Nasal resistance—i. e., the difference in pressure between the nasal introitus and the nasopharynx—is normally between 8 mm and 20 mmH$_2$O. If resistance exceeds 20 mmH$_2$O, the internal nasal valves expand during breathing. Supplemental mouth breathing begins at levels exceeding 40 mmH$_2$O.

Complete exclusion of the nose from breathing leads in the long term to deep-seated mucosal changes. Mechanical obstruction within the nose—e. g., due to septal deviation,

hypertrophy of the turbinates, stenoses from scarring, etc.—can lead to mouth breathing and the resulting deleterious effects (see p. 184), as well as causing mucosal diseases of the nose and the paranasal sinuses.

Computational fluid dynamics (CFD)—simulation of nasal airflow. CFD is the most recent digital method for fluid examination. It can be used to analyze airflow phenomena in the nose (**Fig. 2.12a, b**). It provides data on the important value of integral pressure loss, as well as extensive information about flow, involving velocity vectors, pressure, and turbulences with high resolution, providing detailed information about the fluid flow.

CFD requires five working steps:

1. Creating a geometric model (computed tomography).
2. Generating a computational grid.
3. Preprocessing (physical modeling).
4. Executing calculations (mathematical modeling, equation solving).
5. Postprocessing (graphic and quantitative analysis of results).

In the future, CFD may become an important tool for testing and designing prototypes for the shape of the nasal airway before surgical correction.

Nasal patency. *Nasal patency* can be influenced by many different factors, including the temperature and humidity of the surrounding air; the position of the body; physical activity; changes in body temperature; the effect of cold on different parts of the body, such as the feet; hyperventilation; and psychological stimuli. The state of pulmonary function and of the heart and circulation, endocrinologic conditions such as pregnancy, hyperfunctioning or hypofunctioning of the thyroid gland, and some topical, oral, or parenteral drugs may have a considerable influence on the patency of the nose (see

p. 135). Methods of measuring nasal patency are described on p. 135.

During normal nasal respiration, the inspired air is warmed, moistened, and purified as it passes through the nose.

The *warming* of air inspired through the nose is very effective, and the constancy of the temperature in the lower airways is remarkably stable. The nasal mucosa humidifies and warms the air. The temperature in the nasopharynx during normal (exclusively nasal) respiration is constant at 31–34°C, independently of the external temperature. The heat output of the nose increases as the external temperature falls, so that the lower airways and lungs can function at the correct physiologic temperature.

The *optimal relative humidity* of ambient air for subjective well-being and function of the nasal mucosa lies between 50 % and 60 %. The water vapor saturation of inspired air in the nasopharynx is 80–85 %, and in the lower airway it is fairly constant at between 95 % and 100 %, independent of the relative humidity of the surrounding air. The amount of water vapor secreted by the entire respiratory tract per 1000 L of air can reach 30 g, most of it supplied by the nose. On the other hand, the mucosal blanket makes the nasal mucosa watertight, preventing the release of too much water into the air and consequent drying of the mucosa.

The *cleansing function* of the nose includes firstly, clearing the inspired air of foreign bodies, bacteria, dust, etc.; and secondly, cleansing the nose itself (see below). About 85 % of particles larger than 4.5 μm are filtered out by the nose, but only ≈ 5 % of particles less than 1 μm in size are removed.

Foreign bodies entering the nose come into contact with the moist mucosal surface and the mucosal blanket, which continually sweeps foreign bodies away. The details are described below.

!
Note: The nose warms, moistens, and cleanses atmospheric air as the most important preconditions for normal breathing.

■ **The Nasal Mucosa as a Protective Organ**

In addition to warming, humidifying, and cleansing the inspired air, the nose also has a protective function, consisting of a highly differentiated, efficient, and polyvalent resistance potential against environmental influences on the body. A basic element of this defensive system is the *mucociliary apparatus* (**Fig. 2.13a, b**)—i. e., the functional combination

of the secretory film and the cilia of the respiratory epithelium, by which the colloidal secretory film is transported continuously from the nasal introitus toward the choana. A foreign body is carried from the head of the inferior turbinate to the choana in ≈ 10–20 min. The efficiency of this cleansing system depends on several factors, such as pH, temperature, the condition of the colloids, humidity, the width of the nose, or the presence of toxic gases. Disturbances in the composition or physical characteristics of the mucosal blanket or of ciliary activity can markedly influence the physiology of the nasal cavity. The nasal mucosa protects the entire body by making contact with and providing resistance against animate and inanimate foreign material in the environment.

Local specific immune defense of the nasal mucosa is ensured by humoral and cellular mechanisms (antibodies and immunologically competent cells).

Humoral defense mechanisms. Paraglandular plasma cells produce antibodies—immunoglobulin A (IgA), IgM, and IgG. The glands of the lamina propria absorb the immunoglobulins (e. g., IgA) and then release them as secretory antibodies (sIgA) at the epithelial surface.

Cellular defense mechanisms. The main forces of cellular defense are neutrophilic, basophilic, and eosinophilic granulocytes, macrophages, mast cells, and T and B lymphocytes. B lymphocytes are able to differentiate into plasma cells, which can secrete immunoglobulins. Neutrophils are increased in chronic rhinosinusitis, eosinophils predominate in chronic rhinosinusitis with polyposis, and degranulating mast cells and basophils are important in type I allergic reactions. Intercellular adhesion molecule-1 (ICAM-1) is expressed by the epithelium of the nasal mucosa; it serves as a receptor for viruses (rhinoviruses). Cells of the vascular endothelium are stimulated by inflammation mediators such as tumor necrosis factor-α (TNF-α) and interleukin-1 (IL-1) to express adhesion molecules that ensure diapedesis by immunologically competent cells.

■ **The Nose as a Reflex Organ**

Specific nasal reflex mechanisms can arise:
- Within the nose and affecting the nose itself.
- In other parts of the body or organs and affecting the nose.
- In the nose and affecting other parts of the body.

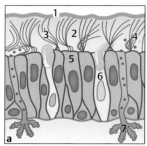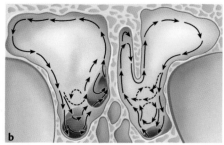

Fig. 2.13a, b a The mucociliary apparatus is the most important defense mechanism in the respiratory epithelium. Goblet cells and seromucous glands produce a two-layered film consisting of a low-viscosity sol phase and a higher-viscosity gel phase. The cilia beat in the sol phase to transport the gel along distinct pathways across the mucosa of the nose and paranasal sinuses toward the choana. The mucociliary apparatus simultaneously facilitates secretion and absorption, and it is the region where initial nonspecific and specific immunological responses to antigens and allergens occur. **1**, Gel layer; **2**, sol layer; **3**, cilia (beating); **4**, cilia (recovering); **5**, ciliated epithelial cell; **6**, goblet cell; **7**, seromucous gland.
b Mucociliary transportation of secretions in the frontal sinus (adapted from Messerklinger).

The *nasal cycle* is a reflex system that is obviously confined to the nose, but its purpose is unknown. One cycle lasts between 2 and 6 hours. If both halves of the nasal cavity are of normal patency, the lumen widens and narrows alternately, lowering or increasing respiratory resistance in each half of the nose. Ideally, the resistance of the entire nose remains constant. This reflex phenomenon is controlled by the action of the autonomic nervous system on the cavernous spaces of the vascular system of the nasal mucosa.

Nasopetal reflexes arise in situations such as cooling of the extremities, which changes the respiratory resistance. They may also arise from the lungs and bronchi and from other autonomic control points.

Important *nasofugal* communications exist between the nose and the lung, the heart and circulation, the metabolic organs, and the genitals.

In addition, there are sneezing, lacrimal, and cough reflexes, and in certain emergency situations, reflexive respiratory arrest.

■ Influence of the Nose on Speech

The nose influences the sound of speech. During the formation of the resonants "m," "n," and "ng," for example, the air streams through the open nose, whereas during the formation of vowels the nose and nasopharynx are more or less closed off by the soft palate from the resonating cavity of the mouth.

■ Function of the Nasal Sinuses

The function of the paranasal sinuses is one of the oldest and most fascinating controversies in medicine. Many theories have been proposed—e. g., that they serve to reduce the weight of the facial skull, provide resonation spaces for the voice, absorb facial trauma forces, moisturize and warm inspired air, provide olfactory function and thermic insulation, are functionless hollows, or provide a source of secretions for the main nasal cavity.

In an experimental study, one important question was answered in 1990. The mucosa of the paranasal sinuses plays a role in secretion production and control of the nasal mucosa. In other words, when the human organism needs higher humidity to moisten the incoming air, such as during sports activity, the sinuses increase secretion and convection through the ostium to the lateral wall mucosa.

The presence of the *ostia* causes particular pathophysiologic problems affecting ventilation and drainage. Ostial obstruction interrupts the self-cleansing mechanism of the affected sinus, causing the secretions to stagnate and change in composition. The retained secretions are an ideal medium for saprophytic bacteria, which are often present in normal sinuses. Ostial obstruction can lead to a vicious circle, as illustrated in **Fig. 2.14**.

The main cause of closure of the ostium is rhinogenous swelling due to a reaction or infection in

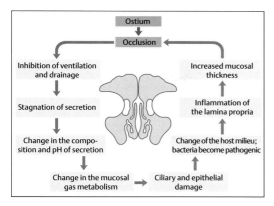

Fig. 2.14 Pathophysiology of the sinus ostium.

the nasal mucosa. Ninety percent of all sinusitis cases begin in the anterior ethmoid *(ethmoidal infundibulum, facial recess, and middle meatus)*. The closure mechanism can be induced by viral or bacterial infection of the nose, barotrauma, hyperreactivity, environmental factors such as relative dryness of the nose, toxic gases, or airborne toxic agents. Other causes include localized congenital or acquired anomalies such as deviation of the septum, scars, lesions of the turbinates, infections of the nose or nasal cavities, allergic diseases of the nose or nasal sinuses (particularly in children), vasomotor dysfunction due to neurogenic or hormonal factors, metabolic diseases such as vitamin deficiencies, diabetes, electrolyte disorders, mechanical obstruction due to crusts, ethmoidal polyps, foreign bodies, prolonged use of a nasogastric tube or prolonged nasal tracheal intubation, and benign and malignant tumors.

The vicious circle of ostial occlusion can only be broken in the long term by treating the causative factors with appropriate medical or surgical measures (**Fig. 2.14**)

The nasal sinuses are only minimally involved in respiratory phases in the nasal cavity. Only slight changes in pressure are recorded in the sinuses during respiration. When the ostium is occluded, a relatively small drop in pressure in the sinuses (from –20 to –50 mmH$_2$O) occurs, which is enough to elicit the symptoms of what has been inappropriately termed *vacuum sinusitis*. The symptoms include moderately severe headaches, which disappear when ventilation of the sinus is restored.

Methods of Examining the Nose, Paranasal Sinuses, and Face

■ External Inspection and Palpation

During external examinations, attention is given to the following points:
- The properties of the overlying skin—e. g., hardness, firmness, discolorations, inflammatory swellings, and tenderness to pressure.
- Externally visible changes in shape of the cartilaginous or bony structure due to congenital or acquired deformities—e. g., saddle nose, hump nose, broad nose, or scoliotic nose; the early or late results of trauma; painful swelling due to inflammation; nonpainful swelling due to tumor.
- Palpable masses in neighboring structures—e. g., the forehead, cheeks, upper lip, or eyelids; proptosis, displacement of the bulb or limitation of its movement.
- The nasal alae during respiration, inspection for indrawing or flaring of the ala.
- The nasal vestibule, the anterior border of the nasal septum, the roof of the vestibule, and the internal part of the nasal cavity, inspected by lifting the tip of the nose.
- Crepitation and mobility of the nasal bony framework.
- The sites of exit of the various nerves (**Fig. 2.15a, b**).
- Sensitivity to pressure on the forehead, cranial vault, or cheek.

■ Anterior Rhinoscopy

Anterior rhinoscopy using a nasal speculum, a strong light source, and a head mirror or headlamp is only carried out after inspection without instruments (**Fig. 2.16 a, b**). The method of using the nasal speculum is shown in **Fig. 2.17 a, b**. Usually, the left hand holds the speculum when inspecting both nasal cavities. Anterior rhinoscopy alone is now considered insufficient, but it is the first step in examining the nose.

Technique. The speculum is introduced into the nasal vestibule with its blades together. The point of the speculum is directed slightly laterally in the nasal vestibule.

The speculum blades are then spread within the nasal vestibule and fixed to the nasal ala with the index finger. The instrument is held slightly open when it is being removed, to prevent pain due to avulsion of vibrissae. The right hand is used to adjust the position of the face and head. As shown in **Fig. 2.17a**, the patient's head is initially in the vertical position, so that the examiner's gaze is parallel to the floor of the

nose and along the inferior turbinate and the inferior meatus (position I). If the nasal cavity is wide, the choana and the posterior wall of the nasopharynx can be seen in this position. To allow inspection of the upper part of the nasal cavity, the patient's head is tilted slightly backward. The middle meatus, which is very important clinically, and the middle turbinate are thus brought into view (position II) (**Fig. 2.17b**). If the head is tilted far backward, the olfactory cleft may also be visible.

Small children and infants, it is advisable to use an otoscope rather than a nasal In speculum for anterior rhinoscopy.

When the head position has been adjusted satisfactorily, the hand holding the speculum can be used simultaneously to fix the head, leaving the right hand free for manipulating instruments, performing aspirations, etc., within the nasal cavity.

!

> **Note:** The nasal mucosa is often so turgescent that the view of the nasal cavity is minimal. In such cases, a decongestant spray is introduced into the nose and allowed to act for 10 min, after which a good view is usually possible.

The following are noted during anterior rhinoscopy:
- Nasal secretions, their color, quantity, and properties; mucus, pus, and crust formation.
- Location of abnormal secretion.
- Swelling of the turbinates, narrowing or widening of the nasal meatus.

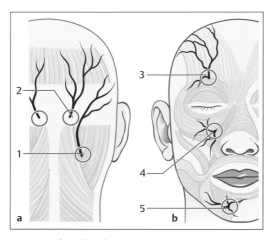

Fig. 2.15a, b   Clinically important nerve exit sites.
a At the occiput: **1**, lesser occipital nerve; **2**, greater occipital nerve.
b On the face: **3**, supraorbital nerve; **4**, infraorbital nerve; **5**, mental nerve.

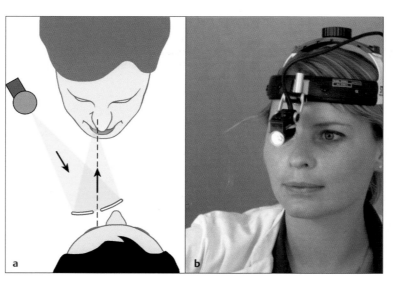

Fig. 2.16a, b   a Traditional rhinoscopy, using a head mirror. **b** Head lamps with cold-light or light-emitting diode (LED) illumination have now largely replaced mirrors.

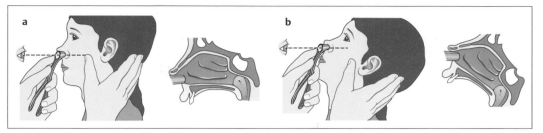

Fig. 2.17a, b   Anterior rhinoscopy.   **a** Position I. **b** Position II.

- Properties of the mucosal surface (including its color)—e. g., whether it is moist, dry, smooth, cornified, or uneven.
- Position of the nasal septum and septal deformities.
- Sites of major blood vessels—e. g., Kiesselbach plexus.
- Abnormal pigmentation or color of the mucosa.
- Presence of abnormal tissue.
- Ulcerations or perforations.
- Foreign bodies.

The clinically important region of the middle meatus may be anatomically narrow and difficult to examine. It can be visualized by using a long Killian nasal speculum, provided that local anesthesia of the nasal mucosa has been induced (e. g., by local application of lidocaine (Xylocaine); or 1 % pantocaine with 1 : 1000 epinephrine, one drop to 1 mL of anesthetic solution; or with a 5 % lidocaine and 0.5 % phenylephrine spray). Gustav Killian (1860–1921) developed this instrument for the medial rhinoscopy technique, having recognized as early as 100 years ago that the lateral nasal wall is important in pathogenesis. The technique of anterior rhinoscopy using nasal endoscopy was added more recently.

■ Posterior Rhinoscopy

Figure 2.18a, b shows the method of examining the nasopharynx with a mirror, with a composite view of the inspected region. Posterior rhinoscopy is used to examine the posterior part of the nasal cavity: the choana, the posterior ends of the turbinates, the posterior margin of the septum, and the nasopharynx, including its roof and the ostia of the eustachian tube.

Nasal endoscopy, including the nasopharynx, should nowadays be an integral part or an adjunctive measure in any examination assessing an otorhinolaryngology patient. It has superseded posterior rhinoscopy and can be regarded as the gold standard for obtaining nasal findings, regardless of the further management.

Technique. Posterior rhinoscopy requires a considerable amount of practice on the part of the examiner, as well as cooperation by the patient. A tongue depressor is placed on the center of the base of the tongue with one hand, and the base of the tongue is pressed slowly downward, increasing the distance between the surface of the tongue and the soft palate and posterior pharyngeal wall. The glass side of a small mirror is warmed and then tested on the hand to make sure it is not too hot. The other hand is used to introduce the mirror into the space between the soft palate and the posterior pharyngeal wall. The mirror must not touch the mucosa, otherwise it will elicit the gag reflex. If the soft palate remains tense, the patient is asked to breathe gently through the nose, to sniff, or to say "ha," causing the palate to relax and providing an unobstructed view into the nasopharynx. A view of the various parts of the nasopharynx is obtained by moving and tilting the mirror (**Fig. 2.18b**). The vertical posterior edge of the septum is used for orientation to locate the normal structures. If a satisfactory view cannot be obtained due to the gag reflex, a successful examination can often be achieved by applying a local anesthetic—e. g., a 1 % lidocaine spray—to the oropharynx, particularly to the soft palate and posterior wall of the pharynx.

If it is not possible to examine the nasopharynx with this method, either endoscopy (see p. 133) or palatal retraction (or both combined) can be carried out, although endoscopy has now made palatal retraction largely obsolete.

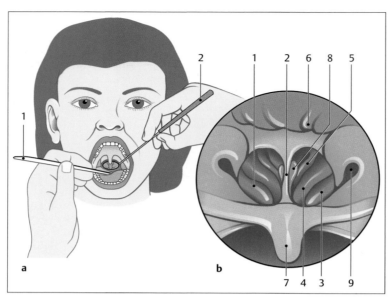

Fig. 2.18a, b Posterior rhinoscopy.
a The method of holding the tongue depressor (**1**) and mirror (**2**).
b Composite picture of the nasopharynx composed of individual views: **1**, choana; **2**, posterior edge of the septum; **3**, inferior turbinate; **4**, middle turbinate; **5**, superior turbinate; **6**, adenoid; **7**, uvula; **8**, septum padding; **9**, tubal ostium.

The following should be noted during posterior rhinoscopy (**Fig. 2.19**):

- The opening and width of the choanae.
- The shape of the posterior end of the inferior and middle turbinates.
- Scars or deformities in the nasopharynx—e. g., due to trauma.
- The shape of the posterior part of the nasal septum.
- Nasal polyps.
- The shape of both tubal ostia and the Rosenmüller fossa (pharyngeal recess).
- Obstruction of the nasopharynx by enlarged adenoids in children.
- Tumors of the nasopharynx.
- Abnormal secretions in the choanae.
- The properties of the mucosa of the posterior part of the nose and the nasopharynx—e. g., for moisture, dryness, thickening, and color.

Computed tomography (CT) is used to evaluate the spread of paranasal sinus lesions to adjacent structures, particularly the skull base, cranial cavity, retromaxillary space, and orbits. Also used in trauma patients, CT is indispensable for differentiated evaluation of bony structures. It is supplemented by magnetic resonance imaging (MRI) for soft-tissue investigations.

■ Nasal Endoscopy

The principle used in the rod lens system was submitted to the Patent Office in the United Kingdom by its inventor, the English physicist Harold Horace Hopkins (1918–1994), on July 16th, 1959. The rod lens system uses precision-polished glass rods with optically processed ends instead of conventional lenses. The system has substantial advantages over conventional lens systems: better resolution and contrast, a wider angle of view, and extremely clear and bright images that resolve even the smallest details throughout the entire field of view.

The German inventor Karl Storz (1911–1996) introduced the system into otorhinolaryngology and developed cold light illumination. This marked the beginning of a new era in otorhinolaryngology—the era of endoscopy.

The Austrian physician Walter Messerklinger (1920–2001) studied mucociliary transport in the paranasal sinus mucosa over a period of several years. He used the new scopes to explore the lateral nasal wall and obtained significant pathogenetic findings:

- The vast majority of cases of recurrent and chronic sinusitis are rhinogenous in origin.
- Inconspicuous signs of mucosal disease or anatomical configurations predisposing to sinusitis are detectable with endoscopy.

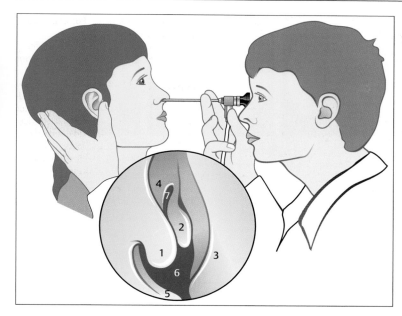

Fig. 2.19 The examination setting for nasal endoscopy. The inset shows typical landmarks when viewing the interior of the right side of the nose through a 0° lens. **1**, Inferior turbinate; **2**, middle turbinate; **3**, nasal septum, **4**, agger nasi; **5**, floor of the nose; **6**, inferior nasal meatus, **7**, middle nasal meatus.

- The endoscope is thus an important optical device for elucidating the spreading pathway of spread of rhinogenous sinusitis.
- Endoscopic devices have therefore made new surgical approaches possible. Endoscopic surgery can be directed at the central pathogenetic mechanism of recurrent or chronic sinusitis (see functional endoscopic sinus surgery, p. 171).

Nasal endoscopy is the most important method for evaluating intranasal findings (**Fig. 2.20a–d**).

Clinical indications for nasal endoscopy. These include acute, recurrent and chronic sinusitis; head and facial pain; chronic nasal catarrh; epistaxis; epiphora; chronic pharyngitis and laryngitis; epipharyngeal disease; chronic otitis media; hyposmia and anosmia; suspected or known cerebrospinal fluid (CSF) rhinorrhea; foreign-body removal; sample biopsies; and sleep disorders.

Normal mucosal findings during nasal endoscopy. The mucosa has a pale pink color and a moist consistency.

Note: The nasal mucosa is continually responding to numerous antigens or allergens via humoral and cellular reactions. Mucosal color, swelling, and secretory status are therefore subject to continuous change.

The *diagnostic evaluation criteria in nasal endoscopy* are shown in **Table 2.3**.

Technique. The examination is carried out with the patient in a sitting, semireclining, or fully reclined position, without premedication. If the mucosa is severely swollen, vulnerable, or sensitive, it can be decongested and anesthetized with a 5% lidocaine and 0.5% phenylephrine spray, or with a single puff of tetracaine plus epinephrine. It is useful to soak a few cotton swabs in a solution of this type for 5 min before the examination. Swabs should be inserted under endoscopic guidance to prevent mucosal injury.

The endoscopic examination should follow a systematic approach in which different regions are explored (**Figs. 2.19, 2.21**). The 0° wide-angle scope (4 mm) is the standard instrument for all endoscopic nasal examinations. Small-diameter endoscopes should be used only if access is limited due to substantial deviation of the anterior septum, or in small children (2.7 mm, 1 mm).

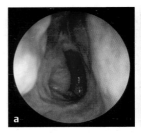
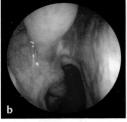
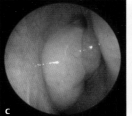
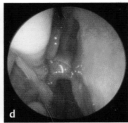

Fig. 2.20a–d   Findings in nasal endoscopy.
a View of the posterior nasal cavity on the right side, 2 cm from the choana. The eustachian tube orifice is at the center of the image, and the posterior end of the lower turbinate is on the left side of the image.
b The insertion of the middle turbinate, lateral to the choana and anterior–cranial to the tubal ostium.

c A solitary polyp in the nasal meatus (right side). (**a–c:** 0° lens, 4 mm.)
d View of the sphenoethmoidal recess, showing a polyp in the ostium of the sphenoid cavity. A stream of mucoid pus is visible from the posterior ethmoid to the eustachian tube orifice (30° lens, 4 mm).

Table 2.3   Nasal endoscopy: diagnostic evaluation criteria

Mucosal surface	Moist, dry (e. g., rhinitis sicca), crusted (e. g., postoperative after FESS, diseases of the mucociliary apparatus), telangiectasia (e. g., Rendu–Osler–Weber disease), perforation (with multiple etiologies), petechiae (vascular disease)
Color of mucosa	Pink (normal appearance of the mucosa), livid (e. g., allergic rhinitis, nasal hypersensitivity), pale (e. g., chronic hyperplastic rhinosinusitis)
Track of pus	Present / absent (e. g., in acute inflammations, in semilunar hiatus or sphenoethmoidal recess)
Secretions (rheologic changes)	Viscous (chronic rhinosinusitis with polyps; the Sampter triad—asthma, NSAID sensitivity, and nasal polyps; fluid (anterior or posterior rhinorrhea)
Swelling	Hyperplasia of the inferior (anterior/posterior) turbinate (e. g., nasal hypersensitivity)
Anatomical variations that may predispose to recurrent sinusitis	Septal deviations, vomer crest deviation, spurs, prominent premaxilla, concha bullosa, paradoxically curved middle turbinate, medialized uncinate process
Early indications of chronic inflammation of the ethmoid infundibulum	Mucosal hyperemia of in region of infundibulum, prolapse of medial wall of infundibulum, localized edema or polypoid mucosa

FESS, functional endoscopic sinus surgery; NSAID, nonsteroidal anti-inflammatory drug.

Step 1: 0° scope: Initially, the nasal vault and nasal isthmus are inspected. Positioning the endoscope in front of the nasal cavity or the isthmus region—without deforming the nostrils by using a nasal speculum—makes it possible to evaluate the functional condition as well as low-pressure phenomena of the alar cartilages during normal and forced nasal breathing, in physiological conditions.

The endoscope is advanced into the nasal cavity to visualize the nasal floor. It is then carefully positioned between the septum and body of the lower turbinate, to advance toward the choanae. The lower turbinate and pharyngeal tubal ostium have the same orientation. The nasopharynx, soft palate motility, and function of the pharyngeal tubal ostium should be inspected. In children, the size and status of the adenoids need to be evaluated.

Step 2: 0° scope: The endoscope is now moved backward to visualize the middle nasal meatus, the "window to the ethmoid." This is particularly important, as sinusitis may originate here. The middle turbinate may be pneumatized by a system of ethmoidal cells and may be quite large (in the case of concha bullosa); it may also be the site of origin for recurrent sinusitis.

Step 3: 0° scope: Gentle medialization of the middle turbinate using a Freer elevator provides a view of the typical relief structure of the lateral nasal wall. The uncinate process is situated ventral to the ethmoidal bulla, the size of which varies depending on its degree of pneumatization. The inferior semilunar hiatus is situated between the posterior margin of the uncinate process and the anterior surface of the ethmoidal bulla. The ethmoidal infundibulum extends in a sagittal direction and opens into the inferior semilunar hiatus. Advancing cranially from the semilunar hiatus, one approaches the frontal recess.

Step 4: 30° or 45° scope: The sphenoethmoidal recess and sphenoid sinus ostium can be inspected with a 30° or 45° scope. The endoscope is advanced along the nasal floor in a cranial direction until the choana is reached. A 45° or 70° scope can be inserted underneath the entire middle nasal meatus; it is used to inspect this area endoscopically in a cranial direction. The olfactory cleft can also be inspected—e.g., to distinguish sensorineural from respiratory hyposmia or anosmia. Angled endoscopes are suitable for inspection of the nasal ostium, which contains the nasolacrimal duct. The ostium is oval in shape and is located just a few millimeters dorsal to the anterior insertion of the lower turbinate.

■ **Assessment of Nasal Patency**

Rhinomanometry. During spontaneous respiration, the nasal airflow ($\dot{V}$, cm^3/s) is measured using a flowmeter (pneumotachograph, mass flowmeter) attached to a mask. Simultaneously, the differential pressure between choana and the mask (ΔP, Pa) is determined. Various resistance values can be calculated from the directly measured results for pressure and flow. In addition, comparison of the ascending and descending inspiratory and expiratory breathing phases in standard graphs makes it possible to assess the influence of the elasticity of the nasal structures. Further information can be obtained by performing rhinomanometry before and after decongestion with nose drops (temporary or permanent nasal resistance), or by provocation of the nasal mucosa with allergens (nasal provocation test) (**Fig. 2.22a, b**).

Measurements are usually performed during spontaneous respiration. The volume of air passing through the nose during active nasal respiration is recorded at the same time as the pressure differential across the nose. The results can be recorded either using a pair of curves or as an *xy* function (**Fig. 2.22a**), and they provide information about unilateral or bilateral nasal patency (**Fig. 2.22b**) (see p. 126).

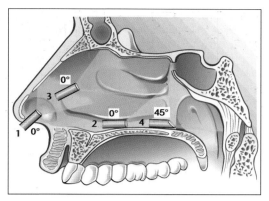

Fig. 2.21 Systematic nasal endoscopy using scopes with different angles of view. **1**, Nasal vestibule; **2**, nasal floor and inferior meatus; **3**, middle meatus; **4**, sphenoethmoidal recess.

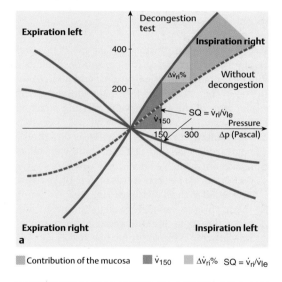

Obstruction	Partial nose	Entire nose
No	> 500	> 800
Light	300–500	500–800
Medium	180–300	300–500
Severe	60–180	100–300
Near-complete	< 60	< 100

b

Fig. 2.22a, b **a** Principle of computer-supported rhinomanometry.
b Reference values in adult patients (flow at 150 Pa, in cm^3).

Acoustic rhinometry. This method uses acoustic reflection for separate measurement on each side of the cross-sectional area of the nose, from the vestibule to the nasopharynx. In contrast to rhinomanometry, it assesses the cross-sectional area of various parts of the nose, rather than flow parameters in the nose. Another difference is that it also serves to determine static parameters without the need for patient cooperation.

A rough *qualitative* test of nasal patency can be achieved by holding a polished metal plate in front of the nose during inspiration and expiration. The surface area of the resulting fogging gives an approximation of the patency of the two sides of the nose.

In *infants,* nasal patency is tested by holding a wisp of cotton wool or a feather in front of the nose.

■ Olfactometry

First, a precise case history is taken that includes triggering events, associated symptoms, relevant illnesses, operations, medications, and noxious influences. This is followed by nasal endoscopy, with exploration of the nasopharynx and the olfactory cleft.

Assessment of olfactory function is based on a standardized, validated test. The following olfaction tests are available and widely used:

- *Sniffin' Sticks:* Sixteen scents on felt-tip pens are presented to the patient, who is asked to identify them. This test is widely used in Europe. It combines threshold, identification, and discrimination of scents; the identification test is suitable for screening.
- *University of Pennsylvania Smell Identification Test (UPSIT):* Forty scents in microcapsules are deposited on paper, where they can be released mechanically by rubbing. The individual scents have to be identified from a list, with four alternatives each. The cross-cultural smell identification test (CCSIT) is a simplified version of this.
- *Connecticut Chemosensory Clinical Research Center Test (CCCRC):* This is a combination of a threshold test for butanol and an identification test for ten scents. The scents are contained in polypropylene flasks that can be pressed open. A disadvantage with this test is low validation.
- *Evoked response olfactometry (ERO):* Objective assessment of olfactory disorders is possible by analyzing the potentials evoked by olfactory stimuli. Derivation of olfactory evoked potentials is the only validated method of confirming a loss of the sense of smell objectively. ERO involves application of chemosensory stimuli via a tube inserted into the middle nasal meatus, at intervals averaging 20–40 s. Each stimulation lasts 250 ms. Phenylethyl alcohol or hydrogen sulfide can be used as scents.

The ability to identify different substances may be of importance in neurologic differential diagnosis (**Table 2.4**).
Two different parameters can be tested:
1. The *threshold* at which the substance is *perceived.*
2. The *threshold* at which it is *recognized.*

The former threshold is lower than the latter. Apart from ERO, all of the methods mentioned above depend on cooperation from the patient, and the results are therefore largely subjective. Objective results can only be obtained with ERO.

Tests for simulation include ERO and the cinnamon test. The taste of cinnamon is mediated by the olfactory nerve. Cinnamon cannot be recognized in the absence of the ability to smell.

Anosmia is complete loss of the ability to smell; *hyposmia* is a reduced ability to smell; and *parosmia* refers to a state in which the subjective impression does not correspond to the substance offered. In *cacosmia,* all smells appear to be offensive. Cacosmia is often an indication of a central nervous system lesion (see also Table 2.1).

> **Note:** Ideally, the sense of smell should always be tested thoroughly before any surgery in the nose or sinuses, for medicolegal reasons.

■ Diagnostic Imaging of the Nose and Sinuses

Diagnosis of diseases of the nasal sinuses is hardly possible without the use of radiology.

Conventional radiology. *Radiographs of the nose* in the lateral projection are necessary to demonstrate a fracture of the nasal bone. They can also be used if an intranasal foreign body is suspected.

Plain sinus radiography (**Fig. 2.23a, b**)*:* The diagnostic value of plain sinus radiographs is controversial today. Proponents of plain sinus radiography say the films provide rapid, noninvasive evaluation of the lower third of the nasal cavity and the maxillary, frontal, sphenoid, and posterior ethmoid sinuses. Plain films are neither useful nor cost-efficient for evaluating the anterior ethmoid air cells, the upper two-thirds of the nasal cavity, or the infundibular, middle meatal, and frontal recess air passages. The clinical role of plain films is thus at best limited to documenting acute maxillary or frontal sinusitis and, if baseline films are available, to following the course of infection and the response to treatment. Detection of air–fluid levels warrants evaluation by CT or nasal endoscopy.

Computed tomography. A CT scan in the coronal plane is the imaging modality of choice for confirming the anatomy and extent of pathology. It helps in understanding the functional sinus anatomy of the individual patient and supports the identification and evaluation of the frontal sinus, frontal recess, uncinate process, ethmoidal infundibulum, maxillary sinus, maxillary sinus ostia, ethmoidal bulla, lateral sinus, middle meatus, posterior ethmoidal sinus cell, sphenoid sinus, and sphenoid recess.

Indications: Patients with a history of chronic, recurrent sinusitis despite repeated medical therapy, independent of normal or pathologic findings at the lateral nasal wall (**Fig. 2.24**), and patients with suspicious space-occupying lesions.

!
> **Note:** Nasal endoscopy should always be done before CT scanning.

Magnetic resonance imaging. MRI is not the primary imaging modality in chronic rhinosinusitis. It is usually reserved (in combination with CT) for investigating more serious conditions, such as neoplasia (**Fig. 2.25a, b**). It is indicated in the diagnosis of intracranial complications (e. g., epidural or subdural abscess, brain abscess) and orbital complications (e. g., orbital infection).

Magnetic resonance angiography. This helps clarify the hemodynamic activity of a tumor.

Table 2.4   Some known olfactory substances

	Stimulation of olfactory nerve	Stimulation of sensory part of trigeminal nerve	Stimulation of chorda tympani (cranial nerve VII) and glossopharyngeal nerve (cranial nerve IX)
Coffee	+		
Wax	+		
Vanilla	+		
Lavender oil	+		
Turpentine oil	+		
Birch tar	+		
Cinnamon	+		
Benzaldehyde	+	+	
Menthol	+	+	
Turpentine	+	+	
Petroleum	+	+	
Peppermint	+	+	
Camphor	+	+	
Alcohol	+	+	
Formaldehyde	+	+	
Acetic acid	+	+	
Ammonia		+	
Chloroform	+		+
Pyridine	+		+

Angiography/digital subtraction angiography. In addition to visualization of the blood vessels, this allows preoperative embolization of the arteries that supply a tumor. This is a prerequisite for endonasal endoscopic surgical resection of angiofibromas.

Ultrasound in A or B mode. This can also be used to investigate the nasal sinuses. The advantage of this method is that the patient is spared exposure to radiation. Its disadvantage is that the findings are less detailed and technical errors more likely.

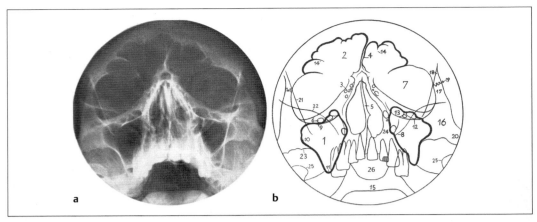

Fig. 2.23a, b   Radiographic anatomy of a plain film of the paranasal sinuses. **1**, Maxillary sinus; **2**, frontal sinus; **3**, ethmoidal air cells; **4**, interfrontal septum; **5**, nasal septum; **6**, infraorbital foramen; **7**, floor of the orbit; **8–11**, medial, cranial, lateral, and caudal walls of the maxillary sinus; **12**, orbital floor; **13**, cranial part of maxillary sinus; **14**, interfrontal septa; **15**, tongue; **16**, zygomatic bone; **17–19**, frontozygomatic suture; **20**, zygomatic arch; **21**, innominate line (orthograde projection of part of the greater wing of sphenoid); **22**, small sphenoid wing; **23**, lower border of zygomatic bone; **24**, round foramen; **25**, head of the mandible; **26**, sphenoid sinus.

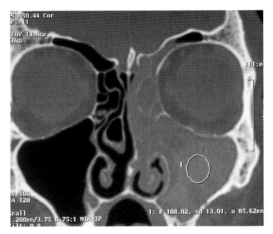

Fig. 2.24   Coronal CT of the paranasal sinuses. On the left side of the image, there is good visualization of the bony structures of the lateral nasal wall. On the right side, there is pansinusitis, with hyperplastic mucosa in the cavities and ethmoidal air cells and destruction of septa between cells.

1. For *diagnostic purposes,* to allow aspiration and lavage of abnormal secretions, bacteriologic and cytologic examination of the secretions, and possibly the introduction of a contrast medium for radiography.
2. The sinuses can be irrigated for *therapeutic purposes,* to allow drainage of abnormal secretions and introduction of locally active substances into the sinuses.

Although lavage of the sinuses was commonly used to treat maxillary empyema up until just a few decades ago, it is rarely done today. Drainage of the frontal sinus using the Kümmel and Beck method is now practically obsolete, having been replaced by endoscopic endonasal microsurgery. However, the otolaryngologist should be familiar with these techniques, to avoid inflammatory complications in case the modern approaches fail: *ubi pus, ibi evacua.*

Lavage of the maxillary antrum. Two methods are routinely used:
1. Access via the *inferior meatus* (sharp puncture)
2. Access via the *middle meatus* (blunt puncture) after fenestration during functional endoscopic surgery.

■ Lavage of the Sinuses

The maxillary sinus, frontal sinus, and sphenoid sinus can be irrigated, but not the ethmoid sinuses. There are two reasons for irrigating the sinuses:

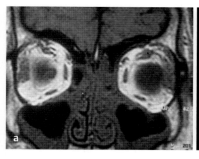

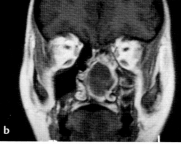

Fig. 2.25a, b Coronal MRI of the paranasal sinuses.
a Good visualization of brain, soft tissues, and mucosal pathology, poor visualization of bony structures.
b Positive enhancement on the surface of a vascularized tumor (T1-weighted with contrast medium).

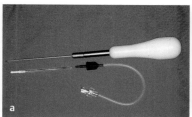

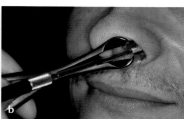

Fig. 2.26a, b A modern lavage system (Atos Medical, Hörby, Sweden; Bess, Berlin, Germany) for the paranasal sinuses. Puncture is performed in the inferior nasal meatus.

Principle of lavage via the inferior meatus: Local anesthesia of the inferior meatus is induced. A Lichtwitz trocar is placed against the lateral nasal wall beneath the origin of the inferior turbinate. After the cannula has been pushed through this part of the lateral nasal wall, which is usually thin, it can be used for aspiration, lavage, or the introduction of drugs.

A long-term drain can be introduced for conservative treatment, especially in children (see p. 180).

The SinuTroc lavage system for the maxillary sinus (**Fig. 2.26a, b**) is an optimized drainage system. During puncture of the maxillary sinus with a trocar in the middle nasal meatus, a 3-mm plastic tube equipped with a plastic hull (1 cm long, 1.5 mm thick) is inserted into the maxillary sinus. The trocar is then removed; two small barbs keep the self-retaining catheter from slipping away from the wall of the maxillary sinus. For repeated lavage, the self-retaining catheter is attached to an adapter tube (19 cm long, Luer-Lok or cone connection).

Complications during blunt puncture are very unlikely if it is performed expertly. During sharp puncture, the point of the cannula may be pushed inadvertently into the soft tissues of the cheek, pterygopalatine fossa, or orbit if the technique is incorrect.

Note: Air should never be used to clear the irrigated sinus, as it can lead to an air embolism. The symptoms are collapse, loss of consciousness, cyanosis, possibly hemiplegia, amaurosis, and sudden death.

Lavage of the frontal sinus. *Puncture* (as described by Kümmel and Beck) (see also p. 140) can be performed using a fine drill under local anesthesia. This allows irrigation for both diagnostic and therapeutic purposes, and also prolonged drainage of the frontal sinus for 1–2 weeks, allowing daily administration of drugs. The principle of puncture is shown in **Fig. 2.27a–d**.

Technique: Anteroposterior and lateral radiographs of the sinuses have to be obtained first. If the frontal sinus has not developed or is very shallow, there is a risk that the frontal lobe may be punctured.

Irrigation of the sphenoid sinus can be performed by a specialist, using special cannulas.

The ethmoidal labyrinth does not have a defined ostium and therefore cannot be irrigated. However, pathologic secretions can be evacuated using suction.

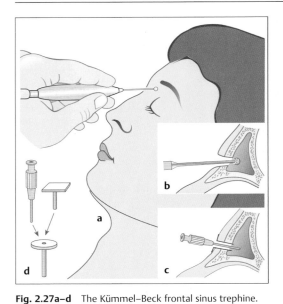

Fig. 2.27a–d   The Kümmel–Beck frontal sinus trephine.
a Access and positioning of the drill.
b The bore hole in the anterior wall of the frontal sinus.
c The guide tube and lavage cannula have been placed.
d The guide tube with the lavage cannula and occlusion plate.

■ Specific Diagnostic Methods

Cytology. Smears of secretions or swabs taken from the mucosa can be assessed cytologically. This is useful for differentiating between catarrh, bacterial infection, allergic rhinitis, and mucosal mycoses.

Allergy studies. Investigations performed on patients include skin tests (scratch, prick, intracutaneous, or friction) and provocation tests (conjunctival and intranasal). Laboratory studies include total immunoglobulin E (IgE) in serum (paper radioimmunosorbent test, PRIST) and specific IgE in serum (radioallergosorbent test, RAST). Eosinophil counts in the blood and nasal secretions are less informative.

Biopsy. This is the method of choice whenever it is unclear whether a disease is benign or malignant.

β_2 Transferrin test. Evidence of CSF rhinorrhea is provided by a positive β_2 transferrin test. In this laboratory test, the ratio of β_1 to β_2 transferrin in the nasal secretions and blood serum is determined. As high β_2 transferrin levels occur only in CSF, they are proof of a CSF leak.

> **Note:** Whenever the diagnosis is not clear, and particularly if a tumor is suspected, a biopsy provides the diagnosis. If the results of the biopsy are negative but a clinical suspicion of malignancy persists, the biopsy needs to be repeated several times, with specimens taken from different sites.

Dermatologic Principles for the Otolaryngologist

Otolaryngologists see dermatologic disorders in the head and neck region every day. They therefore need to understand the basics of dermatologic diagnosis and topical therapy. In some areas, such as the external ear canal, the otorhinolaryngology specialist serves as a "head and neck dermatologist."

Before the conclusion is drawn that a skin finding is a localized change limited to the head and neck region, it needs to be considered whether it might be a regional manifestation of a systemic disease such as lupus erythematosus, systemic sclerosis, or pemphigus vulgaris, or whether it is part of a cutaneous–mucosal disease such as lichen planus or erythema multiforme, to cite but a few dramatic examples.

■ Skin Type

Certain disorders may be more or less common, depending on the skin type. For example, acne vulgaris with follicular comedos, papules, and pustules is more common in those with oily skin (the *seborrheic* skin type), as is rosacea, which features facial erythema, papules, pustules, and sebaceous gland hyperplasia. Rosacea appears in adult life and is occasionally called "adult acne"—an incorrect oversimplification. Atopic dermatitis is more common in those with dry skin (the *sebostatic* skin type). In our experience, healing in oily skin is poorer than in normal or dry skin, an important consideration when planning surgery. The skin type can help one decide to perform a flap rather than primary closure in an oily area.

In describing the skin, a distinction is made between the condition of the skin and its vascular supply. The *skin status* describes turgor, seborrhea, xerosis, atrophy, actinic damage, hyperhidrosis, and hypohidrosis; while the *vascular status* includes factors related to blood supply, such as cyanosis, paleness, cold, warmth, edema, and necrosis.

■ Types of Lesion

Just as the multiplication tables are one of the cornerstones of arithmetic, the terminology and precise description of lesions is a central part of dermatologic knowledge that is necessary for achieving a logical diagnostic approach. Even if the working diagnosis proves to be incorrect, it is easier to advance to the correct diagnosis if the lesions have been precisely and correctly described. If the initial lesions have been poorly described, then it is very difficult to reconstruct a case. The way to describe the different lesions simply has to be learned, therefore—much like learning the words of a foreign language. Describing lesions correctly is extremely important.

A distinction is made between *primary* and *secondary* lesions (**Fig. 2.28a–k**).

Primary lesions

- Macule (spot), urtica (hive), papule (small raised lesion), nodule (larger raised lesion), vesicle (small blister), bulla (large blister), pustule (primary pus-filled blister)

Secondary lesions

- Pustule (vesicle with secondary pus), crust (mixture of pus and scales), scales, erosion (superficial defect of epidermis), excoriation (self-induced defect in the epidermis and upper dermis), rhagades/fissure (linear tear), ulcer (deeper defect), scar, atrophy, cyst (fluid-filled lesion), and necrosis

Primary lesions are fresh lesions that appear as the first sign of a skin disease. Secondary lesions are less sharply defined. They may result from secondary changes in primary lesions (a vesicle becomes a pustule), from exogenous damage (erosion or excoriation), or over time (atrophy, scales). It is more important to describe the lesion correctly than to decide whether it is primary or secondary. It should always be possible to identify a pustule; whether it is primary or secondary can remain an open question.

Along with the type of lesion, the pattern of distribution is also of diagnostic significance. The distribution may be strikingly asymmetrical, segmental, symmetrical, or generalized, as well as fitting light-exposed, hypostatic, or other known patterns. The pattern often facilitates the diagnosis and should therefore always be documented.

Dermatologic differential diagnosis requires a logical approach, as one develops a sense or feeling for the process. At the start, one should consider all the possible diagnoses that fit the morphologic pattern, but always remembering that the most common disorder is the most likely diagnosis. A second important principle is always to consider the possibility of an unusual variation of a common condition; for example, many disorders are more severe or clinically atypical in patients with human immunodeficiency virus/acquired immune deficiency syndrome (HIV/AIDS).

■ Basics of Topical Dermatologic Therapy

Topical therapy has a special role in treatment. The medication is directly applied to the site of disease, and its effect is easily observed without complex instrumentation. A distinction is made between *vehicle, active ingredient,* and *additives.* Most topical agents contain all three components. The active ingredient is the pharmaceutical agent that is to be delivered to the skin in a vehicle. Additives can play many roles, making the vehicles more attractive (with fragrance) or stable (through preservatives). While in the past many formulations contained multiple active ingredients, today most have one or at most two such agents, reducing the likelihood of drug interactions.

Three different types or phases of vehicle are available: solid, liquid, and semisolid. They can all be combined in various ways. A favorite way of visualizing this is using a phase triangle, in which the corners represent the basic phases, while the sides of the triangle signify mixtures of two classes and the center represents a mixture of all three (**Fig. 2.29**).

The vehicles available for topical therapy can also be divided into two groups:

Primary vehicles (one phase): These are the corners of the phase triangle. They include:

- Solids (powders).
- Liquids (wet soaks, solutions).
- Semisolids (ointments, petrolatum, oils).

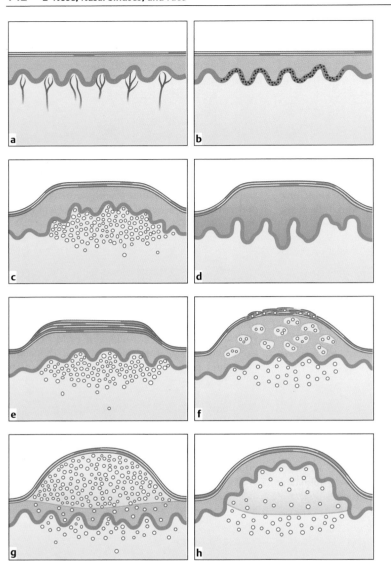

Fig. 2.28a–k The most important types of skin lesion.
a Erythema of a macule, due to circumscribed vasodilation.
b Brown discoloration of a macule, due to a circumscribed increase in pigmentation in the basal layer of the epidermis.
c Dermal papule, due to accumulation of cellular elements in the dermis.
d Epidermal papule, due to thickening of the epidermis.
e Mixed papule, due to thickening of the epidermis, including the stratum corneum, and dermal inflammatory infiltrate.
f Eczema nodules, due to thickening of the epidermis and spongiform edema, with round-cell infiltrates in both the parakeratotic stratum corneum and dermis.
g Subcorneal pustule, in which the stratum corneum is lifted from the rest of the epidermis by edema fluid and leukocytes; there are leukocytic infiltrates in both the epidermis and dermis.
h Subepithelial blister, in which the entire epidermis is lifted by an accumulation of fluid; the dermis contains an inflammatory infiltrate.

Fig. 2.28 i—k ▷

Combined vehicles (two or more phases) fall between the corners, depending on their composition:

- Emulsions (ointments (oil/water, water/oil), creams).
- Shake lotions.
- Pastes.

Principles for Choosing a Vehicle

The correct choice of a vehicle can greatly enhance healing, while an inappropriate vehicle can have adverse effects, even if exactly the correct active ingredient has been chosen. One should try to work with as few vehicles as possible, in order to get to know them well and acquire experience in administering them. The choice of vehicle is based on the skin type, involved area, acuteness of inflammation, and type of lesion.

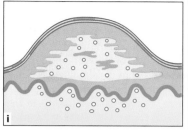

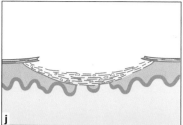

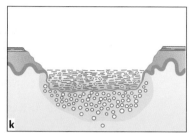

Fig. 2.28 i Intraepithelial blister; acantholysis within the epidermis has led to the formation of an irregular space containing leukocytes and desquamated scales.

j Erosion: a shallow defect in the epidermis, partially filled with serum and leukocyte detritus.

k Ulcer: a defect extending into the reticular dermis and involving destruction of the epidermis and adnexal structures (sweat glands, sebaceous glands and hair follicles), as well as papillary dermis. The defect is partially filled with serum and leukocytic detritus, and the adjacent dermis shows inflammatory infiltrates.

Skin type. *Seborrheic skin:* Powders, alcoholic solutions, shake lotions, creams; no greasy vehicles.

Sebostatic skin: Ointments, ointment emulsions, soft pastes; no drying or only minimally greasy vehicles.

Special body regions. *Scalp:* Aqueous or alcoholic solutions, easily washed emulsion creams; no pure ointments (petrolatum), pastes or shake lotions.

Intertriginous areas: Soft zinc pastes, creams, zinc oils; no shake lotions or thick ointments.

Degree of inflammation. *Acute superficial inflammation:* Dye solutions, moist dressings, powders, shake lotions, creams. Clearly weeping dermatoses should be treated with wet dressings or greasy–wet dressings (slightly greasy dressing covered with wet soaks). Occlusive dressings should not be used for weeping dermatoses, pyodermas, or fungal infections.

Chronic deeper inflammation: Vehicles are required that can ensure penetration of the active ingredients such as ointments, ointment emulsions, soft pastes, and emollient creams, but no powders, shake lotions, or wet dressings.

Morphology of skin changes. *Acute erythema:* Powders, shake lotions, creams, wet dressings.

Vesicles and bullae: Shake lotions, creams, moist dressings, greasy–wet system (greasy vehicle covered by wet dressing).

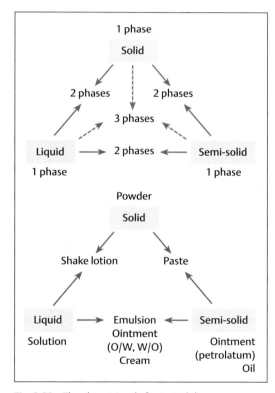

Fig. 2.29 The phase triangle for topical therapy.

Erosions: Wet dressings (wet or greasy–wet), ointments.

Crusts: Wet dressings (wet or greasy–wet), ointments, emollient ointments, soft pastes.

Scales: Ointments, emollient ointments, soft pastes, greasy–wet dressings.

Chronic infiltrates or lichenification: Ointments, emollient ointment, soft pastes.

Atrophy, scars: Ointments, emollient ointments, soft pastes.

Examples of Topical Active Ingredients

Urea: Hygroscopic (binds water), keratolytic, proteolytic, increases penetration, anti-pruritic and weakly anti-proliferative. Non-sensitizing, but irritating, depending on concentration. Indication: dry, pruritic skin.

Salicylic acid: Very keratolytic, weakly anti-inflammatory and antimicrobial, irritating in active inflammation. Usually combined with other active ingredients, such as a topical corticosteroid for pruritic otitis externa. Formulation: acid. salicyl. 3.0, hydroxyquinoline sulf. 0.25, dexamethasone 0.03, ung. alcohol. lanae aquosum ad 100.0.

Corticosteroids: Depending on choice of agent and concentration, varying degrees of effectiveness. Care is also needed on the face, with a preference for lower concentrations and less active agents; in case of infection, corticosteroids should not be used as a single agent, but only as a supplementary anti-infectious therapy. Because they are simply the best topical anti-inflammatory agents, corticosteroids are often used for otorhinolaryngology indications. Formulation (for weeping otitis externa): prednisolone 0.02, ol. zinci oxydat. ad 50.0.

Dyes and antiseptics: Dermatologists nowadays rarely use gentian violet, brilliant green, or Castellani paint (carbolfuchsin topical solution). These products are highly effective, but compliance tends to be poor. From the otorhinolaryngology point of view, these solutions are still valuable because of their good antiseptic, antimycotic, and drying effects. The main difference from dermatologic use is the employment of much smaller amounts at lower concentrations to treat limited areas such as the external ear canal. Formulation of Castellani solution (without phenol): ethanol fuchsin solution 4 % 2.0, chlorocresol 0.02, resorcin 2.0, sodium edetate 0.004, acetone 1.0, aqua purificata ad 20.0.

Our approach to acute otitis externa is to start with a nonspecific dye solution and only to use antibiotics in a targeted or at least calculated way, based on culture results or knowledge of the likely causative agents. One should always avoid indiscriminate use of multiple agents.

Antibiotics: The use of topical antibiotics is somewhat controversial in dermatology. The main reasons for this include the development of resistance and allergic sensitization, which can then leave the individual intolerant to the same or related agents administered systemically. There are many alternatives for most forms of topical antibiotic therapy. The active agents that are still in use after a long period of time and have proved their effectiveness include the following (with examples of representative products):

- *Gentamicin sulfate:* Gentamicin cream 0.1 %, gentamicin ointment 0.1 %.
- *Erythromycin:* Akne-Mycin ointment or solution, Zineryt (solution with zinc acetate), Clinofug gel 2 %/4 %.
- *Oxytetracycline HCl:* Terramycin ointment (with polymyxin B), oxytetracycline ointment 1 %.

Clinical Aspects of Diseases of the Nose, Sinuses, and Face

The main symptoms of diseases of the nose and sinuses are:
- Increased nasal secretion.
- Nasal obstruction.
- Bleeding or hemorrhagic secretion (see **Tables 2.11, 2.12**).
- Fetor.
- Altered or absent sense of smell (see **Tables 2.1, 2.2**).
- Pain in the head or face.
- Disease of neighboring organs—e. g., teeth, the lacrimal apparatus, eyes, mouth, and throat. Important symptoms of eye disease include abnormalities of refraction, limitation of the visual field, acute loss of vision, and displacement of the orbit. Diseases of the mouth and throat may be symptomatic, or a change in the quality of the voice and speech may be noted.

■ Inflammatory Diseases of the Nose and Paranasal Sinuses

■ Inflammations Confined Mainly to the External Nose

The skin of the nose and the face may be affected by the same common typical skin diseases that affect the rest of the skin, such as impetigo, acne, trichophyton, rosacea, and lupus erythematosus. These diseases are treated using the appropriate dermatologic methods.

Other skin diseases that are particularly important in the nasal area are described below.

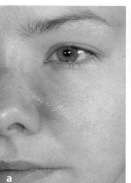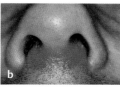

Fig. 2.30a, b   Nasal furuncle.

Nasal Eczema

Clinical Features. The disease is moist in the early phases, with vesicles and pustules. Later, crusts form, followed by painful cracks. In the chronic stage, there is itching, burning, and desquamation. The disease is localized to the external nose and the skin of the nasal vestibule and never affects the nasal mucosa.

Pathogenesis. The disease is often caused by abnormal nasal secretions, but may also be due to a contact allergy (sensitivity testing should be carried out). Promoting factors include diabetes mellitus, generalized eczema, and dietary sensitivity in children.

Treatment. The crusts should be softened with a mild greasy ointment followed by a corticosteroid (hydrocortisone). The use of stronger steroids should be avoided on facial skin. Cracks are treated with 5–10 % silver nitrate solution. The cause should be looked for and treated or eliminated.

Folliculitis of the Nasal Vestibule (Sycosis) and Nasal Furuncle

Clinical Features. Increasing pain, marked sensitivity to pressure, and a feeling of tension in the tip of the nose are followed by reddening and swelling of the tip of the nose, of the nasal ala, and of the upper lip (**Fig. 2.30a, b**). The area becomes edematous, and the patient may have fever. The swelling may begin to resolve before suppuration occurs. Otherwise, a typical furuncle forms, containing pus and a central necrotic core.

Diagnosis. An ascending infection via the facial vein has to be ruled out by testing the medial angle of the eye for tenderness.

Pathogenesis. A pyoderma, usually due to staphylococcal infection, arises from the hair follicles of the nasal vestibule or the upper lip, often close to the nasal tip. The disease is always limited to the skin and never affects the mucosa.

Treatment. Antibiotic creams, such as 2 % mupirocin (Bactroban) or 0.1 % chlorhexidine/0.5 % neomycin (Naseptin) cream or ethacridine lactate solution, are applied to the nasal vestibule as long as the disease remains a circumscribed folliculitis. Manipulation in the nose is contraindicated. If it is suspected that a furuncle is forming, high-dose oral or parenteral antibiotics are given, if necessary in combination with topical antibiotics. The antibiotics of choice for systemic bactericidal therapy are cefadroxil, flucloxacillin (floxacillin), or doxycycline; in severe cases, cefazolin or an aminopenicillin with a β-lactamase inhibitor. Antibiotics must be continued for several days after the symptoms have subsided; they should not be discontinued too early or used at too low a dosage. If an infection is severe, the patient will need hospital admission and intravenous antibiotic and fluid administration.

If there is tenderness in the medial angle of the eye, the facial artery and vein must be ligated.

Note: A furuncle on the nose or upper lip must never be squeezed, due to the risk of spreading the infection and causing complications such as thrombophlebitis and cavernous sinus thrombosis (see p. 117). The veins of the nose and upper lip drain into the venous system of the neck via the facial vein, but also via the angular and ophthalmic veins through the orbit to the cavernous sinus. **Figure 2.2** shows the relevant anatomy, and the point at which the angular vein may be ligated if incipient thrombophlebitis is suspected.

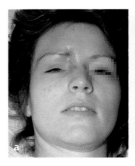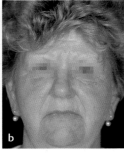

Fig. 2.31a, b   a Acute erysipelas: sharply demarcated erubescence in the vicinity of a skin injury.
b Chronic erysipelas: persistent, edematous, rubescent skin with swelling.

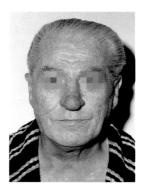

Fig. 2.32   Rhinophyma.

Frostbite and Burns
The nose is particularly at risk for frostbite and sunburn in extremes of weather and temperature. The injury is divided into three degrees of severity, with the most severe being dry or moist tissue necrosis.

Treatment. As for thermal damage to other parts of the body.

Erysipelas
Clinical Features. The incubation period lasts several hours to 2 days. The disease starts with high fever and possibly chills. There is marked pain and sharply demarcated reddening of the edematous skin. Often there is extension on both sides of the nasal pyramid in a butterfly configuration. The disease usually resolves within 1 week with proper treatment. Treatment must be energetic and high-dose, as the disease tends to recur (**Fig. 2.31a, b**).

Pathogenesis. The causative organism is usually a streptococcus. The portal of entry is often a small abrasion on the skin.

Differential diagnosis. Angioneurotic edema, acute dermatitis, and herpes zoster must be considered.

Treatment. Penicillin is the first-line drug. It should be given intravenously to begin with, and continued for 10 days. In severe cases, 10 million IU per day may be required. Alternatively, erythromycin, cephalosporins, or macrolides may be given. Antibiotics are continued for 8 days after the eruptions subside, and local moist dressings are applied.

Prognosis. Good.

Rhinophyma
Clinical Features. The condition starts with coarsening of the skin over the cartilaginous part of the nose. A lumpy, bluish-red pseudotumor develops and slowly progresses to become a markedly protuberant lobular swelling of the anterior part of the nose, which may even obstruct breathing and eating. This disease usually occurs in older men (**Fig. 2.32**).

Pathogenesis. Rhinophyma is due to hypertrophy of the sebaceous glands. It is associated with acne rosacea.

Treatment. The disease is treated surgically. The tissue is removed in layers with a scalpel, CO_2 laser, or by dermabrasion, and is shaved down to the level of the normal nasal contour. The area is then allowed to heal spontaneously, or is covered with a split-skin graft.

Lupus Vulgaris of the Nose
Clinical Features. Fine red nodules are found on the nasal vestibule, the head of the inferior turbinate, and the septum lying opposite to it. The nodular stage is followed by central necrosis of the nodules, with ulceration and formation of granulomas, and finally scarring with deformity of the underlying cartilage. The nasal introitus becomes stenosed, and the cartilaginous framework of the nose collapses (**Fig. 2.33**).

Pathogenesis. The disease is due to tuberculous infection in the presence of relatively robust immunologic resistance (the proliferative form). The organism responsible is *Mycobacterium tuberculosis*, either the human or bovine type.

Diagnosis. The diagnosis is reached by demonstrating the infectious agent and by biopsy. Diagnosis of the disease is notifiable. Characteristic findings are intradermal papules that ulcerate, leaving scars.

Differential diagnosis. Eczema of the nasal introitus, anterior rhinitis sicca, perforating ulcer of the septum, syphilis, mycosis, lupus erythematosus, sarcoid, and malignancy. Tuberculosis usually affects the cartilaginous parts of the nose, whereas syphilis attacks the bony part.

Treatment. Long-term triple combinations of tuberculostatic drugs (see p. 156) and vitamin D_2 are given.

Sarcoidosis (Besnier–Boeck–Schaumann Disease)

Clinical Features. Sarcoidosis is a multisystem disorder of unknown etiology that may occur as an isolated lesion in the nose. Nasal sarcoid presents with nasal obstruction, recurrent epistaxis, crusting, and/or anosmia. Examination may show red nodules within the nasal mucosa giving the appearance of strawberry skin, nasal tenderness, and occasionally infiltration of the facial skin. There may also be a saddle deformity and septal perforation and facial swelling. There may also be associated sinusitis. Regional lymph nodes may be firm and enlarged.

Diagnosis. If nasal sarcoidosis is suspected, a vasculitic screen should be instigated. This should include a full blood count; ESR & CRP; serum biochemistry and calcium; angiotensin converting enzyme (ACE); ANCA and syphilis serology. Urine should be checked for blood and protein and a 24-hour urinary calcium assessment.

The serum ACE diagnosis is usually elevated in active sarcoidosis but is a non-specific non-diagnostic test. The diagnosis relies on obtaining a biopsy that shows non-caseating granulomata. A chest radiograph and/or chest CT should also be requested.

Differential diagnosis. This includes rhinophyma, lupus, gumma, and malignancy.

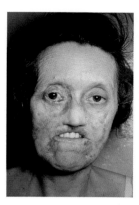

Fig. 2.33 Lupus vulgaris.

Treatment. Systemic steroids are the mainstay of treatment for active disease and should be administered under supervision of a rheumatologist. Immunosuppressive or immunomodulation medication such as methotrexate or an anti-TNF alpha blocker (infliximab) can be helpful in limiting systemic steroid use. Surgery may be considered for sinusitis or to reduce the obstruction from large inferior turbinates, but septal/reconstructive surgery can induce further inflammatory change within the nose and is best deferred until the condition becomes less active.

Syphilis

Syphilis became a rarity after the advent of penicillin, but it has become quite common again and its incidence is increasing.

Clinical Features. *Stage 1* is usually marked by the appearance of a single sore (chancre), but there may be multiple sores. *Stage 2* begins ≈ 9 weeks after the infection. It is characterized by bacteremia, generalized exanthema, mucous membrane lesions, flu-like systemic signs and symptoms, and the production of antibodies. *Stage 3* occurs more than 2 years after the primary infection and shows gummatous infiltration with painful swelling of the bony part of the nose, foul-smelling secretions, formation of sequestra, sharply demarcated ulceration, and usually regional lymphadenopathy. Finally, the typical saddle nose develops, affecting the bony part of the nose, and firm, radiating scars form within the nose (**Fig. 2.34**).

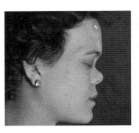

Fig. 2.34 Syphilitic saddle nose.

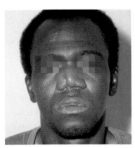

Fig. 2.35 Rhino-scleroma.

Pathogenesis. This illness is due to an infection with *Treponema pallidum*. Intrauterine infection may cause early congenital syphilis within the first months of life, or late congenital syphilis beginning between the age of 3 years and puberty, but accompanied by the triad of interstitial keratitis, Hutchinson teeth, and inner ear deafness. The infection may also be acquired (extrauterine) after birth.

Diagnosis. This is based on the history, serology (which is not always positive in stage 3), Nelson test (*Treponema pallidum* immobilization test, TPI), and biopsy.

Differential diagnosis. Tuberculosis and malignancy must be considered.

Treatment. Antibiotics are administered under the supervision of a venereologist. Local treatment may be required in stage 3. Once the lesion has healed, reconstruction of the defect may be required. The antibiotic of choice is penicillin. In the early stage, benzathine penicillin should be administered intramuscularly at a dose of 2.4 million IU (1.2 million IU in each buttock) as a single dose. In case of penicillin allergy, doxycycline is the usual choice (100 mg b. i. d. p. o. for 14 days); alternatively, erythromycin (500 mg q. i. d. p. o. for 14 days) can be used. In the late stage, the same dose of benzathine penicillin is injected intramuscularly on days 1, 8, and 15. Alternatively, doxycycline (200 mg b. i. d. p. o. for 28 days) or erythromycin (2 g i. v. daily for 21 days) may be given.

Rhinoscleroma

Epidemiology. This disease occurs in eastern Europe, North Africa, Central and South America, and Asia.

Clinical Features. The disease starts with an atypical rhinitis with purulent secretion and crusts. A flat, nodular infiltrate then appears in the nasal mucosa. There is increasing coarsening of the external nose (tapir nose). The lesion heals with extensive scarring (**Fig. 2.35**).

Pathogenesis. The infectious organism is *Klebsiella rhinoscleromatis*.

Diagnosis. This depends on the history, with particular attention to foreign travel, and on the results of biopsy and microbiologic studies.

Differential diagnosis. This consists of tuberculosis, syphilis, sarcoid, mycoses, and Hodgkin disease.

Treatment. Antibiotics are given, as dictated by culture and sensitivity tests.

Prognosis. The outcome is uncertain and recurrence is possible.

Leprosy

Epidemiology. The disease occurs in tropical and subtropical regions.

Clinical Features. A bulbous thickening in the nasal vestibule, obstruction of the nasal cavity, extensive crusting, fetid secretion, ulceration and liquefaction of the nasal framework, and leonine facies may occur.

Pathogenesis. The disease is due to an infection with *Mycobacterium leprae* (Hansen).

Diagnosis. This is based on history of contact, symptoms of infection of other parts of the body, and neurologic lesions that are exclusively sensory. Culture and the lepromin reaction also form part of the investigations.

Treatment. Single skin lesions: rifampicin 600 mg as a single dose. Paucibacillary disease (tuberculoid leprosy): dapsone 100 mg daily and rifampicin monthly for 6 months. Multibacillary disease (lepromatous leprosy): rifampicin 600 mg and clofazimine 300 mg, both monthly for 12 months.

■ Acute and Chronic Inflammations Localized Mainly in the Nasal Cavity

Diseases arising primarily within the nasal cavity are discussed here separately from those arising in the nasal sinuses, although disease of the nose may originate in the sinuses and vice versa.

Acute Inflammations of the Nasal Cavity

Acute Rhinitis

Clinical Features. Since the common cold can be caused by different organisms, the symptoms are not uniform. In the common form, there is a *dry prodromal stage* with generalized symptoms, including chills and a feeling of cold alternating with a feeling of heat, headache, fatigue, loss of appetite, possibly subfebrile temperature, but often a high temperature in children, as well as itching, burning, a feeling of dryness in the nose and throat, and nasal irritation. The nasal mucosa is usually pale and dry. The *catarrhal stage* usually begins a few hours later, with watery secretions, nasal obstruction, temporary loss of smell, lacrimation, rhinolalia clausa, and worsening of the constitutional symptoms. The nasal mucosa is deep red in color, swollen, and secretes profusely. After several days, the disease changes to a *mucous phase.* The generalized symptoms begin to improve, the secretions thicken, the sense of smell improves, and local symptoms gradually regress. Resolution should be achieved within a week. The common cold, or viral rhinosinusitis, is defined as duration of symptoms for less than 10 days.

Secondary bacterial infection may occur. The secretions then turn greenish-yellow, and the disease resolves more slowly. Acute intermittent nonviral rhinosinusitis is defined as an increase of symptoms after 10 days, with a duration of less than 12 weeks (**Fig. 2.36**).

Initial catarrh occurs in influenza and infection with other types of viruses such as parainfluenza virus, adenovirus, reovirus, coronavirus, enterovirus, myxovirus, and respiratory syncytial virus. The symptoms are as described above, but are complicated by other manifestations such as involvement of the entire respiratory tract, the gastrointestinal tract (causing diarrhea), the meninges, the pericardium, the kidneys, and the muscles.

Pathogenesis. The infection is caused by a rhinovirus. More than 100 types belonging to the picornavirus group

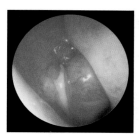

Fig. 2.36 Purulent rhinosinusitis. The mucosa is edematous and hyperemic. A track of pus is seen in the middle nasal meatus.

have been isolated. The disease may also be caused by numerous other viruses. The incubation period of the rhinovirus is from 1 to 3 days. The disease is spread by droplet infection and is exacerbated by cooling of the body.

The most common pathogens in purulent bacterial rhinosinusitis are *Streptococcus pneumoniae, Haemophilus influenzae, Moraxella catarrhalis, Staphylococcus aureus, Streptococcus pyogenes,* and various anaerobes.

Diagnosis. Initially, it is often not clear whether a runny nose is the initial symptom or an accompanying symptom of a severe virus infection.

Differential diagnosis. This can often be made only after a few days. It includes the initial phase of an acute exanthema, allergic or vasomotor rhinitis, congenital syphilis, and nasal diphtheria (usually in children).

Treatment. There is no treatment for the basic cause. Symptomatic treatment includes decongestant nose drops or oral decongestants. Antibiotics should only be given for secondary bacterial infection, and culture and sensitivity tests should be carried out beforehand. Steam inhalations, treatment with infrared lamps, analgesics, and bed rest should be prescribed if necessary.

Prevention. While there is no scientific evidence that prevention is possible, measures to improve general health may be helpful. These include building up the patient's overall resistance using sauna baths, therapeutic regimens at health resorts, hydrotherapy, participation in sports, administration of vitamin C, and scrupulous hygiene, especially in contact with young children. Adenoidectomy may be necessary in children (see p. 243). Immunization against rhinoviruses is not yet possible, but there are vaccines against influenza.

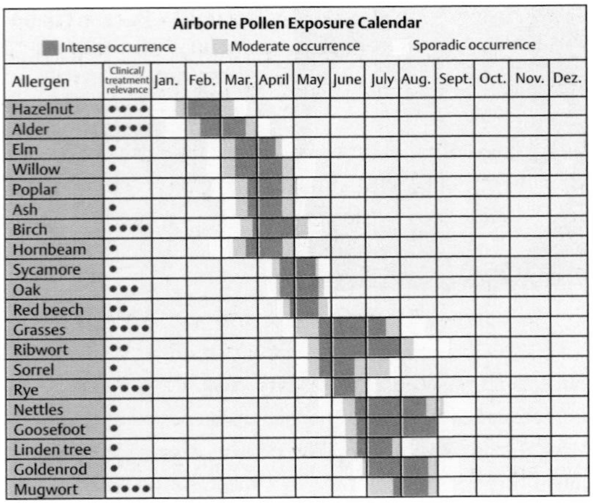

| Airborne Pollen Exposure Calendar |||||||||||||||
Allergen	Clinical/treatment relevance	Jan.	Feb.	Mar.	April	May	June	July	Aug.	Sept.	Oct.	Nov.	Dez.
Hazelnut	••••												
Alder	••••												
Elm	•												
Willow	•												
Poplar	•												
Ash	•												
Birch	••••												
Hornbeam	•												
Sycamore	•												
Oak	•••												
Red beech	••												
Grasses	••••												
Ribwort	••												
Sorrel	•												
Rye	••••												
Nettles	•												
Goosefoot	•												
Linden tree	•												
Goldenrod	•												
Mugwort	••••												

■ Intense occurrence   Moderate occurrence   Sporadic occurrence

Fig. 2.37   Example of airborne pollen exposure calendar.

Allergic Rhinitis

Allergic rhinitis is mainly a type I allergic reaction. In this type of anaphylactic hypersensitivity reaction, cutaneous or mucocutaneous symptoms develop either immediately or within a few minutes after exposure. The most common form is hay fever, but other allergens may be responsible.

Clinical Features. These include itching in the nose, nasal obstruction, sneezing attacks, and a clear, watery nasal discharge. The patient may also have a feeling of stuffiness and irritation of the entire head, possibly conjunctivitis, malaise, temporary fever, loss of appetite, autonomic symptoms, possibly inability to work, and temporary hyposmia or anosmia. Secondary infection is possible.

Pathogenesis. An inhalation allergy is the cause. The shock organ is usually the nasal mucosa, but it may also be the conjunctiva or other mucous membranes. The disease is often hereditary.

Seasonal allergic rhinitis is caused by pollen (**Fig. 2.37**).

Perennial allergic rhinitis is due to an inhaled allergen, regardless of the season. The allergens include fungi, animal hair, house dust mites, houseplants such as primroses and roses, and also foods such as fish, strawberries, nuts, eggs, milk, and flour. There are occupational allergies—e. g., to flour for bakers, to hair and epithelial scales for hair-

dressers, etc.—and other allergies to bacteria and parasites.

Infection and allergy: Bacteria and viruses can act as allergens, but the practical significance of this is still controversial. Three pathogenetic mechanisms are possible:

1. An allergic reaction to bacteria or viruses without clinical infection—e. g., to nasal saprophytes.
2. An allergic reaction to bacterial or viral infection—e. g., chronic bacterial rhinitis or sinusitis with resultant sensitivity to the causative organism.
3. Secondary infection in tissue already altered by allergic reaction. In this case, the infective agent is not the same as the antigen.

The second form corresponds to the term "infection allergy." Its time course classifies it as a *late allergic reaction*.

If an infective allergy is suspected, tests should be carried out for the antigen (i. e., a positive cutaneous late reaction to a bacterial extract), and antibiotics should be given depending on the sensitivity tests. The long-term value of hyposensitization has not yet been confirmed in clinical practice.

Diagnosis. This is made primarily on the basis of the history. Investigations include cytology of the nasal secretions, intracutaneous tests, prick tests, and patch tests, intranasal challenge with rhinomanometry, olfactometry, measurement of serum and secretion IgE, and RAST.

Local findings. The nasal mucosa is livid and pale. In acute stages, the mucosa may also be deep red. The turbinates are swollen, and there are copious amounts of clear secretion.

Differential diagnosis. Nasal hyperreactivity/idiopathic rhinitis and acute rhinitis (coryza) must be considered.

Treatment. *Symptomatic:* The World Health Organization (WHO) has published guidelines on Allergic Rhinitis and its Impact on Asthma (ARIA), which make the following recommendations:

- Mild to moderate symptoms (e. g., first manifestation of allergic rhinoconjunctivitis): a third-generation oral antihistamine (e. g., levocetirizine, desloratadine) or a topical antihistamine (e. g., an azelastine nasal spray), if necessary with concomitant use of antihistamine eyedrops.

Table 2.5 Allergic Rhinitis and its Impact on Asthma (ARIA) guidelines classification of rhinitis

Infectious	Viral, bacterial or due to other pathogens
Allergic	Intermittent, persistent
Occupational (allergic and nonallergic)	Intermittent, persistent
Drug-induced	Intolerance of acetylsalicylic acid or other drugs
Hormonal	
Other causes	Nonallergic rhinitis with eosinophilia syndrome (NARES), irritants, foodstuffs, emotional factors, atrophy, gastroesophageal reflux
Idiopathic	

- Marked nasal symptoms: a combination of an oral antihistamine and a topical steroid (e.g., mometasone, fluticasone, triamcinolone).
- Severe nasal obstruction: brief application of a nasal decongestant containing an α-sympathomimetic drug. Hyposensitization: short-term titration and co-seasonal hyposensitization treatment. Causative therapy: specific immune therapy is the only treatment modality to address the underlying cause. It can prevent the development of allergic asthma.

Principle of specific immune therapy: Standardized allergen extracts of dominant single allergens (major allergens), native or polymerized (chemically modified) extracts—i.e., so-called allergoids—are used. They are bound to a carrier such as aluminum hydroxide, tyrosine, or calcium phosphate. Application may be subcutaneous (subcutaneous immune therapy, SCIT) or sublingual (sublingual immune therapy, SLIT).

Immunologic effects: T lymphocytes are influenced by the activation of regulatory CD4$^+$ T cells (IL-10, transforming growth factor β), inducing immediate hyposensitivity (lowered cytokine production) and replacement of T helper subset 2 (TH2) dominance (IL-4, IL-5, IL-13) with a TH1 response. This in turn affects the production of immunoglobulins by B lymphocytes and inhibits effector cells (e.g., mast cells, basophilic leukocytes, and eosinophilic granulocytes).

Effectiveness: Pollen allergy: symptoms decreased in 30%; grass and birch allergies in 45%; dust allergies in 30%.

Surgery: Indications for surgery have to be established in septal deviation, turbinate hyperplasia, nasal polyps, rhinosinusitis, or adenoids.

Prognosis. This is generally good. The disease gradually regresses as the patients get older, but progression to bronchial asthma (or vice versa) is possible.

Complications. Involvement of the nasal sinuses and the lower respiratory tract, and polyps of the nose and sinuses are possible.

Idiopathic Rhinitis (Nasal Hyperreactivity, Vasomotor Rhinitis)
The WHO's ARIA guidelines recommend that the term "idiopathic rhinitis" should be used instead of noninfectious and vasomotor rhinitis. The synopsis of classifications in the ARIA report and the consensus report on nasal hyperreactivity defines idiopathic rhinitis as a group of nasal oversensitivity syndromes due to unknown pathomechanisms. Idiopathic rhinitis is a diagnosis of exclusion; it is considered present if the forms of rhinitis and differential diagnoses listed in **Table 2.5** can be ruled out.

Clinical Features. The International Consensus Report on the Diagnosis and Management of Rhinitis (1994) requires at least two symptoms from the group *urge to sneeze, runny nose, nasal obstruction, and/or itching,* lasting for more than 1 h per day. Healthy individuals may sneeze or wipe their noses up to four times daily.

Pathogenesis. There are three pathomechanisms:
1. *Neuronal dysfunction* (**Fig. 2.38**): Neurogenic inflammation is mediated by neurotransmitters and interacts in many ways with the immune system. Activation of *neurokinine-1 receptors* in the airways causes contraction of smooth muscles, dilation of blood vessels, glandular secretion, and extravasation of plasma proteins. Activation of *neurokinine-2 receptors* causes bronchoconstriction and stimulates afferent nerves. Hyposympathicotonia or hyperparasympathicotonia leads to obstruction and hypersecretion.
2. *Immune inflammatory disorders*: Among others, CD3$^+$, CD25$^+$, CD8$^+$, CD45RA$^+$, and T cells, eosinophils, and mast cells are increased.
3. *Mucosal damage,* with increased permeability for irritants.

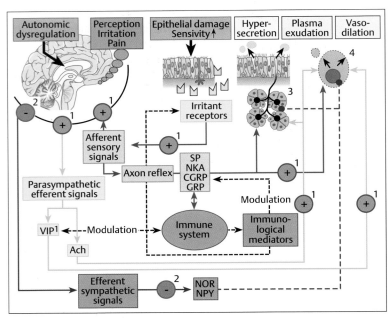

Fig. 2.38 Diagram of neural regulation of the nasal mucosa and its disorders in idiopathic rhinitis. **1**, Enhanced, **2**, reduced neural activity; increased density of innervation or release of neurotransmitters; **3**, glands of the nasal mucosa; **4**, blood vessels, vasodilation. **SP**, Substance P; **NKA**, neurokinin A; **CGRP**, calcitonin gene-related peptide; **GRP**, gastrin-releasing peptide; **NOR**, norepinephrine; **NPY**, neuropeptide Y; **Ach**, acetylcholine; **VIP1**, vasoactive interstitial peptide + VIP-like peptide (adapted from Damm M. Idiopathic Rhinitis. Laryngo-Rhino-Otol. 2006; 85:365).

Diagnosis. History, nasal endoscopy, rhinomanometry, acoustic rhinometry, allergy tests.

Treatment. *Medical:*
1. Ipratropium bromide (anticholinergic, 80–100 mg/day) is effective against rhinorrhea.
2. Topical corticosteroids are effective against symptoms such as obstruction, rhinorrhea, and postnasal drip.
3. Azelastine (antihistamine, 1.1 mg/day) works well against rhinorrhea, sneezing, obstruction, and postnasal drip.
4. An isotonic salt-water spray may be an effective treatment in mild cases.

Surgical: Invasive and surgical measures are considered only after conservative treatment has failed. Severing the nerve of the pterygoid canal (vidian nerve) used to be done to interrupt the parasympathetic innervation of the nose. This treatment option should first be simulated by reversible and repeatable blockade of the sphenopalatine ganglion. To reduce the cavernous tissue in the lower turbinate to counteract both obstruction and hypersecretion, several options such as partial excision, submucosal resection with a microdebrider, caustic agents, radiofrequency therapy (Coblation), or laser therapy, can be considered.

Foreign Bodies in the Nose
Foreign bodies are found in children in most cases and may have been retained for a very long time (**Fig. 2.39**). They include coins, metal fragments, peas, etc.

Clinical Features. These include unilateral nasal obstruction, worsening chronic purulent rhinitis or sinusitis, unilateral fetid secretions, and formation of a rhinolith due to deposition of calcium and magnesium salts around the foreign body.

Diagnosis. This is based on anterior rhinoscopy, nasal endoscopy, and radiology. A foreign body is often an incidental finding. The nose is inspected and probed using an endoscope after decongestion and induction of local anesthesia.

Treatment. The foreign body is removed instrumentally, if necessary under brief general anesthesia, as foreign bodies that have been present for a prolonged period are often firmly attached and provoke brisk bleeding when mobilized.

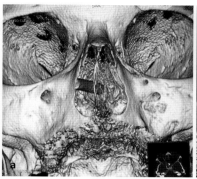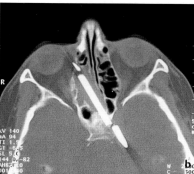

Fig. 2.39a, b In this patient, a pencil had perforated the paranasal sinus system and anterior skull base between the carotid artery and the optic nerve. It was removed 55 years later.

Note: Unilateral chronic purulent rhinorrhea in a small child should suggest the diagnosis of a foreign body, and the child must be examined by a specialist.

Chronic Inflammations of the Nasal Cavity

Rhinitis Sicca Anterior

Clinical Features. These include a feeling of dryness, irritation, formation of crusts in the nose, and also occasional mild nasal bleeding (**Fig. 2.40a, b**).

Pathogenesis. Several factors are responsible, such as injury to the exposed parts of the anterior nasal mucosa, dust, nose-picking, extremes of temperature, etc.

Diagnosis. The nasal mucosa on the anterior part of the nasal septum immediately posterior to the mucocutaneous junction is dry. The mucosal surface is raw, roughened, and granular. Crusts form, followed by ulceration and at times a subsequent septal perforation.

Differential diagnosis. Included here are chemical injury in chromium workers, iatrogenic septal perforation after surgery or incorrect cauterization, trauma, lupus, leprosy, and syphilis.

Treatment. Mild nasal oils that adhere well to the mucosa are applied. Saline spray is also useful. Septal perforation is discussed on p. 201.

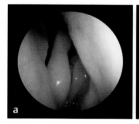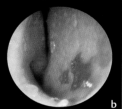

Fig. 2.40a, b The mucosa in chronic rhinitis sicca (0° lens, 4 mm).
a Normal mucosa
b Dry mucosa without a mucus layer, with bleeding at the anterior deviated septum.

Chronic Rhinitis (Nonspecific Inflammation of the Nasal Mucosa)

Chronic rhinitis is one of the most common health-care problems, with a severe impact on lower airway disease and overall health. It is characterized by hypertrophy of the nasal mucosa, especially around the nasal turbinates, as well as by either hyperemia and edema, or true tissue hypertrophy.

Clinical Features. The main symptom is nasal obstruction, which fluctuates markedly in the early stages and also alternates from side to side. Later, it becomes continual and severe, and usually affects both sides. The secretions are viscous, stringy, colorless, and only rarely purulent. Postnasal catarrh is particularly prominent, with sniffles and compulsive throat clearing. Other symptoms include rhinolalia clausa, epiphora, secondary dacryocystitis, and secondary pharyngitis. In severe cases, fatigue, insomnia, an unsteady or woozy feeling in the head, and, occasionally, headache and a feeling of pressure in the head may occur. There is a general loss of psychological and physical well-being.

Pathogenesis. The nasal mucosa is the human immunologic "front line." It is constantly forced to react to countless allergens and antigens. The most important prerequisite for this function is an intact mucociliary apparatus, which supports a wide range of reactions—e. g., absorption, secretion, transportation, cellular or humoral defenses (see p. 127). So-called inflammatory cells (macrophages, granulocytes, leukocytes, and mast cells) are always found on histopathological examination.

Chronic inflammation occurs when the normal capacity to react is overstrained, and it has many etiologies. On the one hand, recurrent inflammatory exacerbations (viral or bacterial) may cause progressive damage to the mucociliary apparatus; on the other hand, variations in anatomic shape (e. g., septal deviation, vomer spur, maxillary crest, polyps, papillomas, adenoids) may elicit chronic rhinopathy.

Cellular changes are described on p. 127.

Chronic inflammation may be due to tobacco smoke and dust, chemicals, environmental toxins, persistent extremes of temperature, abnormal humidity, pregnancy, menstruation, menopause, endocrine disorders (e. g., of the thyroid and adrenal glands, diabetes mellitus), diseases of the heart and circulation, side effects of drugs (see below), or infective allergy.

Diagnosis. The disease is long-standing, and the history often reveals one or more of the toxins named above. Examination shows a dark red and partially bluish-violet swelling, affecting the inferior turbinate especially. The nasal lumen is narrowed or obstructed. The thickened mucosa responds to decongestant nose drops in simple chronic rhinitis, but true tissue hypertrophy in chronic hyperplastic rhinitis does not.

In the later stages, the mucosa over the turbinates develops a slightly granular surface, which gradually becomes nodular and demonstrates micropolyps. These edematous processes can develop into single or multiple *nasal polyps*, especially around the inferior turbinate. Often, this true tissue hypertrophy begins at the posterior ends of the turbinates, usually of the inferior turbinate. The choanae are then blocked by mulberry-shaped masses, which can be seen only on endoscopic examination of the nasopharynx or on indirect examination with a mirror.

Differential diagnosis. This includes sinusitis, foreign bodies, specific infections of the nasal mucosa (see pp. 147, 156), adenoidal hypertrophy, allergy, Wegener granulomatosis, and tumors. Biopsy should be performed if appropriate.

Treatment. *Conservative:* Any known or suspected etiologic agents should be dealt with. Some medicines may need to be curtailed, drug overuse controlled, and the patient may need endocrinology studies by a specialist physician. Attention to the environment and occupation may prove valuable. Symptomatic medical treatment by decongestant nose drops is only of short-term benefit (see p. 159). In the long term, uncritical symptomatic treatment is not only valueless but may be damaging. Topical steroids (e. g., triamcinolone, mometasone, fluticasone) are the treatment of choice in chronic hyperplastic rhinitis. These drugs are suitable for long-term use.

Surgical treatment, in increasing order of extent:
1. *Reduction of the inferior turbinate* is performed with the use of various lasers, radiofrequency surgery (Coblation), and submucosal diathermy.
2. *Turbinectomy* includes a limiting resection of the lower edge of the inferior turbinate, occasionally of the middle turbinate, and from the enlarged posterior ends of the turbinate. The purpose is to reduce the volume of the turbinate, but atrophic rhinitis can occur if too much tissue is removed (see p. 155).

Rhinitis of Pregnancy

Increasing swelling and obstruction of the nose may occur during pregnancy, especially in the second half. The symptoms resolve after delivery.

Rhinitis Medicamentosa

Reversible or irreversible damage to the mucosa may be caused by topically or systemically applied drugs.

Mucosal swelling, potentially leading to hyperplastic rhinitis, may be caused by:
- Antihypertensives such as β-blockers, reserpine, clonidine, or angiotensin-converting enzyme inhibitors.
- Phosphodiesterase type 5 inhibitors such as sildenafil.
- Hormones such as exogenous estrogens, oral contraceptives.
- Pain relievers such as aspirin or nonsteroidal anti-inflammatory drugs (NSAIDs).

- Psychotropic drugs such as chlordiazepoxide–amitriptyline.
- Miscellaneous drugs such as cocaine or gabapentin.

Dryness of the nasal mucosa is caused by atropine, belladonna preparations, corticosteroids, imidazoline, or catecholamine derivatives.

Toxic rhinopathy may result from abuse of decongestant nose drops (see p. 159).

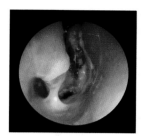

Fig. 2.41   Ozena. Atrophy of the nasal epithelium and the turbinates, with crusts on the epithelial surface and bacterial infection.

Atrophic Rhinitis and Ozena

Atrophic rhinitis is sometimes accompanied by a foul smell from the nose, and in these cases it is known as ozena.

Clinical Features. This disease occurs mainly (but not only) in women, often beginning at puberty. The face is typically flattened and broad. The nasal cavity usually is filled completely with greenish-yellow or brownish-black crusts. Once the crusts are removed, it can be seen that the cavity is very spacious. The mucosa is atrophic and dry due to fibrosis of the subepithelial layer, and the inferior turbinate is atrophic. In ozena, a fetid secretion and crusts are present. The repulsive smell considerably hinders social contact. The patients have anosmia, making them unaware of the unpleasant smell that they produce. However, they do have a sensation of nasal obstruction. There are often severe mucosal changes, including dryness and dry, thick crusts affecting the entire pharynx, larynx, and trachea.

Pathogenesis.   This is not known with certainty, but it is probably multifactorial. Important accepted etiological factors are malnutrition, iron deficiency, vitamin A deficiency, immunodeficiency, and low IgA. The disease is more common among Asians than Caucasians, and more common in Caucasians than in people of African origin. There are geographic concentrations—e. g., in eastern Europe and India. The nasal cavity is abnormally wide due to atrophy of the mucosa and of the bony nasal skeleton. The mucosal glands and the sensory nerve fibers degenerate, the respiratory epithelium undergoes squamous metaplasia, and the mucociliary cleansing system is destroyed. The thick, gluey secretions are decomposed by bacterial proteolysis (**Fig. 2.41**) of *Klebsiella ozaenae, Staphylococcus aureus, Proteus mirabilis.*

Secondary atrophic rhinitis is caused by trauma or excessively extensive surgery of the nose and sinuses, as well as occupational exposure to glass, wood, asbestos, or extensive cocaine consumption.

Treatment. *Conservative:* The nose is cleansed by irrigating it several times a day with dilute salt water and by inserting large cotton-wool tampons impregnated with greasy ointments. Local applications include oily nose drops, emulsions, or ointments, and possibly vitamin A supplements. Steam inhalations with saline solution are given, and osmotically active powders—e.g., dextrose—are sniffed into the nose.

Surgical treatment can be used to prevent the nose from drying out by narrowing the nasal cavity. Two main procedures are used:
1. Bolstering of the nasal mucosa with autologous or homologous tissue (cartilage or bone chips)
2. Median displacement of the lateral nasal wall by mobilizing and rotating it toward the midline, then fixing it in its new position to produce narrowing of the nasal cavity.

Nasal Diphtheria

This usually occurs in children older than 6 months. The secretions may be hemorrhagic and purulent, or exclusively purulent with crusts and cracks around the nostrils. The disease is rare in adults. Nasal diphtheria can occur alone or in combination with pharyngeal diphtheria (see p. 264).

Diagnosis.   Made by culture. *This is a notifiable disease.*

Treatment.   With antitoxic serum (see p. 264).

Tuberculosis of the Nasal Cavity

Two forms can be distinguished: 1, lupus (see p. 147) and 2, exudative ulcerative mucosal tuberculosis. This is usually the result of hematogenous or intraluminal spread in pulmonary tuberculosis. The mucous membrane shows moth-eaten ulcerations.

Diagnosis. This is determined by bacteriology and biopsy.

Syphilis of the Nasal Cavity

Stage 1 (caused by infection from instruments) and stage 2 are very rare. In the middle of the 19th century, stage 3 was more common and was the main reason for saddle nose deformities. Nowadays, cases of syphilis are increasing in numbers again, but nasal manifestations continue to be rare. The diagnosis is made by serology and biopsy, and possibly by identification of the organism.

Sarcoidosis

See page 390.

Scleroma of the Nasal Cavity

See page 148.

Leprosy of the Nasal Cavity

See page 148.

Glanders

Epidemiology. This disease occurs mainly in Eastern Europe and North America. The causative organism is *Malleomyces mallei*. It is transmitted by ungulates.

Clinical Features. Purulent, foul-smelling nasal secretions, granulations, and ulcers are found on the nasal mucosa. The disease may extend to the external nose and surrounding areas.

Diagnosis. This is made by culture, an agglutination test, and biopsy. *The disease is notifiable on suspicion.*

Treatment. Antibiotics are administered.

Blastomycosis

Epidemiology. This disease occurs in North, Central, and South America and is caused by several types of *Blastomyces* (yeasts).

Clinical Features. Crusts and mucosal ulcers are found, which may extend to the external nose. The regional lymph nodes are usually enlarged.

Diagnosis. Culture and biopsy provide the diagnosis.

Treatment. Amphotericin B is given, and may be followed by excision of the diseased skin or mucosa.

Rhinosporidiosis

Epidemiology. The disease occurs in India, Sri Lanka, Africa, and North and South America and is caused by *Rhinosporidium seeberi*.

Clinical Features. These include polypoid, reddish, nodular granulations of the anterior part of the nasal cavity that bleed easily. The disease may extend to the nasal sinuses and pharynx.

Diagnosis. This is made by culture and biopsy.

Differential diagnoses. Mycoses that can also cause nasal symptoms include moniliasis, aspergillosis, mucormycosis, and coccidioidosis.

Treatment. The polyps are removed and the base is cauterized, but there is a danger of bleeding.

Wegener Granulomatosis

This necrotizing granulomatous inflammatory condition preferentially affects the airways and the renal parenchyma. Without treatment, it can progress to a generalized necrotizing vasculitis.

Clinical Features. This nasal disease presents with increasing nasal obstruction, epistaxis, nasal discharge, a combination of crusts, mucosal granulations, and in later stages septal perforations and saddling of the cartilaginous skeleton. There is progressive loss of tissue. In addition, the patient has pulmonary symptoms (chronic bronchitis) and generalized symptoms such as malaise, fatigue, night sweats, and intermittent limb pain (**Fig. 2.42**).

Pathogenesis. The cause of the disease is not clear. It may be an autoimmune condition with granulomatous arteritis, perivasculitis, and necrotizing vasculitis. There is an association with HLA-B8 and HLA-DR2 antigens, related to a family predisposition. Generalized manifestations affect other parts of the body, such as the lungs, kidneys, liver, middle ear, larynx, and trachea.

Diagnosis. The diagnosis is based on the clinical picture, the local findings, the course of the disease, and biopsy. The erythrocyte sedimentation rate (ESR) is usually markedly elevated. Electrophoresis shows reduced albumin and increased globulin. Antineutrophil cytoplasmic antibodies (ANCA) and cytoplasmic-staining antineutrophil cytoplasmic antibodies (c-ANCA; proteinase 3, PR3) are very specific and relatively sensitive tests for Wegener granulomatosis. The lungs should be investigated carefully with a chest radiograph and a CT scan if changes are present. Renal investigations and laboratory tests should also be done.

Differential diagnosis. This includes midline granuloma, leukemia, malignant lymphoma, and sarcoid.

Treatment. This depends on the extent of the disease. It includes local nasal treatment with oils and steroids. In patients with systemic disease, methotrexate 0.3 mg/kg weekly i. v., or prednisolone, and when appropriate high-dose co-trimoxazole (Septrin), or monoclonal antibody (rituximab).

Prognosis. Poor. Death is often due to renal failure.

Lethal Midline Granuloma/T-Cell Lymphoma

Lethal midline granuloma is a clinical term that describes some diseases with an aggressive and progressive destruction of the midface. The nasal prodromes are similar to those of Wegener granuloma. After exclusion of Wegener granuloma, almost all remaining cases that present as lethal midline granuloma are peripheral sinonasal angiocentric T cell and/or natural killer (NK) cell lymphomas. Progressive ulceration of the central part of the face also extends to the maxilla (**Fig. 2.43a, b**).

Pathogenesis. The cause is unknown. The disease may be due to an immune deficiency, but may also be related to a malignancy of the reticulohistiocytic system.

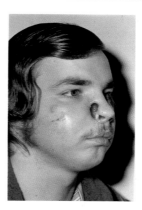

Fig. 2.42 A young patient with Wegener granulomatosis.

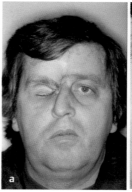
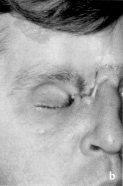

Fig. 2.43a, b A patient with a midline granuloma. The clinical situation 3 months after a frontal sinus operation.

Diagnosis. Typically, the disease is localized to the central part of the face. The ESR is elevated, and there is a hypochromic anemia.

Differential diagnosis. This includes Wegener granuloma, glanders, scleroma gumma, noma, blastomycosis, and histoplasmosis.

Treatment. A combination of radiotherapy, steroids, chemotherapy, immunosuppressive agents, and antibiotics is applied. Occasionally, extensive excision is required.

Prognosis. With early diagnosis and energetic treatment, the outlook is not necessarily unfavorable.

■ Local Conservative Treatment in the Upper Respiratory and Digestive Tracts

The following factors facilitate the treatment of diseases of the upper respiratory and digestive tracts:
- Easy accessibility for local medical treatment.
- Possibility of combining local and systemic medical treatment.
- Easy accessibility for physical methods of treatment such as inhalation, infrared or microwave thermotherapy, treatments in a health resort, change of climate, ionizing radiation for malignancy, etc.

Physical Treatment

Inhalation. Two main methods are possible:

1. *Steam inhalation:* Steam is used for its own therapeutic merits or to carry active agents. A steam kettle or tent can be used. The droplet size is greater than or equal to 30 μm, so the vapor is unstable and rapidly precipitates. Steam is often supplemented by the addition of salts, volatile oils, active agents, detergents, wetting agents, or agents that act on mucopolysaccharide secretions. Precipitation occurs mainly in the nose, mouth, pharynx, and larynx.
2. *Aerosol inhalation:* A true aerosol is used, with a droplet size of less than 30 μm in a quasi-stable suspension of liquid in air. The smaller the particles, the deeper they travel into the airways. The optimal droplet size for the nose and pharynx is 10–15 μm (up to 50 μm), for the trachea 5–10 μm, and for the bronchi and alveoli less than 5 μm. Jet nebulization is better for the upper and middle airways than ultrasound or a gas-driven steam. Drugs used in the aerosol include vasoactive substances to decongest the mucosa, secretolytic agents, antiallergic substances, steroids, antibiotics, chemotherapy, antiasthmatic drugs, and vitamin preparations.

Rules for inhalation therapy:
- The aerosol's droplet size should be sufficient to reach the principal sites of disease in the respiratory tract.

- Medications used should have a pH of around 7.0 and be water-soluble, approximately isotonic, nontoxic and nonirritating, well-retained, and capable of being atomized.
- An inhalation session should last 10–15 min.

Local thermal treatment. The nasal mucosa reacts to warmth with decongestion and swells when exposed to cold. The decongestant effect of applying external warmth is used to treat inflammatory swelling.

The currently preferred warming methods involve the use of microwaves with a wavelength of less than 1 m for the sinuses, larynx, etc. Infrared rays with a wavelength of less than 760 nm are used to treat superficial soft-tissue inflammation. They are generated by an electric lamp with a carbon filament that emits infrared-rich light, and are particularly effective in chronic catarrhal rhinosinusitis. Light in the visible spectrum, especially red light with a wavelength of between 760 and 400 nm, is used to treat superficial soft-tissue inflammations, as are moist warm dressings, mud packs, and heating pads.

Warmth elicits hyperemia by both direct and reflex action on the deep tissues, accelerating and intensifying anti-inflammatory processes in the tissues. Application of cold, on the other hand, inhibits the inflammatory process by retarding the circulation.

Spa treatment. This form of treatment is popular in Europe. In patients with chronic mucosal diseases of the upper respiratory tract, the following are indicated: exposure to the sun or bathing in sulfur springs; exposure to the dry stimulating climate of the high mountains (for chronic catarrh with increased secretions); exposure to a moist, stimulating climate (for dry chronic catarrh). Treatment in spas or health resorts should last for at least 4–6 weeks, and even several months in children.

Medical Treatment

Principles of topical drug application
- Drugs that are active only on the surface of the mucosa (e.g., drugs soluble in oil) need to be distinguished from those that are absorbed and act within the mucosa (e.g., water-soluble drugs).
- Occasionally, water-soluble solutions are absorbed through the mucosal surface as rapidly as an intravenous injection.

- The drug must not damage the ciliary action, the mucosa, or the superficial film of secretions.
- The pH of the drug should be around 7.0, and its osmotic pressure should be between 0.5 and double isotonic; hypertonic solutions dry out the nasal mucosa.
- Locally applied drugs should not have generalized effects, and should be neither antigenic nor carcinogenic.

Groups of drugs. *Vasoactive substances*—e. g., epinephrine, or imidazoline derivatives such as naphazoline and xylometazoline—cause the mucosa to shrink due to vasoconstriction. Uncritical persistent use involves a risk of habituation, leading to rhinitis medicamentosa and resistant mucosal swelling, failure of the autonomic vascular regulation, and organic mucosal damage. Local or systemic decongestants of any type should therefore be used for a brief period only—i. e., for a maximum of 1–2 weeks at a time.

Note: In infants and small children, there is a risk of acute intoxication due to the use of nose drops. Special preparations should therefore be used for children.

Antibiotics: The prerequisites for antibiotic treatment are a correct diagnosis, a clear indication for antibiotic use, and selection of the most appropriate antibiotic and duration of treatment. Swabs and cultures, white blood counts, erythrocyte sedimentation rate (ESR), C-reactive protein (CRP) assay, and in certain cases procalcitonin values are important for diagnosis and assessment of the course. Usually, several antibiotics are equally suitable. The final choice depends on the severity of the disease, the patient's immune status, age, allergies, impairment of liver or kidney function, the activity spectrum of the antibiotic, potential undesired reactions, and price.

Specific information on the most common pathogens and recommended antibiotics is discussed under the headings for the individual clinical entities.

Corticosteroids: These are a double-edged sword. Although they have strong antiallergic and antiinflammatory effects on the upper airways, they also elicit inflammation at other sites, especially in the gastrointestinal tract. Modern topical corticosteroids—e. g., mometasone, fluticasone, or triamcinolone—have marked anti-inflammatory and antiallergic effects on the nasal mucosa, but very low biological availability. Because they are absorbed only to a very slight extent, they appear in minimal concentrations in serum, thus avoiding side effects and allowing long-term administration.

Treatment is usually empirical at first. Ideally, it should be reconsidered after reexamining the patient 48–72 hours later in the light of results for cultures, resistance testing or blood cultures, and should then be continued with the most suitable drug. If possible, a narrow-spectrum antibiotic is preferable to a broad-spectrum one.

Mild bacterial rhinitis in an immunologically competent patient does not require antibiotic therapy.

Oral corticosteroids should be given in single, decreasing (tapered) doses in the morning over a period of up to 3 weeks.

Secretolytic agents: In Germany, standardized Myrtol has been shown to be effective in acute sinusitis and acute bronchitis. It has various effects on inflamed mucosa in the nose and paranasal sinuses. It alkalizes the acidic mucosal environment and has secretolytic, secretomotoric, and antimicrobial effects. Standardized Myrtol may be given for mild bacterial infections or can be used to supplement an antibiotic.

Antihistamines, leukotriene antagonists, cromons: See pp. 150, 168.

■ **Acute and Chronic Rhinosinusitis**

The European Position Paper on Rhinosinusitis and Nasal Polyps (2005) recommends use of the term "rhinosinusitis"—firstly because every infection of the nose involves the mucosa of the paranasal sinuses, which reacts in various ways and at various intensities, and secondly because the great majority of acute and chronic inflammations of the paranasal sinuses are rhinogenous.

This section is based on the following international consensus statements and position papers, and as far as possible on evidence-based criteria:
- European Position Paper on Rhinosinusitis and Nasal Polyps (2005, 2007).
- The World Health Organization (WHO) guidelines on Allergic Rhinitis and its Impact on Asthma (ARIA) (2001).

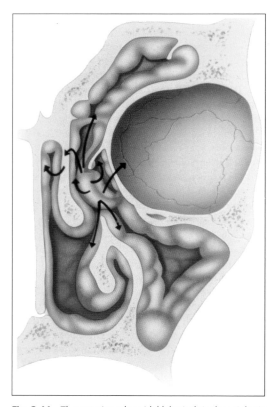

Fig. 2.44 The anterior ethmoidal labyrinth is the etiologic center for acute, recurrent, and chronic inflammations of the maxillary and frontal sinuses. The mucosal disease spreads radially from the ethmoid to the large sinuses, olfactory rim, and inferior turbinate. Inflammation may spread to the orbit through the lamina papyracea.

- International Conference on Sinus Disease: Terminology, Staging, Therapy (Princeton, 2003).
- Recommendations of the European Academy of Allergology and Clinical Immunology (EAACI).
- The European Rhinology Society (ERS) EP3OS document (2007).
- The European Position Paper on Rhinosinusitis and Nasal Polyps (EP3OS), published by the European Rhinologic Society (ERS) (2007).

Pathogens and Antibiotics (Initial Empirical Therapy)

Acute rhinosinusitis: Pathogens include *Streptococcus pneumoniae, Haemophilus influenzae, Moraxella catarrhalis, Staphylococcus aureus, Streptococcus pyogenes*, and anaerobic bacteria. Antibiotics: ami-

nopenicillin with or without a β-lactamase inhibitor; second- and third-generation cephalosporins, macrolides, and quinolones. In severe disease, intravenous administration, otherwise orally.

Chronic rhinosinusitis: Pathogens: *Staphylococcus aureus, Streptococcus pneumoniae, Haemophilus influenzae, Pseudomonas*, anaerobic bacteria, fungi; beware of mixed infections. Antibiotics: aminopenicillin with or without a β-lactamase inhibitor; macrolides, quinolones, second- and third-generation cephalosporins, and clindamycin. In severe disease, intravenous administration.

Acute Rhinosinusitis

Acute and intermittent rhinosinusitis is defined as sudden onset of two or more of the following symptoms: *blockage/congestion, discharge, anterior/postnasal drip, facial pain/pressure, reduction/loss of smell for up to 12 weeks.*

Ethmoidal Sinusitis

The anterior ethmoid bone is the morphologic connection between the nose and the maxillary and frontal sinuses. Both paranasal sinuses drain through the anterior ethmoid to the nose (**Figs. 2.44, 2.45**). Viral, bacterial, or allergic infections of the nasal mucosa or nasopharynx spread immediately to the ethmoidal sinus. Mucosal swelling, edema, and subsequently hyperplasia lead to obstruction of the drainage routes (ethmoidal infundibulum, frontal recess), backup of secretions, and infection of the frontal and maxillary sinuses.

Clinical Features. Impaired nasal breathing, hyposmia or anosmia, sensation of pressure between the eye and nose, subfebrile temperatures, acute inflammation; depending on severity, a feeling of pressure and pain in frontal and maxillary sinuses (**Figs. 2.46, 2.47a,b**).

Diagnosis. Routine otorhinolaryngology examination; inspection (attention to edema of the upper eyelid); palpation of the medial angle of the eye, exclusion of diplopia; nasal endoscopy (critical): mucosal edema, track of pus in the middle nasal meatus; swabs for culture and resistance testing.

Diagnostic imaging: Paranasal sinuses (occipitomental and/or occipitonasal projections), coronal CT in case of recurrent exacerbations or chronic sinusitis and always before surgery.

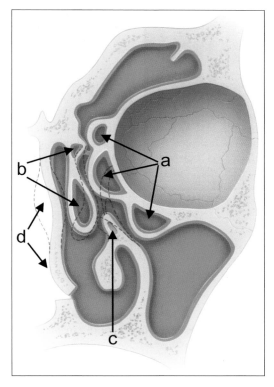

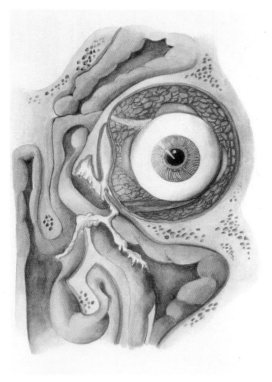

Fig. 2.45   Schematic illustration of typical cell formations causing recurrent sinusitis. **a,** Cell formations in the medial orbital wall, with a large ethmoidal bulla and orbitoethmoid cells (Haller cells); **b,** pneumatized sections of the middle turbinate; **c,** the uncinate process, which varies in size, length, and point of insertion; **d,** deviated nasal septum.

Fig. 2.46   Schematic illustration of ethmoidal sinusitis. Children are at particular risk for orbital complications, due to the thinness of the lamina papyracea. (Illustration courtesy of A. Muecke, Berlin, Germany.)

Olfactometry, allergy tests (prick test, RAST) in chronic and recurrent forms.

Differential diagnosis. Charlin neuralgia, cluster headaches.

Complications. Especially in children, rapid spread to the orbital cavity (due to thinness of the lamina papyracea) and development of orbital complications (see p. 186).

Treatment. *Acute ethmoidal sinusitis:* Decongestant nose drops, high tamponades, decongestion and aspiration of the middle nasal meatus. Application of infrared light or microwave or short-wave therapy, secretolytic agents; administration of antibiotics in case of failure of conservative therapy or purulent infection (see maxillary sinusitis). Possibly oral corticosteroids, or medialization of the medial turbinate. In some countries, supplementing antibiotics with simple antral lavage in severe acute purulent sinusitis has been found to be often effective. Surgery is indicated for recurrent sinusitis with involvement of the maxillary and/or frontal sinuses, orbital, or central complications.

Chronic ethmoidal sinusitis: Topical corticosteroids, antibiotics. Surgery is indicated if conservative therapy has failed, for recurrent sinusitis (maxillary and/or frontal), for nasal and paranasal polyposis, for chronic sinusitis with or without bronchial asthma, or for suspected tumor. The surgical techniques depend on endoscopic and CT findings: infundibulotomy; anterior or complete ethmoidectomy, possibly with supraturbinate fenestration of

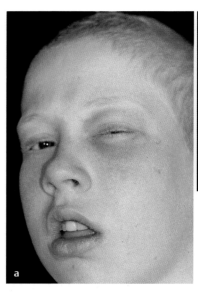

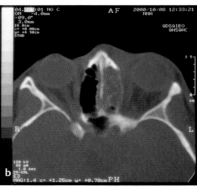

Fig. 2.47a, b   a A 9-year-old boy with palpebral edema as a sign of incipient orbital complications. **b** The axial CT shows ethmoid sinusitis.

the maxillary cavity or enlargement of the frontal recess; pansinus operation.

Maxillary Sinusitis
Acute or chronic bacterial, fungal, or allergic rhinogenous, or (more rarely) odontogenic inflammation. The vast majority of cases originate at the lateral nasal wall and the anterior ethmoid. The maxillary and frontal sinuses are functionally downstream from the ethmoid.

Symptoms of acute maxillary sinusitis. These include acute pain in the central and ipsilateral parts of the face, hyperesthesia of the facial skin, but occasionally only a sensation of pressure or fullness. Sensitivity to tapping over the cheek, ipsilateral swelling of the turbinates, and a stream of pus in the middle meatus and on the floor of the nose are other findings (**Figs. 2.48, 2.49**).

Odontogenic sinusitis: Pathogens are *Streptococcus intermedius* and *Streptococcus constellatus*, often mixed with anaerobes (e. g., *Fusobacteria, Peptostreptococcus,* or *Prevotella*).

Symptoms of chronic maxillary sinusitis. Pain is often slight, and there may be only a sensation of pressure. Symptoms also include headache that increases on bending head forward, swollen cheeks, palpebral edema, chronic nasal obstruction, mucoid or purulent secretion, painful trigeminal nerve exit,

and neuralgia in the distribution of the infraorbital nerve, disorders of smell including cacosmia, nasal fetor, chronic rhinitis, and hypertrophic turbinates, streams of secretion, and possibly polyps.

Diagnosis. Case history, routine otorhinolaryngology examination, inspection, palpation (cheek, facial wall of maxillary sinus), nasal endoscopy, examination for pain on bending head forward and of nerve exits, pain on tapping, percussion of the teeth, dental status.

Sonography: A-mode ultrasound reveals partial or total echo at the back wall of the maxillary sinus.

Radiography: Plain radiography shows partial or total clouding, or an air–fluid level in the maxillary sinus. CT is appropriate in severe cases, in chronic sinusitis, when complications are present, and if surgery is indicated.

Allergy testing: Prick test, RAST, intranasal provocation.

Treatment of acute rhinogenous sinusitis. *Conservative.* Nasal detumescence by use of decongestant nose drops, heat application (infrared light at a distance of 30 cm from the face and nose) or deep heat (short wave), steam inhalation with chamomile or volatile oils.

Herbal secretolytic agents (e. g., standardized Myrtol, which has bacteriostatic, mucolytic, secretomotoric, and deodorizing effects); analgesics (paracetamol, ibuprofen).

> **Note:** Acetylsalicylic acid (ASA, aspirin) must be used with caution, due to the high rate of ASA intolerance among sinusitis patients.

Antibiotics: The first choice is an aminopenicillin in combination with a β-lactamase inhibitor, or a second- or third-generation cephalosporin. Alternatives are macrolides, ketolides, or third- or fourth-generation fluoroquinolones, as indicated by resistance testing.

Lavage or drainage of the maxillary sinus is indicated in persistent empyema (swabs should be taken first).

In patients with allergies, a third-generation antihistamine (see p. 151), steroids (topical or oral), or hyposensitization are indicated.

In suspected *Aspergillus* infection, a search should be made for a foreign body (overstuffed root canal; endoscopy of the maxillary sinus). For *Aspergillus* sinusitis, see p. 182.

Treatment of acute odontogenic sinusitis. In patients with odontogenic sinusitis, the first-line treatment is dental repair, root canal treatment, or extraction.

Antibiotics: The first choice is penicillin (phenoxymethyl penicillin, aminopenicillin plus a β-lactamase inhibitor); alternatives (after resistance testing) are metronidazole, lincosamide, cephalosporins, or macrolides; reserve antibiotics are carbapenems (imipenem, meropenem).

Surgical treatment is indicated when conservative treatment fails (e. g., in chronic rhinosinusitis with or without bronchial asthma, fungal infections, recurrent empyema, or polyposis).

Treatment of chronic maxillary sinusitis. Antibiotics are used as described above.

Surgical treatment: Infundibulotomy, anterior or complete ethmoidectomy with supraturbinate fenestration of the maxillary sinus, if necessary with intracavitary repair (removal of polyps, cysts, or fungal concrements).

Frontal Sinusitis
This is an acute or chronic rhinogenous infection of the frontal sinus involving viral, bacterial, or allergic inflammation and obstruction of the anterior ethmoid (frontal recess). The spectrum of pathogens is

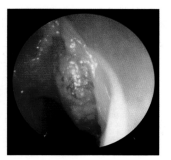

Fig. 2.48   A track of pus along the lateral nasal wall—a typical finding in purulent maxillary sinusitis.

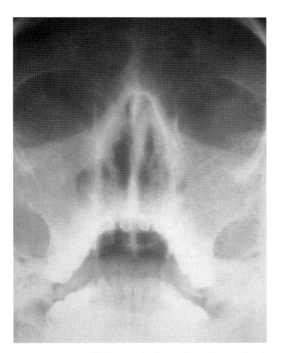

Fig. 2.49   Mucosal edema in both maxillary sinuses, visualized on a plain film.

described above. It may also occur in the form of diving sinusitis or barosinusitis. Usually, anatomic variations that impede ventilation and drainage of the frontal sinus are present (e. g., high septal deviation, pneumatization variations of the ethmoid air cells; see p. 161).

Clinical Features. These include severe pain in the forehead, sensitivity of the forehead to pressure or

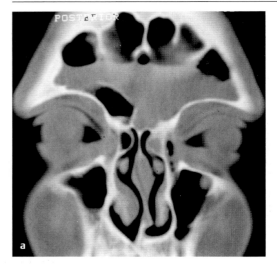

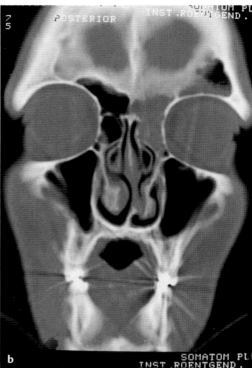

Fig. 2.50a, b   a Empyema of both frontal sinuses.
b Occlusion of the anterior ethmoid by hyperplastic, edematous mucosa.

tapping, tender sites of exit of the supraorbital nerve, and tracks of secretions or pus on the anterior part of the middle meatus. The mucosa of the middle meatus is often glazed, swollen, and red (**Fig. 2.50a,b**).

Complications. Orbital complications (see p. 186), osteomyelitis of the frontal bone with abscess formation (Pott puffy tumor), meningitis, epidural abscess, brain abscess, thrombosis of the sagittal sinus, mucocele.

Diagnosis. *Routine otorhinolaryngology examination; inspection:* edema of forehead and eyelids, conjunctivitis; palpation: floor of frontal sinus painful, exit of the first trigeminal nerve (supraorbital branch), tender pain on bending the head forward.
Nasal endoscopy: Edema, pus and mucoid pus in middle nasal meatus; inflammatory redness. Swabs: culture, resistogram. Radiography of the paranasal sinuses shows mucosal hyperplasia or empyema.
Further diagnostic measures: Coronal CT in case of recurrent exacerbations or preoperatively.
Laboratory investigations: CRP, white blood count, ESR.
Allergy tests: Prick tests, RAST.
Depending on the clinical findings, an ophthalmologist or neurologist should be consulted (lumbar puncture if meningitis is suspected).

Treatment. Decongestion and aspiration of the middle nasal meatus. Application of infrared heat or deep heat by microwave or short wave, endoscopically guided placement of high tamponade in the middle nasal meatus—e. g., using a sponge soaked with tetracaine and epinephrine. "High fillings" in the middle meatus.
Antibiotics: Start empirically, then assess effectiveness after 3 days; if necessary, adjustment according to the resistogram (see maxillary sinusitis, p. 162).
If empyema is present, the frontal sinus is drained with endoscopic surgery; in the age of endoscopic microsurgery, puncture using the Kümmel and Beck method has become less important (see p. 140).
Surgical intervention: Indications are recurrent or chronic exacerbations or orbital or central complications (e. g., subperiosteal abscess, orbital phlegmon, meningitis, epidural abscess, brain ab-

scess, sinus thrombosis, failure of conservative therapy, osteomyelitis, mucocele). The principles of endonasal and external surgery of the frontal sinus are explained on pp. 171, 177.

Sphenoid Sinusitis

Acute, chronic, rarely allergic inflammation of one or both sphenoid sinuses, usually due to morphologic or inflammatory obstruction of the ostium. Drainage of the sphenoidal cavity proceeds via the sphenoethmoidal recess, rather than through the anterior ethmoid to the nose as in the maxillary and frontal sinuses (**Fig. 2.51a, b**).

Pathogenesis. This disorder may develop independently and alone, or in association with other forms of sinusitis (pansinusitis). Acute and chronic sinusitis in ventilated patients (usually in intensive-care units) starts with sphenoid sinusitis, due to the patient's constantly supine position.
   For the pathogen spectrum, see page 160.

Clinical Features. Signs of infection are largely lacking; overall, the symptoms are vague. The patient may report pain or a feeling of pressure within the skull, radiating to the occiput or the temple. Deep pain in the eyes is also possible. Nasal respiration is usually not obstructed. Secretions usually drain into the nasopharynx, causing postnasal drip and coughing. There is a stream of pus on the posterior wall of the pharynx or in the superior meatus.

Anatomy. Several nerves run along the lateral wall of the sphenoid sinus—e. g., the optic, abducent, and maxillary nerves. The posterior ethmoidal air cells may invade the body of the sphenoid in a cranial direction, interfering with pneumatization; they may project above the ethmoidal cavity. If they achieve a typical pyramidal configuration (i. e., with the tip pointing dorsally) with prominence of the optic nerve, they are termed Onodi cells (posterior sphenoethmoidal air cells).

Complications. Orbital complications, spread of inflammation to the optic nerve, visual impairment, paralysis of the abducent nerve; central complications: meningitis, brain abscess, thrombosis of the cavernous sinus; osteomyelitis.

Diagnosis. Routine otorhinolaryngology examination, nasal endoscopy, swabs of free pus for culture and resistance testing, coronal CT.

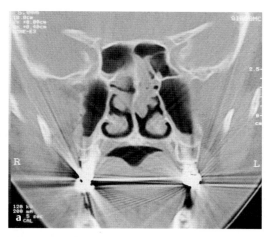

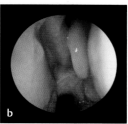

Fig. 2.51a, b   Sphenoid sinusitis, caused by occlusion of the sphenoidal ostium by a polyp.

If diagnosis of the pathogen is equivocal, especially before surgery, vascularization has to be studied (e. g., by magnetic resonance angiography or angiography). Consultation with an ophthalmologist and a neurologist, and a radioisotope bone scan, are indicated if osteomyelitis is suspected. Allergy tests: prick test, RAST.

Differential diagnosis. Mucocele, benign or malignant tumors, fungal disease, pituitary tumor, meningioma of the sphenoid wing.

Treatment. *Conservative:* Localized decongestion and aspiration of the sphenoid, tamponade of the sphenoethmoidal recess with a pointed swab containing, e. g., tetracaine/epinephrine; antibiotics (see pp. 159, 160); antiinflammatory agents; in appropriate cases, antiallergic therapy (see p. 150); oral steroids.
   Surgery: Indications are failure of conservative treatment and incipient or overt complications.
   Principle of the operation: The method of choice is endoscopic or microscopic transnasal (via the sphenoethmoidal recess) or transethmoidal enlargement of the ethmoidal cavity ostium, or trep-

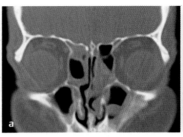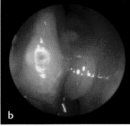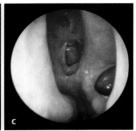

Fig. 2.52a–c   Endoscopic pansinus surgery.
a The preoperative CT, showing polypoid mucosa in all of the paranasal sinuses.
b The preoperative endoscopic view, showing polyposis of the nose and paranasal sinuses.

c Endoscopic view of the cleared, spacious ethmoid, showing an open, epithelialized window to the maxillary and sphenoid sinuses (0° lens).

anation of the anterior wall. Alternatively, a transseptal or transmaxillary route can be used. For surgery of complications or tumors (see pp. 226, 288), midfacial degloving or lateral rhinotomy may be required.

Pansinusitis

Rhinogenous inflammation of all paranasal sinuses on one or (more commonly) both sides, caused by viruses, bacteria, or allergenic agents. The symptoms are those of disease of the various sinuses combined, and may be bilateral.

> **!**
> **Note:** In patients with diffuse mucosal edema or hyperplasia of all the paranasal sinuses, one should always check for acetylsalicylic acid intolerance and asthma.

Diagnosis. See Ethmoidal Sinusitis, above.

Treatment. *Conservative,* in the acute phase. Topical steroids, depending on findings; oral corticosteroids; antibiotics.

Surgery, when there is a chronic course and in severe symptoms. Ethmoidectomy with supraturbinate fenestration of the maxillary sinus, enlargement of the frontal recess, and/or removal of the floor of the frontal sinus (Draf I–III), or pansinus operation (**Fig. 2.52a–c**).

Chronic Rhinosinusitis

Chronic rhinosinusitis is one of the most common health problems, with a serious impact on lower airway disease and overall health. The condition is diagnosed when symptoms persist for more than 12 weeks.

Whereas acute sinusitis is an inflammatory rhinogenous process caused by obstruction of ventilation and drainage of the paranasal sinuses located functionally downstream from the ethmoid, in chronic rhinosinusitis the postulated cause involves gradual obstruction of the ostiomeatal complex by edema, induration, hyperplasia, and polyposis of the mucosa.

The role of anatomic blockage in the origin of chronic rhinosinusitis is controversial. The spectrum of pathogens involved in chronic rhinosinusitis differs from that in acute sinusitis. There has been a change in the way in which bacterial infection is assessed. In addition to biomechanical and bacterial factors, other pathomechanisms for inflammation of the nasal and sinonasal mucosa are now being considered. In the mucosa and secretions of patients with chronic rhinosinusitis, increased numbers of neutrophilic granulocytes are found, as well as eosinophils, mast cells, basophils, and mononuclear cells (T lymphocytes, CD8$^+$ suppressor cells, cytotoxic T cells, and CD4$^+$ T-helper cells). Raised concentrations of histamines and leukotrienes and prostaglandin D have been found in the nasal secretions of patients with chronic rhinosinusitis.

Chronic Hyperplastic Rhinosinusitis with Nasal Polyps
Eosinophils and fungi are considered to be of particular importance in chronic hyperplastic rhinosinusitis with nasal polyps. The granules of eosino-

philic granulocytes contain cytotoxic proteins, which are released when degranulation occurs: eosinophil cationic protein (ECP), major basis protein (MBP), eosinophil peroxidase (EPO), and eosinophil-derived neurotoxin (EDN). It has been suggested that eosinophils migrate from the epithelium into the mucus, where they dock onto T cells. When they degranulate within the supraepithelial mucus blanket, they release their cytotoxic cytokines, in particular MBP, which docks onto fungal elements to form so-called "horseshoes." This leads to a toxic–inflammatory reaction on the surface epithelium, paving the way for secondary invasion by bacteria, infection, and eventually chronic rhinosinusitis. The most common fungi involved are *Alternaria, Penicillium, Candida,* and *Aspergillus.* The term "eosinophilic fungal rhinosinusitis" has been proposed for rhinosinusitis induced by fungi.

Immune and Tissue-Specific Reactions

In contrast to the biomechanical and infectious pathomechanism involved in acute sinusitis, immune and tissue-specific inflammatory reactions play a critical role in chronic rhinosinusitis. This explains why patients and physicians face further inflammatory exacerbations and recurrences of mucosal disease, even after surgical improvement of ventilation and drainage. Surgical repair based on the principles of functional endoscopic surgery of the paranasal sinuses (the Messerklinger concept) can therefore only form part of the therapy. It is equally important to institute targeted and individualized follow-up, oriented toward the clinical findings, with long-term administration of anti-inflammatory agents (topical steroids, oral corticosteroids in appropriate cases, antibiotics for purulent inflammation; see p. 160).

Nasal Polyps

Two types of chronic rhinosinusitis can be distinguished, depending on whether neutrophilic or eosinophilic leukocytes predominate. Nasal polyps tend to occur mainly in the eosinophil-dominated type, in which they form a subgroup of chronic rhinosinusitis.

Nasal polyps appear as grape-like structures in the upper nasal cavity, originating from within the ostiomeatal complex. They are characterized by loose connective tissue, edema, inflammatory cells, and a few glands and capillaries, and are covered with various types of epithelium—mostly respiratory pseudostratified epithelium with ciliated cells and goblet cells. Eosinophils are the most common inflam-

Table 2.6 Classification of polyps (adapted from Stammberger)

I	Antrochoanal polyps
II	Large single polyp
III	Polyps associated with chronic rhinosinusitis (CRS) (not eosinophil-dominated)
IV	Polyps associated with CRS (eosinophil-dominated)
	Diffuse polyposis in patients with aspirin intolerance, allergic fungal CRS, or asthma
V	Polyps associated with specific diseases (cystic fibrosis, malignancies)

matory cells in nasal polyps, but neutrophils, mast cells, plasma cells, lymphocytes, and monocytes, as well as fibroblasts, are also present. IL-5 is the predominant cytokine in nasal polyposis, reflecting activation and prolonged survival of eosinophils. The reason why polyps develop in some patients, but not in others, remains unknown. There is a definite relationship in patients who have what is known as the Sampter triad—asthma, NSAID sensitivity, and nasal polyps.

In the general population, the prevalence of nasal polyps is 4%; in patients with asthma, a prevalence of 7–15% has been noted, whereas nasal polyps are found in 36–60% of patients with NSAID intolerance. Epidemiological data provide no evidence for a relationship between nasal polyps and allergy. In children, the presence of polyps should suggest the possibility of cystic fibrosis.

The clinical picture of polyps is highly variable (**Table 2.6**). All gradations are possible, ranging from solitary polyps to diffuse nasal and paranasal polyposis. Nasal polyps hardly ever originate within the nose itself, but rather in the anterior ethmoidal air cells, when inflamed areas of mucosa are subjected to pressure. From there, they follow gravitational pull along the path of least resistance through the middle nasal meatus to the nasal cavity (**Fig. 2.53**).

Nasal polyps are benign, pedicled, or sessile masses of nasal or sinus mucosa caused by inflammation.

Clinical Features. These include mechanical obstruction of nasal breathing, mechanical anosmia,

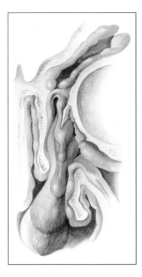

Fig. 2.53 Phases in the development of a nasal polyp from the anterior ethmoid: mucosal inflammation, edema, polyp growth, obstruction of the middle meatus and anterior ethmoid due to compression by the polyp tissue, leading to complete nasal obstruction.

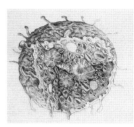

Fig. 2.54 The eosinophilic granulocyte.

epiphora, colorless stringy or purulent secretion, postnasal catarrh, headache, snoring, and rhinolalia clausa. Abnormal growth of the facial skeleton in children leads to a broad, bony nose, with an appearance known as 'frog face'. Chronic rhinosinusitis may be caused by obstruction of the sinus ostia. Polyps can also arise in one or all sinuses even if the nasal cavity is free.

Choanal polyps have a long pedicle and usually arise in the antrum. They may completely block the choana or the nasopharynx.

Pathogenesis. Immunohistochemical evidence shows that chronic rhinosinusitis with and without nasal polyps are two distinct diseases. In both types, the numbers of neutrophils, T cells, B cells, NK cells, and mast cells are increased. In polyposis, eosinophilic granulocytes, plasma cells, and macrophages are present in addition.

Biomarkers: Acute rhinosinusitis: activation of lymphocytes. Chronic rhinosinusitis: proinflammatory cytokines. Polyposis: in addition, high concentrations of nasal IgE and

IL-5, derived from T cells and eosinophils and indicating a self-enhancing eosinophilic inflammatory reaction.

It has also been suggested that eosinophils migrate from the epithelium into the mucus, where they dock onto T cells. In the process of degranulation, they release cytotoxic cytokines—e. g., MBP. MBP docks onto fungal elements present in the nasal secretion, forming so-called horseshoes (**Fig. 2.54**). The latter cause a toxic–inflammatory reaction on the epithelial surface, which becomes infected with bacteria secondarily.

Leukotrienes: The role of leukotrienes in the pathogenesis of bronchial asthma is undisputed, and increased levels of these mediators have been detected in patients with rhinosinusitis and nasal polyps.

Patients with *ASA intolerance* are a critical group. Aspirin and other nonsteroidal anti-inflammatory drugs that inhibit the enzyme cyclooxygenase interfere with metabolism of arachidonic acid to prostaglandins. This in turn leads to relative overproduction of leukotrienes.

Staphylococcus superantigens: In nasal polyposis, but not in chronic rhinosinusitis, *Staphylococcus*-derived superantigens may at least modulate the severity and expression of disease.

United airways: The particular features of the eosinophil-dominated inflammatory reaction in nasal polyps resemble inflammation of the bronchial mucosa. Both involve an immune response in which TH2 predominates, and there is a high degree of comorbidity involving nasal polyposis and bronchial asthma or ASA intolerance. This helps explain the danger of a change in level from the upper to the lower respiratory tract in chronic hyperplastic rhinosinusitis (**Fig. 2.55a–d**).

Diagnosis. The typical findings on anterior rhinoscopy are solitary or multiple, glazed, transparent, smooth-walled, whitish-yellow masses, mobile to pressure with a probe, usually located in the middle meatus or the choana. They are often bilateral. Other studies include nasal endoscopy, CT, C-reactive protein, nasal cytology, and allergy tests.

C-reactive protein (CRP) is one of the acute-phase response proteins. The CRP value is useful in the diagnosis of bacterial infections. However, in patients in whom there is a suspicion of infectious disease, CRP levels of up to 100 mg/L are compatible with all types of infection (bacterial, viral, fungal, and protozoan).

> **Note:** Polypoid sinusitis often develops in addition to nasal polyps. In patients with nasal polyps, the sinuses should therefore always be investigated by radiography and possibly by endoscopy (see pp. 132, 137).

Differential diagnosis. This includes encephalomeningocele (excluded by radiography and probing), a bleeding polyp of the septum (see p. 194), malignant nasal tumors, and a pituitary tumor—e. g., an adenoma.

Treatment. Treatment of polyposis requires a stepwise approach consisting of medical and surgical modalities. Because of the great tendency of polyps to recur, a long-term strategy involving endoscopy is necessary. The recommendations of the EAACI and European Position on Polyposis and Sinusitis (EPOS) are as follows.

Topical steroids: Owing to their strong anti-inflammatory effect, these are the first-choice drugs (e. g., mometasone, fluticasone) (**Fig. 2.56a, b**).

Antibiotics: Targeted antibiotic administration for inflammatory exacerbations (beware of *Staphylococcus* superantigens; empirically: amoxicillin plus clavulanic acid). Conclusive studies are still lacking for long-term treatment with antibiotics (evidence level III, level of recommendation c).

Leukotriene antagonists: These drugs have not been tested in controlled trials for rhinosinusitis and nasal polyps. A few case-controlled trials indicate that antileukotriene treatment may have a beneficial effect on nasal symptoms in patients with chronic persistent rhinosinusitis and nasal polyposis.

ASA deactivation: Adaptive deactivation by means of long-term administration of 100 mg orally has been shown to improve the chances of avoiding recurrence. A prerequisite for deactivation is in-hospital surveillance of the patient during the induction phase.

Surgery: Pretreatment with topical steroids is expedient; perioperative medication with methylprednisolone (starting at 125 mg and then gradually tapering off over 3 weeks). Functional endoscopic repair of the ethmoidal and paranasal sinuses depends on the individual endoscopic and CT findings. Procedures range from infundibulotomy to bilateral pansinus operations (shavers). An operation does not affect the cause of the mu-

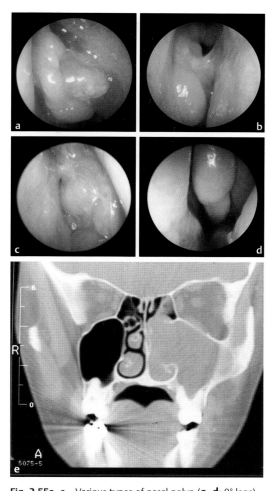

Fig. 2.55a–e Various types of nasal polyp (**a–d**: 0° lens).
a Chronic hyperplastic (noneosinophilic) rhinosinusitis.
b The triad of acetylsalicylic acid (ASA) intolerance, bronchial asthma, and nasal polyposis: typical color of the mucosa, rheologic changes, and thickening of the mucus.
c Induration and scarring after repeated polypectomies.
d, e An antrochoanal polyp; this is the only polyp that originates in the maxillary sinus.

cosa's tendency toward a TH2-shifted immune response. However, it does provide a better situation for effective treatment with topical steroids. Long-term postoperative anti-inflammatory treatment with endoscopic monitoring is essential (**Fig. 2.57**).

Although nasal polyps shrink or disappear completely with steroids, this treatment is not appropriate, as the polyps recur when the steroids are discontinued. If an allergen can be demonstrated, it should be eliminated.

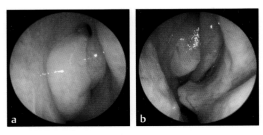

Fig. 2.56a, b   The effect of topical corticosteroids on a large polyp in the middle nasal meatus, **a** before and **b** after steroid therapy.

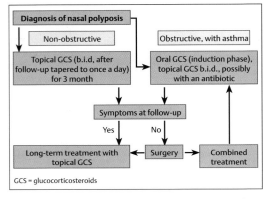

Fig. 2.57   Decision algorithm for the treatment of polyposis nasi (adapted from C. Bachert, *Allergologie* 2004;12: 484–94).

Polypectomy: So-called blind polypectomy is no longer indicated. The method of choice is functional endoscopic surgery of the ethmoid (ethmoidectomy) and the paranasal sinuses. Microdebriders have the advantage of allowing efficient and atraumatic surgery with little bleeding, preventing postoperative adhesions (**Fig. 2.58a, b**).

Churg–Strauss Syndrome

The Churg–Strauss syndrome is a necrotizing vasculitis classically characterized by hypereosinophilia and bronchial asthma.

Clinical Features. Otorhinolaryngology manifestations include sinusitis initially, and later asthma.

Diagnosis. Required diagnostic criteria are asthma, eosinophilia, sinusitis, pulmonary infiltrate, histologic proof of vasculitis, and mononeuritis multiplex.

Treatment. Corticosteroids alone or with cyclophosphamide and/or plasma exchange.

Prognosis. Favorable in the long term.

Rhinosinusitis and HIV

Rhinosinusitis is very common in HIV patients. Nasal obstruction may be due to rhinosinusitis, allergy, neoplasm or adenoid hypertrophy.

Clinical Features. Kaposi sarcoma or lymphoma present with nasal obstruction, epistaxis, and rhinorrhea. Adenoid hypertrophy in adults raises a concern regarding HIV.

Pathogenesis. Acute sinusitis pathogens are similar to those in normal patients. *Staphylococcus, Pseudomonas,* anaerobes, and fungi are found in chronic rhinosinusitis in HIV patients.

Diagnosis. Swabs from the middle nasal meatus, and determination of the current viral load.

Treatment. CD4 counts > 200/mm^3: amoxicillin plus clavulanic acid, systemic decongestants, guaifenesin 1200 mg b. i. d. for 3 weeks; topical decongestant spray for 1 week. CD4 counts < 200/mm^3: add coverage for *Staphylococcus, Pseudomonas,* and anaerobes—e. g., with ciprofloxacin plus clindamycin; severe infections require hospitalization, intravenous antibiotics, and endoscopic drainage; in selected patients with HIV, endoscopic sinus surgery is effective, although less so than in immunologically competent patients.

■ Rhinogenous Headache

The quality of rhinogenous headache depends on the underlying cause. Sinus inflammation is characterized by a dull, nagging, position-dependent headache that is associated with a sensation of pressure over the affected sinus (**Fig. 2.59**). Headache is a late symptom of tumors of the nose and paranasal sinuses. Adenoid cystic carcinoma grows

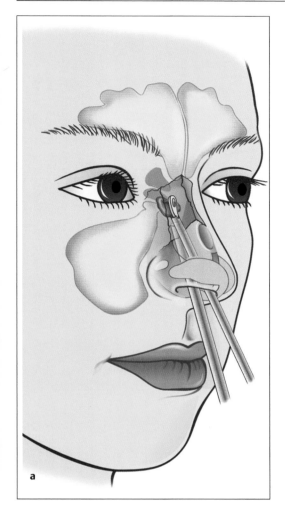

a

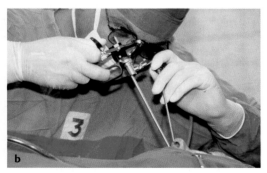

b

Fig. 2.58a, b **a** Endoscopic microsurgery with paraendoscopic preparation is now the standard surgical treatment for polyposis of the nose and paranasal sinuses.
b Microdebriders ensure smooth wound surfaces, little bleeding, and rapid healing.

along nerve fibers and is associated with pain. A neoplasm that reaches the dura mater will produce intense, unremitting pain. Mucoceles, which almost always occur in surgical or posttraumatic cavities, lead to pressure erosion of the adjacent bone. Typically, the pain subsides when the mucocele can expand by eroding through the lamina papyracea or orbital roof toward the globe.

■ **Facial Neuralgias**

Trigeminal nerve: Idiopathic trigeminal neuralgia is marked by paroxysms of intense, stabbing pain on one side of the face (*tic douloureux*).

Nasociliary nerve: Severe, unilateral, paroxysmal pain that is maximal at the medial canthus of the eye, epiphora with marked conjunctival injection, and edematous swelling of the ipsilateral nasal mucosa are features of nasociliary neuralgia (Charlin neuralgia).

Pterygopalatine ganglion: Unilateral, aching nocturnal pain centered in the lower half of the face ("lower-half head-ache"), combined with variable rhinorrhea and sneezing attacks, may be symptomatic of pterygopalatine ganglion neuralgia. It is caused by tumors and inflammations of the nose, sinuses, orbit, or pterygopalatine fossa.

Post-Caldwell–Luc syndrome: Inflammatory exacerbations in a previously operated maxillary sinus, scar traction on the infraorbital nerve, severe maxillary deformity, or scar-related infiltrates and abscesses can cause an aching or stabbing pain of variable and sometimes agonizing intensity. Anesthetic blockades may provide clues as to the nasal or sinogenic origin of the head and facial pain. If the pain is relieved by local mucosal anesthesia or conduction anesthesia of the trigeminal nerve branch and recurs after the anesthesia subsides, this confirms the origin of the pain.

■ **Principles of Surgery of the Paranasal Sinuses**

Endoscopic Endonasal Microsurgery of the Paranasal Sinuses and the Anterior Base of Skull
Endonasal surgery of the paranasal sinuses developed at the beginning of the 20th century. During the past 30 years, thanks to the introduction of optical systems and endoscopes in particular, it has become the international state of the art. Today, radical procedures on the paranasal sinuses (e. g., the Caldwell–Luc, Riedel, and Ritter–Jansen methods) are indicated only in selected cases or for revision surgery.

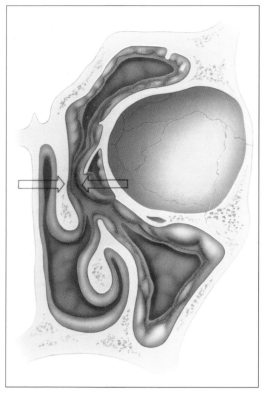

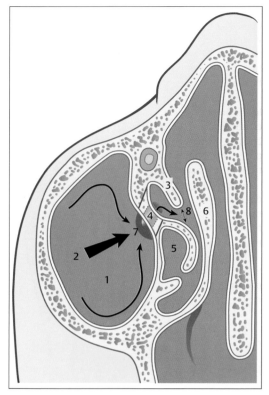

Fig. 2.59   Rhinogenic headache often starts when drainage and ventilation of the ethmoid sinus are obstructed.

Fig. 2.60   Mucociliary transportation of secretions through the lateral nasal wall, illustrated with the maxillary sinus as an example. **1**, Maxillary sinus; **2**, secretion tracks in the maxillary sinus; **3**, uncinate process; **4**, ethmoidal infundibulum; **5**, ethmoidal bulla; **6**, medial concha; **7**, natural ostium of the maxillary sinus; **8**, semilunar hiatus.

The philosophy and details of endonasal surgery are described in numerous publications representing various schools of thought (Messerklinger, Stammberger, Wigand, Kennedy, Draf, Simmen, and others).

Concept. The concept of *functional endoscopic sinus surgery (FESS)*, the Messerklinger technique—spread throughout the world through the efforts of Stammberger and Kennedy—was broadly accepted in the 1980s and has been evaluated in numerous prospective and retrospective case-controlled studies and nonrandomized clinical trials. The original idea involved a concept of endoscopic diagnosis for the nose and lateral nasal wall; the development of an endoscopic surgical strategy was secondary. One of the

essential aims of this strategy is to restore the mucociliary apparatus (**Figs. 2.60, 2.61**).

In the functional approach to rhinosinusitis, it was hypothesized that recovery of the diseased sinus mucosa could be achieved by allowing ventilation through the natural ostia and restoring mucociliary clearance, using a minimally invasive endoscopic technique (**Fig. 2.62a–c**).

Depending on the findings, endoscopic surgery can be limited to the removal of the uncinate process for wider access to the ethmoidal infundibulum (infundibulotomy), or used for anterior or complete ethmoidectomy, with or without supraturbinate fenestration of the maxillary cavity and enlargement of the access to the frontal sinus (Draf I–III), or extended into a bilateral pansinus operation.

The range of indications for endonasal microsurgery in the hands of specialized surgeons has expanded enormously as a result of several decades' experience with endoscopic microsurgery and constant advances in endoscope and instrument technology, the incorporation of navigation systems, and completely new interdisciplinary developments (such as interventional radiology, endocrinology, and ophthalmology).

Indications. The *main indications* for endonasal microsurgery are acute (frontal sinus empyema), recurrent, and chronic sinusitis; nasal and sinus polyposis; and supportive measures (at the nasal septum, in surgery of the turbinates).

Extended indications include postsaccal tearduct stenosis, CSF leaks, decompression of the optic nerve, tumor operations (e.g., pituitary tumors, meningiomas, osteomas, and certain angiofibromas).

Mucosa-sparing microtherapy is based on the following pathophysiologic and histopathologic presuppositions:

- The transportation of secretions into and out of the paranasal sinuses proceeds along defined pathways.
- The maxillary and frontal sinuses are functionally downstream from the ethmoidal sinus.
- Chronically inflamed mucosa has a strong capacity for self-repair.
- Restoration of ventilation and drainage are the most important prerequisites for recovery of the epithelium.

Preoperative diagnostic requirements. Nasal endoscopy, coronal CT, allergy tests.

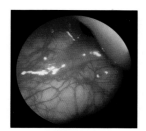

Fig. 2.61 The confluence of the secretion tracks in front of the ostium of the right-sided maxillary sinus (0° scope).

Balloon Sinuplasty and Biostatic Endoscopic Ethmoid Surgery (BESS)

Catheter-based balloon sinuplasty is a new procedure to restore ostium patency without removing tissue. For selected indications, it seems especially suited to open blocked ostia: acute recurrent sinusitis, barosinusitis, sinus empyema, primary or secondary stenosis. *Biostatic endoscopic ethmoid surgery (BESS)* is a new surgical strategy. The surgeon has to distinguish between biostatic and nonbiostatic cell formations to keep the ethmoidal space wide and open in the long term and to avoid shrinking by scarification. Both procedures can also be combined in a *hybrid operation*.

Maxillary Sinus Surgery

Infundibulotomy

The three-dimensional space of the ethmoid infundibulum, which runs in a sagittal direction through the lateral nasal wall, is approached using a crescent-shaped incision and resection of the uncinate process (**Fig. 2.64**). After this, the natural ostium in the caudal part of the infundibulum can be entered endoscopically and enlarged (supraturbinate fenestration). Intracavitary manipulations (e.g., removal of cysts or polyps, aspiration of secretions) can now be performed under vision using a 30°, 45°, or 70°

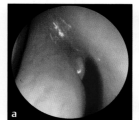
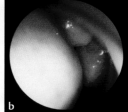
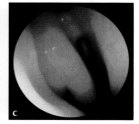

Fig. 2.62a–c With the aid of nasal endoscopy, even minimal mucosal pathology can be identified (0° scopes).
a Edema of the middle nasal meatus.

b Polyps in the ethmoidal infundibulum.
c Prolapse of the medial infundibular wall in chronic inflammation.

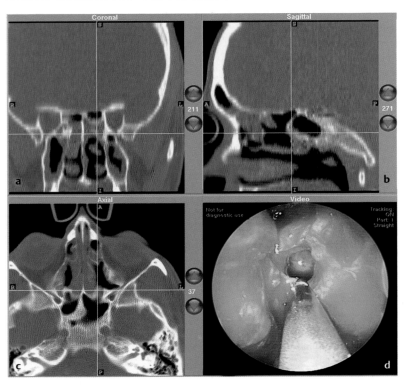

Fig. 2.63a–d Navigation-supported endoscopic surgery of the sphenoid sinus.
a Coronal view.
b Sagittal view.
c Axial view.
d Intraoperative endoscopic view of the anterior wall of the sphenoid sinus.

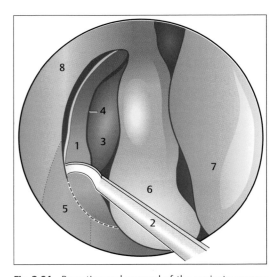

Fig. 2.64 Resection and removal of the uncinate process for access to the ethmoidal infundibulum of the nose (ethmoidal infundibulotomy). **1**, Uncinate process; **2**, sickle knife; **3**, ethmoidal bulla; **4**, semilunar hiatus; **5**, ethmoidal infundibulum; **6**, middle turbinate; **7**, nasal septum; **8**, agger nasi.

lens (**Fig. 2.65a–d**). However, there are still a few blind spots, so that in some cases access to the maxillary sinus cavity has to be completed using an infraturbinate trepanation or puncture of the canine fossa (**Fig. 2.66**).

Note: Infraturbinate fenestration for therapeutic purposes is inappropriate, as the secretions are transported past it toward the natural ostium.

Anatomical definitions: The ethmoidal infundibulum is the space enclosed by the uncinate process (medially), the lamina papyracea, and possibly the frontal process of the maxilla and lacrimal bone (laterally), and the ethmoid bulla (dorsally). The infundibulum can be accessed via the inferior semilunar hiatus.

The inferior semilunar hiatus (the gateway to the infundibulum; see **Fig. 2.62**) is a sagittal, crescent-shaped slit between the free posterior border of the uncinate process and the anterior surface of the bulla.

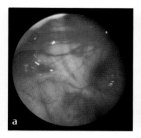 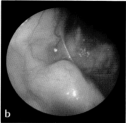 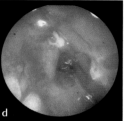

Fig. 2.65a–d Mucosal findings in the maxillary sinus (0° and 30° scopes).
a Normal mucosa in the maxillary sinus.
b Dental root in the maxillary sinus.

c What is known as a "cobblestone relief" is left to heal by itself.
d Edematous mucosa in acute inflammation, with obstruction of the natural ostium.

Caldwell–Luc Radical Antrostomy

Radical surgery is nowadays no longer a primary procedure, and it is indicated only for revision surgery (**Fig. 2.67**).

Local or general endotracheal anesthesia is used. Access is obtained via the oral cavity. The soft tissues of the cheek are elevated from the canine fossa, and a window is created in the anterior wall of the antrum. After the diseased antral mucosa is removed, a large window is created in the lateral nasal wall, leading from the antrum into the inferior meatus.

Intranasal Antrostomy

This is a palliative procedure for recurrent catarrhal maxillary sinusitis. Local or general anesthesia may be used. A large window is created between the inferior meatus and the antral cavity, with the physician working from the nasal cavity.

Frontal Sinus Surgery

Endonasal Methods

The types of endonasal drainage of the frontal sinuses as defined by Draf (1991) are as follows (**Fig. 2.68a–c**):

- Type I. Simple drainage: opening of the frontal recess by removal of the anterior ethmoid and dissection to the anterior base of the skull (**Fig. 2.69a**).
- Type IIa. Extended drainage: enlargement of the route of access without touching the middle turbinate (**Fig. 2.69b**).
- Type IIb. Expanded drainage: removal of the medial floor of the frontal sinus from the lamina papyracea to the nasal septum, including the anterior vertical lamella of the middle turbinate.
- Type III. Endonasal median drainage: removal of both the floor of the frontal sinus, as in type II,

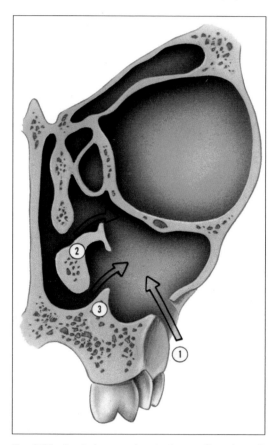

Fig. 2.66 Surgical approaches to the maxillary sinus. **1**, Supraturbinal access route; **2**, infraturbinal route; **3**, canine fossa route.

and of the nasal septa and frontal sinus septa adjacent to the floor of the frontal sinus (**Fig. 2.69c**).

Table 2.7 shows the indications for endonasal frontal sinus drainage types I–III using the Draf methods.

External Methods

Bicoronal incision with osteoplastic sinusotomy. The bicoronal incision divides the skin and epicranial aponeurosis behind the frontal hairline (**Fig. 2.70**). The plane of dissection is supraperiosteal and suprafascial and extends past the supraorbital margins. A bone flap is elevated and fractured inferiorly, leaving it attached on a hinge of periosteum. This technique provides good exposure of all recesses in well-pneumatized frontal sinuses. The

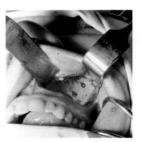

Fig. 2.67 Radical surgery of the maxillary sinus. This used to be one of the most common operations, but today it is done only when very strictly indicated, or as a revision procedure.

surgeon can dissect through the frontal infundibulum into the cranial part of the ethmoid bone (**Fig. 2.71a, b**).

Indications: Large osteomas; mucoceles in large sinus; central rhinogenous complications (brain abscess); treatment of defects, fractures, and CSF leaks involving the posterior wall of the frontal sinus; osteomyelitis (Pott puffy tumor). The bone should be burred away to a level that extends past the frontal sinus boundaries. Defect reconstruction is carried out with bioceramic glass implants made using computer-aided design/computer-aided manufacturing (CAD/CAM), or with autologous bone.

Contralateral, ipsilateral, and median (CIM) drainage concept for external revision surgery. Patients with a history of persistent frontal sinus disorders and often several previous operations, or of skull base fractures, often suffer from mucociliary drainage disorders as well as morphological problems in the lateral sinus (**Fig. 2.72**). Unfortunately, frontal sinuses that are less well pneumatized are especially susceptible to inflammatory disease, making the osteoplastic approach problematic in these cases. Typical problem areas in previously operated frontal sinuses are the lateral recess, the frontal sinus roof, the orbital roof, and the frontal infundibulum.

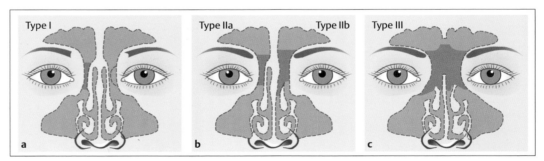

Type I   Type IIa   Type IIb   Type III

a   b   c

Fig. 2.68a–c Drainage pathways from the frontal sinus according to Draf.

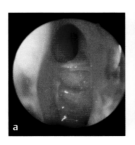
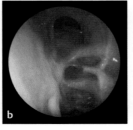
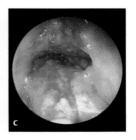

a   b   c

Fig. 2.69a–c Endoscopic drainage of the frontal sinus.
a Draf type I.
b Draf type II.
c Draf type III.

Table 2.7 Indications for endonasal frontal sinus drainage (Draf types I–III)

Indications for type I drainage

Acute sinusitis: failure of conservative surgery, orbital and endocranial complications

Chronic sinusitis: first-time surgery, absence of risk factors (e. g., aspirin intolerance, asthma triad), revision after incomplete ethmoidectomy

Indications for type IIa drainage

Serious complications of acute sinusitis, medial mucopyocele, tumor surgery (benign tumors), healthy mucosa

Indications for type IIb drainage

All indications for type IIa if the resulting drainage is small, when drilling is necessary

Indications for type III drainage

Primary procedure in patients with prognostic risk factors (asthma triad, cystic fibrosis), Kartagener syndrome, ciliary immotility syndrome, benign and malignant tumors

CIM is a surgical strategy that uses an open approach. Depending on the local situation, an ipsilateral, contralateral, or median drainage pathway to the nose can be reconstructed. In many cases, it is necessary to involve all of the pathways at once. It is very important to rebuild the bony defect of the sinus floor using ear cartilage. To achieve an inconspicuous scar and a good esthetic outcome, a special dermis-everting suture is used (**Figs. 2.73, 2.74a, b**).

Beck trephine. The principle of the *Beck trephine* is shown in **Fig. 2.27a–d** and described on page 140. A burr hole is made in the anterior wall of the sinus in the supraorbital region. A short blunt cannula is introduced, through which the cavity of the frontal sinus can be aspirated, irrigated, and filled with antibiotics. The cannula should not be retained for more than 8 days, due to the foreign-body response of the sinus mucosa.

The use of the Kümmel and Beck technique for frontal sinus trepanation has now declined to the point of near-obsolescence in the age of endoscopic microsurgery of the paranasal sinuses. The appropriate approach to relieve frontal sinus empyema is endoscopic surgery.

Principle of the Traditional Frontal Sinus Operations
The following surgical procedures are described here because they were the most commonly used otorhinolaryngology operations for several decades. Even today, patients present to otorhinolaryngologists with operations of this type in their medical history, or with late complications of these types of surgery. The operations are no longer indicated as primary procedures (**Fig. 2.75**).

1. **Jansen–Ritter method.** A curved incision is made near the medial canthus and extended into the eyebrow. Through a window created in the floor of the frontal sinus, the mucosa is cleared completely from the sinus. Next, a wide drainage opening is created into the nasal cavity. A permanent communication between the nose and the frontal sinus is secured using an Uffenorde mucosal flap or a large synthetic stent for at least

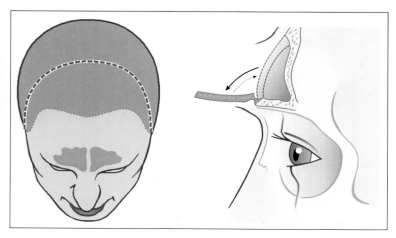

Fig. 2.70 Osteoplastic surgery in the frontal sinus.

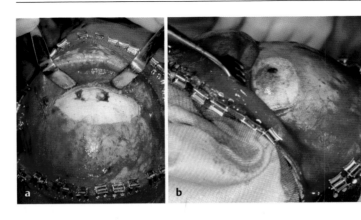

Fig. 2.71a, b Surgical approaches to the frontal sinus and frontal bone.
a For a large osteoma.
b For an intraosseous hemangioma.

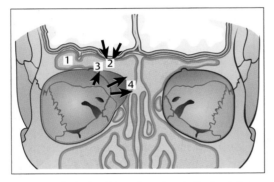

Fig. 2.72 Typical problematic regions in the frontal sinus following trauma or previous surgery. **1**, Lateral recess; **2**, roof of the frontal sinus; **3**, floor of the frontal sinus; **4**, frontal infundibulum/frontal recess.

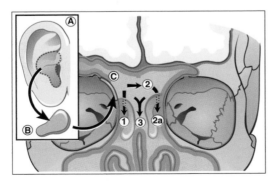

Fig. 2.73 The contralateral, ipsilateral, and median (CIM) concept of drainage and reconstruction of the frontal sinus floor (according to Behrbohm). **A**, Cartilage is harvested from the auricular concha; **B**, a suitable cartilage graft is prepared; **C**, the frontal sinus floor or lamina papyracea is reconstructed. **1**, Ipsilateral transethmoidal route; **2**, contralateral route through the interfrontal septum; **2a**, adjunctive endoscopic clearance or enlargement of the frontal recess; **3**, median drainage.

8 days. The advantage of this procedure is that it allows a cosmetically acceptable external incision. The disadvantage is that it can only be used for relatively small frontal sinuses. The procedure is not suitable for dealing with trauma to the anterior base of the skull.

2. **Killian method.** Access is obtained as in method 1 above. In addition, a window is created in the anterior wall of the frontal sinus, with retention of the bony orbital arch to preserve the profile. The operation then proceeds as in method 1. This procedure is indicated for very large frontal sinuses, as it guarantees access to all the loculi of the sinuses and thus allows removal of all parts of the mucosa. The contour of the forehead is preserved.

3. **Riedel method.** Access is obtained using method 1 above. The floor and anterior wall of the frontal sinus are removed, and the operation continues as in method 1. The advantage of this procedure is that it ensures clearance of the sinus and postoperative obliteration of the frontal sinus area. Its disadvantage is the resulting cosmetic deformity in the face due to sinking in of the forehead, requiring subsequent correction using a synthetic implant.

Sphenoid Sinus Surgery

The method of choice is endoscopic sphenoid sinus surgery. Depending on the indications—e. g., large, well-vascularized tumors—access may be via a transmaxillary or transseptal route, lateral rhinotomy, or midfacial degloving.

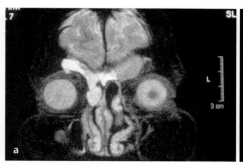

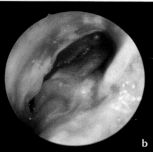

Fig. 2.74a, b **a** MRI showing mucoceles in both frontal sinuses following several previous operations.
b Endoscopic view of the frontal sinus after repair (45° lens).

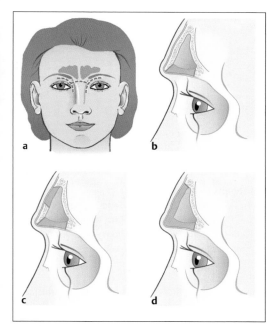

Fig. 2.75a–d The principle of external frontal sinus operations.
a Incisions.
b Bone removal with the Jansen–Ritter method.
c Killian operation.
d Riedel operation.

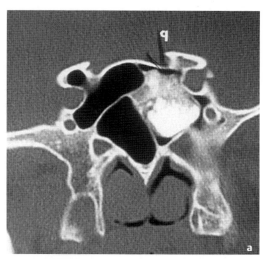

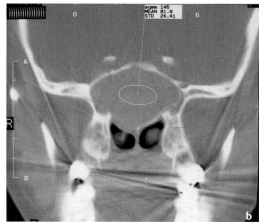

Fig. 2.76a, b **a** Osteoma of the left-sided sphenoid.
b Mucocele of the sphenoid sinus.

Endoscopic Sphenoid Sinus Operations

The ostium of the sphenoid sinus is identified in the sphenoethmoidal recess, ≈ 10 mm above the vertex of the choanae (nasal part) in the anterior wall of the sphenoid; or the anterior wall of the sphenoid sinus is identified and trephined in the ethmoidal part via posterior ethmoidectomy (**Fig. 2.76a, b**).

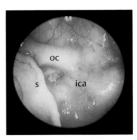

Fig. 2.77   View into an operated sphenoid sinus. **s**, Intersphenoid septum; **oc**, optic canal; **ica**, internal carotid artery (0° lens).

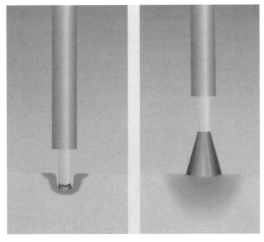

Fig. 2.78   The principle of contact and noncontact techniques in laser application.

The anterior wall of the sphenoid sinus (sphenoid bone) is thicker and harder than the septa separating the air cells of the ethmoid bone. The possibility of anatomic variations (e. g., Onodi cells) means that secure orientation is needed in this region.

> **Note:** If the nature of a tumor is uncertain, preoperative exclusion of a vascular tumor using MRI or magnetic resonance angiography (MRA) is always required. Blind use of sharp instruments in the sphenoid sinus is strictly prohibited, due to the risk of injury to the carotid artery and the optic nerve (**Fig. 2.77**)

Lasers in Rhinology

The various lasers differ in the way they are generated and in their wavelengths, their specific absorptions, the depth to which they penetrate biological tissues, and thus in their range of surgical applications (**Fig. 2.78**).

Physical properties (Table 2.8)
- *CO_2 lasers:* The rays are absorbed in the outermost layers of tissue. These work very well for ablation and cutting, but not for coagulating.
- *Neodymium:yttrium-aluminum-garnet (Nd:YAG) and diode lasers:* The effects are practically the converse of the CO_2 laser. Depending on the power, the rays can penetrate deeper than 4 mm into tissue and are strongly diffracted. The coagulation effects are marked.
- *Holmium:yttrium-aluminum-garnet (Ho:YAG) lasers:* Generated in pulses. Coagulation and ablation are possible.
- *Potassium titanyl phosphate (KTP) lasers:* These are basically Nd:YAG lasers that work at double frequency.
- *Nd:YAG and argon lasers:* A unique feature of this type is absorption by hemoglobin, allowing special effects in well-vascularized tissue (e. g., "optical purse-string suture").

■ Rhinosinusitis in Children

Rhinosinusitis in childhood is anatomically, immunologically, and clinically different from that in adults.

Pathogens of acute infections. Rhinoviruses, coronaviruses, adenoviruses, myxoviruses, and respiratory syncytial viruses may be implicated. The most important pathogens for acute bacterial rhinitis in children are *Pneumococcus*, *Haemophilus influenzae*, *Moraxella catarrhalis*, and *Staphylococcus aureus*.

Anatomy. The child's skull is different from that of an adult in many respects. In a toddler, the floor of the maxillary sinus is at a higher level than in an adult, never extending below that of the floor of the nose; the alveolar process is not yet developed. Thus, the ethmoid bone is longer than the maxillary sinus. The infundibulum is short and narrow. The distance between the medial wall of the infundibulum and the lamina papyracea is only a few millimeters. The lamina papyracea is particularly thin, facilitating the spread of rhinogenous infections to the orbit. Diseases of the maxillary sinuses may occur at any age. Pneumatization of the frontal sinus does not take place until the fourth year of life, and frontal sinusitis seldom occurs before the age of 6 years. Approximately the same age data apply for the sphenoid sinus (**Fig. 2.79**).

Table 2.8   Characteristics and biological effects of some important laser types

Type of laser	Wavelength	Operating mode	Depth of tissue penetration (mm)	Effects	Applications
CO_2	10.6 µm	CW	≈ 0.15	Cutting, ablation coagulation (to a limited extent)	No contact
Argon	488/514 nm	CW	≈ 2.0	Cutting, coagulation	No contact
KTP	532 nm	CW	≈ 2.0	Cutting, coagulation	No contact
Ho:YAG	2.1 µm	Pulsed	≈ 0.4	Cutting, coagulation	No contact
Nd:YAG	1064 µm	CW	1.5–4.0	Cutting, coagulation	No contact, in contact
Diodes	805, 950, 980 nm	CW	1.5–4.5	Cutting, coagulation	No contact, in contact

CW, continuous wave; Ho:YAG, holmium:yttrium-aluminum-garnet; KTP, potassium titanyl phosphate; Nd:YAG, neodymium:yttrium-aluminum-garnet.

Immunology. An infant has immunity, acquired through transplacental transfer of maternal immunoglobulin G (IgG), allowing it to ward off respiratory infections. This immunity is gradually replaced by the infant's own production of IgG. The production of IgA contributes additionally to the defense against infections. With its ability to achieve rapid production of IgM, the lymphatic tissue in the nasopharynx further supports specific immune defenses against respiratory infections.

Clinical Features. In infants and toddlers, nonspecific, generalized symptoms such as fever and lymphadenitis predominate (**Table 2.9**). Younger children react with generalized mucosal disease of the airways. Only as the children grow do the symptoms become limited to various levels of the airways. The main symptoms of acute sinusitis include dry cough and nasal congestion and discharge. Nocturnal coughing may indicate sinusitis. Chronic sinusitis may remain concealed behind vague symptoms such as loss of appetite, malaise, low-grade fever, recurrent coughing, and pharyngitis.

Diagnosis

Note: The history usually depends on statements made by the parents, who are likely to have already interpreted the symptoms.

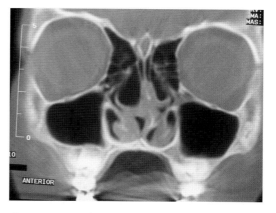

Fig. 2.79   Coronal CT in a child with bilateral concha bullosa, missing alveolar recesses, and narrow ethmoid infundibula.

The diagnosis is based on the history, inspection, and nasal endoscopy. Allergy test, nasal cytology, immune status (IgG, IgA, IgM), A-mode sonography, and nasal secretion studies (bacteriology, mycology, cytology) may also be useful investigations. If chronic rhinosinusitis is suspected, a CT examination is necessary.

Therapy. *Acute rhinosinusitis:* Supportive measures consist of decongestant nose drops, heat or short-wave application, aspiration of the nose with a simple suction apparatus, administration of an iso-

Table 2.9 Symptoms of acute and chronic rhinosinusitis in children

Acute rhinosinusitis	Acute rhinitis, purulent rhinorrhea, nasal obstruction, fever, lymphadenitis
Chronic rhinosinusitis	Coughing, mouth breathing, pharyngitis, serous otitis media

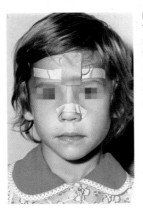

Fig. 2.80 A child with Thornwald drains in both maxillary sinuses. This treatment option is now more or less obsolete in the era of targeted antibiotic therapy and endoscopic microsurgery.

tonic salt solution as nose drops or inhaled, and secretolytic agents.

Antibiotics: The first-line agent is amoxicillin, 50 mg/kg/day, in three divided doses. Children who have been started on amoxicillin (e.g., in case of infection with *Moraxella catarrhalis* or *Haemophilus influenzae*) should be given amoxicillin plus clavulanic acid, 50 mg/12.5 mg/kg/day, in two divided doses; alternatively, clarithromycin, 15 mg/kg/day in two divided doses, may be given. Treatment should be continued for 10–14 days (**Fig. 2.80**).

Chronic rhinosinusitis: Supportive measures such as decongestant nose drops (beware of long-term use), secretolytic agents, adenoid removal with or without antral lavage, and possibly FESS are useful.

Antibiotics: Amoxicillin plus clavulanic acid, 50 mg/kg/day in three divided doses, or clindamycin, 40 mg/kg/day in three divided doses. Children older than 14 years of age may be given doxycycline, 5 mg/kg/day in one dose.

Mycotic infections: Amphotericin B, ketoconazole, or 5-flucytosine.

Complications. Orbital complications are more common in children than in adults, because of the thinness of the lamina papyracea (for staging, see p. 186). Intracranial complications are less common; they may consist of subdural or epidural abscesses, meningitis, brain abscesses, cavernous sinus thrombosis, or osteomyelitis (see the individual disease entities). Pathogens and antibiotics are described given on page 188 (**Fig. 2.81a, b**).

■ **Fungal Diseases of the Paranasal Sinuses**

Fungi are ubiquitous and are frequently being inhaled. Detection of fungi within the nose is therefore a normal finding in the healthy nose. However, in the pathological sense, fungal disease can be considered as:

• Noninvasive—the most common group of disorders.
• Invasive—rarely seen.

Fungi have also been implicated in the pathogenesis of eosinophilic fungal rhinosinusitis (EFRS), characterized by extensive polyps with eosinophilic mucus. The current understanding is that high numbers of eosinophils migrate to the nasal mucosa and pass into the overlying mucus, where they cluster around fungal hyphae and spores. The eosinophils try to destroy the fungi by degranulating and releasing major basic protein (MBP), which is highly toxic to the mucosal cellular surface. As more fungi are inhaled, the cycle continues and MBP increases.

Some patients also have an IgE-mediated allergy to fungi, but these patients do not always have MBP within the mucus. It has recently been noted that the IgE component is neither causative nor a major factor in the pathogenesis of this disease, and the previously accepted diagnosis of "allergic fungal sinusitis" is a misconception (Stammberger, personal communication, 2008).

Noninvasive Forms

Saprophytic Forms

Fungi can colonize the surface of mucus crusts, inspissated debris, foreign bodies, internal splints, stents and nasogastric tubes. The treatment consists of removing the mucus, crusts, or foreign body. Localized unilateral crusts may form over abnormal mucosa, and malignant change has to be excluded.

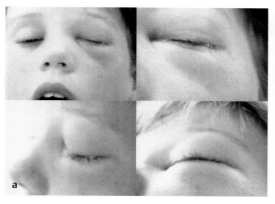
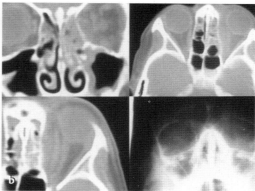

Fig. 2.81a, b **a** A 10-year-old boy with marked soft edema of the upper and lower eyelids.
b Subperiosteal abscess, visualized on coronal and axial CTs.

Fungus Ball

Fungal masses occur within a sinus air cell or sinus lumen and act as an irritant foreign body.

Clinical Features. These resemble those of chronic sinusitis. Portions of the fungal conglomerate may reach the nose, causing bloody secretions and a fetid odor. The most frequently affected sites are the maxillary and frontal sinuses.

Diagnosis. Nasal endoscopy reveals chronic rhinosinusitis. MRI and CT show characteristic opacification. CT often shows hyperdense central areas that look calcified due to high concentrations of calcium sulfate, phosphate, and metals, which are metabolized by the fungi.

Treatment. This consists of endoscopic cleansing of the affected paranasal sinus and establishment of unobstructed ventilation. The fungal concretions must be removed completely, but mucosa can be preserved.

Samples should be sent for fungal culture and histology. Antimycotic therapy is not indicated (**Fig. 2.82**).

Invasive Forms

Acute Fulminant Form

Clinical Features. Acute illness with fever, abnormal fatigue, and facial pain, followed later by visual impairment and somnolence to the point of coma.

Pathogenesis. Usually occurs in patients receiving immune suppression or individuals with impaired immunity (e.g., those with diabetes mellitus, AIDS, or wasting diseases). Fungi such as *Mucor*, *Absidia*, or *Aspergillus* invade the tissues, including blood vessels, leading to hematogenous spread to the central nervous system or the orbit.

Treatment. Immediate, complete excision of all affected tissue, following the principles of cancer surgery. Systemic administration of amphotericin B, ketoconazole, itraconazole, or the more recent voriconazole for long periods is needed. There is recent evidence that long-term itraconazole is effective for invasive *Aspergillus* infection. The prognosis is serious.

Chronic Indolent Granulomatous Form

This is rarely seen in industrialized countries, but is more common in north Africa. In contrast to the acute form, patients are not usually immunocompromised.

Clinical Features. A slowly progressive disease over many years. Invasion beyond the paranasal sinuses may affect the orbit, with subsequent orbital swelling. The infratemporal fossa or infratemporal fossa may also be affected. Cranial nerve defects may occur.

Diagnosis. Samples should be sent for both fungal culture and histology. CT and MRI scans should be obtained.

Treatment. The diseased area should be debulked and long-term antimycotic therapy instigated. The prognosis with this regimen is good.

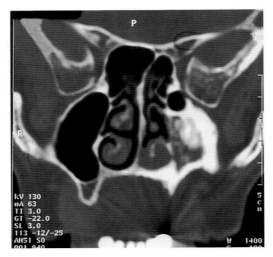

Fig. 2.82 A left-sided hypoplastic maxillary sinus, with fungal conglomeration and appositional growth of bone in reaction to the inflammation.

■ **Pathophysiologic Relationship between the Sinuses and the Rest of the Body**

United Airways Syndrome (Sinobronchial Syndrome)

The upper and lower airways form a functional unit. The mucosa, submucosa, and vascularization are similar in the two regions, and biochemical regulatory mechanisms involve the same mediators. The mucosa of both the upper and lower airways reacts to stimuli from allergic, physical, or chemical irritants or microbial infection with eosinophilic infiltration, mucosal edema, and endocrine malfunction.

The WHO's Allergic Rhinitis and its Impact on Asthma (ARIA) guidelines emphasize the importance of consistent treatment of allergic rhinitis (see above) in preventing allergic bronchial asthma.

Note: One child in three with allergic rhinitis develops asthma by the age of 7 years.

Cystic Fibrosis

This is the most common congenital disorder in children. The function of the exocrine glands is abnormal, causing a constant increase in chloride and sodium in the sweat and saliva, and abnormally viscous secretions. The main symptoms are pulmonary (progressive bronchial obstruction) and abdominal (due to deficiency of pancreatic enzymes), rectal prolapse, and liver cirrhosis. Nasal manifestations include sinusitis and polyps of the nose and sinuses.

Primary Ciliary Dyskinesia

Immotile cilia syndrome (ICS) is an autosomal-recessive disease with genetic heterogeneity, characterized by abnormal ciliary motion and impaired mucociliary clearance. In 1933, Kartagener described a syndrome characterized by the triad of situs inversus, chronic sinusitis, and bronchiectasis. Later, it was noted that these patients have defects in the ultrastructure of the cilia.

■ **Mucoceles and Cysts**

A *mucocele* is characterized clinically as a benign but locally destructive epithelial space-occupying lesion that arises within an anatomical cavity, but almost extends beyond its boundaries, compressing and eroding neighboring structures (**Fig. 2.83a, b**).

Whereas the classic signs of inflammation, such as redness, heat, and pain are absent with mucoceles, the clinical presentation of which depends entirely on space-occupying effects, a *pyocele* usually presents as an inflammatory condition with conspicuous symptoms such as eyelid swelling, pain, fever, and generalized manifestations (**Fig. 2.84**).

Mucoceles and pyoceles are caused by obstruction of sinus drainage and the resulting retention of secretions in the sinus. The frontal, ethmoid, sphenoid, and maxillary sinuses are affected, in decreasing order of incidence. The cause may be inflammation, trauma, surgery, or tumor. In the absence of spontaneous drainage, the increasing internal pressure gradually converts the bony sinus wall into a fibrous capsule extending in the direction of least resistance, such as the floor of the frontal sinus or the lamina papyracea.

Frontal sinus mucoceles: Three factors are critical in the pathogenesis of frontal sinus mucoceles: damage to the mucoperiosteum, displacement of the drainage zone, and retention of secretions. The rising intrasinus pressure leads to erosion of the bony sinus wall and formation of a fibrous capsule. The pressure may act in all directions, affecting the orbit, the anterior cranial fossa, and the ethmoid bone.

Solitary mucoceles can often be treated by *marsupialization*. This involves partial removal of the lower part of the mucocele sac, allowing the mucocele to drain to the nose while preserving the epithelial lining of the frontal sinus. This procedure is often facilitated by the fact that years of mucocele growth and expansion into the ethmoid bone will have caused widening of the frontal infundibulum. The endonasal endoscopic approach using the 45° scope is very advantageous in these cases.

Clinical Features. The main symptoms include displacement of the orbit externally or interiorly and limitation of movement of the bulb, leading to disorders of vision and double vision. Optic atrophy and amaurosis can occur in extreme cases. Mucoceles of the posterior sinuses can cause an orbital apex syndrome (see p. 187) or simulate a hypophyseal or cerebral tumor. Lesions arising in the maxillary sinus cause increasing distension of the cheek, but ocular symptoms are unusual.

Diagnosis. This is by coronal or axial computed tomography.

Differential diagnosis. Early inflammatory complications, malignancy, and meningocele must be considered.

Treatment. Clearance of the affected sinus and creation of a wide communication with the nasal cavity must be attained.

Cysts

Cysts are relatively common in the paranasal sinuses, especially in the maxillary sinus. They may produce clinical symptoms or may be noted as incidental findings. Unlike a mucocele or a pyocele, a cyst does not extend beyond the anatomical boundaries of its cavity. A cyst forming a tense, convex mass impinging on the apposed bony walls of the sinus may cause a pressure sensation or headache.

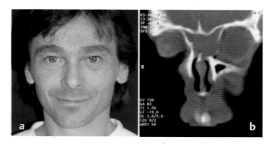

Fig. 2.83a, b   A patient with extensive bilateral frontal sinus mucoceles and mild swelling at the medial canthus of the left eye.

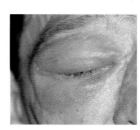

Fig. 2.84   Pyocele of the right frontal sinus.

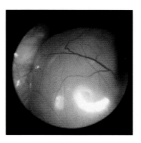

Fig. 2.85   A cyst in the maxillary sinus (0° scope).

Mucous retention cysts (small and yellowish, with thick walls) can be distinguished from true cysts (larger, with thin walls and fine vascular markings) by endoscopic examination (**Fig. 2.85**).

Cysts arising in the maxillary sinus may be *dental radicular* (arising from a tooth root) or *follicular* (arising from a displaced tooth germ). They produce typical radiologic findings.

Treatment. This is by removal of the cyst, either via the antral cavity or via the mouth; radicular cysts are removed by a maxillofacial surgeon.

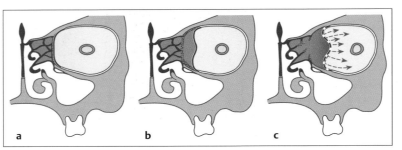

Fig. 2.86a–c The clinically most important orbital complications arising from the ethmoid: **a**, periorbital cellulitis; **b**, subperiosteal abscess; **c**, orbital abscess.

■ **Complications of Sinus Infections**

Extension to the External Soft Tissues
This may be due to frontal sinusitis (causing swelling of the soft tissues of the forehead or the upper eyelid), ethmoiditis (causing swelling of the eyelids, especially the lower one), or maxillary sinusitis (causing swelling of the cheek and edema of the lower eyelid). The cause is usually acute sinusitis or an acute exacerbation of chronic sinusitis. The soft tissues over the point of rupture show a boggy swelling that is usually reddened and painful on pressure.

Diagnosis. This is based on the history, clinical findings, and CT or sometimes MRI.

Treatment. Appropriate antibiotic therapy and surgical drainage of the affected sinus in suitable cases are essential.

Orbital Complications
These are relatively common and potentially very serious. They usually originate in the ethmoidal or frontal sinuses, and less frequently from the maxillary sinus. The term "periorbital cellulitis" is often used to refer to all degrees of orbital infection and is imprecise. However, a system of grouping the various stages of infection according to severity has been described (Chandler 1970) (**Fig. 2.86a–c**):
• Periorbital cellulitis (preseptal edema).
• Orbital cellulitis.
• Subperiosteal abscess.
• Orbital abscess or phlegmon.
• Cavernous sinus thrombosis (see p. 189).

Clinical Features. Orbital complications, especially in children, often occur without pain. Orbital involvement is initially manifested by edema and erythema of the medial aspects of the eyelid, and later by swelling, exophthalmos, and impaired extraocular eye movements. Periorbital or orbital cellulitis may result from direct or vascular spread of the sinus infection.

Periorbital Cellulitis
This is the most common complication of rhinosinusitis in children. The inflammation involves tissue anterior to the orbital septum.

Clinical Features. Orbital pain, blepharal edema, and high fever are typical; eye movement is not impaired. The sclera will be white and not red.

Diagnosis. Nasal endoscopy and/or axial CT reveal soft-tissue swelling anterior to the orbital septum.

Therapy. This should be started with empirical antibiotic therapy, which should be as targeted as possible and cover upper respiratory tract anaerobes.

Orbital Cellulitis
This implies spread of the inflammation to the orbital septum, leading to limitation of ocular movements and possibly exophthalmos.

Clinical Features. Chemosis, exophthalmos, ocular pain, and tenderness are accompanied by decreased action of the extraocular muscles.

Diagnosis. Axial CT can distinguish between an orbital and a subperiosteal abscess.

Therapy. This is based on ophthalmologic assessment of visual acuity and intravenous administration of antibiotics. Conservative therapy is appropriate if an abscess can be excluded. Supportive measures—e.g., so-called "high tamponade" or spreading of the middle turbinate, depend on the endoscopic and CT findings.

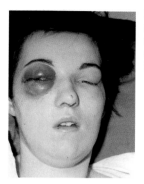

Fig. 2.87 Right orbital abscess with "board-like" swelling, visual impairment, and loss of eyeball mobility.

Subperiosteal Abscess

Clinical Features. Swelling of the eyelids, pain, and lateral and inferior bulb displacement are noted. Protrusion of the bulb may be present. Depending on the extent, diplopia or limitation of eyeball movement, chemosis, or fever may occur in children. If the abscess spreads to the eyelid there is pain, redness, and firm swelling of the eyelid.

Diagnosis. This requires inspection, nasal endoscopy, consultation with an ophthalmologist, and axial CT.

Treatment. At first calculated high-dose intravenous antibiotic therapy with ampillicin and sulbactam, or clindamycin, or ceftazidim; later targeted antibiotic therapy depending on the resistogram.

Absolute indication for endoscopic surgical drainage of the abscess and sinus of origin.

Orbital Abscess or Phlegmon

An orbital abscess or phlegmon is the most serious immediate threat to the eye. The most important symptom distinguishing it from other orbital complications is the hard swelling that surrounds the bulb, visibly limiting its range of motion (**Fig. 2.87**).

Clinical Features. Marked edema and discoloration of the lids, chemosis, marked protrusion of the bulb, rapid loss of visual acuity, severe pain that increases when pressure is applied to the bulb or on movement of the eye, and limitation of movement of the eye due to damage to the ocular muscles and their nerves. Later features include complete paralysis of the orbit, congestion of the retinal veins, papilledema, and possibly panophthalmitis. Secondary intracranial extension to the cavernous sinus is possible.

Treatment. In addition to the treatment as for a subperiostal abscess, wide fenestration of the lamina papyracea is important to drain the abscess or phlegmon from the orbit to the nose.

Differential diagnosis. This depends on radiographic, CT, and ophthalmologic findings. Malignancy of the orbit, mucoceles, benign tumors (e. g., osteoma), inflammation of the lacrimal drainage system, cavernous sinus thrombosis, noninflammatory orbital diseases, and erysipelas must be excluded.

Orbital apex syndrome occurs when a lesion of the orbital apex affects the nerves and vessels that cross the optic foramen and the superior orbital fissure. The main symptoms are loss of vision, ptosis, double vision, severe temporoparietal headache, and exophthalmos due to compression of cranial nerves II, III, IV, V, and VI. Causes include trauma, neoplasms, and extension of ethmoidal or sphenoidal sinusitis. Treatment is by immediate decompression, because of the danger of amaurosis.

Rhinogenous retrobulbar optic neuritis is due to extension of inflammation of the sphenoidal air cells or posterior ethmoidal sinuses into the retrobulbar space. It is rare. Symptoms are primarily ophthalmologic. Treatment is by surgical drainage of the appropriate sinus, provided there is clear evidence of the presence of infection of that sinus.

Malignant exophthalmos (dysthyroid eye disease) due to thyrotoxicosis can be managed using a nasal operation (see p. 171). Edema of the soft tissues of the orbit, with resulting effects on the circulation and an actual increase in tissue, leads to increased intraorbital pressure and consequent injury to the bulb and the optic nerve. Decompression can be achieved by removing the bony floor of the orbit, the ethmoidal air cells, and the lamina papyracea, while preserving the infraorbital nerve.

Note: Any unilateral or bilateral loss of vision or oculomotor disorder causing double vision requires thorough rhinologic investigation.

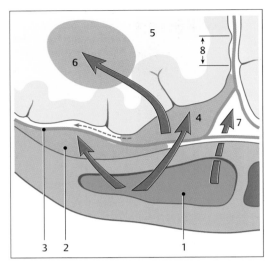

Fig. 2.88 Genesis of the intracranial complications of sinusitis. **1**, Frontal sinus with empyema; **2**, epidural abscess; **3**, dura mater; **4**, subdural abscess with marginal adhesion (**8**) or with extension as meningitis in the direction shown by the small dashed arrow; **5**, brain; **6**, abscess; **7**, extension to the sagittal sinus.

Intracranial Complications

Intracranial complications include epidural or subdural abscesses, brain abscess, meningitis, cerebritis, and cavernosus sinus thrombosis. All endocranial complications begin as cerebritis, but as necrosis and liquefaction of brain tissue progress, a capsule develops, resulting in a brain abscess (**Fig. 2.88**).

Diagnosis. A CT scan is essential for diagnosis, as it allows accurate assessment of bony involvement. MRI is essential when there is any soft-tissue involvement—e. g., in cavernous sinus thrombosis. Abscesses and tumors are best visualized using MRI or CT scans with contrast administration. Lumbar puncture may be useful if meningitis is suspected.

Figure 2.88 shows the principal pathways of spread of rhinogenous (usually sinus) infections into the intracranial cavity. These can be explained anatomically as follows:

- Direct extension after destruction of the bone by circumscribed osteitis, and necrosis of the bony wall of the sinus, possibly due to trauma.

- Extension via osteomyelitis (see p. 190).
- Extension via blood vessels, usually the veins in the bone, which communicate between the sinus and the intracranial cavity.
- Extension via the general circulation (hematogenous metastasis).

Epidural Abscess

Clinical Features. There are no typical symptoms of this disease. Symptoms may include subfebrile temperatures, headache and pressure in the head, and fatigue. Usually there are no signs clearly indicating the local disease. The findings in cerebrospinal fluid are unremarkable. Epidural abscess is often only discovered incidentally during surgery on the sinus of origin, in which osteitis or bony necrosis—e. g., of the posterior wall of the frontal sinus—may be found.

Supplementary diagnostic procedures. MRI; CT scans with contrast medium may be useful.

Differential diagnosis. Epidural hematoma.

Treatment. This consists of drainage of the sinus of origin with wide exposure of the inflamed dura until healthy tissue is exposed on all sides, and drainage into the nasal cavity.

Subdural Abscess

Clinical Features. As with epidural abscess, there are no typical symptoms. The patient may occasionally report headache and show increasing signs of meningeal irritation—e. g., pleocytosis of the CSF. The symptoms of meningitis or brain abscess—e. g., clouding of consciousness, neurologic irritation, neurologic signs, convulsions, or hemiparesis—develop gradually. The CSF may be normal or may show inflammatory changes, and CSF pressure may be raised. Meningitis with an unfavorable prognosis may develop.

Diagnostic methods. These include CT scans of the sinuses, MRI, or cerebral CT (with contrast medium); neurologic examination; electroencephalography; and carotid angiography.

Differential diagnosis. Subdural hematoma, in which there is blood in the CSF.

Treatment. Drainage of the sinus of origin and of the subdural abscess (via the pathway of spread) must be carried out, supported by administration of high-dose antibiotics.

Rhinogenous Brain Abscess
This usually arises from the frontal sinus, and only rarely from the ethmoid air cells. Even rarer is a hematogenous *frontal lobe abscess.*

Clinical Features. Frontal lobe abscesses cause relatively few localizing symptoms. Four stages of a rhinogenous frontal lobe abscess can be distinguished: initial, latent, manifest, and terminal. Generalized symptoms, symptoms typical of increased intracranial pressure, and focal symptoms are usually pronounced. Confirmatory signs include a deteriorating overall condition, occasionally fever, increasing boring headache and sensitivity to pressure on the vault of the skull, nausea, vomiting, bradycardia, papilledema, unilateral anosmia, confusion, increasing somnolence, decreasing awareness of the surroundings, loss of concentration, overall mental torpor, altered behavior such as inappropriate joking and excessive euphoria, restlessness, coma, and cranial nerve paralysis (particularly of cranial nerves I, III, and VI).

Supplementary diagnostic methods. These include MRI or CT scans (with contrast medium) and assessment by a neurosurgeon.

Treatment. Therapy depends on the stage of the disease and the size and site of the abscess. The mainstay of treatment of abscesses arising from the nose or sinuses is combined neurosurgery and nasal surgery to excise the abscess, accompanied or followed immediately by drainage of the appropriate sinus.

Sinus Thrombosis
Cavernous Sinus Thrombosis
Clinical Features. These include edema of the upper and lower lid, oculomotor disorders, proptosis, papilledema, increasing loss of vision, possibly leading to blindness, chemosis, a septic temperature course with chills, a high continuous or remitting irregular fever, headache, variable pulse rate, and increasing clouding of consciousness. Examination of the CSF shows an increased cell count and increased protein content. The generalized symp-

toms of sepsis, with splenomegaly and a typical blood picture, may also be found.

Pathogenesis. Causes include propagated thrombophlebitis arising from a furuncle of the upper lip or nose and spreading via the angular vein, septal abscess, sphenoiditis with adjacent osteomyelitis, acute osteomyelitis of the frontal bone, orbital phlegmon, or petrositis with extension to the cavernous sinus.

Differential diagnosis. This covers orbital abscess, dental or tonsillar phlegmons and septicemia, otogenic sinus thrombosis, and hematogenous spread from elsewhere (i.e., of staphylococcal sepsis).

Treatment. Broad-spectrum antibiotics should be given at *high dosages* for a *prolonged period* at the earliest suspicion of thrombophlebitis, if possible selected according to culture and sensitivity tests after blood cultures. Treatment also includes bed rest, fluid balance, and the use of heparin anticoagulation. If there is a furuncle of the nose or upper lip, the angular vein should be divided with electrocautery or partially resected, depending on the local findings.

In some advanced cases, an attempt to drain the cavernous sinus surgically may be justified.

Prognosis. Very poor.

Complications. These include meningitis and septic metastases in the pulmonary and general circulation (**Fig. 2.89**).

Rhinogenous Meningitis
Symptoms of typical purulent meningitis. High fever, hyperesthesia, photophobia, variable pulse rate, nuchal stiffness, headache, vomiting, Jacksonian attacks, and symptoms of motor irritability (floccillation) are present. The Kernig and Lasègue sign and Brudzinski signs are all positive, and later there is opisthotonus and scaphoid abdomen.

The cranial nerves, especially III and IV, are affected. Examination of the CSF shows high-grade pleocytosis (normal: ≤ 12/3 cells/mL), markedly elevated pressure (normal: 7–12 cm H_2O), increased protein (normal: 25–40 mL/100 mL), and decreased sugar (normal: 40–90 mg/100 mL). The causative organism may also be isolated.

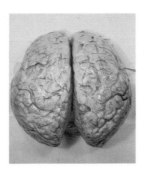

Fig. 2.89 Severe purulent leptomeningitis following frontal sinusitis. There are waxy, layered deposits of pus, hypervascularization, and ectasia of the cerebral blood vessels.

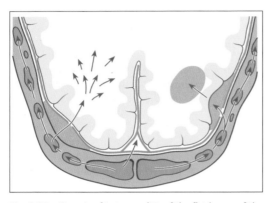

Fig. 2.90 Genesis of osteomyelitis of the flat bones of the skull. There is extension from a frontal sinus empyema to the diploë and marrow spaces of the vault, followed by an epidural or subdural abscess, sinus thrombosis (sagittal sinus), diffuse or circumscribed encephalitis, and brain abscess.

Supplementary diagnostic procedures. These include lumbar or suboccipital puncture, neurologic investigation, bacteriologic examination of the CSF, MRI, or CT (with contrast medium) to rule out a brain abscess.

Differential diagnosis. Nonrhinogenous meningitis—e.g., epidemic meningitis, viral meningitis, subarachnoid hemorrhage, and other cerebrospinal diseases—must be considered (**Fig. 2.89**).

Treatment. Therapy consists of immediate surgical drainage of the sinus of origin and exposure and closure of any defects found in the dura mater. High-dose antibiotics are given, and lumbar puncture is repeated frequently until the cell count falls below 100/mL. Recurrent episodes of meningitis

may be due to an anterior skull base defect, which needs to be excluded or identified and repaired.

Bony Complications

Osteomyelitis of the Flat Bones of the Skull (Pott Puffy Tumor)

This life-threatening disease may spread directly from frontal sinusitis due to inflammatory disease or trauma, but may also be due to hematogenous spread (**Fig. 2.90**).

The course is often fulminating, because the diploë of the vault of the skull (spongiosa, medullary space, diploic veins) does not have any anatomic barriers. Infection that has broken through into the diploë thus spreads rapidly in all directions and then breaks out of this layer into the intracranial cavity, allowing the development of typical intracranial complications (see p. 188). External rupture, giving rise to a subperiosteal abscess, is also possible.

Clinical Features. Adolescence is the most susceptible age. The course may be stormy or indolent.

Main symptoms. High fever, chills, deteriorated overall condition and fatigue, severe headache, clouding of consciousness, tenderness of the frontal region and the vault of the skull, and a boggy soft-tissue swelling over the diseased part of the bone may occur. In addition, there may be clear symptoms of the development of an intracranial complication, over a longer or shorter period (see p. 188).

Diagnosis. In a patient with a painful, boggy swelling on the forehead, the physician must consider a Pott puffy tumor if the swelling exceeds the boundaries of the frontal sinus and if its peripheral borders are difficult to define. Important information is provided by CT and radioisotope bone scans, and by alkaline phosphatase as a laboratory parameter (**Fig. 2.91a, b**).

Differential diagnosis. Erysipelas and other septic diseases have to be excluded.

Treatment. The critical steps in the management of frontal bone osteomyelitis with a subperiosteal abscess (Pott puffy tumor) are early diagnosis and initiation of radical surgical therapy, supported by targeted antibiotic therapy with an antibiotic that can penetrate bone (e.g., fosfomycin).

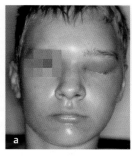
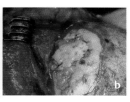

Fig. 2.91a, b   a A young patient with osteomyelitis of the frontal bone. **b** After removal of the entire osteitic bone via an osteoplastic access route, the defect is covered with bone from the cranial vault.

The bone of the vault of the skull should be exposed widely with a healthy margin, with removal of the external table, decortication, and removal of the diploë and, occasionally, the internal table of the vault of the skull. If necessary, an already manifest intracranial complication has to be managed surgically.

Osteomyelitis of the Upper Jaw

This condition is not common. It is usually caused by dental disease; more rarely, it may be due to hematogenous spread, or may originate from the sinuses—e. g., in trauma. It may also arise from bony necrosis after infectious fevers—e. g., typhus, measles, or scarlet fever, or from radionecrosis following radiotherapy.

Clinical Features. These include swelling of the cheek, pain in the face, abscesses pointing into the mouth, the antrum, or externally.

Treatment. Removal of the (dental) cause is indicated. Antibiotics are administered, and the diseased bone is removed.

Osteomyelitis of the Upper Jaw in Infants

This condition is accompanied by acute swelling of the cheek, signs of local infection, and an abscess pointing either into the mouth or externally.

Cause. Possibly infection of the antral cavity, which is still very small in infants.

Treatment. This consists of high-dose antibiotics, and possibly careful drainage from the vestibule of the mouth, with care being taken not to damage the follicles of the teeth.

The causes of swelling of the face are shown in **Table 2.10**.

▪ Epistaxis

Epistaxis is one of the most frequent emergencies in otolaryngology, and other specialty disciplines may be involved in the clinical management.

Although the course is usually innocuous and the cause often banal and nonspecific, epistaxis may be a serious disease that is extremely difficult to treat, with a cause that may not be remediable, and that may lead to death. Epistaxis should therefore not be regarded as harmless, either from the diagnostic or therapeutic point of view. The most common sources of bleeding are shown in **Fig. 2.10**. Depending on the etiology, epistaxis due to local causes is distinguished from symptomatic nosebleeds with a generalized cause. The most important etiologies are summarized in **Table 2.11**. Two important causes that should be considered are:

1. By far the most common source of bleeding (in ≈ 90 % of cases) is the Kiesselbach plexus (see **Fig. 2.10**), located on the anterior portion of the septum. The mucosa in this area is very fragile and adheres tightly to the underlying cartilage, thus offering little resistance to mechanical or functional stress.

2. Capillary hemangioma is another source of bleeding that is found occasionally on the anterior third of the septum. This type of circumscribed, dark red, benign angiomatous neoplasm is thought to result from mechanical irritation.

Diagnosis. Table 2.12 shows the necessary diagnostic steps. In some patients, it may be very difficult or even impossible to localize the source of bleeding with certainty. Bleeding from the posterior part of the nasal cavity or from the middle and superior meatus (see **Fig. 2.10**) is never innocuous, and requires immediate expert investigation and treatment. It may arise from the anterior or posterior ethmoidal artery or the sphenopalatine artery.

Table 2.10 Facial swelling

Site	Cause	Typical symptoms
Forehead and upper lid	Frontal sinusitis and complications	Soft-tissue edema, sensitivity to pressure, reddening
	Osteomyelitis of the frontal bone	Boggy soft tissue swelling, sensitivity to pressure on the vault of the skull, rapidly progressive edema, chemosis, swelling of the lids, swinging temperature chart. Typically, the edema is not confined to the borders of the frontal sinus
	Mucocele of the frontal sinus or the ethmoidal sinus	Resilient, nontender, noninflamed swelling that grows slowly
	Encephalocele	Noninflammatory, pulsating swelling at the root of the nose
	Tumors	Noninflammatory, firm, usually immobile swelling; maybe edema and pain on pressure
	Trauma	Edema and often hematoma of the upper lids, signs of fracture, pain on pressure
Upper jaw, cheek, and lower lid	Maxillary and ethmoidal sinusitis	Soft tissue edema of the cheek, lower lid, and medial canthus; pain on pressure; reddening
	Mucocele of the antrum or ethmoids	Resilient, noninflammatory swelling of the cheek or the medial canthus, not tender and not inflamed
	Osteomyelitis of the upper jaw due to sinusitis, dental causes, or radiotherapy	Painful inflammatory swelling and redness
	Zygomatic abscess due to otitis media	Painful inflammatory swelling of the temple and zygoma with edema of the lid and ear symptoms
	Parotitis	Inflammatory swelling of the preauricular area and cheek, severe pain, and tenderness
	Sialadenosis of the parotid gland	Painless, occasionally fluctuating, marked preauricular swelling
	Parotid tumors	Benign: slow-growing, no pain, no facial nerve paralysis Malignant: rapid growth, pain, and possibly facial paralysis
	Inflammatory dental disease	Painful swelling of the cheek, edema of the lids, and possibly trismus, disappearance of the mucosal reflection between alveolar process and cheek
	Odontogenic cysts	Painless swelling of the cheek and slow growth
	Dacryocystitis	Very sensitive to pressure; inflammatory swelling, possibly fluctuation in the medial canthus, drainage of pus from the lacrimal duct
	Tumors	Firm, usually poorly mobile swelling, usually not very tender
	Trauma	Edema, often hematoma of the lower lids, possibly signs of fracture, sensitivity to pressure
	Angioedema	Allergic edema with a sensation of tension and pruritus, facial swelling, particularly of the lip and the lid, sudden onset and tendency to recur

Table 2.10   Facial swelling (continued)

Site	Cause	Typical symptoms
Mandible	Osteomyelitis due to dental diseases or radiation	Inflammatory painful swelling, possibly with trismus
	Inflammatory dental disease	Painful swelling and possibly trismus
	Odontogenic cysts	Painless, slow-growing swelling
	Masseteric hypertrophy	Painless thickening of the masseter muscle on mastication
	Sialadenitis of the submandibular gland	Inflammatory swelling in the submandibular region
	Sialadenosis of a major salivary gland	Painless swelling, slow growth
	Tumors	Firm, usually poorly mobile swelling
	Trauma	Swelling, often a hematoma on the injured area and possibly signs of a fracture

Diffuse facial swellings may also occur in nephrosis, chronic nephritis, endocrine disorders (e. g., myxedema), and Cushing disease

---

Differential diagnosis. This includes bleeding that does not arise in the nose, but in which the blood escapes through the nose—e. g., due to tumors of the nasopharynx or the larynx, hemoptysis, bleeding esophageal varices, and escape of blood due to injury to the vessels around the base of the skull (e. g., the internal carotid artery) via the sphenoid sinus or the eustachian tube.

Treatment of Epistaxis (Table 2.13)
Supportive measures in treatment of severe nosebleeds
- Maintain a calm atmosphere.
- The patient should sit with the upper part of the body tilted forward and the mouth open so that blood can be spit out rather than swallowed.
- Cold compresses are applied to the nape of the neck and to the dorsum of the nose.
- Mild pressure is applied to both nasal alae for several minutes.

Local Procedures
Coagulation and chemical cauterization of the Kiesselbach plexus. Several methods can be used to stop bleeding that has been localized to the Kiesselbach plexus. In everyday practice, bipolar coagulation after local anesthesia has become the favored method for obliterating a bleeding vessel. Traditionally, chemical cauterization with silver nitrate ($AgNO_3$) or chromic acid beads was widely used; application of either of these chemicals is still an acceptable alternative.

Lasers offer another modality for managing recurrent epistaxis, but they are not suitable for treating acute epistaxis. Their method of action is determined according to the wavelength: argon and Nd:YAG lasers are absorbed selectively by hemoglobin, resulting in a photothermolytic effect that makes them suitable for the so-called "optical purse-string sutures" used to treat recurrent hemorrhage in areas of the skin or mucosa—e. g., in Rendu–Osler–Weber disease. Other lasers (CO_2 lasers, diode lasers) produce coagulation.

Anterior nasal packing and balloons. *Technique:* First, topical anesthesia of the nasal mucosa is induced (see p. 195). Strips of ointment-saturated gauze, 2–4 cm in width, are introduced into the nasal cavity in layers from above downward, or from behind forward. The pack should produce sufficient pressure to compress the bleeding source. Pneumatic packing with an inflatable balloon can be used as an alternative.

The following procedures may be required to achieve hemostasis if anterior packing fails to stop profuse hemorrhage—e. g., following trauma or vascular rupture in hypertension, or if the source of bleeding is concealed and lies far posteriorly.

Table 2.11   Epistaxis

Local causes of epistaxis	
Idiopathic	This refers to mild, recurrent nosebleeds in children and adolescents
Vascular	Microtrauma to Kiesselbach plexus
Anterior rhinitis sicca	Due to chemical or thermal injury to the nasal mucosa or to septal perforation, this condition frequently involves minor bleeding or blood-stained nasal discharge, accompanied by a feeling of dryness or crusting in the nose
Environmental influences	E.g., living at high altitudes, reduced air pressure, or drying due to air-conditioning may be implicated
Trauma	E.g., fractures of the nasal bone or the nasal septum, injuries to the facial skeleton or the anterior base of the skull. There is usually severe, profuse hemorrhage as a direct result of the trauma. Injury to the internal carotid artery may pose an immediately life-threatening problem, or there may be an interval before the formation of an aneurysm and attacks of bleeding
Foreign body in the nose, or rhinolith	This may cause unilateral mild bleeding and fetor, and purulent secretion in the long term
Bleeding polyp of the septum	This refers to a histologically telangiectatic granuloma or hemangioma, with a marked tendency to bleed when it is disturbed
Tumors	Malignant tumors of the nose or sinuses in particular often cause blood-tinged secretions only
	Lesions in the nasopharynx, especially nasopharyngeal angiofibroma, may cause massive life-threatening hemorrhage
Causes of secondary epistaxis	
Infection	Acute contagious diseases such as influenza, measles, typhus, and catarrh, may be involved. The epistaxis usually involves minor, brief bleeding episodes, principally in children and adolescents
Vascular and circulatory diseases	E.g., arteriosclerosis and hypertension. The bleeding is arterial, often pulsating and spurting. It affects middle-aged and elderly individuals and tends to recur
Blood diseases and coagulation diseases	Thrombopathy, e. g., in thrombocytopenic purpura or idiopathic thrombocytopenic purpura (Werlhof disease), sickle-cell anemia, leukemia, thromboasthenia (Glanzmann disease), and von Willebrand–Jürgens constitutional thrombopathy, or myeloproliferative diseases—e. g., essential thrombocythemia
Coagulopathy	E.g., hemophilia, Waldenström disease, prothrombin deficiency or overdosage with anticoagulants, fibrinogen deficiency, and deficiency of vitamins K and C
Vasculopathy	E.g., scurvy, infantile scurvy (Möller–Barlow disease), and Henoch–Schönlein purpura. The bleeding in this group is usually a superficial trickle of relatively dark blood
Uremia and liver cell failure	
Endocrine causes	E.g., vicarious menstruation due to endometriosis, epistaxis during pregnancy, and pheochromocytoma, which causes hypertensive crises due to circulating catecholamines
Hereditary hemorrhagic telangiectasia with typical mucosal lesions (Osler–Rendu–Weber disease)	This causes recurrent, mild to moderate, treatment-resistant, and often multifocal bleeding, principally in the anterior and posterior part of the septum

Gauze or a swab soaked with an ointment containing panthenol, an antibiotic, tetracaine with epinephrine or thrombin solution are used to stanch nosebleeds. In the United Kingdom, bismuth–iodoform–paraffin packs are widely used. An alternative is a tamponade consisting of a finger-stall filled with polyvinyl alcohol, which is a compressed foam polymer (Merocel). Hygroscopic tamponades containing oxidized cellulose (Oxycel), cellulose, or synthetic material—e. g., hydrocolloid fabric (Rapid Rhino)—that expand when moistened can also be applied. Other options are gelatin sponges, hyaluronic acid packings, or packings containing hemostyptic additives—e. g., thrombin. Fibrin glue can also be used. In the inflatable balloon designed by Masing for tamponing the nasal cavity and the nasopharynx, the pressure is fully controllable. Other products that work on a similar principle include epistaxis catheters (e. g., Epi-Max), choanal balloon catheters, epistaxis balloon catheters, and Foley catheters.

Posterior nasal packing. This procedure is very painful and requires, if possible, general anesthesia and intubation, or at least very good topical anesthesia.

Principle: A gauze or sponge pack attached to a string is used to close off the choana and is fixed in the nasopharynx to prevent the blood escaping from the nose into the nasopharynx. Anterior packing is then performed. The original packing method described by Bellocq was quite stressful for the patient and required skill on the part of the surgeon, as well as satisfactory anesthesia (**Fig. 2.92**). The posterior part of the nasal cavity can be closed off from the nasopharynx more easily and efficiently using a catheter with an inflatable cuff.

Technique: A catheter with an inflatable cuff is passed into the nasopharynx through the side of the nose that is bleeding, with the patient under general anesthesia or, if necessary, with topical anesthesia. The cuff is then filled with water until the nasopharynx is occluded securely and the flow of blood posteriorly has been stopped. The anterior part of the nose then is packed, and the end of the catheter emerging from the nose is fixed.

An inflatable catheter of this type should always be at hand in every hospital and otorhinolaryngology practice.

A severe septal deviation or prominent spur may necessitate surgical correction of the septum.

Table 2.12   Epistaxis: diagnostic steps

1	History
2	Localization of the source of bleeding and determination of its cause
	Anterior bleeding: nose-picking, idiopathic epistaxis, rhinitis anterior, infectious diseases
	Posterior or middle bleeding: hypertension, arteriosclerosis, fractures, tumors
	Superficial bleeding: hemorrhagic diatheses, coagulation disorders, Osler–Rendu–Weber disease
3	Measurement of blood pressure and assessment of the circulation
4	Analysis of blood coagulation
	In appropriate cases:
5	Computed tomography of the nose and paranasal sinuses (e. g., if a tumor is suspected)
6	Examination by a general physician to exclude generalized causes (see **Table 2.8**)

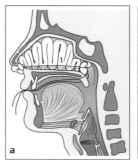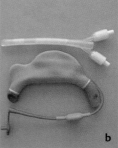

Fig. 2.92a, b   a Nasal packing. **1**, Anterior nasal packing in vertical layers. **2**, Completion of the packing (Bellocq tamponade).
b Two inflatable nasal balloons for tamponading the nasal cavity and nasopharynx.

Complications: Although balloon tamponades are effective for hemostasis, they may—depending on the cuff pressure—occlude circulation, leading to mucosal necrosis and consequent infection, ulcerations, and finally scars and adhesions.

Table 2.13 Epistaxis: treatment

Supportive measures

Calm patient (if necessary with medication)

Have the patient sit upright

Apply cold to the nape of the neck

Lower the blood pressure if hypertension is present

Administer fluid and plasma expanders

Blood transfusions are needed if hemoglobin (hematocrit) falls below 50%

Do coagulation studies and check levels if the patient is on anticoagulants

Local measures

Occlusion of the bleeding source by:

Local application of hemostatic substances, e. g., thrombin, gelatin tampons, oxycellulose, or fibrin

Injection of vasoconstricting agents into the bleeding area

Cautery, galvanocautery, or laser applied to a small bleeding point

Endoscopic ligation/coagulation of the sphenopalatine artery and the anterior and posterior ethmoidal artery is now commonly performed and is the surgical procedure of first choice

Anterior packing or inflatable tampons

Posterior packing (balloon catheter)

Selective embolism during angiography or digital subtraction angiography; alternatively, vascular ligation may be performed

Depending on the source of the bleeding, and provided the bleeding cannot be arrested by any other means, the following blood vessels may be divided:

Internal maxillary artery

Anterior and posterior ethmoidal arteries

External carotid artery

Replacement therapy in bleeding disorders:

Fresh blood transfusions, vitamin C, and systemic hemostatic agents in thrombopathies

Coagulation-promoting plasma, transfusion of fresh blood, Cohn fraction, in appropriate cases administration of vitamin K for coagulopathy or ACTH, steroids, calcium, vitamin C, and estrogens for vasculopathy.

For Osler–Rendu–Weber disease: "optical purse-string suture" using photocoagulation with an argon or Nd:YAG laser

Septal dermoplasty (Saunder plasty)

Another effective means of controlling recurrent bleeding in this condition is closure of the nasal airway using the Young procedure

ACTH, adrenocorticotropic hormone; Nd:YAG, neodymium: yttrium-aluminum-garnet.

A catheter left in the nose or a string attached to a postnasal pack must not exert pressure on the nasal alae or the columella. Necrosis can occur rapidly, causing scars at the tip of the nose and in the anterior part of the nasal cavity. A posterior nasal pack should not be left in for longer than necessary, and never for more than 5–7 days. Antibiotic coverage should be given while the pack is in place, as there is a risk of sinusitis or otitis media due to blockage of the pharyngeal ostium of the eustachian tube if the pack is in the correct position.

> **Note:** All nasal packing must be visibly secured to prevent aspiration. Caution must be exercised in the use of ointments and oils, as disfiguring lipogranulomas or paraffinomas that require surgical removal may develop even years later.

Endoscopic location and control of bleeding. This is done either under local anesthesia or in theater under general anesthesia, combined when necessary with septal surgery and occasionally ethmoid dissection.

Endoscopic ethmoidal and sphenopalatine artery occlusion can be carried out using bipolar diathermy.

Embolization. Interventional radiologic embolization is indicated for recurrent bleeding that cannot be stanched using conservative methods. The most recent method for obliterating an actively or recurrently hemorrhaging artery is selective embolization during digital subtraction angiography. Selective embolization can also be achieved with less technical apparatus using conventional angiography. Examples of target vessels are the maxillary and facial arteries.

Vascular ligation. This procedure has to be performed in cases of uncontrolled, life-threatening epistaxis if the methods described above fail. Depending on the source of the bleeding, it may be necessary to ligate the internal maxillary artery in the pterygopalatine fossa, the anterior and posterior ethmoidal arteries (**Fig. 2.93**), or the external carotid artery at the anterior border of the sternocleidomastoid muscle above the origin of the lingual artery.

However, it should be noted that these techniques were developed at a time when endoscopic location and cautery and endoscopic sphenopalatine artery occlusion were not yet possible.

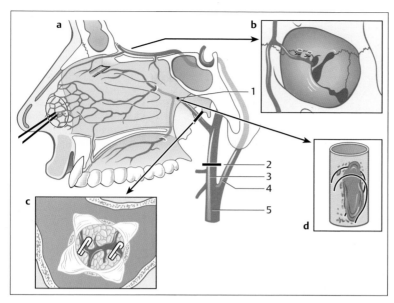

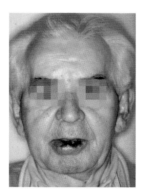

Fig. 2.93a–d Sites for ligation in severe epistaxis.
a Overview. **1**, Internal maxillary artery; **2**, ligation of the external carotid artery; **3**, external carotid artery; **4**, internal carotid artery; **5**, common carotid artery.
b Ligation or embolization of the ethmoidal arteries.
c Ligation or embolization of the internal maxillary artery or sphenopalatine artery in the pterygopalatine fossa.
d Embolization with a coil.

Hereditary telangiectasia (Osler–Rendu–Weber disease) (Fig. 2.94). Homozygotic carriers of this trait suffer from recurrent hemorrhaging even during childhood, in part precipitated by transfusions. Trauma to the mucosa must be avoided as much as possible, and the mucosa should be cared for with oils and isotonic solutions or loose, mildly antibiotic packing.

A modern method of symptomatic treatment for hereditary telangiectasia is known as the "optical purse-string suture." A noncontact technique is used to irradiate the submucous venous plexus in a given area of skin or mucosa using an argon or Nd:YAG laser, until a delicate, whitish discoloration—not coagulation—of the spot appears. At first, there is a marked tissue reaction, with some renewed bleeding. As scar formation and obliteration proceed, the incidence and intensity of the bleeding decreases.

In Saunders dermoplasty, the mucosa of the anterior septum is removed and replaced with split skin from a distant site.

Complete occlusion of a nasal cavity using flaps in the region of the internal nasal valve (Young procedure) has been used effectively in patients with severe, frequent bleeding in whom the above techniques have not been successful.

Fig. 2.94 A patient with Rendu–Osler–Weber disease. Hereditary telangiectasia of the lips and nasal mucosa.

■ Diseases of the Septum

Few people have a perfectly straight, perpendicular nasal septum. The septum usually shows slight bends and spurs. Provided these do not obstruct nasal respiration, they should not be regarded as abnormal.

Deviation of the Nasal Septum

This may be *developmental,* due to unequal growth of the cartilage and bone of the nasal septum; or it may be *traumatic,* due to facial fracture, fracture of the nose or septum, or possibly due to injury at birth. The parts of the septum may either be too large for the available skeletal space, or may have

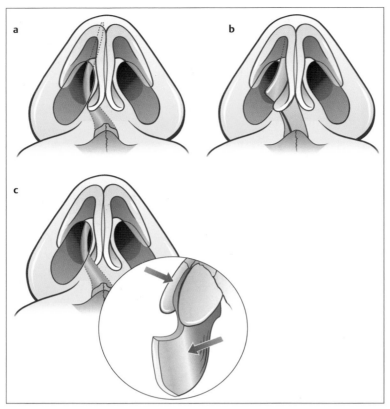

Fig. 2.95a–c The most common types of septal deviation.
a The dorsobasal extension of the septum is too long.
b Vomeral crest.
c The craniocaudal extension of the septum is too long. *Inset:* A septal deviation causes stenosis on both sides of the septum.

dislocated and healed in an incorrect position. These situations lead to deviations, spurs, and crests that reduce the patency of the nasal cavity (**Fig. 2.95**)

Clinical Features. These include nasal obstruction, which is often unilateral and may be intermittent, hyposmia or anosmia, and headaches that may vary depending on the condition of the nasal cavity. Subluxation of the septum—i.e., displacement of the ventral edge of the septum and obstruction of the nasal introitus to one side and septal deviation with obstruction of the nasal cavity on the other side—is especially likely after trauma. This combination of factors can lead to complete bilateral obstruction of the nasal cavity

Tension septum: The septum is too large for the available space, subjecting it to tension and constricting the nasal valve to less than 15°. The nares are often unrounded and slit-like, potentially causing nasal obstruction and headaches.

Diagnosis. The diagnosis is based on rhinoscopy, nasal endoscopy, and computed rhinomanometry.

Treatment. *Surgery:* **Figure 2.96** illustrates the principles involved in septoplasty. It is possible to remove all parts of the septum and reimplant them if necessary after shifting and remodeling. However, the function of the nasal cavity may often only be restored satisfactorily with simultaneous correction of the external nasal pyramid (see the section on septorhinoplasty, p. 212).

Principles of submucous septoplasty: Maurice H. Cottle (1896–1981) introduced his cartilage-preserving operation as an alternative to the Killian septal resection. The Cottle operation strives to preserve the supporting function of the septal cartilage and the physiological function of the nasal mucosa. After the margin of the septum has been exposed, the mucoperichondrium is undermined to create a superior tunnel on the left side and an inferior tunnel on both sides. The mucosa remains adherent to the septal cartilage on the right side.

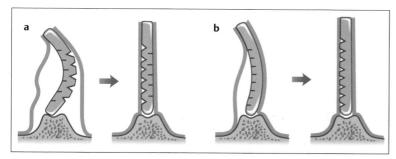

The classic Cottle operation has been continually modified over the years. One modification involves the "swinging door" technique, in which the septal cartilage is detached just anterior to the perpendicular plate to increase the mobility of the cartilage during the operation. The anterior septal cartilage can be trimmed using incomplete and complete incisions until it can be positioned in the midline without tension (**Figs. 2.97, 2.98**)

Complications of septoplasty include septal perforations (see below). If too much cartilage is resected, the cartilaginous part of the nose may collapse, causing an anterior or inferior saddle, or duckbill nose (see p. 213). In both cases, reconstructive procedures are available and indicated. Patients should also be warned about possible loss of sensation in the incisor teeth.

The Pediatric Nasal Septum

The septum, maxilla, and premaxilla develop independently of each other. Strict criteria have to be applied in selecting children for septal operations. Nevertheless, even small children can successfully undergo surgery for traumatic deformities or malformations of the septum that cause significant nasal obstruction. Deformities of the anteroinferior septum are the most common problem. It is important that the surgery should preserve the perichondrium, the growth zones (e. g., the caudal septum), the premaxilla, and the sutural junctions with the perpendicular plate and vomer. The aim in pediatric septal operations should be a chondroplastic mode of surgery.

Septal Hematoma and Septal Abscess

These are usually caused by trauma, and usually occur in children. Blunt nasal trauma with a shearing effect leads to elevation of the mucoperiosteum from its cartilaginous or bony attachment. A hematoma forms in the newly created perichondrial—

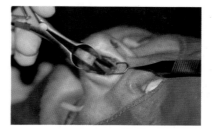

Fig. 2.97   Exposure of the border of the anterior septum via a hemi-transfixion incision.

periosteal space, and it is often bilateral. Infection leads to a septal abscess.

Clinical Features. These include increasing nasal obstruction, tenderness, and pain. If an abscess forms, local pain increases, and the patient complains of headaches, fever, pain on pressure, and reddening of the bridge of the nose. In the long term, the cartilaginous part of the nose undergoes necrosis and sinks in.

Diagnosis. The history reveals an incident of trauma. Examination shows that the hematoma is usually located to the most anterior part of the septum. There is also evidence of swelling of the septum, which occludes the lumen of both nostrils and feels cystic when palpated with a probe.

Treatment. Wide incision and drainage of the hematoma is performed, followed by splinting (with Doyle splints) of the nostrils to encourage the mucoperichondrium and mucoperiosteum to re-adhere. If infection is found, the incision must be held open with a drain to prevent cartilaginous necrosis, which would lead to deformity of the ex-

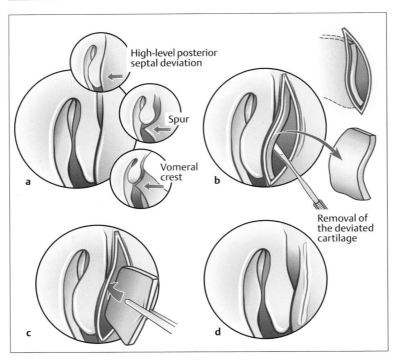

Fig. 2.98a–d Surgical steps in adjunctive endoscopic septal surgery.
a Indications for adjunctive septal surgery.
b Removal of the deviated posterior septum, external straightening with cross-hatching, morselization or incomplete cartilage incisions.
c Reimplantation of the cartilage.
d Straightening of the septum, with decompression of the middle turbinate.

ternal nose or septal thickening due to fibrosis. Antibiotic coverage is given. If necrosis occurs, the nonviable fragments are removed, and it may be necessary to implant preserved cartilage to support the nose.

Complications. If an infection is not drained, it may extend to the meninges or the cavernous sinus.

Septal Perforation

This condition is usually the result of trauma, nasal surgery, rhinitis sicca anterior, frequent nose picking, cocaine sniffing, infection (e. g., lupus, syphilis, leprosy, rhinoscleroma), or an occupational injury.

Clinical Features. These include crusting, fetor (possible but rare), slight recurrent nosebleeds, and a whistling noise on inspiration and expiration if the perforation is small. Large perforations located posteriorly may cause no symptoms whatsoever.

Diagnosis. A biopsy of the edge of the defect may be helpful to rule out generalized disease (e. g., Wegener granulomatosis). The consensus in the

United Kingdom is that biopsy is not necessary in most patients. However, if the perforation edge is obviously abnormal or granulomatous, then a biopsy may be helpful.

Treatment. *Surgical treatment:* Various methods have been proposed, based on reconstruction of the cartilage defect (e. g., with turbinate, cartilage, or occasionally prosthetic material such as porcine intestinal submucosa or bioglass), covering it with mucosal flaps, and inducing epithelization. **Figure 2.99** shows the principle of bilateral bridge flaps developed by Schulz-Coulon. More important than the size of the perforation is the extent of the remaining septum and the mucosa surrounding the defect.

Conservative treatment: The local symptoms of crusting and epistaxis may be alleviated by daily nasal douches and mild ointments. Occlusion of the defect with a Silastic collar stud–shaped button may be effective, but patients may remain symptomatic. An obturator is a foreign body, and plastic reconstruction is therefore preferable.

■ Trauma to the Nose, Paranasal Sinuses, and Facial Skeleton

Trauma to the Nose

Clinical Features. These include a visible deformity, lateral dislocation or depression of the nasal pyramid, hematoma of the soft tissues, orbital hematoma, swelling of the overlying soft tissue, septal hematoma, pain on application of pressure to the nasal pyramid, possibly headaches, epistaxis, nasal obstruction, and disorders of olfaction.

Fractures of the nasal bone are among the most common midfacial fractures.

Pathogenesis. This is circumscribed trauma to the nose from the front or from the side. Nasal injuries may also be part of a severe trauma to the face and skull. Depending on the intensity of the impact, the cartilaginous and/or bony nasal skeleton may be broken. In addition to the nasal bones, the frontal process of the maxilla as well as the nasal septum are often fractured.

Causes include traffic accidents, occupational accidents, blows, brawls, falls, etc. The injuries can be divided into closed and open. In *closed* injuries due to blunt trauma, the injury is not penetrating and the nasal skeleton is covered completely by soft tissues, with no external communication. In *open* injuries due to abrasions, cuts, or stab wounds, the cartilaginous or bony part of the nasal skeleton is exposed.

Diagnosis. This begins with the history and an examination, which reveals deformity and abnormal mobility of the external nose, soft-tissue injuries across the nose, and crepitation of the fragments on lateral pressure to the nose. Radiography of the nasal pyramid should be done (**Fig. 2.100**), and rhinomanometry and olfactometry may be useful after a few days. Involvement of the paranasal sinuses and the anterior base of the skull must be excluded.

> **Note:** A greenstick fracture in young patients, or an apparently harmless soft-tissue swelling, may initially conceal a fracture and severe skeletal injury. If fracture of the nasal bone is suspected, thorough investigation should always be carried out for functional, cosmetic, and medicolegal reasons.

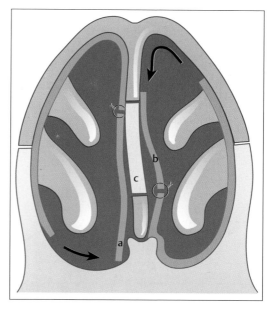

Fig. 2.99 Closure of a septal perforation using the Schulz-Coulon bridge-flap technique. **a**, Caudal flap; **b**, cranial flap; **c**, septum perforation.

Treatment. An open injury is first carefully cleaned. The wound edges and the nasal bones are checked, the displaced fragments are repositioned, and the soft tissues are repaired with atraumatic sutures. Antibiotic cover is necessary.

Repositioning of Fractures of the Nasal Bone

Simple, Closed Fracture

Repositioning should be carried out *within the first 48 h*, as the fracture can be most easily reduced in the early stages. However, in some cases it may be advantageous to wait for resolution of severe edema of soft facial tissue, before reducing the fracture on the fourth or fifth day. In theory, reduction is possible up to 10 days after an injury, but delay may have considerable cosmetic and functional sequelae if the fragments heal in a displaced position.

Technique. Short-acting intravenous or intubation anesthesia is used. The deviated part of the skeleton is repositioned, and the depressed part of the skeleton elevated as shown in **Fig. 2.101a**. If the fragments are already fixed or wedged, they must be refractured in the direction opposite

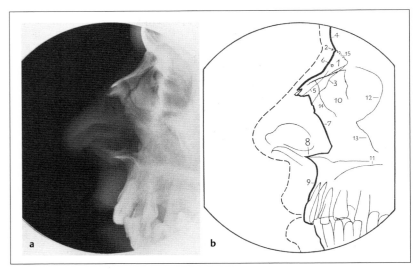

Fig. 2.100a, b Radiographic anatomy of a plain film of the nasal bone. **1**, Nasal bone; **2**, root of nose; **3**, nasomaxillary suture; **4**, frontal bone; **5**, ethmoidal sulcus; **6**, nasal foramen; **7**, piriform aperture; **8**, anterior nasal spine; **9**, alveolar process; **10**, frontal process of maxilla; **11**, hard palate; **12**, lateral border of orbit: **13**, zygomatic bone; **14**, anterior border of ethmoidal perpendicular plate; **15**, nasofrontal suture.

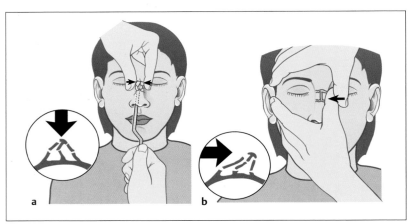

Fig. 2.101a, b Fracture of the nasal bone.
a By a blow from the front, and reposition by elevation of the fragments
b By a blow from the side, and subsequent reposition.

that of the original trauma (**Fig. 2.101b**), or even repositioned by osteotomies. The septum must be checked and corrected if necessary. Anterior nasal packing is introduced, and an external splint is worn for 8 days to ensure fixation.

Management of a Compound Fracture of the Nasal Bone or Nasal Pyramid

The affected part of the skeleton is examined and debrided carefully through the soft-tissue wound, which may need to be extended. The fragments are replaced and fixed, if necessary, with wires. The soft tissues are sutured, packing is introduced, and a splint is applied. Antibiotic cover is given.

If the soft tissues have been extensively damaged and show evidence of contamination, swelling, or necrosis, treatment of a compound fracture of the nasal bone may have to be delayed for 8–14 days until the acute tissue reaction has settled. The decision about the timing of surgery for a fracture of the nasal bone must be made by the rhinologic surgeon (**Fig. 2.102**).

Open repositioning of fractures of the nasal bone and/or septum is indicated in the following cases:
- Fractures that cannot be repositioned without open surgery.
- Penetration of the skin by bony fragments or perforation of soft tissues.
- Fractures requiring immediate reconstruction.
- Severe simultaneous injuries with a vital or absolute indication for surgery.

Supportive treatment includes antibiotics (if indicated), analgesia, prevention of nose blowing, internal or external splinting, and hemostyptic packing.

Complications. These include septal deviation (see p. 197), septal hematoma, and abscess (see p. 199). Long-term cosmetic defects may be caused by poor initial management or secondary infection. Elaborate and difficult plastic surgery is then needed, often in several stages. For a discussion of injuries to the nasolacrimal system, see p. 210.

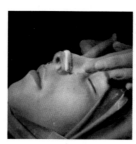

Fig. 2.102　A fracture of the nasal bone is immobilized with a splint or cast for a total of 10 days.

■ **Trauma of the Middle Third of the Face and the Sinuses**

Figure 2.103 shows typical examples of the mechanism.

Maxillary Fracture

Sagittal, vertical fractures are unusual, whereas transverse fracture involving both sides of the face and in all cases the antral cavity is most common. It may also involve the other nasal sinuses and the anterior base of the skull. **Figure 2.104** shows the three typical horizontal fractures of the middle third of the face. These are usually classified using the Le Fort system.

Symptoms

1. In *Le Fort class I* (low maxillary horizontal fractures), the alveolar process is detached. The patient has abnormal occlusion and a hematoma or fracture of the wall of the antrum.
2. In *Le Fort class II* (pyramidal fractures), the upper jaw is detached, and the fracture passes through the nasal bone, the frontal process of the maxilla, the medial orbital floor, and the zygomatico-maxillary suture. In this form of fracture, there is often considerable dislocation and depression of the central part of the face, with involvement of the ethmoids, the orbital contents, and the lacrimal apparatus, and an increase in the interpupillary distance, causing hypertelorism.
3. In *Le Fort class III* fractures, the facial skeleton is separated from the base of the skull. The fracture usually runs along the zygomaticofrontal, maxillofrontal, and nasofrontal sutures. The ethmoids, sphenoids, and often the frontal sinus and the orbit and its contents are involved, as

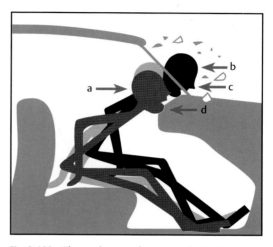

Fig. 2.103　The mechanism of trauma to the facial skeleton and base of the skull in a traffic accident. The following regions are frequently affected: **a,** cervical spine (whiplash injury); **b,** forehead and anterior base of the skull; **c,** midfacial structures; **d,** chin.

are all the structures of the central part of the facial skeleton, often with massive depression of the middle third of the face and multiple fractures of the bones of the face, producing a so-called "dish face." This type of fracture also usually extends to the anterior part of the base of the skull (**Fig. 2.104**).

The typical symptoms of shock, concussion, and cerebral contusion almost always occur immediately after the injury.

For facial swelling as a symptom, see **Table 2.10**.

Pathogenesis. Central middle-third fractures are typical high-speed injuries, mainly due to traffic accidents and more rarely to occupational injuries.

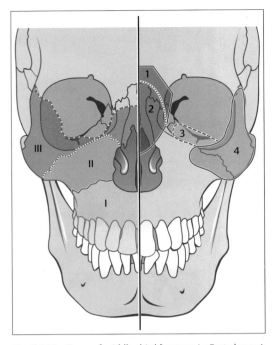

Fig. 2.104   Types of middle-third fracture. Le Fort classes I, II, III; **1**, naso-orbito-ethmoid complex; **2**, nasomaxillary complex; **3**, orbital floor; **4**, zygomatic bone.

Diagnosis. A history is taken to obtain information about the type, direction, and force of the trauma. Inspection often shows massive skeletal fractures, dislocations, and depression, with little soft-tissue injury. The symmetry of the central middle third of the face and frontal area should be noted. The inside *and* outside of the nose must be inspected. The orbit and its contents also have to be examined, with attention being given to unilateral or bilateral hematoma, eye movements, and the possibility of double vision. Vision is assessed. Palpation is used to assess tenderness on pressure, abnormal movement of the upper jaw, a break in the normal facial contour, steps and defects in the bony skeleton, especially of the orbital rim, trismus, and crepitation of the root of the nose (**Fig. 2.105**). The movement of the mandible in all directions, occlusion, and the condition of the teeth are assessed, and defects of sensory or motor innervation, any CSF rhinorrhea, and prolapse of brain tissue are looked for.

Radiography: CT scans are best for diagnosis of bony injury and dislocations. In certain cases, MRI, angiography, or functional diagnostic studies (e. g., olfactometry) may also be needed.

A maxillofacial surgeon, an ophthalmologist, a neurologist, or a neurosurgeon may need to be consulted. If multiple injuries are present, advice from a general or orthopedic surgeon may be necessary before treatment is started. The timing sequence of the various procedures should be agreed.

> **Note:** Skeletal asymmetry or deformity in middle-third fractures is often concealed by rapid soft-tissue swelling or bloody effusion. In addition, harmless-looking soft-tissue injuries in the region of the base of the skull may conceal serious life-threatening skeletal injuries.

Treatment. Before a patient is removed from the setting in which the injury occurred, the ABC of traumatology has to be observed:

A: The **a**irway is secured and **a**spiration is prevented.

B: **B**leeding must be controlled.

C: **C**irculatory shock must be treated.

> **Note:** Every patient with a fracture of the middle third of the face must be hospitalized. The department to which the patient is to be admitted is decided on the basis of the extent and type of the injury to the skull and other injuries to the extremities, thorax, and abdomen. Since patients with head injuries very often require immediate treatment by special trauma teams consisting of a neurosurgeon, a rhinosurgeon, a maxillofacial surgeon, and an ophthalmic surgeon, immediate admission to a suitably equipped large trauma center is indicated.

The purpose of definitive surgery is to restore normal anatomy and function by debridement, ventilation, and drainage. The specific duties of the rhinologic surgeon are:

1. Treatment of the soft-tissue injury and management of the nose and sinuses by debridement, drainage, and ventilation.
2. Assessment of the base of the skull (because of the frequent combination with a fracture of the anterior cranial fossa and the pterygopalatine fossa).
3. Correction of the facial skeleton and bony orbit (see p. 206).

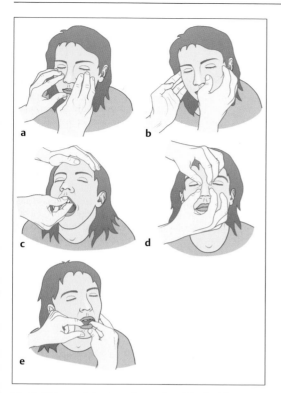

Fig. 2.105a–e Palpation of central middle-third fractures.
a Bony orbital rim.
b Zygomatic bone.
c Maxilla.
d Nasal pyramid.
e Mandible.

Definitive surgery for middle-third fractures should be performed as quickly as possible, as the fracture may heal very rapidly in the wrong position due to the callus formation. The management of simultaneous frontobasal injuries is described on p. 207.

Fractures of the Zygoma and Bony Orbit

Combined fractures involving the trifurcate zygoma with the zygomatic arch, and also the orbital rim with the orbital floor (lateral midface fracture), are frequent. Isolated blow-out fractures of the orbital floor and isolated fracture of the zygomatic arch may also occur. Fractures of the zygoma and orbit may also form part of a more severe midfacial fracture or frontobasal fracture. The antrum is almost always involved (**Fig. 2.106a, b**). The mechanism of fracture is usually blunt violence to the lateral part of the face by a blow from a fist, a traffic accident, or a

fall down stairs. The fracture is almost always depressed. Dislocation of the fragments may be minimal, but there may be extensive comminution, with multiple fragments that can only be repositioned and fixed with great difficulty (**Fig. 2.106a, b**).

Clinical Features. These include orbital hematoma, swelling of the eyelids, asymmetry of the middle third of the face with a sunken contour of the cheek on the side of the fracture, inferior displacement and possibly enophthalmos on the side of the fracture, a step in the bony wall of the orbit inferiorly or laterally, rarely of the upper rim, and possibly trismus. The soft tissues in the zygomatic area swell initially, but the underlying bony outline is flattened. Sensation may be lost in the infraorbital nerve. In a blow-out fracture, there is partial limitation of the movements of the eye, with double vision due to trapping of the inferior rectus or inferior oblique muscles.

Diagnosis. This is based on the history of the type and direction of trauma, inspection, and bimanual palpation, which shows asymmetry of the facial skeleton, a step in the orbital wall, or limitation of movement of the lower jaw. Radiography includes standard views of the nasal sinuses, special views for the zygomatic arch, and tomograms. An ophthalmologic examination should be performed.

> **!**
>
> **Note:** Fractures of the zygoma are relatively commonplace. They are often overlooked initially because of the soft-tissue swelling of the cheek and of the lateral part of the face. They are therefore recognized late, after bony consolidation in an incorrect position. Even after relatively mild trauma to the middle third of the face, from in front or from the side, asymmetry of the facial skeleton or a step in the orbital wall or loss of sensation of the infraorbital nerve should always be looked for using bimanual palpation, to allow comparison of the two sides.

Treatment. Several operations are available for repositioning and stabilizing fractures of the zygoma (**Fig. 2.107a, b**):
1. Access from the vestibule of the mouth and from the maxillary antrum.
2. Access from the temporal region.
3. Access directly through the overlying soft tissues.

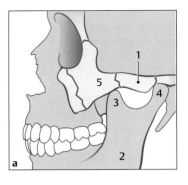

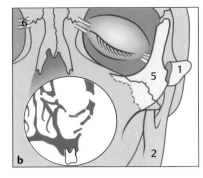

Fig. 2.106a, b Zygomatic fracture.
a Lateral view. **1**, Zygomatic arch; **2**, mandible; **3**, coronoid process; **4**, head of mandible; **5**, body of zygomatic bone.
b Anterior view. **1**, Zygomatic arch; **2**, mandible; **5**, body of zygomatic bone; **6**, medial palpebral ligament. The inset shows involvement of the orbit, antral cavity, and ethmoids.

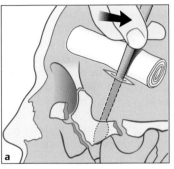

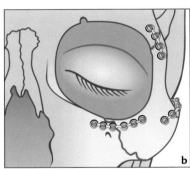

Fig. 2.107a, b Management of a typical zygomatic fracture.
a Soft-tissue incision to allow repositioning of the fragments and access for elevation.
b The condition after repositioning and osteosynthesis with microplates.

The use and combination of repositioning and methods of stabilization—e. g., single-pronged retractors, osteosynthesis with microplates, or wiring—depend on the type and severity of the fracture. If there is loss of sensation of the infraorbital nerve, the nerve must be exposed and decompressed.

Isolated Blow-out Fracture

Fracture of the orbital floor with descent of the orbital contents into the maxillary cavity, caused by blunt force acting on the ocular bulb in an axial direction; it may be accompanied by fracture of the medial zygoma or the infraorbital rim.

Such fractures are caused by violence localized to the orbital contents by a blow—e. g., from a fist, a tennis ball, or a champagne bottle cork. The thin bony floor of the orbit breaks and prolapses into the antral cavity (**Fig. 2.108a–c**). This can lead to trapping of the orbital contents (fat, ocular muscles such as the inferior rectus and inferior oblique muscles) by the fragments and to prolapse of the fractured floor of the orbit into the antral cavity. A blow-out fracture can also occur in the ethmoid, caused by a defect in the lamina papyracea.

Clinical Features. These include enophthalmos, double vision, limitation of movement of the eye (most obvious when the patient is looking upward, due to trapping of the lower ocular muscles), and disorders of sensation of the infraorbital nerve.

Diagnosis. Precise documentation of the course of the accident, routine otorhinolaryngology examination, inspection (enophthalmos, abnormal position of the bulb), palpation (step formation at the infraorbital rim, cutaneous emphysema), bulbar movement (double vision, especially on looking upward), comparison of sensory perception on both sides (especially of the infraorbital nerve), nasal endoscopy, CT, and ophthalmologic examination.

Indications for surgery are dislocated fractures (double vision, sensory deficiencies) or orbital herniation, with or without impaired motility of the bulb (**Fig. 2.109**).

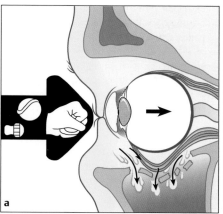
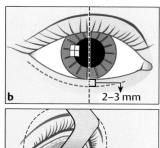
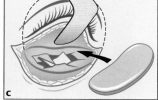

Fig. 2.108a–c Blow-out fracture.
a Mechanism.
b Subciliary approach to the orbital floor
c Stabilization of the orbit with an implant (septal cartilage, titanium).

2–3 mm

Treatment. The antral cavity must be explored as early as possible, preferably using the endoscopic endonasal supraturbinal approach. (For differentiation between a mucosal hematoma or edema and an orbital hernia, see p. 208). The bony fragments are exposed and the prolapsed part is replaced, possibly combined with bridging or stabilization of the bony defect with lyophilized dura, fascia, or autologous septal cartilage. Alternative or supplementary measures include access via the orbit through an incision in the lid and introduction of a septal cartilage transplant, lyophilized dura, or fascia to support the orbital contents. If the fracture heals in an incorrect position, the resulting enophthalmos can be corrected by supporting the orbital contents with an implant, preferably using autologous rather than synthetic material. Decompression of the infraorbital nerve and possibly osteosynthesis of the orbital limbus may be required.

Supportive treatment: Prohibition of nose blowing; administration of analgesics, antibiotics, and nose drops; application of cold.

Barotrauma of the Sinuses

This is caused by the considerable difference between the air pressure in the sinus and that of the environment if rapid equalization of pressure is not possible due to anatomic abnormalities. Aviators, divers, and parachute jumpers are most often affected.

Clinical Features. These include sudden, severe, stabbing pain in the region of the nasal sinuses, usually the frontal and rarely the antrum, during and after a temporary marked pressure difference. The result may be a nosebleed or sinusitis due to severe mucosal damage to the affected cavity.

Treatment. This includes decongestion of the nasal mucosa, treatment of symptoms, possibly antibiotics, and surgery to the nose and sinuses, such as septal correction, conchotomy, or functional endoscopic sinus surgery (FESS) as a preventive measure.

Frontobasal Injury to the Anterior Cranial Fossa and the Neighboring Sinuses

Trauma to the frontal area and the root of the nose usually occurs in traffic accidents, but occasionally also in occupational injuries. It causes a fracture that first affects the upper sinuses (the frontal, the ethmoid, and the sphenoid sinuses), and from there extends into the anterior cranial fossa. Alternatively, the fracture may primarily affect the upper part of the frontal bone, together with the dura mater and the intracranial structures, and the fracture line may extend from there into the nasal sinuses. Frontobasal fractures occur in 70% of all fractures of the skull base. There are typical fracture lines in the anterior cranial fossa and the rhinobase, similar to the fracture lines in laterobasal fractures (see pp. 208, 209, **Fig. 2.110a–d**).

Dural tears and brain injuries, which may be open or closed, thus often arise in the anterior cranial fossa. Infection may ascend to the intracranial cavity through the fracture line from the nose or the sinuses, either immediately after the acci-

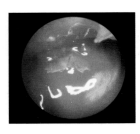

Fig. 2.109 Endoscopic view of a blow-out fracture through a supraturbinal window (45° lens).

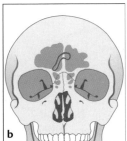

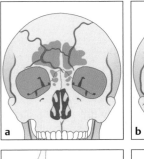

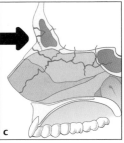

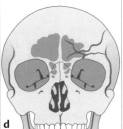

Fig. 2.110a–d Frontobasal fractures.
a High fracture (Escher type I).
b Middle fracture (Escher type II).
c Deep fracture (Escher type III).
d Latero-orbital fracture (Escher type IV).

dent (early infection) or years later (late infection), leading to meningitis or a brain abscess.

Clinical Features. Cardinal symptoms include CSF rhinorrhea, brain tissue prolapsing from the nose or from the external wound of the nasofrontal area, extensive facial hematoma, possibly surgical emphysema, proptosis with or without loss of vision, and frontal pneumoencephalocele.

Symptoms also include cerebral concussion or contusion, unilateral or bilateral ocular hematoma, which is *not* conclusive evidence of frontobasal injury, and occasionally severe bleeding from the pharynx, mouth, and nose. Cere-

brospinal fluid rhinorrhea is a definite sign of a dural tear, but dural tears are possible without a CSF leak. Anosmia occurs in 75% of patients, and cranial nerve II and, more rarely, cranial nerves III IV, V, and VI may be injured. External soft-tissue injuries are minor or absent in 20% of all patients. Occasionally, signs of incipient increased intracranial pressure are present—e. g., bleeding, pulse rate alteration, homolateral dilation of a pupil, and fixed pupil.

Diagnosis. This is based on the history and type of accident, radiographs of the skull in two planes, radiographs of the sinuses in several different projections (occipitomental, occipitofrontal, axial, and overextended axial), and computed tomography (**Fig. 2.111**).

Evidence of CSF rhinorrhea is provided by a positive β_2 transferrin test. In this laboratory test, the ratio of β_1 to β_2 transferrin in the nasal secretions and blood serum is determined. As high β_2 transferrin levels occur only in CSF, they are proof of a CSF leak. Sodium fluorescein can be used to locate a dura lesion with a CSF leak. Although this drug is not approved for intrathecal use, it has proved useful for locating CSF fistulas in thousands of cases. It is applied via lumbar puncture at least 10 min before surgical dissection of the base of the skull. It is very important to use a highly purified solution; the recommended dose is 1.5 mL of a 0.5% solution.

Use of indicator paper to determine the glucose content of nasal secretions, which are elevated in the presence of CSF, does not offer conclusive proof of a CSF leak.

Another option is radioisotope scanning of the cerebrospinal space.

Treatment. As soon as the patient has been stabilized by treatment for shock, the anterior cranial fossa and the affected nasal sinus should be exposed to allow debridement and watertight closure of the intracranial cavity with dural repair. The procedure is performed via the nasal sinuses. Injuries to the nasal sinuses are repositioned.

Three groups of indication for surgical intervention include:
1. *Vital indications* requiring immediate surgical intervention:
   - A life-threatening increase in intracranial pressure due to intracranial hemorrhage.
   - Life-threatening hemorrhage into the sinuses, nasopharynx, or base of the skull.

2. *Absolute indications* mandating surgical intervention as soon as possible:
   - Evidence of a dural tear—e. g., CSF rhinorrhea or pneumoencephalocele.
   - Open brain injury.
   - Early or late intracranial complications—e. g., meningitis, extradural abscess, subdural abscess, or cerebral abscess.
   - Impacted foreign body.
   - Orbital complications.
   - Osteomyelitis of the frontal bone.
   - Depressed fracture with a suspected dural tear.
   - Cranial nerve lesions requiring decompression.
   - Impalement injuries.
3. *Relative indications* requiring surgical intervention within 1–2 weeks:
   - Fractures affecting the frontal, ethmoid, or sphenoid sinus in which dura involvement is suspected, but not proved with certainty.
   - Depressed fractures and fractures with obvious displacement of fragments, with or without suspicion of a dural tear.
   - Injuries to the nasal sinuses with penetrating soft-tissue injuries.
   - Infection of the nasal sinuses already present at the time of injury.
   - Posttraumatic sinusitis and mucopyocele.

The purpose of the operation is to achieve wide exposure of the injured area together with the dura, to allow removal of fragments and management of injury to the brain and the base of the skull. This is followed by closure of the dura with fascia or galea and establishment of free drainage of the affected sinus using one of the typical rhinologic sinus operations (see pp. 171 ff.).

The four typical routes of access are shown schematically in **Fig. 2.112**:
1. Endoscopic, endonasal.
2. Fronto-orbital.
3. Transfrontal–extradural.
4. Transfrontal–intradural.

The choice of procedure and the sequence of the surgical steps depend on the individual patient and on joint treatment planning by a neurosurgeon, rhinologist, and maxillofacial surgeon, possibly with the addition of an ophthalmic surgeon, and a general surgeon or traumatologist in patients with multiple injuries.

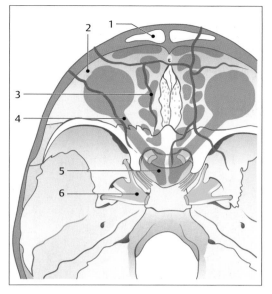

Fig. 2.111 Typical fracture lines in the anterior base of the skull. **1**, Frontal sinus; **2**, orbit; **3**, ethmoid; **4**, optic nerve; **5**, sphenoid sinus; **6**, Gasserian ganglion.

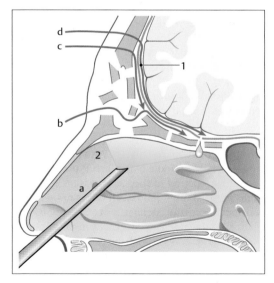

Fig. 2.112 Routes of access for management of frontobasal fractures. **a,** Endoscopic, endonasal approach; **b,** fronto-orbital approach; **c,** transfrontal–extradural approach; **d,** transfrontal–intradural approach. **1**, Dura mater; **2**, nasal cavity.

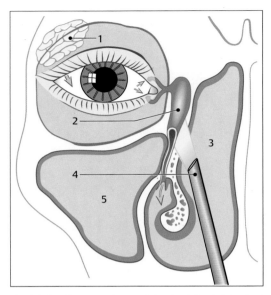

Fig. 2.113 The eye and nose. **1**, Lacrimal gland; **2**, lacrimal sac with lacrimal ducts; **3**, nasal cavity; **4**, site for dacryocystorhinostomy; **5**, antral cavity.

Complications. These include CSF fistula, recurrent late meningitis, early or late brain abscess, osteomyelitis of the flat bones of the skull (see p. 190), and formation of mucoceles or pyoceles (see p. 184).

Other Possible Injuries to the Facial Skeleton
Injury to the facial nerve. See page 112.

Injuries to the lacrimal system (Fig. 2.113). These are quite commonly combined with injuries to the sinuses and the middle of the face. If possible, they should be repaired in the same session as the injuries to the sinuses and face. If this is not possible, or is not successful, stenosis or complete obstruction of the lacrimal sac or nasolacrimal duct may occur (see **Fig. 2.113**), requiring correction (dacryocystorhinostomy; see **Fig. 2.113**) either by an ophthalmic or rhinologic surgeon.

Injuries to the mandible and temporomandibular joint. These injuries are managed by a maxillofacial surgeon, who is also responsible for restoring correct occlusion.

The main symptoms of mandibular fractures include swelling of the lower part of the face, abnormal movement or deformity of the mandible,

anomalies of occlusion, pain on movement, compression or torsion of the mandible, and possibly trismus.

Immediate first aid measures should be undertaken for comminuted fractures, particularly fractures of the chin with extensive soft-tissue injury. The patient should be intubated, or a tracheotomy should be performed, due to the danger of respiratory obstruction. Profuse bleeding should be arrested, if necessary with a pressure dressing. Soft-tissue defects or scars are dealt with in the usual way using plastic surgery reconstructive procedures.

■ Congenital Anomalies and Deformities of the Nose

■ Congenital Anomalies of the Nose

Development of the embryonic face involves nine processes. Due to the complexity of these processes, congenital anomalies are relatively common, although many of them are only slight. Anomalies incompatible with life—e. g., arhinia—are extremely rare.

Cleft Face and Nose
Oblique facial clefts, even in a rudimentary form, are rare, as are *transverse facial clefts,* in which the angle of the mouth is located near the tragus, causing macrostomia.

Median clefts are more common, but are usually only rudimentary. They range in extent from hypertelorism, with or without a true median facial cleft and with or without meningoencephalocele, to dog nose, proboscis, or even double nose.

Treatment. Plastic surgery.

Cleft Lip, Jaw, and Palate
These anomalies are relatively common, affecting 1 % of Caucasians.

Treatment. Reconstructive surgery, occasionally in stages, and orthodontic and prosthetic procedures. In addition, speech therapy may be needed. Treatment planning is described on page 281.

Cleft lip and palate present the rhinologist with several problems: firstly, anomalies of the external nose, such as a flattened nasal ala, and anomalies

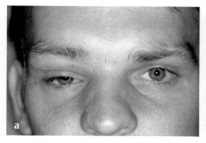

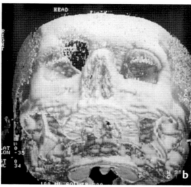

Fig. 2.114a, b Post-traumatic meningoence-phalocele following fronto-basal fracture with a large frontal bone defect.
a Caudal displacement of the eyeball.
b Bony defect in the anterior base of the skull.

within the nose, such as dislocation of the septum; secondly, speech disorders, such as rhinolalia aperta of varying degrees of severity; and thirdly, abnormalities of tubal aeration which are regularly present, causing seromucotympanum or chronic otitis media.

Nasal Fistulas, Nasal Cysts, Dermoid Cysts, and Gliomas

Median nasal fistulas, from which a cloudy secretion may drain, usually end blindly at the level of the glabella or in the ethmoidal–septum region. This is also true of *congenital nasal cysts*, which develop at the same site, but also may arise in the nasal vestibule or nasal septum.

Dermoid cysts are more common. They often contain hair and accessory structures, such as ectodermal inclusions, which lie above, below, or within the frontal bone.

Gliomas are tumors of the frontal region or the root of the nose in the midline; they consist of solid glial tissue.

All of these anomalies must be removed surgically.

Meningoencephalocele

Dural and brain herniations (hernias and celes) may be found in the nose, where they are easily mistaken for nasal polyps. They may also be located extranasally and be related to the frontal bone, ethmoid, or nasal septum. The causes are incomplete closure of the neuropore during the third week of embryonic development, and trauma (**Fig. 2.114a, b**). Meningoencephaloceles and gliomas can often be removed and the defect can nowadays be repaired endoscopically.

Diagnosis. MRI with contrast medium and CT.

Treatment. Surgical removal, closure of the dura, and osteoplastic correction of any existing hypertelorism, if required.

Stenosis and Atresia of the Nostrils

These are usually congenital, but may also be acquired—e.g., due to trauma or destructive infections.

Treatment. Plastic surgery.

Choanal Atresia

This is a bony or membranous occlusion of the posterior nasal opening, and may be bilateral. Girls are more often affected than boys. Hereditary factors have been demonstrated. The disorder is usually congenital, but it may also be acquired due to trauma. Incomplete atresia (stenosis) also occurs.

Clinical Features. Newborn babies with bilateral choanal atresia present with intermittent cyanosis, especially during feeding. Other symptoms include chronic purulent nasal discharge, inability to breathe through the nose or to sneeze, and anosmia.

Note: Bilateral atresia in the newborn is a life-threatening condition. As the infant is unable to breathe satisfactorily through the mouth due to the relatively high position of the larynx, it has to rely on nasal respiration during feeding. This poses a risk, in bilateral atresia at least, of asphyxia, cyanosis, atelectasis of the lungs, or aspiration pneumonia. Spontaneous feeding is difficult or impossible.

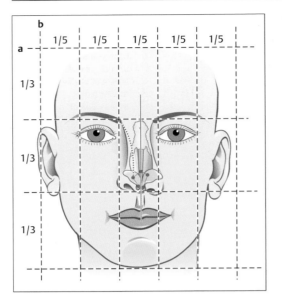

Fig. 2.115a, b Facial proportions and symmetry.
a Lines dividing the face into vertical thirds (Leonardo da Vinci).
b Lines dividing the face into horizontal fifths (Powell and Humphreys). Right half of face, features of symmetry: esthetic eyebrow-tip line, facial midline, nasal tip rhomboid. Left half of face, major causes of asymmetry: asymmetrical eyebrow-tip line, hypoplasia of maxilla, midface or mandible (usually with a crooked mouth), slanted nasal base (cleft lip and palate), asymmetry of specific structural elements such as the upper lateral or alar cartilage).

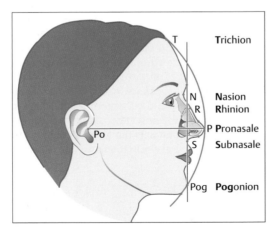

Fig. 2.116 Geometric points and lines used in profile analysis.

Diagnosis. The most reliable and simple test is to hold a cold metal spatula just beneath the nose and look for misting. Further tests include probing the nose with a smooth catheter and endoscopy of the nose and nasopharynx.

Differential diagnosis. This includes any disorders that cause nasal obstruction, especially polyps, foreign bodies, encephalocele, and tumors.

Treatment. When *bilateral atresia* has been recognized, the airway obstruction can be relieved by inserting an oropharyngeal airway until surgical correction can be arranged. Transpalatal surgery has now been largely superseded by dilation under direct vision of the posterior choana using a 120° endoscope in the pharynx.

In *unilateral atresia*, surgical correction can be deferred to a later date.

■ **Disorders of Shape of the External Nose**

Anomalies of the shape of the external nose often require rhinoplasty, both for esthetic reasons and because of impaired function.

Anomalies of the shape of the nose may be due to the cartilaginous or bony parts of the internal or external nose skeleton being too large or too small, or being improperly positioned in relation to each other or to surrounding structures. Analysis of the deformities is based on certain parameters, as illustrated in **Figs. 2.115** and **2.116**, on standardized photographs. Certain angles in the facial contour also have to be taken into account.

Fundamentals of Rhinoplasty
Rhinoplasty has two purposes:
1. It should restore a normal shape to the nose, so that it harmonizes with the rest of the face.
2. The function of the nose and nasal sinuses with regard to respiration, olfaction, etc., should be maintained, improved, and returned to normal.

This dual character of modern nasal surgery often requires correction of both the outside and inside of the nose—i.e., *septorhinoplasty.* These operations must be performed by a suitably trained rhinologist.

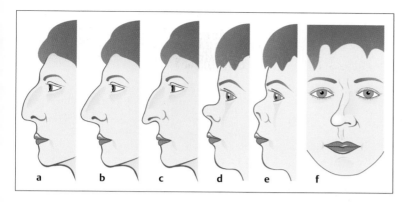

Fig. 2.117a–f Different nasal types.
a Hump nose.
b Overprojecting nose, functional tension nose.
c Drooping nasal tip.
d Saddle nose.
e Short nose.
f Deviated nose.

A distinction is made between *corrective* and *reconstructive* operations. In corrective rhinoplasty, and particularly for correction of the supporting framework of the nose, all of the surgical steps are performed from inside the nose, without an external incision (**Fig. 2.117**).

The principal steps in rhinoplasty are:

- An incision in the nasal vestibule or at the medial columella.
- Elevation of the soft tissue covering the nasal skeleton.
- Exposure, mobilization, and correction of all skeletal elements.
- Union of the mobilized and corrected skeletal parts to form a pleasing nasal framework and a functionally competent nasal cavity.
- Fixation of the mobilized, corrected skeletal elements in the required position.

Anomalies of the cartilaginous part of the nose include anomalies of the shape of the base of the nose—e. g., a hanging nasal tip, or a tip that is too flat or too wide, cleft, too long, or too short; nasal alae that are flaccid, too arched, or asymmetrical; a nasal columella that projects too much, is too retracted, too thick, too short, or too bent. The entire nose may also be too long or too short.

Anomalies of the bony part of the nose include anomalies of the shape of the bridge of the nose—e. g., hump nose, saddle nose, twisted nose, broad nose, or narrow nose; of the root of the nose; and of the nasal septum. The bony and cartilaginous parts of the nose usually need to be corrected together.

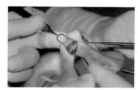

Fig. 2.118 The splitting approach for cranial volume reduction of the alar cartilage.

Approaches. Three approaches have proved valuable for rhinoplasty:

- The splitting approach (**Fig. 2.118**).
- The delivery approach (**Fig. 2.119**).
- The open approach (**Fig. 2.120**).

Which approach is used depends on the specific morphologic problems. Other decisive factors are types of skin and connective tissue. Thick skin predisposes to healing problems, whereas thin skin limits the selection of surgical techniques—e. g., using tip or shield grafts that might remain visible through the skin.

Reconstructive rhinoplasty deals with partial loss of the soft tissue, of the skeleton of the nose, or total loss of the nose, and reconstruction of a complete nose. Local or distant flaps are used, depending on the type and extent of the defect (see p. 217).

Hump Nose

This is due to an excess of the bony or cartilaginous nasal skeleton. Usually, it does not cause any marked functional disturbance.

Treatment. Rhinoplasty is performed, with removal of the hump and narrowing of the nasal bridge. The principles of the procedure are shown in **Figs. 2.121a,b** and **2.122**.

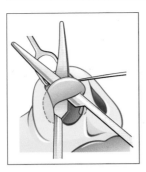

Fig. 2.119 The delivery approach for shaping the nasal tip.

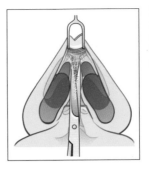

Fig. 2.120 The open approach for correction of difficult asymmetries of the tip and nasal dorsum.

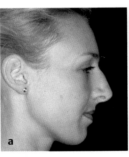

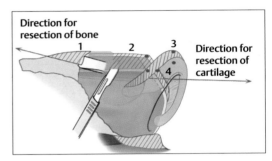

Fig. 2.121a, b **a** A young woman with dorsal hump, overprojecting nasal tip, recessed chin, and effaced nasolabial angle.
b The appearance 3 years after septorhinoplasty. The dorsum has been lowered and projection decreased, the chin appears normal, and the upper lip and nasolabial angle are relaxed.

Fig. 2.122 The principle of nasal hump correction. **1**, Bony resection; **2**, cartilaginous resection; **3**, shaping of the nasal tip; **4**, correction of the anterior nasal septum.

Saddle Nose

The term "saddle nose" denotes a multifactorial condition that is associated with destabilization or destruction of the bony or cartilaginous structures of the nose. Osseous forms of saddle nose are nowadays rare and usually result from dysplasia of the nasal bones or from nasal midfacial trauma.

Cartilaginous saddle nose is a more frequent concern for rhinologists. The central problem in this condition is the serious structural compromise caused by a loss of anterior septal cartilage between the rhinion (keystone area) and what is known as the septal pedestal at the level of the premaxilla and the anterior nasal spine.

Pathomechanism. The septal cartilage is partly or completely absent due to trauma, an incorrectly executed septoplasty, a septal abscess, or an infection; the condition may also be congenital.

There is considerable functional disturbance due to ballooning—i.e., expansion of the nasal valve caused by collapse of the ala (**Figs. 2.123a, b** and **2.124a–c**).

Clinical Features. The profile of the nose is typical. The patient may also report nasal obstruction due to absence of support for the nasal valve and introitus.

Treatment. A reconstructive procedure is needed for surgical treatment of a saddle nose. Rhinoplasty is performed, with implantation of several struts and implants to restore the cartilaginous framework of the nose, particularly the important central structure of the anterior nasal septum.

Deviated Nose

The cartilaginous *and* bony nasal skeleton and nasal septum are most often involved here. The cause is usually trauma, but a deviant nose may be congenital. Deviation usually causes considerable interference with function (**Fig. 2.125**).

Analysis. Assessment of the axial deviation is important in order to determine whether the deviation is due to cartilaginous or bony factors, whether it has a C or an S shape, and whether the condition is a pseudodeviation caused by differences in the esthetic eyebrow lines.

The *esthetic eyebrow line* is a theoretical line connecting the medial end of the eyebrow with the point that defines the tip of the nose (the pronasal or tip-defining point).

Treatment. This consists of septorhinoplasty with correction of the skeletal parts of the external nose and of the septum. The principles are shown in **Figs. 2.119, 2.120,** and **2.122** and the septal operation in **Fig. 2.96.**

Reconstruction of the bony nasal pyramid requires osteotomy. Spreader grafts are slender implants taken from the septal cartilage and used subcutaneously for various indications, one of which is correction of a deviant nose.

Other Deformities of the Nose

A *broad nose* is usually due to trauma, particularly if initial treatment has been incorrect, whereas a *narrow nose, large nose,* or *long nose* are all congenital. Interference with function can be expected, especially in cases of narrow nose and posttraumatic wide nose. A large nose and a long nose usually only cause esthetic problems.

Treatment. Septorhinoplasty is performed.

Anomalies of the Nasal Alae

Nasal alae that are too weak and prolapse on inspiration, or that are too flared, are corrected by strengthening or reducing the nasal cartilage. The lateral alae can be stabilized by autologous transplantation of cartilage taken from the septum or a turbinate (**Fig. 2.126**).

The profile of the forehead and the chin have to be included in an esthetic analysis of the face as a whole, in addition to the shape of the nose. A profile plasty may sometimes be required, with reduction or building up of the chin or forehead.

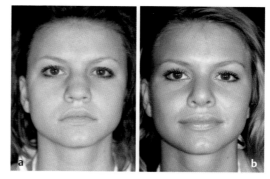

Fig. 2.123a, b **a** A young woman with a broad, saddled nasal dorsum. **b** Three years after septorhinoplasty.

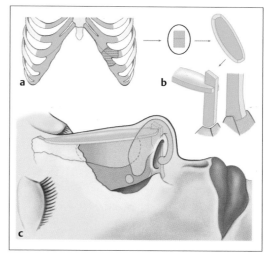

Fig. 2.124a–c Reconstruction of saddle nose with costal cartilage.
a Harvesting of the transplant.
b Shaping of a balanced costal graft.
c Tongue-and-groove connection of the grafts.

■ **Basic Plastic Reconstruction Procedures in the Head and Neck**

Soft-tissue and skeletal defects in the head and neck due to trauma, mutilating tumor operations, or congenital anomalies are encountered frequently; they require reconstruction for functional and esthetic reasons. This type of operation requires special surgical techniques and a thorough understanding of the complex anatomy and physiology of the structures of the head and neck. Such oper-

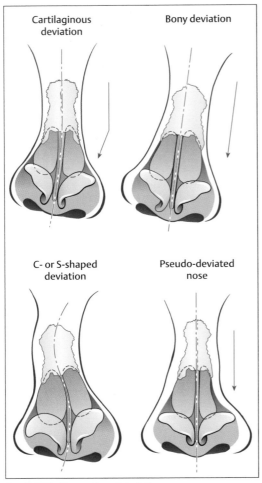

Fig. 2.125 Types of nasal deviation.

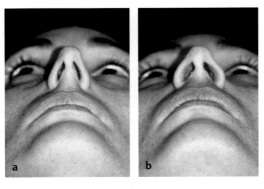

Fig. 2.126a, b   **a** Functional tension nose, with obstruction of the nasal valve.
b Enlargement of the nasal valve angle by shortening the height of the nasal septum.

ations therefore have to be performed by surgeons who are well trained in this area and who are able to combine preservation of function with reconstruction. The principles of regional plastic surgery also have to be taken into account in preoperative planning of reconstruction when a mutilating resection has to be performed.

Priority in treatment of defects in the head and neck regions is given to reconstructing them as soon as possible. The British plastic surgeon Sir Harold Gillies (1882–1960) stated the principle "Replace like with like." Although that is not always feasible, the principle emphasizes that autologous tissue should be used to the greatest possible extent for closure of defects.

Numerous reconstructive procedures are available, but they can be reduced to a few basic ones that can be modified and combined, depending on the type and site of the defect. This applies to planning and execution of the incision, wound closure, and wound care. Defects in overlying soft tissue can be closed using several different operations, depending on the site and size. A fundamental principle is that the relaxed skin tension (RST) lines need to be observed when making incisions, including incisions for taking flaps; in the face, the direction of most of these lines is perpendicular to that of the muscles.

Simple Incisions

Z-plasty can alter the direction of tension on a scar, pulling it more in the direction of the main RST lines. Continuous Z-plasty can be used to achieve "optical resolution" of visible scars (**Fig. 2.127**).

VY-plasty can be used to achieve elongation or slackening of an area of skin.

Free Transplants

In principle, autologous grafting is the method of choice for the face, particularly the nose. Free skin grafts of various thicknesses are used to cover superficial defects in the skin at different sites. A distinction is made between full-thickness and split-skin grafts (**Fig. 2.128**).

Composite grafts have the advantage that they are able to replace two layers of skin and one of cartilage (**Fig. 2.129**). They are taken from the auricle and are used for reconstruction of the nasal alae or the columella, for example (**Fig. 2.130a–c**).

Grafting of autologous or homologous tissue can be used for structural reconstruction—of a saddle

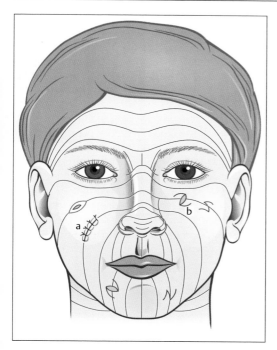

Fig. 2.127 Relaxed skin tension lines and the principles of scar correction **(a)** and Z-plasty **(b)**.

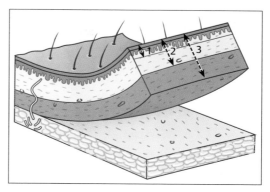

Fig. 2.128 Different types of free skin graft. **1**, Thiersch graft; **2**, split skin graft; **3**, full-thickness graft.

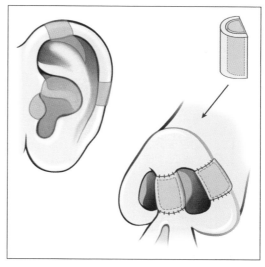

Fig. 2.129 Composite graft from the auricle for reconstruction of an alar nasal defect.

nose, for example—as a *structural graft*, or to fill contour defects as so-called *contour grafts*. Auricular cartilage is particularly well suited as a biomaterial for this, as it is available in a wide variety of shapes. Alternatives include rib cartilage and fascia. Alloplastic implants may either be enclosed in fibrin or overgrown by connective tissue; silicone remains biologically inert, whereas porous Gore-Tex is incorporated into the body tissues.

Flaps

Local flaps: As they are developed from the tissue immediately adjacent to the defect, the circulation in local flaps is intact, so that they can be set into their final position using advancement or rotation techniques.

Advancement flaps: These must run parallel to the relaxed skin tension lines. Good elasticity of the skin is a prerequisite. Excision of *Burow triangles* at the base of the flap prevents buckling due to excess tissue. With regard to the blood supply, a distinction is made between *random-pattern* and *axial-pattern flaps* (**Fig. 2.131a, b**). Examples are subcuta-

neous pedicled gliding flaps and island flaps. Advancement flaps have the drawback that they develop tension in a longitudinal direction; they must not be used if there is tension, particularly on the eyelid, lip, or nasal ala.

Transposition flap: The base of the flap is located immediately adjacent to the defect. This type of graft is particularly suitable for covering defects in the glabella, canthus, or lower third of the nose. Examples are bilobed flaps and the Limberg flap, in which the primary defect is trimmed to form an equilateral rhombus (**Figs. 2.132a–d, 2.133a, b, 2.134a–d**).

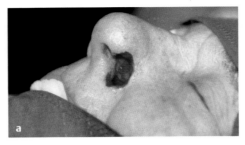
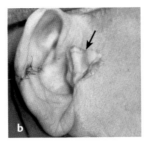
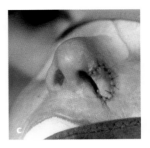

Fig. 2.130a–c   Composite graft (arrow in **b**) for defect repair.

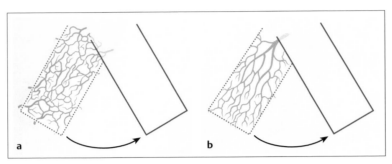

Fig. 2.131a, b   a Random-pattern flap (with random blood supply from the area).
b Axial-pattern flap (with blood supply from a single longitudinal artery).

Rotation flap or sliding flap: The advantage of this type of flap is its broad base, guaranteed blood supply, and great variability of design. It is suitable for covering defects of the cheek, lateral neck region, and forehead, for example (**Fig. 2.135a–c**).

Pedicled regional flaps: By virtue of their axial blood supply, these flaps can bridge long distances for covering defects. An example is the paramedial forehead flap (**Fig. 2.136a–d**).

Distant flaps: In the form of pedicled distant flaps or tunnel grafts (also called tube flaps or rope flaps), this type of graft is an important technique for covering defects caused by oncologic operations. Examples are the deltopectoral graft (**Fig. 2.137**) and the latissimus dorsi flap.

Microvascular grafts: The radial forearm graft is the prototype of a free fasciocutaneous neurovascular graft with microvascular anastomosis to cover defects of the face or neck. The advantages of this transplanted flap are that it has large blood vessels and good vascularization (**Fig. 2.138**).

Customized flaps: These flaps are not available in normal anatomy. They range from enlargement of the skin surface (possibly including several tissue appendages) using an expander to embedding of cartilage for reconstruction of deformities of the auricle.

Prostheses

In certain cases, it may be more reasonable to replace a defect with a prosthesis rather than embarking on protracted multistage reconstructive procedures—e. g., after total loss of the auricle or the orbital contents.

■ Tumors of the Nose and Sinuses

■ Benign Tumors

These are relatively unusual in the nasal cavity and sinuses. In addition to rare tumors, benign tumors include osteoma, ossifying fibroma, papilloma, hemangioma, lymphangioma, chondroma, fibroma, and giant cell tumor.

Osteoma

This condition is relatively common in the frontal and ethmoid sinus, but rare in the maxilla and sphenoid bones. Its etiology is unknown; there is an association with Gardner syndrome.

Clinical Features. Headache and pressure in the head predominate. Recurrent sinusitis or mucocele may occur due to obstruction of drainage. Displacement of the eye and later intracranial complications may arise. Many osteomas are asymptomatic and are found incidentally.

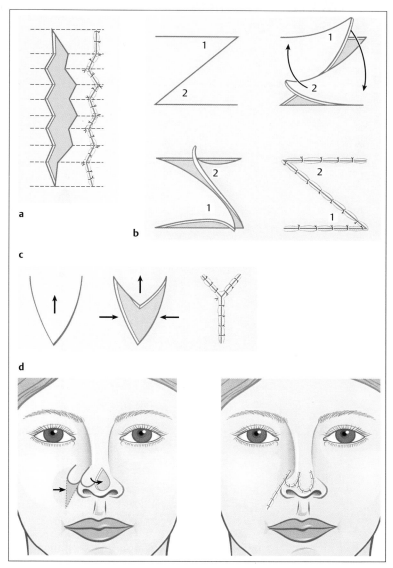

Fig. 2.132a–d Techniques used in plastic surgery of the face.
a Continuous W-plasty for correction of a scar.
b Tissue transposition with a Z-plasty.
c Tissue elongation or release of tension with a VY-plasty.
d Coverage plasty using a bilobed flap.

Diagnosis. CT scans of the paranasal sinuses typically show a calcified, well-demarcated tumor, which can be diagnosed clinically and then treated by surgery if necessary.

The differential diagnosis needs to distinguish between osteomas (which often have a slender pedicle) and ossified fibromas (which involve extensive laminar bony metaplasia). Whereas removing an osteoma using appropriate methods is uncomplicated, ossified fibromas tend to recur (**Fig. 2.139**).

Treatment. Small asymptomatic tumors may not require intervention. Small medial tumors can be removed endoscopically. Larger osteomas of the frontal sinus invariably require external surgery. The tumor fragments should be sent for histology (see **Fig. 2.71a**).

Metaplastic Osteogenesis
Bone is formed not only by osteoblasts normally present in bony tissue, but also by cells derived from pluripotent precursors (usually fibroblasts)

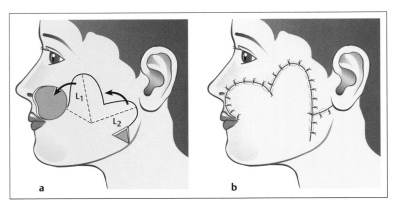

Fig. 2.133a, b Coverage of a defect with a bilobed flap.

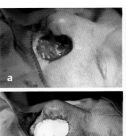
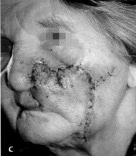
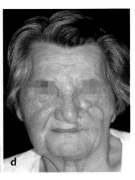

Fig. 2.134a–d Reconstruction of a large defect with a bilobed flap following resection of a malignant skin tumor.
a Defect.
b Dermoplasty with alloplastic material (after histologic control of wound margins).
c Three days postoperatively.
d Six months later.

that have undergone transformation (metaplasia) into osteoid-producing osteoblasts. Bony metaplasia occurs in numerous tumors of bony and soft tissues—e.g., fibrous dysplasia, ossifying fibroma of the facial skeleton, or malignant fibrous histiocytoma.

Ossifying Fibroma

A more comprehensive term is "benign fibro-osseous lesion." This includes fibrous dysplasia, ossifying fibroma, and cementifying fibroma.

Ossifying fibromas are considered to be a localized form of fibrous dysplasia of the facial skeleton. They occur principally in the middle third of the face and at the base of the skull in children and adolescents.

Clinical Features. These include unilateral expansion of the facial skeleton, headaches, and possibly visual field loss and lesions of other cranial nerves.

Diagnosis. CT scans show a fairly radiopaque tumor arising from normal skeletal structures. A biopsy can also be performed.

Treatment. Usually only partial removal is possible. There is a tendency for the lesions to recur.

Papilloma

Inverted papillomas are the most common sinonasal papillomas, accounting for ≈ 70 % of such tumors and ≈ 3 % of all neoplasias of this region. Because of their strong tendency to recur, destructive growth, the possibility of multicentric lesions, and the danger of malignant transformation, surgical treatment of inverted papillomas is very challenging. A radical surgical procedure involving transfacial block resection via lateral rhinotomy or midfacial degloving was therefore favored for many years. Today, the high standard of endonasal endoscopic microsurgery makes it possible to remove papillomas with comparable results. Even lower rates of recurrence than after transfacial operations

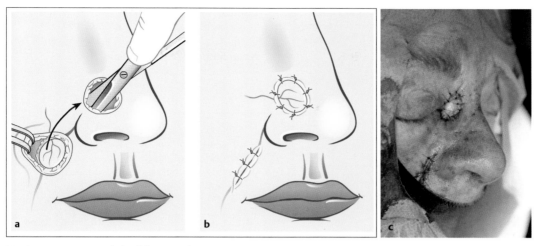

Fig. 2.135a–c Regional island flap transplantation.

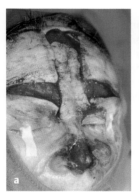
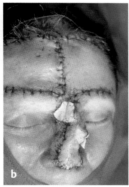
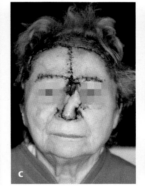
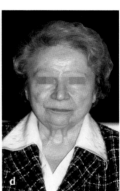

Fig. 2.136a–d Reconstruction of the tip of nose using a forehead flap.
a Elevation of the flap.

b Temporary wound closure.
c Four weeks later, before severing the pedicle.
d Six months after the operation.

have been reported several times in the recent literature.

Clinical Features. Nasal obstruction and epistaxis are typical. Endoscopically, papillomas appear as solid tumors with a lobed surface. On CT scans, they are seen unilaterally more frequently than polyposis. Macroscopically, inverted papillomas are often indistinguishable from nasal polyps (**Fig. 2.140**).

Diagnosis. This is established by histological examination of biopsy material.

Note: Tumors of the nose and paranasal sinuses are always masked by mucosal edema and inflammation. Complete and careful inspection of all regions of the nose and lateral nasal wall is therefore essential.

Treatment. Because of the tendency to malignant degeneration and recurrence, surgical excision is indicated. Papillomas do not respond to radiotherapy.

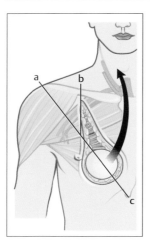

Fig. 2.137 Myocutaneous pectoralis major island flap. **a–c,** Acromion–xiphoid process line; **b,** midclavicular line.

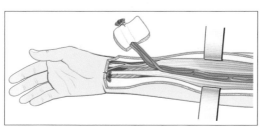

Fig. 2.138 Radial forearm flap for tissue grafting with microvascular anastomosis.

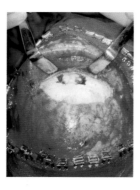

Fig. 2.139 A large osteoma of the frontal sinus; open approach, osteoplastic flap.

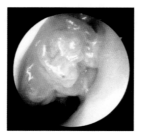

Fig. 2.140 Inverted papilloma in the nasal cavity—distinguishable from a polyp due to its solid, lobulated structure.

Glioma

This condition is described on page 288.

Nasopharyngeal Angiofibroma

This condition is described on page 288.

■ Malignant Tumors of the External Nose

Primary tumors of the external nose include *basal cell carcinoma, squamous cell carcinoma,* and *malignant melanoma. Senile keratoma* and *xeroderma pigmentosum* are included in the group of *precancerous lesions. Keratoacanthoma* is actually benign, but may be very difficult to differentiate from a squamous carcinoma.

Basal Cell Carcinoma

Basal cell carcinoma is a malignant epithelial skin tumor with a locally destructive growth pattern, but with a very low tendency to metastasize. It is the most common malignant cutaneous tumor worldwide in white populations, and its incidence is increasing. The most common exogenous risk factors are lifetime cumulative exposure to ultraviolet light and frequent sunburns. Further risk factors are chemical carcinogens, ionizing radiation, genetic predisposition, and immunosuppression. The tumor is predominantly located in the central face. Eighty-six percent of these tumors are localized on the head: 26% on the nose, 19% in the frontal or temporal area, 16% on the cheek, 14% near the eye, especially the medial canthus, and 11% on the auricle. Basal cell carcinoma is the most common malignant tumor of the external nose (**Fig. 2.141**).

Clinical Features. Initially, there is a small single nodule with telangiectasia. The nodule often has a dimpled center, which grows slowly. Later, it ulcerates and infiltrates superficially into the underlying tissue. There is no predilection for either sex, and the tumor usually first appears between 60 and 70 years of age. The superficially recognizable skin lesion has a diameter of less than 1 cm in 70% of patients, but extension into the surrounding tissue is very often considerable, with the tumor often occupying an area of more than 20 cm². A true basal cell carcinoma does not metastasize, and transition to squamous cell carcinoma is very rare. However, malignant degeneration may occur in tumors that have previously been irradiated or insufficiently excised, producing a very aggressive malignancy that may seed to other sites (e. g., the lung) via the bloodstream.

Clinical types of basal cell carcinoma:

- Nodular type: convex, shiny nodules, often with central ulceration.
- Rodent ulcer: ulcerating basal cell carcinoma; convex tumor with flat ulcerations.
- Invasive basal cell carcinoma: rapid, deep invasion over a wide area.
- Sclerodermiform basal cell carcinoma: atrophic lesions, spreading to the corium, with a bead-like limbus.

> **!**
>
> **Note:** The extent of spread is always greater than it appears clinically.

- Superficial basal cell carcinoma: flat, spreading, often light brown, squamous plaques with a finely beaded edge.

Diagnosis. The most common site is the center of the face and the auricle. Diagnosis should be confirmed by biopsy (punch biopsy) if there is any doubt as to the diagnosis.

Differential diagnosis. Squamous carcinoma and precancerous lesions must be considered.

Treatment. The treatment of first choice is complete, histologically controlled excision.

The initial treatment should consist of complete excision with a histologically controlled margin. The defect is then closed with an alloplastic skin graft (e. g., an alloplastic synthetic skin substitute for temporary wound coverage). Reconstruction using regional rotational or transposition flaps or a free graft is performed after complete tumor resection has been confirmed histologically. In selected cases of superficial basal cell carcinoma, radiotherapy, topical immunotherapy with imiquimod (5 % cream), or photodynamic therapy may be therapeutic alternatives.

Mohs surgery: Frederic E. Mohs (1910–2002) described a special technique of skin tumor surgery in 1941. The Mohs technique consists of stepwise removal of small layers of skin along with immediate microscopic control of the skin cancer

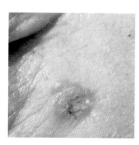

Fig. 2.141 Basal cell carcinoma: a centrally ulcerated, raised nodule.

margins. The advantage of this technique is that it allows a controlled tumor resection with minimal resection volume and wound surfaces. Frozen skin sections are used for microscopic analysis.

Prognosis. This is good if the initial resection is complete, with histologic checking of the margins and immediate further resection if necessary. Basal cell carcinoma does not metastasize unless it undergoes malignant degeneration.

Squamous Cell Carcinoma

This is the second most common tumor of the external nose.

Clinical Features. After beginning as a precancerous lesion or as a nodular, firm, nonhealing lesion of the skin, squamous cell carcinoma then grows rapidly, soon ulcerating to form a crater. Regional lymph-node metastases occur relatively early.

Diagnosis. The most common site is the lower third of the face. The diagnosis is confirmed by biopsy and lymph-node staging.

Differential diagnosis. This includes precancerous lesions, keratoacanthoma, and basal cell carcinoma.

Treatment. Histologically controlled excision of the tumor is the treatment of choice. Other treatment options are radiotherapy and cryotherapy. Laser or photodynamic therapy and polychemotherapy are only indicated in inoperable tumors.

Prognosis. This is favorable if the tumor is removed immediately with histologic control, and depending on the lymph-node stage.

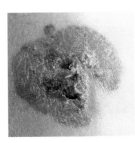

Fig. 2.142 A superficially spreading melanoma, 6 mm in diameter.

Malignant Melanoma

The most common malignant skin tumor, malignant melanoma affects females, with a 2 : 1 preponderance over males. The maximum incidence is between the twentieth and sixtieth years of life. Ten percent of malignant melanomas occur on the head and neck, affecting the face and the scalp.

Clinical Features. The tumor often arises from a pigmented mole, but also may arise from apparently normal skin.

Suspicious symptoms include an increase in surface area, increased prominence, and darkening of color of a pigmented mole, possibly with a black-berry type of surface, formation of satellites in the neighboring tissue, or enlargement of the regional lymph nodes. *Clinical forms* include:

- Superficial spreading melanoma (60%): irregularly pigmented spots and plaques with blurred and polycyclic borders.
- Primary nodular malignant melanoma (20%): regular, dark brown, rarely pink or skin-colored nodules lacking a halo.
- Malignant lentigo (≈ 10%) (**Fig. 2.142**).
- Acrolentiginous malignant melanoma (≈ 5%), which is rarely found on the head and neck.
- Primary nodular malignant melanoma (≈ 40%).

The most unfavorable type is nodular melanoma, which grows deeply and metastasizes rapidly from the start, whereas superficial spreading melanoma, malignant lentigo, and acrolentiginous melanoma initially spread horizontally on the surface. The site is often the face, or scalp and head, or the ear and neck. It is rare on the external nose, but more common on the anterior part of the septum, where it leads to epistaxis, nasal obstruction, and formation of crusts. The tumor can also occur on the oral and pharyngeal mucosa.

Diagnosis. A dermatologic consultation is necessary. Biopsy should be avoided, as it may activate and spread the tumor. Total removal with a wide margin of healthy tissue is indicated immediately on well-founded suspicion of malignant melanoma. Amelanotic melanomas also may occur. There are also numerous pigmented tumors that are not malignant melanoma, and an absolute diagnosis without biopsy therefore is very difficult.

Sentinel node: If the tumor is more than 1 mm thick, excision of the sentinel node is recommended. The sentinel node is a regional lymph node that is fed directly by the lymphatic vessel draining the tumor. Radioisotope scans of lymphatic drainage and the histologic findings are of critical importance for prognosis and treatment.

Differential diagnosis. This includes juvenile melanoma, papilloma, telangiectatic granuloma, pigmented basal cell carcinoma, and blue nevus.

> **Note:** Manipulation of a malignant melanoma should be avoided if at all possible, and immediate surgery is indicated.

Treatment. The mainstay of treatment is rapid and extensive excision by three-dimensional surgery with a macroscopic margin of 5 cm, although this cannot always be obtained on the face. Frozen sections of the margins should be examined immediately so that further resection can be undertaken if necessary. The defects should be reconstructed immediately with advancement flaps or free skin grafts. Conservative lymph-node surgery or radical neck dissection is indicated, depending on the histology of the sentinel node, at least for high-risk malignant melanomas of the head and neck. However, the value of this is controversial, because of occasional widespread early metastasis. Supportive immunotherapy, chemotherapy, or endolymphatic radioisotope therapy by a dermatologist or radiotherapist may be helpful. Convincing benefit has not been shown with conventional radiotherapy, immunotherapy with bacillus Calmette–Guérin (BCG), or currently available forms of chemotherapy.

Prognosis. This depends on early diagnosis and is determined by Clark levels (**Fig. 2.143**) of growth depth and the presence or absence of metastases. With adequate early surgery in stage I, the 5-year survival rate is 70%, and in

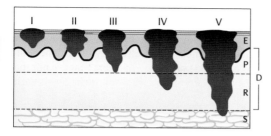

Fig. 2.143 Invasion levels of primary malignant melanoma of the skin as defined by Clark. Level **I**, limited to the epidermis; level **II**, into the underlying papillary dermis; level **III**, to the junction of the papillary and reticular dermis; level **IV**, into the reticular dermis; level **V**, into the subcutaneous fat. **E**, epidermis; **D**, dermis; **P**, papillary dermis; **R**, reticular dermis; **S**, subcutaneous tissue.

stage II, 30–40 % lower. The poor prognosis depends less on the superficial extent of the lesion than on its total thickness, depth, and metastatic spread. A depth of extension of 0.76 mm marks the boundary between high-risk and low-risk malignant melanoma.

■ **Malignant Tumors of the Nasal Cavity and Nasal Sinuses**

The most common tumors of the nasal cavity and nasal sinuses are *squamous cell carcinoma, adenoid cystic carcinoma,* and *adenocarcinoma.*

Mesenchymal tumors such as spindle cell sarcoma, round cell sarcoma, chondrosarcoma, osteosarcoma, and malignant lymphoma, are rare. Malignancies arising in the nasal cavity or sinuses represent less than 1 % of all malignant tumors. Histologically, the relative incidence is as follows: squamous cell carcinoma, ≈ 57 %; adenocarcinoma and similar forms, ≈ 18 %; undifferentiated carcinomas, ≈ 10 %; and mesenchymal tumors (malignant lymphoma, sarcoma, and melanoma), ≈ 15 %.

In children, histiocytosis X (eosinophilic granuloma) and rhabdomyosarcoma are relatively common.

Olfactory Neuroblastoma

This is the most typical olfactory tumor, originating from deep inside the olfactory epithelium. This tumor is malignant, aggressive, and forms metastases. The incidence curve of the tumor shows two peaks, one in the second and one in the sixth decade of life.

Tumors in patients between 20 and 30 years of age have a stronger tendency to metastasize.

Clinical Features. Loss of olfaction and taste, obstruction of nasal breathing, bloody or blood-tinged secretions, and—depending on the extent of the tumor— headache or CSF leakage may occur.

Therapy. The therapy of choice is radical surgery combined with irradiation. One of the main factors affecting the prognosis is the histological grade (types I–IV). Tumors with an intracranial localization—i. e., mainly meningiomas—or tumors of the olfactory sulcus may also affect the olfactory system, as may tumors of the medial and posterior sections of the frontal base. Surgical treatment of such tumors requires a combination of otolaryngologic procedures and neurosurgical techniques, to provide optimal access to the cribrous lamina and ensure a high degree of radical functional surgery.

Symptoms of Malignant Tumors of the Nose or Sinuses

Tumors of the nasal cavity are often clinically silent for a long period, making early diagnosis often difficult.

Suspicious symptoms, especially in persons over 50 years of age, include unilateral nasal obstruction, unilateral chronic nasal discharge, hemorrhagic nasal secretion, fetid secretion, loss of sensation of one of the branches of the trigeminal nerve, swelling of the cheek or of the medial canthus, pressure in the head or face, and a feeling of fullness in the nose. Marked headache only occurs in later stages, when the tumor extends to the dura, causing treatment-resistant pain. Signs of invasion of neighboring tissue include restriction of eye movements, displacement of the eye or proptosis, swelling of the soft tissue of the medial canthus, the eyelids, the cheek, the palate, and the alveolus, loosening of the teeth, interference with mastication, cranial nerve palsies, epiphora, and regional lymphadenopathy.

Prognosis. The further cranially and dorsally a tumor of the paranasal sinuses is located (**Fig. 2.144**), the poorer the prognosis. This is the implication of the levels defined by Sebileau and the plane of Ohngren, although these are rarely used today.

Diagnosis. This is based on the history and on inspection and palpation of the oral cavity, nose, and

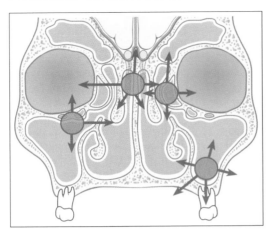

Fig. 2.144 Typical directions of extension of tumors of the nose and sinuses.

oropharynx. Endoscopy can also be used. Axial radiographs of the sinuses and of the base of the skull show a diffuse opacity destroying and obscuring the normal bony contour. CT scans are also obtained. The patient should be examined by a neurologist and an ophthalmologist. If necessary, a biopsy is taken after the suspect sinus has been opened. If invasion of the base of the skull is suspected, angiography should be performed and the CSF examined. Regional lymph-node metastases and distant metastases to the lung, skeleton, brain, and liver are looked for.

Differential diagnosis. This includes infection of the sinuses and the associated complications, and benign tumors (see pp. 186–193).

The TNM system is used for staging to determine treatment and prognosis and to allow recording and analysis of the results (**Table 2.14**).

■ Principles of Management of Malignant Tumors of the Nose and Paranasal Sinuses

Three methods of treatment are available: surgery, radiotherapy, and chemotherapy (cytotoxic drugs, administered intra-arterially if required). In some situations, combinations of the three methods may be appropriate.

Surgery. Three standard methods of removing the tumor are in use: 1, partial maxillectomy and, if necessary, resection of the frontal bone; 2, total

Table 2.14 TNM classification: nasal cavity and paranasal sinuses

Maxillary sinus	
T1	Mucosa
T2	Bone erosion or destruction, hard palate, middle nasal meatus
T3	Posterior bony wall maxillary sinus, subcutaneous tissues, floor or medial wall of orbit, pterygoid fossa, ethmoid sinuses
T4a	Anterior orbit, cheek, pterygoid plates, infratemporal fossa, cribriform plate, sphenoid or frontal sinuses
T4b	Orbital apex, dura, brain, middle cranial fossa, cranial nerves other than V2, nasopharynx, clivus
Nasal cavity and ethmoid sinus	
T1	One subsite
T2	Two subsites or adjacent nasoethmoidal
T3	Medial wall or floor orbit, maxillary sinus, palate, cribriform plate
T4a	Anterior orbit, skin of nose or cheek, anterior cranial fossa (minimal), pterygoid plates, sphenoid or frontal sinuses
T4b	Orbital apex, dura, brain, middle cranial fossa, cranial nerves other than V2, nasopharynx, clivus
All sites	
N1	Ipsilateral single ≤ 3 cm
N2	a. Ipsilateral single ≥ 3 cm to 6 cm
	b. Ipsilateral multiple ≤ 6 cm
	c. Bilateral or contralateral ≤ 6 cm
N3	>6 cm
Distant metastasis	
MX	Distant metastasis cannot be assessed
M0	No distant metastasis
M1	Distant metastasis

maxillectomy; and 3, exenteration of the orbit, combined with procedures 1 or 2. The principles are shown in **Fig. 2.145a–c**. The operation is determined by the type, site, and size of the tumor (**Fig. 2.146**).

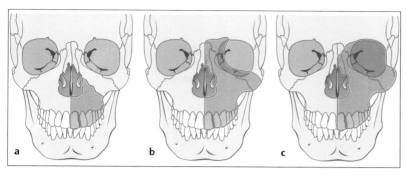

Fig. 2.145a–c Resection of the upper jaw.
a Partial resection.
b Total resection.
c Total resection with exenteration of the orbit.

Since the operation almost always needs to be extensive, secondary reconstruction or provision of a prosthesis to cover both external and palatal defects is necessary.

Only ≈ 10 % of these patients have lymph-node metastasis, and only 5 % have hematogenous metastasis. Suspicious lymph nodes must be sought out, using MRI and sonographic monitoring. Neck dissection is usually performed when lymph-node metastases are suspected, or for certain other oncologic considerations.

Radiotherapy. This can be administered alone or following surgery. The survival rate following radiotherapy of the nasal cavity and the sinuses as the sole treatment for squamous carcinoma is not as good as that for surgery, depending on the stage and site of the disease. Radiotherapy is therefore usually reserved for highly radiosensitive tumors— e. g., mesenchymal tumors—and for inoperable tumors. For all other tumors, a combination of surgery and radiotherapy, possibly supplemented by chemotherapy, is preferred. As a rule, the operation precedes radiotherapy, but preoperative radiotherapy can also be used, particularly for very large tumors. What is known as sandwich treatment— i. e., half the dose of radiotherapy, then surgery, followed by the second half of the radiotherapy—is also practiced. Radiotherapy is usually administered with cobalt-60 or supervoltage therapy (e. g., with the betatron) to deliver a tumor dose of 58–70 Gy. Radiotherapy may be the treatment of choice for certain small tumors of the external nose with no invasion of the skeleton.

The dose and volume of postoperative radiotherapy and the decision to combine radiotherapy with chemotherapy (chemoradiotherapy) depend on

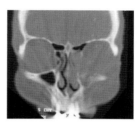

Fig. 2.146 Coronal CT, showing destructive tumor growth with invasion of the orbit. The orbital floor and parts of the orbital lamina have been destroyed by destructive tumor growth.

whether the resection is complete. If the tumor has been completely resected, all of its margins are histologically free of tumor (R0 resection, low risk). In an R1 resection (high risk), microscopic residual disease is left behind.

In brachytherapy, small radioactive rods are implanted directly into the tumor or placed next to the area requiring treatment. This ensures a high and selective tumor dose.

Chemotherapy. At present, chemotherapy still does not have an established role as a primary curative treatment for epithelial malignancies of the face, nose, and sinuses—especially with regard to the long-term results. Depending on the tumor stage and the histology of the tumor, an interdisciplinary, individual therapeutic strategy needs to be determined, including surgery, radiotherapy, chemotherapy, and combinations of these.

Prognosis. With suitable treatment, 5-year average survival rates of 40 % can be achieved. This is only an overall figure, and it may be more or less, depending on numerous oncologic factors.

3   Mouth and Pharynx

Applied Anatomy and Physiology

■ Basic Anatomy

■ Oral Cavity

The oral cavity is bounded anteriorly by the lips, posteriorly by the anterior faucial arch, inferiorly by the floor of the mouth, and superiorly by the hard and soft palates. It is continuous with the oropharynx through the anterior faucial arch (**Figs. 3.1, 3.2a**).

The faucial arch and the base of the tongue form the *faucial isthmus.* The oral cavity is divided into two parts by the upper and lower alveolar process

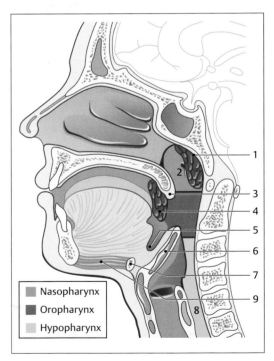

Fig. 3.1   Anatomy of the mouth and pharynx. **1**, Roof of the nasopharynx; **2**, ostium of the eustachian tube; **3**, soft palate; **4**, palatal tonsil; **5**, vallecula; **6**, epiglottis; **7**, hyoid bone; **8**, hypopharynx; **9**, floor of the mouth.

Nasopharynx
Oropharynx
Hypopharynx

and the teeth: first, the *vestibule of the mouth,* lying between the lip and cheek on one side and the teeth and the alveolar process on the other and second, the *oral cavity proper,* limited externally by the alveolar process and the teeth.

The *vestibule of the mouth* communicates directly with the oral cavity proper on both sides, even when the teeth are in apposition, between the ascending ramus of the mandible and the last molar tooth.

This is of practical importance: in intermaxillary wiring, the patient is able to ingest a fluid diet using this route, even when the teeth are fixed in occlusion.

The *tongue* fills the oral cavity almost completely when the mouth is closed (**Fig. 3.2b, c**). The surface tension force ensures that the tongue adheres to the hard and soft palate, thus maintaining closure of the mouth.

The following parts of the tongue are distinguished: the *tip,* the *margins,* the *body,* the *base,* the *dorsum,* and the *ventral surface.*

The dorsum of the tongue is covered with a modified epithelium containing the filiform papillae at the tip, the fungiform papillae at the tip and margins, the foliate papillae on the posterolateral part of the tongue, and the vallate papillae on the dorsum. The boundary between the body of the tongue and the base of the tongue is formed by the V-shaped *terminal sulcus,* the central point of which is the foramen cecum, a remnant of the thyroglossal duct.

The base of the tongue contains the *lingual tonsil,* which can be a site of inflammation and abscess due to an impacted foreign body and can cause mechanical difficulty in swallowing when it is hypertrophic. The base of the tongue is limited inferiorly by the edge of the *epiglottis.* The two *valleculae* lie in the angle between the epiglottis and the base of the tongue. They are sometimes difficult to inspect and may be a site for cysts, foreign bodies, and malignant tumors. In supine unconscious patients or patients under general anesthesia, the base of the tongue may fall backward to occlude the entrance to the larynx, and together with the epiglottis may lead to respiratory obstruction. This is prevented by pulling the tongue forward and by introducing an oropharyngeal airway.

The arrangement of the musculature of the tongue provides it with extreme mobility. Two groups of muscles can be distinguished: firstly, those without any bony attach-ments, running free in the body of the tongue—i.e., the transverse, superior, and inferior longitudinal muscles, and the vertical muscles; and secondly, muscles that are attached to fixed points—i.e., the styloglossus, the genioglossus, the hyoglossus, and the palatoglossus muscles (**Fig. 3.3**).

The *floor of the mouth* is formed mainly by the mylohyoid muscle, which is stretched between the U-shaped mandible like a diaphragm and which is inserted into the hyoid bone and the median raphe. On the *oral surface,* with the tip of the tongue elevated, the plica sublingualis with the sublingual caruncle can be found on both sides of the *lingual frenulum.*

In the caruncle and the immediate neighborhood lie the efferent ducts of the submandibular gland, the submandibular duct (Wharton duct), and the sublingual gland and sublingual duct (Bartholin duct). The efferent duct of the parotid gland (Stensen duct) opens into the cheek at the level of the second upper molar, and that of the anterior lingual gland (Blandin gland) in the region of the fimbriated fold on the ventral surface of the tongue.

The *mandible* consists of two separate bones at birth, but these consolidate to form one bone during the first year of life. **Figure 3.4a** shows the most important anatomic details and the typical sites of fracture. The third branch of the trigeminal nerve runs in the body of the mandible, together with the blood vessels that supply the lower teeth. The mandibular nerve enters the mandible at the mandibular foramen and exits at the mental foramen.

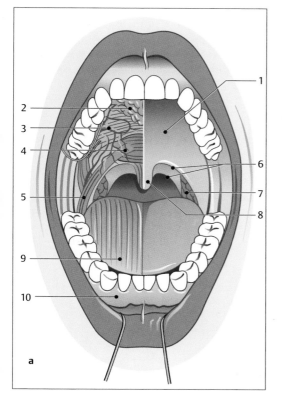

a

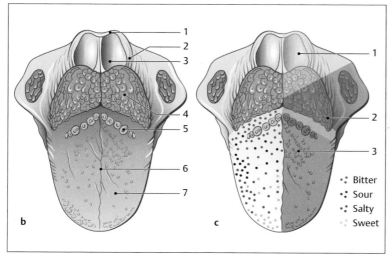

b

c

* : Bitter
* : Sour
* : Salty
* : Sweet

Fig. 3.2a–c Oral cavity and tongue.
a Topographic anatomy of the oral cavity. **1**, Hard palate; **2**, palatine glands; **3**, palatine arteries and nerves; **4**, veli palatine muscles; **5**, palatoglossus; **6**, palatoglossal arches; **7**, palatine tonsil; **8**, uvula; **9**, tongue; **10**, gingiva.
b Anatomy of the tongue. **1**, epiglottis; **2**, lateral glossoepiglottic fold; **3**, epiglottic vallecula **4**, lingual tonsil; **5**, vallate papillae; **6**, median sulcus of the tongue; **7**, body of the tongue.
c Innervation and distribution of qualities of taste on the tongue. **1**, Vagus nerve (X); **2**, glossopharyngeal nerve (IX); **3**, lingual nerve (mandibular nerve, V3).

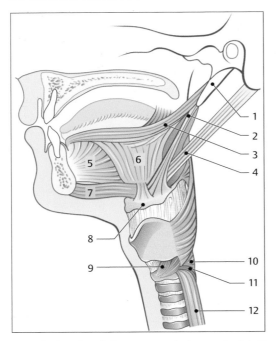

Fig. 3.3 Muscles of the tongue and pharynx. **1**, Styloid process; **2**, stylohyoid muscle; **3**, styloglossus muscle; **4**, digastric muscle; **5**, genioglossus muscle; **6**, hyoglossus muscle; **7**, geniohyoid muscle; **8**, hyoid bone; **9**, cricothyroid muscle; **10**, Killian triangle; **11**, inferior part of the cricopharyngeus; **12**, esophagus.

The *temporomandibular joint* is of considerable clinical interest, as it may be involved in dental diseases, in trauma of the facial skeleton and skull, in otologic diseases, and in generalized arthropathies. In addition, it may be the cause of headache in Costen syndrome. **Figure 3.4b** shows the anatomic relationships. Its proximity to the auditory meatus and mastoid, the lateral part of the base of the skull, the parotid gland, and the lateral wall of the oropharynx and nasopharynx should be noted.

The *epithelial lining of the oral cavity* consists of nonkeratinized stratified squamous epithelium that is thickened in certain points such as the alveolar edges and hard palate, where it unites with the underlying periosteum to form a mucoperiosteum. Subepithelial collections of minor salivary glands are found all over the oral cavity, and are more common in some parts than others (see **Fig. 7.2**).

Vascular supply. The external carotid artery supplies the tongue via the lingual artery; the floor of the mouth via the sublingual artery; the cheek via the facial artery; and the palate via the ascending pharyngeal artery and descending palatine artery. The latter arises from the internal maxillary artery. Venous drainage is through the veins of the same names to the facial vein, the pterygoid venous plexus, and the internal jugular vein. There is also

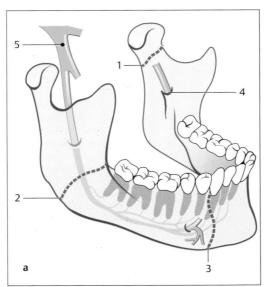

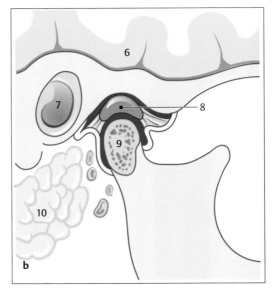

Fig. 3.4a, b   a Mandible with typical fracture lines. **1**, Fracture of the neck; **2**, fracture of the angle of the jaw; **3**, fracture of the chin; **4**, mandibular foramen; **5**, mandibular nerve.

b Temporomandibular joint and surrounding structures. **6**, Middle cranial fossa; **7**, external auditory meatus; **8**, articular disk; **9**, head of the mandible; **10**, parotid gland.

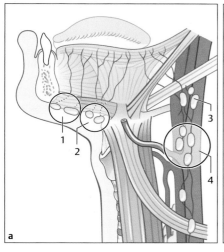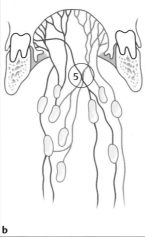

Fig. 3.5a, b   Lymph drainage of the tongue.
a Groups of lymph nodes. **1**, Submental; **2**, submandibular; **3**, upper deep cervical, with lymph nodes at the superior venous angle (**4**).
b Contralateral lymphatic drainage of the tongue. **5**, Crossing of the lymphatic drainage.

a connection to the cavernous sinuses via the pterygoid plexus.

The lymph drains via the regional submental, submandibular, and parotid nodes to the internal jugular chain. The lymph drainage of the base of the tongue and the floor of the mouth is to the same side *and* to the opposite side (**Fig. 3.5a, b**). This is important for the development of contralateral lymph-node metastases (see pp. 285, 399).

Nerve supply. The tongue derives its motor supply from the hypoglossal nerve. Its sensory supply comes from the lingual nerve and the vagus nerve, which innervates the posterior part of the base of the tongue. Taste fibers come from the glossopharyngeal nerve to the base of the tongue and from the chorda tympani fibers of cranial nerve VII, accompanying the lingual nerve for the anterior two-thirds of the tongue (see **Fig. 3.2c**).

The floor of the mouth derives its motor supply from the mylohyoid branch of the mandibular nerve and its sensory supply from the trigeminal nerve. Parasympathetic secretory fibers from the salivary glands are supplied from the chorda tympani and branches of the submandibular ganglion. Sympathetic fibers for blood vessels of the glands come from the carotid plexus.

The masticatory muscles derive their motor supply from the mandibular branch of the trigeminal nerve, but the buccinator muscle is supplied from the facial nerve.

The teeth of the upper jaw receive their sensory supply from the maxillary nerve and those of the lower jaw from the mandibular. These are both branches of cranial nerve V.

The temporomandibular joint derives its nerve supply from the auriculotemporal branch of the mandibular nerve.

The soft palate derives its motor innervation from the glossopharyngeal, vagus, and trigeminal nerves, and probably the facial nerve as well.

■ Nasopharynx, Oropharynx, and Hypopharynx

The pharynx is a muscular tube, 12–13 cm long in the adult; it narrows from above downward, is covered with mucosa, and is divided into three compartments, each of which has an anterior opening (**Fig. 3.6**).

The *nasopharynx* is limited superiorly by the base of the skull and inferiorly by an imaginary plane through the soft palate, and it opens into the nasal cavity. The most important anatomic structures are as follows: anteriorly, the choanae; superiorly, the floor of the sphenoid sinus; postero-superiorly, the adenoid; laterally, the pharyngeal ostium of the eustachian tube and the cartilaginous torus tubarius, immediately posterior to which is the Rosenmüller fossa (pharyngeal recess) and the tubal tonsil; and anteriorly and inferiorly, the soft palate. The embryonic pharyngeal bursa (**Fig. 3.7**) may persist in the posterior wall of the nasopharynx, causing chronic inflammation and retention of secretions. The posterior wall of the nasopharynx is

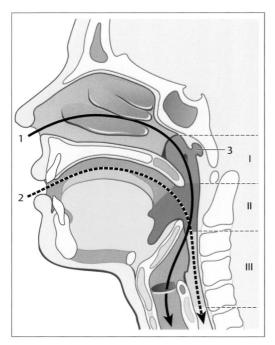

Fig. 3.6 Divisions of the pharynx. **I**, Nasopharynx; **II**, oropharynx; **III**, hypopharynx. Crossing of the upper airway (**1**) and the upper food passage (**2**). Site of the pharyngeal bursa (**3**).

The valleculae (see **Fig. 3.1**), the base of the tongue, the anterior surface of the soft palate, and the lingual surface of the epiglottis are usually described as being part of the oropharynx.

The epithelial lining consists of nonkeratinizing stratified squamous epithelium.

The *hypopharynx* extends from the upper edge of the epiglottis superiorly to the inferior edge of the cricoid cartilage (see **Fig. 3.6**). It opens anteriorly into the larynx. On each side of the larynx lie the funnel-shaped piriform sinuses. Important anatomic structures and relationships include: on the anterior wall, the marginal structures of the laryngeal inlet and the posterior surface of the larynx; on the lateral wall, the inferior constrictor muscle and the piriform sinus, the latter being bounded medially by the aryepiglottic fold and laterally by the internal surface of the thyroid cartilage and the thyrohyoid membrane. Immediate relationships of the hypopharynx at the level of the larynx include the common carotid artery, the internal jugular vein, and the vagus nerve. Relationships of the posterior wall, apart from the pharyngeal constrictor muscle (see below), include the prevertebral fascia and the bodies of the third to the sixth cervical vertebrae. Inferiorly, the hypopharynx opens into the esophagus, the boundary being the superior sphincter of the esophagus. The epithelial lining consists of nonkeratinized stratified squamous epithelium.

The muscular tube of the entire pharynx consists of two layers with different functions:

1. A circular muscle layer consisting of the three pharyngeal constrictor muscles: the superior constrictor, inserted into the base of the skull; the middle constrictor, inserted into the hyoid bone; and the inferior constrictor, inserted into the cricoid cartilage (see **Figs. 3.3, 3.7**). Each of these funnel-shaped muscular segments is overlapped at its lower end by the segment below. All of the segments are inserted posteriorly into a tendinous median raphe.

The inferior constrictor muscle is of particular clinical importance. It is divided into a superior thyropharyngeal part and an inferior cricopharyngeal part. **Figure 3.7** shows how the triangular dehiscence *(Killian triangle)* is formed from the posterior wall of the hypopharynx between the superior oblique and the inferior horizontal fibers. A pharyngoesophageal pouch (Zenker diverticulum) may develop at this weak point in the hypopharyngeal wall.

separated from the spinal column by the tough prevertebral fascia, which lies on the longus capitis muscles, the deep muscles of the neck, and the arch of the first cervical vertebra.

The shape and width of the nasopharynx show marked individual variation. The epithelial lining consists of respiratory ciliated and stratified squamous epithelium, with transitional epithelium at the junction with the oropharynx.

The *oropharynx* extends from the horizontal plane through the soft palate described above to the superior edge of the epiglottis (**Fig. 3.7**) and is continuous with the oral cavity through the faucial isthmus. It contains the following important structures: the posterior wall, consisting of the prevertebral fascia and the bodies of the second and third cervical vertebrae; the lateral wall, containing the palatine tonsil with the anterior and posterior faucial pillars; and the supratonsillar fossa, lying above the tonsil between the anterior and posterior faucial arches.

2. Raising and lowering of the pharynx are also carried out by three paired muscles radiating into the pharyngeal wall from outside. These are the stylopharyngeus, the salpingopharyngeus, and the palatopharyngeus muscles. The stylohyoid and styloglossus muscles are also responsible for elevation. A true longitudinal muscle does not occur in the pharynx and only begins at the mouth of the esophagus. The ability of the pharynx to slide over a distance of several centimeters is due to the existence of fascial spaces (parapharyngeal and retropharyngeal) filled with loose connective tissue. The importance of these tissue spaces in the spread of infection is described on p. 270 and in **Fig. 3.45a, b**.

Vascular supply of the pharynx. The *arterial supply* is provided by the ascending pharyngeal artery, the ascending palatine artery, the tonsillar branches of the facial artery, branches of the maxillary artery (i.e., the descending palatine artery), and branches of the lingual artery. These all arise from the external carotid artery. *Venous drainage* is via the facial vein and the pterygoid plexus to the internal jugular vein.

The *lymphatic drainage* is either via an inconstant retropharyngeal lymph node and then to the deep jugular lymph nodes, or directly to the latter group. The inferior part of the pharynx also drains to the paratracheal lymph nodes and is thus connected to the lymphatic system of the thorax. See also page 231.

Nerve supply of the pharynx. The individual pharyngeal muscles gain their motor supply from the glossopharyngeal (IX), vagus (X), hypoglossal (XII), and facial (VII) nerves. The nasopharynx derives its sensory nerve supply from the maxillary division of the trigeminal nerve (V), the oropharynx from the glossopharyngeal nerve (IX), and the hypopharynx from the vagus nerve (X) (see p. 231).

■ Lymphoepithelial System of the Pharynx

Note: The term "lymphoepithelial tissue" is used to indicate the close symbiosis of epithelial and lymphatic cells on the surface of a mucosa.

The epithelial and subepithelial tissue is loosely arranged so that lymphatic cells can enter it in large numbers ("reticulated epithelium"). The reticulo-

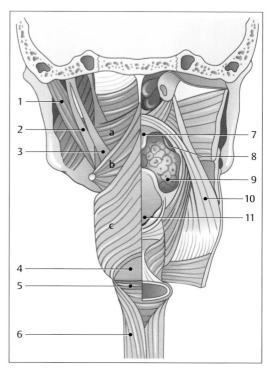

Fig. 3.7 Pharyngeal musculature. **1**, Digastric muscle; **2**, stylohyoid muscle; **3**, stylopharyngeus muscle; **4**, Killian triangle; **5**, inferior part of the cricopharyngeus muscle; **6**, esophagus; **7**, uvula; **8**, palatine tonsil; **9**, tongue; **10**, palatopharyngeus muscle; **11**, epiglottis; **a**, superior pharyngeal constrictor muscle, **b**, middle pharyngeal constrictor muscle, **c**, inferior pharyngeal constrictor muscle.

histiocytic system, more commonly known as the reticuloendothelial system (RES), with its storage cells, is strongly represented in lymphoepithelial tissue. **Figure 3.8** shows the principle of a lymphoepithelial unit. Solitary units of this type, solitary follicles, are found in all parts of the mucosa. The epithelium is also diffusely interspersed with lymphocytes.

A very distinct collection of lymphoepithelial tissue, the Waldeyer ring, lies at the opening of the upper aerodigestive tracts.

The lymphoepithelial organs are called *tonsils*. From above downward, the following are distinguished:

1. The *pharyngeal tonsil,* the adenoids, which is single and lies on the roof and posterior wall of the nasopharynx

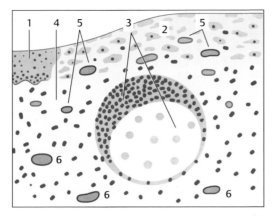

Fig. 3.8 Lymphoepithelial tissue. **1**, Continuous squamous epithelium; **2**, reticular epithelium; **3**, secondary nodes with light centers and a dark zone of small lymphocytes; **4**, basic lymphoid tissue; **5**, arterioles and venules; **6**, postcapillary veins.

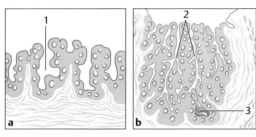

Fig. 3.9a, b   The nasopharyngeal tonsil and adenoids (**a**), and the palatine tonsil (**b**). **1**, Tonsillar lacunae; **2**, tonsillar crypts; **3**, cryptic abscess.

2. The *tubal tonsil,* which is paired and lies around the ostium of the eustachian tube in the Rosenmüller fossa
3. The paired *palatine tonsil,* lying between the anterior and posterior faucial pillars
4. The *lingual tonsil,* which is single and lies in the base of the tongue.

Less constant and obvious are:

5. The *tubopharyngeal plicae,* lateral bands, which run almost vertically at the junction of the lateral and posterior walls of the oropharynx and nasopharynx
6. Lymphoepithelial collections in the laryngeal ventricle

Unlike lymph nodes, lymphoepithelial organs only have efferent lymph vessels and do not have afferent vessels. Differences in the pathology and physiology of the individual collections of lymphoid tissue are due to their different structures. **Figure 3.9** shows the structure of a palatine tonsil and of the adenoids.

The fine structure of a tonsil (**Figs. 3.8, 3.9a, b**) is in principle as follows: the soft-tissue lamellae or septa arise from a basal connective tissue capsule. These serve as a supporting framework in which blood vessels, lymphatics, and nerves run. This fan-shaped supporting framework considerably increases the active surface of the tonsil, as it holds the actual lymphoepithelial parenchyma. In the palatine tonsil, the active surface is sunk into the mucosa, whereas in the adenoids, it projects above the surface. The broad flat niches opening into the oral cavity caused by infolding are called *lacunae,* and the branching clefts running throughout the entire substance of the tonsil are called *crypts.* The actual tonsil tissue consists of a collection of a very large number of the lymphoepithelial units described above (see **Fig. 3.8**). The crypts usually contain cell debris and round cells, but may also contain bacteria and colonies of fungi, collections of pus, and encapsulated microabscesses. (See p. 266 for the description of chronic tonsillitis.)

The tonsils of the Waldeyer ring are present at the embryonic stage, but they only acquire their typical structure with secondary nodes during the postnatal period—i. e., after direct contact with environmental pathogens. They begin increasing rapidly in size between the first and third years of life, with peaks in the third and seventh years.

They involute slowly as of early puberty. Like the rest of the lymphatic system, they atrophy with increasing age.

The arterial blood supply to the pharyngeal tonsil is provided by various branches of the external carotid artery, including the facial artery and/or the ascending palatine artery, the ascending pharyngeal and lingual arteries, and possibly direct tonsillar branches.

The veins of the pharyngeal tonsil usually drain via the palatal vein to the facial vein, and from there to the jugulo-facial venous angle of the internal jugular vein. There is also drainage via the pterygoid venous plexus to the internal jugular vein. This route provides a possible pathway of spread for infection from the tonsils to the cavernous sinus (see **Figs. 3.45a, b; 3.46**).

■ Physiologic and Pathophysiologic Principles

Several functional systems are collected in the mouth and pharynx, including the masticatory system, the swallowing apparatus, the taste organs, the lymphoepithelial ring, pregastric digestion, and articulation. In addition, the respiratory and digestive tracts cross in this area (see **Fig. 3.6**). This requires a reliable reflex protective system. An important prerequisite for this is a well-functioning autonomic and voluntary nervous supply to this region, and a mucosa adapted to this dual function. The mouth is only involved in respiration as a supplementary measure (see p. 232); continuous mouth breathing causes considerable local damage and can also affect the entire body. Typical functional disturbances due to defects of the nervous supply are summarized in **Table 3.1**.

■ Eating, Preparation of Food, and Swallowing

Normal feeding requires a normal masticatory apparatus and teeth, masticatory muscles, and temporomandibular joint. The function of the cranial nerves also has to be normal (see **Table 3.1**). The preparation of food serves to reduce the size of the food bolus by chewing and to moisten the food with saliva, of which 1.0–1.5 L are produced daily. The saliva lubricates the mucosa and makes the food capable of being swallowed. In addition, the enzymes contained in saliva prepare the food by partial chemical decomposition for further digestion in the gastrointestinal tract.

The results of quantitative or qualitative defects of saliva are summarized on p. 416. Satisfactory moistening of the mucosa of the oral cavity and pharynx by saliva is also necessary for normal speech and for normal taste (see discussion of salivary function on p. 415).

The act of swallowing. This an extremely complex sequence of events that is controlled by several cranial nerves (trigeminal nerve, facial nerve with chorda tympani, glossopharyngeal nerve, vagus nerve, superior and inferior laryngeal nerves, hypoglossal nerve) and cervical nerves (cervical plexus, C1–C4). Central coordination is performed in the motoric cortex of the precentral gyrus, the amygdaloid body, nuclear regions of the hypothalamus, and the ventral tegmentum of the midbrain. The deglutition centers are located in the rhombencephalon of the reticular formation and in the medulla oblongata. The "pattern generator" coordinating the interactions of the nerves and muscles is inborn.

Phases of swallowing. *Oral preparation phase:* Food is chewed and mixed with saliva. The lips close, round off, and are retracted. The mandible and the tongue move in all directions, the cheeks tauten, and the soft palate faces anteriorly.

Oral phase: The bolus is pressed along the back of the tongue into the oropharynx, eliciting the swallowing reflex. The corresponding receptors are located in the palatoglossal arch and the base of the tongue.

Pharyngeal phase: This phase of the swallowing reflex consists of a succession of movements that include closure of the larynx and further transportation of the bolus through the pharynx to the esophagus.

Esophageal phase: This phase comprises transportation of the bolus by peristaltic waves through the esophagus and into the stomach.

Pathophysiologic aspects. Closure of the laryngeal inlet by the epiglottis is not strictly necessary for normal swallowing. A patient whose epiglottis has been removed—e.g., in tumor surgery—usually learns to swallow without difficulty. However, the sensory nerve supply to the hypopharynx and the laryngeal inlet from the superior laryngeal branch of the vagus nerve has to be intact, as well as the pharyngeal constrictor for reflex protection of the laryngeal inlet. Increased tone or spasm of the cricopharyngeus is a common autonomic disorder—e.g., in thyrotoxicosis or Plummer–Vinson (Paterson–Kelly) syndrome. This can cause the globus symptom of discomfort on swallowing at the level of the cricoid cartilage, true dysphagia (see **Table 3.1**), and possibly the development of a hypopharyngeal diverticulum.

Disturbances of swallowing may also occur in paralyses of one or more cranial nerves (especially cranial nerve X, but also nerves IX and XII), which affect the tongue, soft palate, or pharyngeal musculature.

Table 3.1 Differential diagnoses of dysphagia

Site	Causal disease
Oropharyngeal	*Inflammatory:* glossitis, abscess of the floor of the mouth, specific and nonspecific pharyngitis, tonsillitis, peritonsillar abscess, retropharyngeal and hypopharyngeal abscess, edema of the uvula and angioneurotic edema
	Neural: lesions of vagus, hypoglossal and glossopharyngeal nerves, glossopharyngeal and vagus neuralgia
	Mechanical obstruction: foreign body, hypopharyngeal diverticulum, pharyngeal stricture, styloid process syndrome, benign and malignant tumors
	Congenital anomalies: macroglossia, clefts of the lip and jaw and palate, cysts of the base of the tongue, lingual thyroid, hyoid anomalies, cervical cysts and fistulas (median and lateral)
	Miscellaneous: results of radiotherapy, xerostomia, humidifying disorders, sialadenitis, fractures of the upper and lower jaw and the hyoid, lesions of the masticatory muscles, burns and scalds, results of surgery
Laryngeal	*Inflammatory:* epiglottitis, specific and nonspecific laryngitis, perichondritis of the larynx
	Neural: neuralgia of the superior laryngeal nerve, paralysis of the superior laryngeal nerve
	Miscellaneous: laryngeal trauma (contusion, distortion, fracture), results of radiotherapy, laryngocele, benign and malignant tumor, foreign bodies, and results of surgery
Esophageal	*Inflammatory or traumatic:* esophagitis including reflux esophagitis, esophageal mycosis, esophageal trauma, caustic burns, results of trauma and surgery, strictures and stenoses, esophageal foreign bodies and esophageal perforation
	Disorders of motility: esophageal spasm, "upper achalasia" (spasm of the cricopharyngeus muscle), external compression by goiter, aortic aneurysm or tumors of the lung and mediastinum, achalasia (cardiospasm), scleroderma, results of vagotomy, esophageal varices, presbyesophagus
	Neighboring organs: goiter
	Congenital anomalies: diverticulum, megaesophagus, hiatus hernia, congenital esophageal stenosis, vascular abnormalities
	Tumors: benign or malignant esophageal tumors (the latter are more common)
Diseases of the cervical spine	Arthritis of the cervical spine, subluxation of the cervical spine, dislocation of the cervical spine, prolapsed disk, spondylolisthesis, cervical rib
Neurologic disorders	Amyotrophic lateral sclerosis, bulbar paralysis, pseudobulbar paralysis, bulbar poliomyelitis, polyneuritis, multiple sclerosis, syringomyelia, cerebral and cerebellar ischemia, thrombosis of the posterior inferior cerebellar artery or basilar artery, brain tumors and brain stem tumors, disorders of cerebrospinal fluid circulation, vertebrobasilar insufficiency, myasthenia gravis, chorea (Huntington–Sydenham disease), Parkinson disease, tabes dorsalis, diabetic and alcoholic neuropathy, Wallenberg syndrome, lead intoxication
General diseases	Infections, botulism, iron-deficiency anemia (Plummer–Vinson or Paterson–Kelly syndrome), megaloblastic anemia, agranulocytosis, tetany, tetanus, goiter, thyroiditis, hypocalcemia, leukemia, vitamin A and B_1 deficiency, mitral valve disease, aortic aneurysms
Skin diseases	Scleroderma, urticaria, lupus erythematosus, erythema multiforme, pemphigus, recurrent aphthous ulcers, hereditary epidermolysis bullosa, dermatomyositis
Autonomic dysphagia	Autonomic dysfunction, psychogenic overlay (globus hystericus)

■ Taste

The basic taste sensations are *sweet, salty, sour,* and bitter. A proposed fifth taste sensation is *umami* (a sensation of savoriness), which applies to specific glutamic acid receptors. All other tastes are mixed sensations in which the sense of smell is also integrated. Many foods are "tasted" by the olfactory nerve. Pure sensory nerve fibers to the tongue and oral mucosa may also be stimulated by sour or spicy foods.

The sensory organs for taste are the taste buds lying in the vallate papillae, foliate papillae, and fungiform papillae on the tongue and on the hard palate (**Fig. 3.10**), the anterior faucial pillar, the tonsil, the posterior pharyngeal wall, the esophageal orifice, and the buccal mucosa. The fine gustatory hair cells have to be bathed in saliva or other fluids to allow the sense of taste to be evoked. **Figure 3.2c** shows the topical arrangement on the tongue of the sites where the different taste qualities are recognized. The sensory nerve supply is provided peripherally by two nerves in particular: the chorda tympani, arising from cranial nerve VII and accompanying the lingual nerve from cranial nerve V, and the glossopharyngeal nerve, arising from cranial nerve IX.

The boundary of the area supplied by each individual nerve in the mouth and pharynx is still not fully agreed upon, but the following is generally accepted (see **Fig. 1.20**). The anterior half of the tongue is supplied by the ipsilateral chorda tympani via the nervus intermedius, with synapses in the sensory geniculate ganglion. The posterior third of the tongue and the walls of the oral pharynx receive their sensory supply from the glossopharyngeal nerve. It is probable that the vagus nerve also has sensory contributions to the epiglottis, the laryngeal inlet (aditus), the upper part of the esophagus, and possibly also a small part of the center of the base of the tongue. Gustatory sensations from the soft palate are transmitted by the palatine nerves via the pterygopalatine ganglion, the greater petrosal nerve, the geniculate ganglion, and the nervus intermedius to the medulla oblongata.

The boundary between the area supplied by the lingual nerve and the accompanying chorda tympani and the glossopharyngeal nerve is still not generally agreed on.

Reflex reactions may affect the sense of taste, as they do the sense of smell. These include alterations in the quantity and quality of salivary secretion, the production of gastric juice, and interference with the course of the swallowing act.

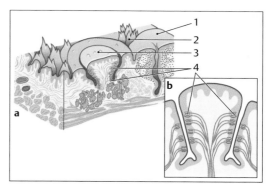

Fig. 3.10a, b   Structure of the sense of taste on the tongue. **1**, Lingual tonsil; **2**, filiform and fungiform papillae; **3**, vallate papilla; **4**, taste buds.

Basic pathophysiology. Although sensory disorders of taste are less common than those of smell, they occur more commonly than is generally thought. Apart from direct, accidental, inflammatory, viral, or iatrogenic causes, they may also be due to neural lesions, certain drugs (see below), endocrine diseases, and deficiency diseases (**Table 3.2**). Disorders of taste may vary in degree and involve different qualities of taste (**Table 3.3**). Usually the threshold is increased—i. e., gustatory function is reduced. Reduction of the threshold is rare, but may occur in mucoviscidosis. The relation of the four senses of taste to each other may be disassociated.

Drugs that have side effects on the sense of taste include acetylsalicylic acid, biguanidine, carbamazepine, lithium, methylthiouracil, oxyfedrine, penicillamine, and phenylbutazone. Side effects may also occur after local use of ether oils, chlorhexidine, and hexetidine.

■ Function of the Tonsils

The tonsils have an immune-specific defense function. They send immunologically marked lymphocytes and immunoglobulins from the organism's "front line" to the various stations in the immune system. This is made possible by the way in which the tonsils are structured. In the crypts and reticular epithelium, intensive contact with the widest variety of antigens in the oral cavity is ensured. The tonsils form lymphocytes and plasma cells; T lymphocytes serve specifically for cellular immune defense, while immunoglobulins (e. g., IgA, IgE, IgM) and B lymphocytes are formed for humoral immunological reactions. At the same time, lymphocytes and immunoglobulins are released directly from

Table 3.2   Classification of disorders of taste

Quantitative taste disorders	
Hypogeusia	Reduced sensitivity—e. g., due to radiotherapy
Hyper-geusia	Increased sensitivity—e. g., in glossopharyngeal neuralgia
Ageusia	Absence of the sense of taste. This may be partial, due to a lesion in the chorda tympani; total, due to toxins; or selective, as in "taste blindness" for certain substances
Qualitative taste disorders	
Parageusia	Faulty taste; may be due to virus infection
Cacogeusia	Unpleasant taste, occurring typically in cerebral sclerosis
Phanto-geusia	Perception of taste sensations in the absence of a source
Gustatory hallucinations	May occur due to drug abuse, psychoses, and disorders of the central nervous system

Table 3.3   Definition of taste disorders

Epithelial origin	Damage to taste buds as a sequela of infection or radiation exposure, deficient oral hygiene, fungal infections, diabetes mellitus, Sjögren disease, adverse drug effects, hepatic and renal diseases, atrophic glossitis, salivary deficiency (e. g., due to antihypertensive drugs, antihistamines, antidepressants), burning mouth syndrome, hyperthyroidism, Cushing syndrome
Neural origin	Damage to cranial nerves VII, IX, X (e. g., following tonsillectomy, basal skull fractures, neurodegenerative disorders)
Central origin	Central nervous disorders of the taste fibers (e. g., posttraumatic anosmia/ageusia syndrome, brain tumors, brain stem lesions, neurodegenerative disease, temporal lobe epilepsy)

the tonsillar crypts into the oral cavity. The tonsils thus have both local and systemic immunological functions.

Basic pathophysiology. The increase in lymphoepithelial tissue during the early years of childhood development is explained by immunobiologic requirements. This increase in size is primarily only an expression of an active defensive function of the infant's organism to antigenic substances in the environment. During this period, tonsillar hyperplasia is therefore a welcome condition and in no way suggests excess inflammation. Since the tonsils lie at a narrow point in the respiratory and digestive tract, the nasopharynx and the faucial isthmus, an increase in their volume beyond a certain point leads to increased narrowing of the diameter of this essential pathway, to the detriment of the rest of the body (**Fig. 3.11a, b**). Obstructive sleep apnea may develop in extreme cases. Removal of the tonsils and adenoids is therefore justified in these circumstances, despite potential immunologic disadvantages. The palatine tonsils alone have slitlike, branching, poorly drained crypts permeating their entire substance. As long as these clefts drain freely into the oral cavity, the function of the tonsil is not endangered. However, if the physiologic content of the crypt stagnates due to

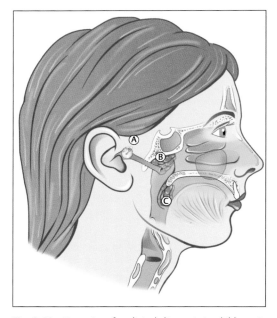

Fig. 3.11   Key points for clinical diagnosis in children. **A,** Otoscopy. Depending on their size and direction of growth, the adenoids (**B**) can block the nasopharynx and the pharyngeal ostium of the eustachian tube. Both the size and the extension of the tonsils (**C**) toward the posterior wall of the pharynx should be assessed. The easiest way of doing this is with an endoscope (4 mm, wide angle).

anatomic or infective stenosis, an ideal culture medium is set up for microorganisms. Colonies of bacteria or fungi become established, leading to chronic suppuration (cryptitis), small abscesses in the crypts, and superficial ulceration of the surface of the crypts. In anatomicopathologic terms, this represents *chronic tonsillitis*. This is in no way related to the size of the tonsil. **Figure 3.8** shows how the superficial tonsillar capillaries are unprotected and course close to the lumen of the crypt, allowing relatively unhindered access for infective or toxic materials to the general circulation.

■ **Formation of Sound and Speech**

The oral cavity and pharynx make an important contribution to the timbre of the speech and voice, due to their action as a variable resonating space. In addition, the tongue, along with the palate, is necessary for the formation of consonants and vowels. Despite this, experience with tumor surgery shows that large parts of the tongue can be removed without loss of comprehensible speech.

With regard to nasality, it is still unclear whether closure of the nasopharynx during the articulation of consonants functions according to an "all or nothing" rule or whether it involves a graded mechanism of muscular obstruction by the soft palate.

Methods of Investigation

■ **Inspection, Palpation, and Examination with the Mirror**

The examination is carried out, with good illumination from a head lamp or head mirror, using two tongue depressors (see **Fig. 2.14b, c; Figs. 3.12, 3.13**). The following should be observed:

- The color and the normal symmetrical mobility of the lips, the condition of the skin and mucosa, and changes in the surface, ulcerations, induration, and tenderness of the lips are inspected.
- The arrangement of the teeth and the occlusion are examined with the lips open. The symmetry of the contour of the jaws, the mobility of the mandible, and the function of the temporomandibular joint are also examined.
- The shape and mobility of the tongue is examined with the mouth open. In hypoglossal pare-

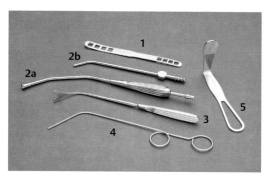

Fig. 3.12 Some traditional instruments for examining the mouth and pharynx. **1**, Bruening tongue depressor; **2a, b**, suction tubes for mouth and oropharynx; **3**, Reichert hook; **4**, long curved cotton applicator; **5**, angled tongue depressor for the base of the tongue.

sis, the tongue deviates slightly to the paralyzed side. The floor of the mouth and the two caruncles are examined using a tongue depressor, with the tongue elevated. The surface and consistency of the tongue and articulation are also assessed.

- The properties of the mucosa of the mouth and cheeks are assessed, with particular attention to color, moisture, dryness, membranes, ulceration, tumors, and disorders of sensation.
- The condition of the hard and soft palate is examined. The innervation of the two sides is compared. In paralysis of the palate, the uvula deviates to the healthy side. The innervation of the pharyngeal musculature is tested.
- The upper and lower vestibule of the oral cavity are examined with a tongue depressor.
- The parotid duct in the cheek opposite the upper second molar tooth is inspected.
- The palatine tonsils, lingual tonsil, and mucosa of the posterior wall of the pharynx are examined using two tongue depressors (**Fig. 3.13e**). Normally, these structures should be pale yellow to pale pink, moist, and shiny. Dryness, coating, glazed crusts, and yellow streams of pus may be noted.

Examination of the tonsils: A tongue depressor is laid carefully with the left hand on the lateral part of the posterior part of the tongue, and the tongue is pressed gently downward. The spatula should not be placed on the base of the tongue, since this elicits the gag reflex. As soon as the tonsillar cleft can be seen, the other hand is used to introduce the second tongue depressor between the ascending ramus of the mandible and the tonsil, and the edge of the tongue depressor is placed gently on the anterior faucial pillar, lateral to the tonsil, to dislocate it from its fossa into the oral cavity. An attempt is made to press material out of the visible crypt opening. The size of the tonsil and its connective tissue fixation to the tonsillar fossa, the color and properties of the surrounding mucosa on the faucial pillars, and the color and properties of the surface of the tonsil, including any exudate and the expressed contents of the crypt, are noted. Differences between the two sides are also looked for. Palpation of the lymph nodes now follows, with particular attention being paid to the nodes at the angle of the jaw and in the submandibular and submental areas (see **Figs. 6.11, 6.16a–e**).

Suspect areas in the oral cavity and base of the tongue should always also be palpated. The index finger, enclosed in a finger cot or glove, is used to palpate the suspicious area carefully for induration, infiltration, ulceration, and tender areas. Most patients tolerate careful examination. In patients with an exaggerated gag reflex, the oral and pharyngeal mucosa—particularly that of the soft palate, the base of the tongue, and the posterior wall of the

pharynx—can be rendered insensitive first by applying a spray or a cotton applicator saturated with 1 % tetracaine or lidocaine (Xylocaine). Local anesthesia of the pharynx is also recommended if satisfactory examination of the nasopharynx, hypopharynx, or larynx is not possible due to a marked gag reflex.

Note: Examination of the mouth with a tongue depressor or with the finger must be performed gently after the patient has received an explanation of the procedure. This is the only way to prevent gagging and allow a satisfactory view of the whole of the mouth and pharynx (**Fig. 3.13**).

The nasopharynx, the hypopharynx, and the larynx are now examined with the mirror (**Fig. 3.14a**). The technique of posterior rhinoscopy is described on page 132 and the technique of indirect laryngoscopy on page 298. The introduction of the loupe endoscope is described on page 298 (**Fig. 3.14b**).

Indirect mirror examination of the hypopharynx may be very difficult in patients with a protruding or infiltrated tongue base, if it is tender, or in those with a sensitive gag reflex. These patients are best examined using transnasal hypopharyngoscopy with a flexible endoscope. Flexible nasendoscopy (FNE) is the standard method now used by speech and language therapists.

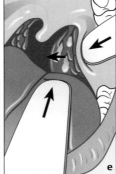

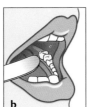
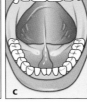
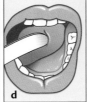

Fig. 3.13a–e Examination of the oral cavity.
a Situation during the clinical examination.
b Inspection of the buccal mucosa and parotid duct orifice, opposite the second upper molar.
c Inspection of the floor of the mouth and submandibular duct orifices.
d Evaluation of the lateral oral floor.
e Examination of the palatine tonsil with two tongue depressors.

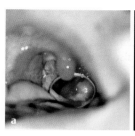
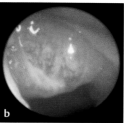

Fig. 3.14a, b **a** Examination of the nasopharynx with a mirror.
b Endoscopy of the nasopharynx in a child with adenoids.

Note: When there is clinical suspicion of a tumor, all lymph-node fields in the head and neck have to be carefully palpated (see p. 385) and appropriate imaging studies performed (B-mode ultrasonography, computed tomography, magnetic resonance imaging). During palpation of the neck, the head should be flexed toward the examination side, to relax the muscles and fascia (see **Fig. 8.13**).

■ Endoscopy

Various endoscopic techniques are available for examining the pharynx and hypopharynx. These include flexible transnasal endoscopy with local anesthesia, and rigid endoscopy in the clinical setting using suspension laryngohypopharyngoscopy (see **Fig. 4.8**) with the patient under general anesthesia.

Rigid endoscopy is an important diagnostic method in oncologic patients for evaluating the size, extension, and precise location of a tumor and for obtaining biopsies from margins of the lesion. The results are important for decision-making regarding the operability of a tumor, the surgical approach, and defect repair.

■ Imaging Studies

Tumors, enlarged adenoids, and other conditions in the *nasopharynx* are well displayed in a lateral view of the skull. This projection is also suitable for imaging the soft tissues of the nasopharynx.

Computed tomography (CT), magnetic resonance imaging (MRI; **Fig. 3.15**), and occasionally radionuclide scanning can be used for demonstrating the limits of a tumor or destruction caused by a nasopharyngeal tumor. Bilateral carotid angiography and superselective angiography to identify individual branches of the carotid artery are used to investigate nasopharyngeal angiofibromas, which are highly vascular, in preparation for embolization (**Fig. 3.16**; see also p. 242).

The *hypopharynx* is best demonstrated after administration of a contrast agent such as Gastrografin or barium. The swallow with contrast is very useful for diagnosing a pharyngeal pouch, stenoses, and swallowing disorders.

Lateral views of the neck and the upper thoracic region can be used to localize the site of radiopaque foreign bodies in the hypopharynx and upper esophagus. This projection is also of great value in inflammatory soft-tissue swelling and surgical emphysema of the parapharyngeal tissues due to pharyngeal injuries, pharyngeal abscess, mediastinal abscess, etc.

Radiographic demonstration of the salivary glands using sialography and scanning is described on page 418.

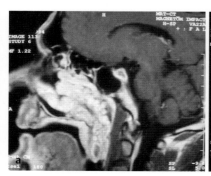
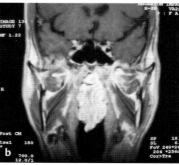

Fig. 3.15a, b A large nasopharyngeal angiofibroma (magnetic resonance images with contrast medium).

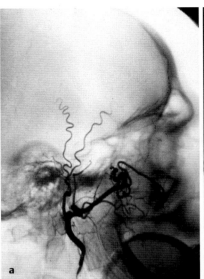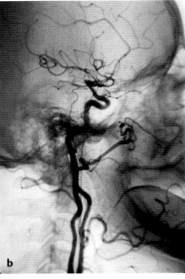

Fig. 3.16a, b Angiography of a nasopharyngeal angiofibroma. Before (**a**) and after (**b**) embolization of the tumor artery.

■ Examination of the Saliva

See page 416.

■ Gustometry

Taste can be tested by applying substances to the tongue that represent the four taste qualities—sweet, salty, sour, and bitter—at increasing concentrations, to assess the lowest concentration that can be recognized.

Examination of overall taste sensation. The three-drop method makes it possible to evaluate the threshold of recognition for the qualities sweet, sour, salty, and bitter. Börnstein's concentrations are used for testing. These are as follows: glucose 4%, 10%, 40%; sodium chloride 2.5%, 7.5%, 15%; citric acid 1%, 5%, 10%; quinine 0.075%, 0.5%, 1% (stale solutions should not be used). The sensation of taste is observed 0.5–4.0 s later, depending on the site tested, the temperature of the solution, and the size of the area tested. The test solution is applied alternately to the right and left sides of the tongue with a pipette, or better with a small piece of blotting paper ≈ 1 cm^2 in size. Confirming the threshold of recognition is usually satisfactory in ordinary practice.

Alternatively, test solutions of substances at concentrations slightly below or above the taste threshold can be administered in a defined sequence as one-drop tests. The sum of the recognized concentration levels of all four taste qualities is taken as a gustatory index. This test has high test–retest reliability—i. e., it is highly reproducible.

Assessing the ability to identify taste qualities. Oral application of sweet, sour, salty, and bitter test solutions, each at a concentration above the threshold that the patient is supposed to identify, is suitable for screening purposes. The test substances can be applied in solid form (known as tasties, taste strips, or wafers) or as fluids (drops, sprays). The patient is asked to identify each taste quality immediately after application.

Electrogustometry. Electric current can also be used to stimulate the taste receptors instead of test solutions. An anode current is used, with a normal threshold in adults between 2 and 7 µA. Electrogustometry has numerous advantages, but it is usually only used in specialist practices or hospital departments.

Objective gustometry can also be used in university hospitals. Reflex changes in the respiratory resistance of the nose or the electrical resistance of the skin are recorded simultaneously in response to a taste stimulus. **Table 3.2** shows the most frequent causes of disorders of taste.

■ Specific Diagnostic Procedures

Bacteriologic, mycologic, and virologic culture. Culture is still the basis of treatment with anti-inflammatory drug agents. The diagnostic methods provided by microbiology, such as culture testing and sensitivity testing, can be frequently used.

Biopsy. Tissue needs to be taken for biopsy if a tumor is suspected and if abnormal findings remain unexplained. Tumors and lesions in the mouth and pharynx are easily accessible, and biopsy in this area is preferable to aspiration or cytology.

Clinical Aspects of Diseases of the Mouth and Pharynx

The main symptoms and disorders that indicate disease of the mouth and pharynx include:
- Pain on eating, chewing, or swallowing.
- Dysphagia (see **Table 3.1**).
- Globus symptoms (see p. 277 and **Table 3.1**).
- Burning of the tongue (see **Table 3.7**).
- Blood in the sputum.
- Oral fetor (see **Table 3.5**).
- Disorders of salivary secretion (see p. 416).
- Disorders of taste (see **Table 3.2**).
- Respiratory obstruction (see **Table 6.2**).
- Disorders of speech.
- Swellings on the head, neck, mouth, floor of the mouth, and swelling of the lymph nodes at the angle of the jaw (see p. 401).

■ Hyperplasia of the Lymphoepithelial Organs

The adenoid, the tonsil, and occasionally the lingual tonsil cause symptoms due to their size.

Hyperplasia of these organs is not in itself a disease, but only the morphologic expression of marked immunobiologic activity. A marked increase in the size of the tonsil produces primary mechanical obstruction of the respiratory or digestive tract and has detrimental effects on the entire body. Inflammation of neighboring organs is secon-

dary. For this reason, tonsillar hyperplasia is here discussed separately from inflammation.

Adenoid Hyperplasia

Clinical Features. These include nasal obstruction, leading to mouth breathing; difficulty in feeding, especially in small children; noisy respiration; snoring; a typical adenoid face—i. e., dull facial expression, open mouth, dilated and flattened nasolabial folds, indrawn nasal alae, protruding upper incisor teeth; enlarged lymph nodes at the angle of the jaw or in the nuchal area; adenoid habitus; and rhinolalia clausa.

Obstruction of the nasopharynx may be responsible for:
1. *Aural diseases,* including obstruction of the eustachian tube, chronic tubal and middle ear catarrh, serous effusion, recurrent acute otitis media, formation of adhesions, and also progression of chronic otitis media and conductive deafness (see p. 58).
2. Diseases of the *nose and paranasal sinuses,* including chronic purulent rhinitis or sinusitis, and even pansinusitis.
3. *Disorders of the masticatory apparatus, including:* maldevelopment of the upper jaw—i. e., arched or "gothic" palate due to absence of the pressure of the tongue on the hard palate, and absence of lateral pressure on the upper jaw and alveolus by the tension of the buccinator muscle and the masticatory muscles because of the open mouth. Also including anomalies of position of the teeth, such as incorrect contact and orientation of the mandibular occlusion, and gingivitis.
4. *Disorders of the lower respiratory system*—i. e., chronic laryngitis, tracheitis, and bronchitis.
5. *Other somatic effects,* including a flat chest, round shoulders, thirst, loss of appetite, poor general development, and sensitivity to attacks of infection.
6. Effects on *intelligence and mental development* due to chronic respiratory obstruction and hypoxia during sleep; increased levels of CO_2 in the blood leading to restless, broken sleep and causing tiredness during the day, apathy, dullness, poor school performance, and "pseudodementia."

Pathogenesis. The disease is caused by above-average hypertrophy of the lymphoepithelial tissue of the pharyngeal ring, which is immunobiologically active during childhood. There is probably a hereditary disposition. Endocrine and constitutional factors and an influence of diet, particularly carbohydrates, have been suggested.

Diagnosis. The main symptoms include chronic mouth breathing, snoring, and proneness to infection. Examination by transnasal endoscopy or posterior rhinoscopy shows the enlarged adenoid (**Fig. 3.11**).

Differential diagnosis. This includes choanal atresia, foreign bodies in the nose, and other causes of nasal obstruction such as nasopharyngeal angiofibroma and malignant tumors of the nasopharynx, possibly of mesenchymal origin, especially in children. Dental causes should be looked for to explain positional anomalies of the teeth and malocclusion.

Treatment. Conservative treatment, with a change of climate, diet, drugs, and so forth is *not* satisfactory.

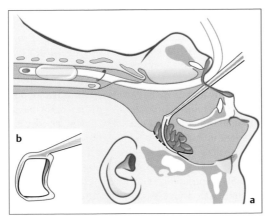

Fig. 3.17a, b   Adenoidectomy with the head extended (**a**), using a Beckmann ring curette (**b**).

Surgical treatment consists of adenoidectomy (**Figs. 3.17a, b, 3.18a–c**). Endotracheal anesthesia should be used to prevent aspiration and to ensure optimal operating conditions. However, the operation can be performed under a brief anesthetic without a tube, provided that the neck is extended. Adenoidectomy is usually performed with the head in the hanging position. A Beckman ring adenotome is usually used to remove the adenoid. The instrument separates the adenoid at its base.

Tonsillar Hyperplasia

Clinical Features. This is usually combined with hypertrophy of the adenoid (see above). In addition, there is increased difficulty in swallowing and eating because of obstruction of the faucial isthmus. Considerable respiratory obstruction may also occur when only the tonsils are hyperplastic.

Diagnosis. See the section on adenoid hyperplasia. The local findings are obvious.

Differential diagnosis. This is similar to that for adenoid hypertrophy. It is important to determine whether the tonsils alone are hypertrophic, or whether there is coexisting adenoid hypertrophy.

> **Note:** Unilateral hyperplasia of the tonsil in an adult must always lead to a suspicion of malignancy. Rapid hyperplasia of the lymphatic pharyngeal ring indicates a disease of the entire lymphatic system.

Treatment. The modern practice for the treatment of tonsillar hyperplasia is tonsillotomy. This can be performed using different types of laser, radiofrequency surgery, or Ultracision. In patients with a history of recurrent or chronic inflammation, a tonsillectomy is indicated.

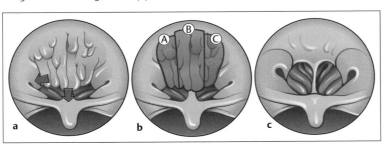

Fig. 3.18a–c   a Obstruction of the pharyngeal ostium of the eustachian tube.
b Typical adenoidectomy in three portions.
c Decompression of the ostia.

!

Note: Not every enlargement of the tonsil or adenoid in a child is an indication for removal. There must be considerable hyperplasia with obvious mechanical obstruction of the nasopharynx or oropharynx, and the appropriate clinical effects and disorders must be present.

Course and prognosis. The symptoms usually resolve rapidly after removal of the mechanical obstruction. The child usually returns surprisingly rapidly to normal physical, psychological, and intellectual health. The prognosis is very good; recurrence after correctly performed adenoidectomy is unusual. The main complications are postoperative bleeding and aspiration. These are only to be feared if hemostasis is not achieved during surgery, if postoperative care is inadequate, or if tissue has been left behind.

!

Note: To avoid overlooking a pathologic bleeding tendency, the following investigations should be performed *before* adenoidectomy or tonsillectomy:
1. A history and family history relative to bleeding and coagulation disorders should be taken. This is the most important diagnostic step for avoiding pathologic bleeding.
2. The bleeding time should be determined if the history is consistent with a bleeding problem.
3. Further tests include the partial thromboplastin time (PTT) and the thrombocyte count.
4. The individual coagulation factors and the thrombocyte function should be investigated if the history and the routine tests indicate a disorder of hemostasis. In addition, analgesics such as salicylates should not be given for at least 10 days before the operation, as they inhibit the function of thrombocytes.

Adenoidectomy or tonsillectomy may still be performed in patients with manifest coagulation disorders if there are convincing indications. However, the operation should be performed with the appropriate substitution therapy, in a special unit.

Other postoperative complications include a change in the sound of the voice, which is usually only temporary, although occasionally rhinolalia aperta may persist. Rare complications include adhesions in the nasopharynx, injuries to the ostium of the eustachian tube, and, very rarely, injuries to the cervical spine.

Relative contraindications include cleft palate, either corrected or not. A speech therapist consultation must be obtained *before* a decision is made for surgery.

Hyperplasia of the lingual tonsil rarely occurs in children, but may occasionally be seen in adults. Symptoms include a feeling of pressure in the throat, especially on swallowing, and occasionally recurrent inflammation of the base of the tongue. If necessary, the lymphoepithelial tissue can be partially removed. The cryoprobe or the laser are particularly suitable for this.

■ Dysphagia

Diagnosis. The two mainstays of diagnosis are radiographic videography and video endoscopy. Radiographic evaluation of swallowing using fluoroscopy requires the administration of a contrast medium bolus (barium sulfate, provided there is no risk of aspiration; otherwise nonionic, low-osmolar contrast medium containing iodine). Phases and functional disorders can be visualized that elude identification by endoscopy—e.g., pumping movements of the base of the tongue, passage into the larynx, or peristaltic waves.

Etiology. A distinction is made between *neurogenic* and *structural* etiologies. Neurogenic dysphagias occur as sequelae to apoplexy, cerebrocranial trauma, hypoxia, neurosurgical operations, or degenerative disease. Structural dysphagias result from tumors or tumor resection in the aerodigestive tract (see also **Table 3.1**, p. 236).

Pathophysiology. Dysphagia is defined as difficulty in swallowing and may be accompanied by the following symptoms (**Fig. 3.19**):
- *Drooling:* The bolus leaves the mouth through incompletely closed lips (e.g., due to lip defects or facial nerve paralysis).
- *Leaking:* The bolus enters the pharynx during the oral preparation phase (e.g., due to tongue paralysis or soft palate impairments such as clefts or paralysis).
- *Larynx penetration:* The bolus arrives at the entrance to the larynx. Aspiration is prevented only by the vestibular folds and the vocal folds.
- *Regurgitation:* Larynx elevation, which plays an important role in opening the superior sphincter, may be impaired (e.g., after tracheotomy or excision of goiter), causing reflux into the mouth if the closing pressure in the

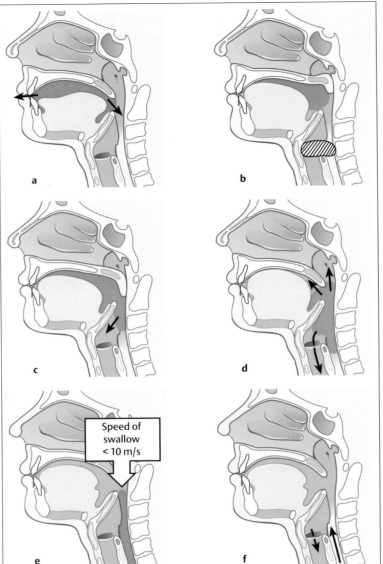

Fig. 3.19a–f Typical swallowing disorders.
a Drooling.
b Globus pharyngeus.
c Laryngeal aspiration.
d Regurgitation.
e Odynophagia.
f Postdeglutitive aspiration.

Speed of swallow < 10 m/s

superior sphincter is too high. Reflux to the epipharynx—e. g., in velopharyngeal insufficiency—is known as nasal regurgitation.

- *Odynophagia:* Pain on swallowing—e. g., due to inflammation.
- *Bolus retention*—e. g., in an epiglottic vallecula, the piriform sinus, or a diverticulum—is possible. Gastroesophageal reflux leads to aspiration at the end of the swallowing act (post deglutition).

Functional treatment. The goal of logopedics or speech therapy is to improve swallowing efficiency and prevent aspiration.

Exercises and facilitation techniques: Dysphagia is treated using techniques that facilitate the sequence of movements and inhibit undesired elevation of muscle tone. Sensibility is stimulated, and the coordination, force, and endurance of motor activity are improved by providing training in target-oriented movements and patterns of motion.

Pathologic reflexes are reduced and pharyngeal contractions improved.

Compensatory techniques: Instead of abolishing the causes, these techniques compensate for deglutition disorders. Their purpose is to facilitate swallowing and prevent aspiration. They include changing the posture of the head by inclination and rotation.

Adaptation methods: This term refers to adjustment of food consistency, positioning the food if there are transportation disorders within the oral cavity, and using special eating and drinking aids.

■ **Inflammatory Diseases**

■ Labial and Oral Mucosa

Internal or dermatologic diseases often present on the lips, oral mucosa, gingiva, and tongue. **Table 3.4** provides an overview of the most common and most important of these disorders. Since changes in the mucosa of the lips, mouth, or pharynx can occur in many disorders, the following description will be confined to the most common ones.

Rhagades of the commissures, along with slight bleeding and pain in the commissures accompanying opening of the mouth. Causes include ill-fitting false teeth, mycotic infection, poor general resistance, diabetes, iron-deficiency anemia, nonspecific pyogenic infections, and syphilis. If possible, the cause should be confirmed and dealt with before treatment is attempted. Carcinoma of the commissure may also simulate rhagades in the early phases. Nonspecific local treatment includes topical corticosteroids, either as a cream or in a special base designed to adhere to mucosal surfaces. In addition, a long-established favorite is gentian violet solution, also known as crystal violet, methyl violet, or pyoktanin. A standardized version is available in Europe using one active ingredient— methylrosaniline chloride 0.1 % aqueous solution (crystal violet). It is recommended to use this form, which is safe and inexpensive.

Cheilitis may be solitary and acute due to trauma, thermal injury (hot food), chemical injury (smoke), actinic damage (sunburn), or exposure to radiation.

Cheilitis granulomatosa, Miescher disease, is a chronic recurring disease which is usually ushered in with a complete *Melkersson–Rosenthal syndrome* of cheilitis, granuloma-

tous glossitis, and facial paralysis. The pathogenesis of this triad is unknown, and the treatment is the same as that of idiopathic facial paralysis (see p. 111).

Although *tuberculosis* or *syphilis,* primary or secondary, may occur on the lips, a chronic or recurrent erosive or hyperkeratotic lesion of the labial mucosa must always be suspected of being premalignant (leukoplakia, Bowen disease). Numerous diseases affecting the oral mucosa also affect the lips.

Stomatitis, often combined with *gingivitis* or *inflammation of the buccal mucosa,* may be a primary disease of many different causes or may be secondary to other diseases. The clinical symptoms and prognosis are thus extremely variable.

Ulceromembranous Stomatitis
Clinical Features. The disease usually begins on the gingival margins with redness, swelling, and sensitivity to pressure. Swelling of the buccal and lingual mucosa, stomatitis simplex, may also occur. The disease often progresses to ulceration with severe pain, presenting with superficial, and occasionally deep, mucosal ulcers with a dirty-gray fibrinous membrane. There are marked constitutional symptoms: oral fetor, sialorrhea, possibly cloudy or purulent saliva, loss of taste, difficulty in eating, and high fever in the initial stages. The disease may spread to the pharynx, and the regional lymph nodes may be enlarged and painful.

Pathogenesis. This includes poor oral hygiene, reduced general resistance, infections from cutlery, dental damage, virus infections with possible secondary bacterial infection, mucosal rhagades, gingival pockets, and dental calculus (**Fig. 3.20**).

Diagnosis. Bacteriologic culture is necessary, and often shows spirochetes and fusiform rods as in Vincent angina (see p. 265).

Differential diagnosis. This consists of mucosal mycosis, excluded by culture, virus infection (herpes simplex, aphthous stomatitis, and herpes zoster), syphilis, tuberculosis, acquired immune deficiency syndrome (AIDS), hematologic diseases including agranulocytosis and leukemia, which can be excluded using a differential white blood count, and carcinoma, which requires a biopsy.

Treatment. This includes appropriate oral and dental hygiene or 1–2 % gentian violet solution. Anti-

Table 3.4 Common lesions of the oral mucosa in generalized and dermatologic diseases

	Cause
Dryness	Febrile infectious diseases, uremia, polyglobulinemia, cachexia, atropine poisoning, Sjögren syndrome and other sialadenoses, vitamin A deficiency, occasionally diabetes mellitus and hyperthyroidism, Plummer–Vinson (Paterson–Kelly) syndrome (iron deficiency), hypertension, prolonged use of certain drugs such as phenothiazines, belladonna and psychotropic drugs
Alterations of pigmentation	
Pallid	Anemia
Cyanotic	Pulmonary congestion
Intense red	Polycythemia rubra vera, reactive polyglobulinemia
Reddish-violet	Right heart insufficiency
Yellow	Jaundice, often as an initial symptom, hepatic congestion, megaloblastic anemia
Red, like lipstick	Hepatic insufficiency
Whitish patches like leukoplakia with dry mucosa	Vitamin A deficiency
Grayish-violet staining of the gingival mucosa	Argyrosis
Grayish-blue to brownish discoloration of the gingiva	Bismuth and lead intoxication
Spotted hyperpigmentation	Oral contraceptives
Punctate or striated, occasionally diffuse pigmentation of the lips, cheeks, gingiva, tongue and palate	Addison disease, of which it is often the first symptom
Bleeding	
From the gingiva, with a dark-red discoloration and swelling of the interdental papillae	Scurvy
Bleeding from cavernous angiectasia on the vermilion border and on the oral mucosa	Hereditary hemorrhagic telangiectasia (Rendu–Osler–Weber disease)

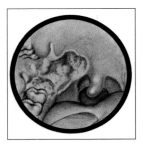

Fig. 3.20 Ulceromembranous stomatitis. Extremely severe ulcerous destruction in the region of the right side of the palate and the gingiva. Swabs often reveal spirochetes and fusiform rods, as in trench mouth.

biotics are given if indicated by culture and sensitivity tests. Local and general antimycotic therapy is given for fungal infections.

Course and prognosis. Both are good if the cause is treated appropriately.

Herpes Simplex Stomatitis and Gingivitis

Clinical Features. These include a burning sensation in the mouth, difficulty in eating, a feeling of being unwell, fever in the early stages, and lentil-sized, clear vesicles at the mucocutaneous junctions of the lip and the nasal introitus, and also in the entire mouth. The vesicles may progress to superficial circular or oval ulcers with a red center. The disease often occurs in conjunction with febrile general infections or overexposure to sunlight. There is marked oral tenderness, oral fetor, sialorrhea, and painful regional lymphadenopathy. The disease is contagious. Serial crops of fresh vesicles may occur. Children are most at risk.

Table 3.4   Common lesions of the oral mucosa in generalized and dermatologic diseases (continued)

	Cause
Punctate lesions	
White spots surrounded by an erythematous zone. The site of predilection is the buccal mucosa opposite the molar teeth, Koplik spots	Measles
Reticular or striated bluish-white membrane and edematous red spots mainly on the lips, but also on the tongue	Lupus erythematosus
Opalescent plaques, often with superficial ulceration	Secondary syphilis
Membranes on the oral mucosa	
Whitish, striated, nonadherent membrane brilliant white punctate spots in infants	Candidiasis
Vesicles, erosions, and cysts	Varicella (the vesicles are the size of hempseed and lie mainly on the palate), erythema multiforme, herpes simplex, herpes zoster, hereditary epidermolysis bullosa dystrophica, pemphigus vulgaris, mucosal pemphigus, AIDS
Aphthous ulcers	Aphthosis and Behçet disease
Stomatitis and necrotic ulcers	Pellagra, agranulocytosis, thrombocytopenia, panmyelophthisis, leukemia, mercury intoxication
Gingival hyperplasia	Pregnancy, possibly the contraceptive pill and hydantoin
Atrophic lesions	
Induration, sclerosis, narrow pale lips, shortened frenulum, microglossia	Progressive scleroderma

Pathogenesis. The cause is infection with the herpes simplex virus and usually occurs first in childhood. The first infection often causes no symptoms. The disease is very infectious: 90 % of the population are said to be carriers of the virus, but clinical manifestations in the form of herpes labialis (**Fig. 3.21**) or stomatitis herpetiformis only occur in 1 %.

Diagnosis. This is made by exclusion. An attempt can be made to isolate the virus from the contents of the vesicle, if possible within the first 24 h of the vesicular stage. The material is inoculated in the rabbit cornea.

Differential diagnosis. Chronic recurrent aphthous stomatitis, varicella, the acute infectious exanthemas, herpangina, foot and mouth disease, Behçet disease, pemphigus, and mycoses must all be considered.

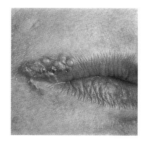

Fig. 3.21   Herpes labialis. Small blisters at the border between lip and skin.

Treatment. Systemic antiviral therapy (acyclovir, valaciclovir, famciclovir) is most effective. It should be used for 72 h for initial infections. Recurrent cases can often be controlled with topical measures including topical anesthetics, 0.1 % methylrosaniline chloride aqueous solution, or topical antiviral agents (acyclovir, penciclovir). If the patient is treatment-resistant, systemic treatment or prophylaxis can be tried. A bland liquid diet and gentle rinsing should also be advised. Steroids must *not* be given.

Course and prognosis. This disease is usually harmless and lasts 1–2 weeks. The vesicles heal to form crusts, but do not form scars. Recurrence is frequent, but herpetic sepsis and herpetic encephalitis are very rare.

Viruses of the Picornaviridae family (coxsackievirus, echovirus) and rarely of the variola group may also cause small oral ulcers.

Metal stomatitis. A stomatitis with discoloration of the gingiva can be caused by either medical or occupational exposure to mercury or bismuth. The same also applies to workers handling lead. The use of gold in the treatment of arthritis can cause a gingival stomatitis. Finally, the mucosa can be damaged by arsenic, chlorine, chromium, fluoride, copper, manganese, nickel, sulfur, thallium, and zinc; by organic substances such as benzol, dimethyl sulfate, tetrachlorocarbons, tetrachloroethylene; and by mixed substances such as corrosive agents, synthetic resins, synthetic materials, enamels, etc., as well as by wood, dyes, hops, wool, and insecticides.

Stomatitis due to drugs. This may be observed particularly after the use of bromides, iodides, salicylates, antibiotics, and sulfonamides, psychoactive drugs that dry the mouth, and antiepileptic agents, and after pyramidone, barbiturates, laxatives such as phenolphthalein, and the contraceptive pill.

Allergic stomatitis. Hypersensitivity reactions on the oral mucosa and the lips, with varying severity, with or without angioneurotic edema, may be observed in response to almost all drugs, dental material, mouthwashes, toothpaste, cosmetics, chewing gum, and also to some foods such as fruit, fish, protein, and milk. The diagnosis can be established by testing, and if the allergen is found it should be withdrawn. Otherwise, antiallergic or local symptomatic treatment are given.

Candidal Stomatitis

Clinical Features. Burning in the mouth and tongue, superficial white foci, and exudates on the mucosa are symptomatic. The exudate can be wiped off with mild pressure.

Pathogenesis. In normal individuals, almost all cases of oral yeast infections are caused by *Candida albicans;* rarely, other agents may be involved in severely immunosuppressed hosts. Candidiasis affect individuals with diabetes mellitus, reduced resistance, and after prolonged administration of antibiotics, chemotherapy, steroids, oral contraceptives, and after radiotherapy. Acute severe infection with ulceration can be a presenting sign of immune deficiency, human immunodeficiency virus (HIV) infection, or acute leukemia.

Diagnosis. This is made on the basis of the characteristic membranous white or gray exudates and very inflamed mucosa. Superficial ulceration occurs. A specimen is taken for culture for fungi.

Differential diagnosis Diphtheria.

Treatment. The standard therapy is nystatin or imidazole solutions or rinses. Options include 0.1 % methylrosaniline chloride aqueous solution or borax–glycerin solution. Good oral hygiene is also crucial.

Course. The prognosis is good if the patient is relatively healthy. Prompt treatment for several weeks, with monitoring by culture, is advised in more severe cases. In immunosuppressed individuals, there is a risk of systemic spread if treatment is not adequate.

Herpes Zoster

Clinical Features. Unilateral rapidly progressive vesicles are quickly followed by fibrinous superficial epithelial defects, affecting the segments of the face innervated by the second and third divisions of the trigeminal nerve. The disease is very painful. Mucosal lesions may occur in the same stage and may be partially confluent and arranged in groups.

Pathogenesis. This is a neurotropic infection with the varicella-zoster virus, which is morphologically identical to the herpes simplex virus.

Diagnosis. The diagnosis is established on the basis of the typical segmental arrangement of the vesicles, severe pain, and culture of the contents of the vesicle (**Fig. 3.22**).

Differential diagnosis. This includes herpes simplex and recurrent aphthous stomatitis.

Treatment. Prompt institution of high-dose regimens of systemic antiviral agents (acyclovir, valaciclovir, famciclovir) within 48 h has been shown to reduce the duration and severity of the acute disease and somewhat reduce the risk of postherpetic neuralgia. In severe cases or immunosuppressed patients, intravenous aciclovir should be considered. A prophylactic vaccine has recently been approved. Good oral hygiene, a bland liquid diet, and topical anesthetics or 0.1 % methylrosaniline chloride aqueous solution, can be used for symptomatic relief.

The disease is often followed by severe, therapy-resistant neuralgias, which may persist for months after resolution of the mucosal lesions. Occasionally, other regions and internal organs may be involved simultaneously. The generalized form in older patients suggests a systemic malignancy or immunosuppression.

Acquired Immune Deficiency Syndrome (AIDS)

Clinical Features. Approximately 35–40 % of HIV infections are associated with otorhinolaryngologic symptoms, including early symptoms such as angular cheilitis and Kaposi sarcoma (**Figs. 3.23, 3.24**). HIV infection has a relatively high association with cervical lymphadenopathies, candidiasis, herpes simplex, and herpes zoster. Other potential manifestations of HIV infection include sinusitis, tonsillitis, gingivitis, pharyngitis, esophagitis, tracheitis, sudden hearing loss, facial paralysis, and facial pain. General accompanying features are fever, anorexia, headache, muscle and joint pain, transient or persistent lymph-node enlargement, diarrhea, and profound weight loss.

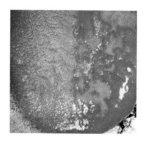

Fig. 3.22 Herpes zoster of the tongue. The oral symptoms are due to involvement of the second or third branch of the trigeminal nerve. The incidence increases in older age groups.

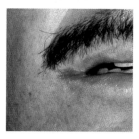

Fig. 3.23 Angular cheilitis, an early sign of human immunodeficiency virus (HIV) infection. The condition is due to *Candida* infection at the corners of the mouth.

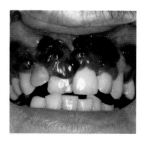

Fig. 3.24 Kaposi sarcoma. The gingiva is the second most common location for oral Kaposi sarcomas. Proceeding from uncharacteristic swelling of the gums, blue-black changes with bleeding develop.

Pathogenesis. HIV infection.

Diagnosis. HIV infection is diagnosed by the detection of HIV antibodies in the serum in a screening test (e.g., enzyme-linked immunosorbent assay, ELISA) followed by a confirmatory blot test.

Differential diagnosis. See the list of symptoms above. HIV infection should be suspected whenever a "classic" disease has an unusual location and presentation, runs an atypical course, and presents in an atypical age group, especially if the patient is in a high-risk group (male homosexuals, intravenous drug users, etc.).

Treatment. The HIV virus cannot be eliminated by any of the current treatment regimens. In addition, no vaccine is available. However, highly active antiretroviral therapy (HAART) using multiple drugs in different therapeutic classes designed to inhibit HIV in different ways has radically improved the outlook for infected patients and altered the spectrum of oral diseases seen. Oral Kaposi sarcoma has become uncommon again, and severe oral candidiasis, oral hairy leukoplakia, and recurrent herpetic infections are all suppressed with HAART.

Chronic Recurrent Aphthae

Aphthae are recurrent oral ulcerations, generally small with an erythematous base. Three types are observed:

1. Minor type (Mikulicz): only two to six oval aphthae in the oral mucosa; also known as canker sores.
2. Major type (Sutton): large mucosal aphtha (> 1 cm), usually occurring on the soft palate, cheek mucosa, tongue or lips.
3. Herpetiform type (Cooke): many very small and painful herpetiform ulcerations on the lateral border of the tongue.

Clinical Features. Aphthae occur intermittently, affecting the buccal mucosa, the tongue, the palate, and the gingiva. They are very painful. The regional lymph nodes may be swollen, and concomitant stomatitis is possible.

Pathogenesis. The cause is unknown. The disease is not thought to be infectious, but instead to represent activation of intrinsic inflammation in susceptible individuals. Aphthae can be triggered by infections, hormonal factors such as menstruation, and certain foods.

Diagnosis. This is made on the basis of the long history of the condition and its tendency to recur. There is no sialorrhea, no oral fetor, and no fever.

Differential diagnosis. Herpes simplex, which occurs with fever, fetor, sialorrhea, a general malaise, and a large number of vesicles which are confluent and arranged in groups must be considered. Behçet disease can present with recurrent multiple aphthous ulcers.

Treatment. Causal or prophylactic treatment is not possible. Symptomatic treatment includes 0.1 % methylrosaniline chloride aqueous solution, borax solution, chlorhexidine, and topical corticosteroids. The major type sometimes responds to antibiotics and oral tetracycline solution may be helpful.

Course. The lesions heal without scarring in 1–3 weeks, but early recurrence is possible. The course may extend over decades, and familial occurrences are known.

Behçet Disease

Clinical Features. Aphthae occur in crops in the mouth and on the genitals. *Eye symptoms* are often monocular and typically wax and wane. They include hypopyon iritis, which is often fleeting, and later papilledema, involvement of the retina, and blindness. Rheumatic symptoms and renal involvement may also occur.

Pathogenesis. The cause is unknown. It may be generalized vasculitis, an autoimmune event, or a virus infection.

Diagnosis. The main, and often the first, symptom is involvement of the eye. Acute cochleovestibular disturbances may also occur.

Treatment. Treatment relies on immunosuppressive medication (cyclophosphamide, cyclosporine) und long-term steroids. Oral mucosal lesions can be treated locally with topical corticosteroids, 0.1 % methylrosaniline chloride aqueous solution, and gentle rinses.

Course. With treatment, the symptoms can be eased, the mucosal infections can be reduced, and the disease can be controlled over a lifetime.

Tuberculosis

Clinical Features. Mucosal lesions may take the form of a mucosal lupus or exudative ulcerative *mucosal tuberculosis.* Round nodules occur in groups in mucosal lupus, and they demonstrate yellowish-brown flecks in the oral mucosa on pressure with a glass spatula. They are not painful. Flat, dirty, exudative, painful ulceration with undermined edges and lymph-node involvement is found in ulcerative mucosal tuberculosis (see p. 265).

Pathogenesis. The oral cavity is nowadays almost never a primary site of manifestation of tuberculosis. The disease is usually due to hematogenous or intraluminal spread from the primary site, usually the lung.

Diagnosis. This is made by biopsy and culture, and chest radiography. Tuberculosis is a notifiable disease.

Differential diagnosis. Syphilis, mycoses, and carcinoma must be excluded.

Treatment. The original focus in the lung is treated by tuberculostatic drugs. Triple therapy consisting of isoniazid, rifampicin, and ethambutol is now usually given, supervised by a chest physician.

Course. This depends on the outcome of the primary lesion. However, the prognosis for mucosal lesions is good with general antituberculous therapy.

Syphilis

Clinical Features. All stages of syphilis can occur in the mouth.

Stage I (primary syphilis): primary chancres occur on the lips, tonsil, anterior part of the tongue, commissure, gingiva, and buccal mucosa (**Fig. 3.25**). A sharply delimited nodule 2–3 mm in diameter grows to the size of a penny. After a few days, a painless ulcer forms, with a very hard edge, and there is painless regional lymphadenopathy in the submandibular or jugulodigastric area. The primary lesion regresses spontaneously after 3–6 weeks.

Stage 2 (secondary syphilis): Eight to 10 weeks after the infection—i. e., 5–7 weeks after the appearance of the primary chancre and at the same time as or before the skin lesions—a superficial exanthema develops in the entire oral cavity. Dark-red mucosal spots a few millimeters in size form, with a tendency to merge. The lesions are of varying severity and last for several weeks. Dark-red papules form gradually, and also flat areas with a cloudy epithelial surface. The surface of the tongue looks like sugar icing with areas of loss of papillae. A very firm indolent lymphadenopathy develops.

Stage 3 (tertiary syphilis): A gumma develops on average 15 years after the primary infection. The sites of predilection in the mouth are the lips, the hard palate, the tongue, and the tonsils. There is a diffuse nodular infiltrate with liquefaction of the center, fetor, a sharp punched-out ulcer, and radiating scars.

Pathogenesis. This infection is caused by *Treponema pallidum*. The pathway of infection is either genital or extragenital. The incubation period is on average 3.5 weeks.

Diagnosis. Demonstration of the organism by culture and dark-ground illumination is used in stages 1 and 2. Serologic tests become positive from the fourth week. The *Treponema* immobilization test (Nelson test) only becomes positive in the ninth week. In stage 3, serologic reactions are positive and the disease can be demonstrated by histology. This is a notifiable disease. (See Syphilitic Tonsillitis for further details.)

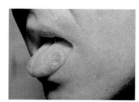

Fig. 3.25 Primary chancre of the tongue.

Differential diagnosis. In stage 1 lesions, tuberculosis, mycoses, and herpes should be considered; in stage 2, erythema multiforme and tuberculosis; in stage 3, malignant tumors and leukemia.

Treatment. Penicillin should be administered by a dermatologist or a specialist in venereal diseases (see also p. 265).

Hyperkeratosis and Leukoplakia

Clinical Features. These include a velvety or nodular, usually sharply circumscribed epithelial lesion, hyperkeratosis, a flat epithelial plaque or white thickening that cannot be wiped off, and leukoplakia usually occurring on the lips, floor of the mouth, or buccal mucosa.

Pathogenesis. This is an epithelial disease with many different causes, including exogenous irritative factors such as chronic mechanical irritation by the irregular edge of teeth, pressure from a denture, smoking, excess alcohol consumption, lichen planus, syphilis, and lupus erythematosus. There may be no recognizable cause.

Two groups of lesions can be distinguished in leukoplakia, depending on the color and surface:
1. *Simple leukoplakia* with sharp edges, occurring in ≈ 50 % of cases. This is only rarely premalignant.
2. *Patchy leukoplakia,* which can be divided into: a) *verrucous leukoplakia* (≈ 25 % of cases), which shows an irregular, wrinkled grayish-red speckled surface and which may be premalignant; and b) *erosive leukoplakia* (≈ 25 % of cases), with a reddish erosive lesion and often an irregular nodular surface—this form becomes malignant in ≈ 35 % of cases and is very similar to Bowen disease.

The probability of malignant degeneration depends largely on the degree of histologic dysplasia. The frequency of progression of a leukoplakia to carcinoma increases with the degree of the dysplasia (**Figs. 3.26, 3.27**).

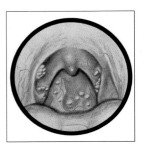

Fig. 3.26 Hyperkeratosis. Whitish-yellow, thorn-shaped or button-shaped structures are located singly or in groups on the tonsils, palatal arch, or posterior wall of the pharynx. Confusion with lacunar pharyngitis is unlikely, as the plaques are firmly attached to the underlying tissue.

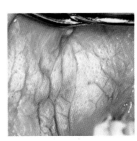

Fig. 3.27 Leukoplakia of the buccal mucosa.

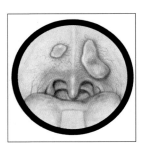

Fig. 3.28 Pemphigus. Two large, isolated serous bullae on the soft palate. The bullous stage is very short, so that this stage is rarely observed. Usually, the ruptured shreds of the blister membrane are all that can be seen.

!

Note: Leukoplakia should be regarded as being potentially premalignant and should therefore be investigated and followed up carefully.

Diagnosis. This is made by histology. The lesion should be entirely removed, if possible with a clear margin.

Differential diagnosis. Ulcerative stomatitis, mycoses, lichen ruber planus, lupus erythematosus, and pemphigus must be considered.

Treatment. This is by generous surgical removal, preferably at the time of biopsy and avoidance of possible causative agents.

Bowen Disease (Erythroplasia, Erythroplakia)

This is a premalignant lesion or carcinoma in situ. It is an intraepithelial squamous cell carcinoma with an intact basal membrane; the tumor has not yet invaded the subepithelial layer. It occurs on the skin or mucosa.

Clinical Features. Sharply demarcated full red foci of varying sizes, with a smooth surface, that occur on the mucosa of the cheek or tongue. It may also take the form of white patches of leukoplakia or verrucous vegetative papillomatous lesions the size of a hazelnut. The disease occurs mainly in men in the fourth to seventh decades of life. Progression to true squamous cell carcinoma is possible at any time and is very common.

Diagnosis. Biopsy distinguishes the lesion from other precancerous lesions of the mucosa such as leukoplakia and pure hyperplasia.

Treatment. The lesion must be excised with a healthy margin.

Inflammations of the Oral Mucosa in Dermatoses
Pemphigus

Clinical Features. The first symptom is often in the mouth and takes the form of flat soft or tense vesicles (**Fig. 3.28**). These give way to superficial epithelial erosions with a fibrin layer and epithelial tags at the edge. The course is episodic, and several stages may be present at any one time. There is oral fetor, often regional lymphadenopathy, and a bullous eruption on the skin. The disease usually begins between age 40 and 60.

Pathogenesis. Pemphigus vulgaris is a well-established autoimmune disease with autoantibodies directed against desmosomal proteins, primarily desmogleins. The main desmoglein of the mucosa is desmoglein 3. Almost all patients with oral involvement have antibodies against this desmoglein. Other components of the desmosome may also be targets.

Diagnosis. Routine histology may suggest the diagnosis by demonstrating acantholysis, but it has to be confirmed using direct and indirect immunofluorescence studies or molecular biological identification of autoantibodies.

Differential diagnosis. This includes stomatitis, hereditary epidermolysis bullosa, erythema multiforme, lichen planus, and mucosal pemphigoid.

Treatment. Systemic corticosteroids and immunosuppressive agents are administered under the supervision of a dermatologist.

Erythema Multiforme

Clinical Features. Fibrinous exudate, crust, and vesicles form on the lips and oral mucosa. There are simultaneous skin and joint lesions, and also fever. The skin lesions may be target-shaped and occur preferentially on the hands and feet. The symptoms are those of severe acute infection, with oral fetor, sialorrhea, pain, and regional lymphadenopathy. Far more common is recurrent disease, which is milder and often confined to the mucosa. Drug-induced or atypical erythema multiforme is more likely to be on the trunk and not to have target morphology, and it can progress to Stevens–Johnson syndrome or toxic epidermal necrolysis.

Pathogenesis. Acute disease is usually caused by *Mycoplasma* infection. Chronic disease is almost invariably caused by recurrent herpes simplex virus infection. A wide variety of drugs have been implicated in atypical erythema multiforme, including allopurinol, carbamazepine, co-trimoxazole, lamotrigine, nevirapine, nonsteroidal anti-inflammatory drugs (of the oxicam type) phenobarbital, phenytoin and sulfonamides.

Diagnosis. This is made on the basis of the generalized disease picture, and possibly by biopsy.

Differential diagnosis. Pemphigus, lichen planus, and enanthema due to drug reactions must be excluded.

Treatment. In severe primary disease, the underlying infection should be sought and treated properly. Most recurrent disease can be suppressed with either long-term low-dose or episodic promptly introduced antiviral drugs (usually acyclovir). Topical corticosteroids may be helpful, as are a bland liquid diet or even parenteral feeding for severe primary disease. A possible drug trigger should be investigated.

Prognosis. Primary disease may be life-threatening. Recurrent disease is annoying and reduces

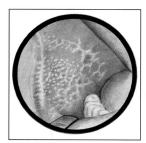

Fig. 3.29 Lichen planus (lichen ruber). Bluish-white papules with a mother-of-pearl shimmer, small and sharply bordered, posteriorly connected by fine lines forming a network. Delicate shapes are seen, usually with a symmetrical distribution. Leukoplakia and mucous plaques need to be included in the differential diagnosis.

quality of life but rarely causes severe problems. Drug-induced disease may be life-threatening, advancing to Stevens-Johnson syndrome or toxic epidermal necrolysis. Ophthalmologic consultation should be obtained.

Lichen Planus

Clinical Features. The mucosal appearance of lichen planus can be specific, with a lacy network of white lines or streaks (Wickham striae). More often, there are nonspecific eroded lesions on the buccal mucosa, gingiva, and tongue. Blue-gray, smooth, tiny papules are sometimes also found on the dorsum of the tongue. The lesions cannot be wiped off and are firm. The ulcerations can be very painful. Pruritic red-brown to pink papules, often polygonal, 2–3 mm in size, may be seen on the skin, preferentially on the volar surface of the wrist (**Fig. 3.29**).

Pathogenesis. The etiology is unknown.

Diagnosis. This is made on the basis of the full clinical picture, at times supported by biopsy. In contrast to the skin, lichen planus in the mouth is a potentially premalignant disease. It may be accompanied by *Candida* infection, which can complicate the clinical picture and diagnosis.

Differential diagnosis. This includes leukoplakia, hyperkeratosis, Bowen disease, mycosis, enanthema of drug reactions, and lupus erythematosus.

Treatment. Possible toxic agents such as sunlight, tobacco, and chemical agents should be excluded. The disease is not curable, but is controllable when significant or symptomatic. Topical corticosteroids or retinoids are the best approach. A cyclosporine oral rinse is expensive but helpful in refractory

Table 3.5   Oral fetor

Site of origin	Cause
Teeth, gingiva, and mouth	Dental caries, parodontosis, gingivitis, stomatitis, erythema multiforme, pemphigus, neglected false teeth, abscesses of the floor of the mouth, ulcerating tumors
Pharynx	Acute tonsillitis, Vincent angina, mononucleosis, peripharyngeal and retropharyngeal abscess, pharyngeal diphtheria, chronic tonsillitis and pharyngitis, foreign body in the nasopharynx, tertiary syphilis
Airway	Atrophic rhinitis, ozena, purulent rhinitis, sinusitis, bronchitis, bronchiectasis, bronchial foreign body, lung abscess, and pneumonia
Digestive tract	Hypopharyngeal or esophageal diverticulum, hiatus hernia, esophagitis, diseases of the stomach and the intestines with or without hiccup and vomiting
Generalized disorders	Diabetes mellitus with ketosis (acetone), renal failure (urine), and hepatic coma, which produces a sweet aromatic smell

cases. Careful follow-up is needed, as this is a premalignant lesion.

Other rare inflammatory lesions of the oral cavity include rhinoscleroma, leprosy, and sarcoidosis (see p. 147), as well as AIDS. See also page 251.

An overview of the common causes of oral fetor is given in **Table 3.5**.

■ Tongue

The inflammatory diseases described above usually also produce symptoms on the tongue. The following inflammatory disorders affect the tongue primarily.

Glossitis (Glossopyrosis and Glossodynia)
Clinical Features. These include burning of the tongue, especially at its tip and edges, and frequent parageusia or hypergeusia. On the tongue itself, only minimal mucosal lesions can be demonstrated, such as circumscribed inflammation or loss of papillae.

Pathogenesis. The cause may lie in mechanical irritation by sharp teeth, dental calculi, pressure from dentures, intol-

erance to dental materials—e. g., denture material or the use of metals that are electrically noninert, mouthwashes, drug sensitivity, vitamin B_{12} deficiency (Hunter glossitis), megaloblastic anemia, iron-deficiency anemia (Plummer–Vinson syndrome), diabetes, and gastrointestinal diseases, including cirrhosis and mycoses.

Diagnosis. The diagnosis is based on the detection or exclusion of mechanical irritation, sensitivity reactions, diabetes, gastrointestinal or hematologic diseases, and also on the mycologic findings. Finally, the diagnosis can be made by exclusion of all other causes. Often it is difficult to classify the symptoms. Fifty percent of cases have a psychosomatic etiology. Neurologic forms based on diseases of the glossopharyngeal nerve, lingual nerve, hypoglossal nerve or chorda tympani produce only localized symptoms. Episodes of pain may be induced by tumors of the brain or skull base. Myofascial pain syndrome (Costen syndrome) may be accompanied by glossodynia.

Differential diagnosis. This should include allergic glossitis or a depressed immune response.

Treatment. The cause should be eliminated if possible. A bland diet (the patient should avoid very hot, cold, or spicy foods and heavy alcohol consumption) is essential. Symptomatic topical treatment with anesthetics or corticosteroids is rarely helpful. Often, systemic psychotropic medications are required for relief of discomfort.

Median Rhomboid Glossitis
This is an anomaly that occurs when the tuberculum impar is displaced into the tongue during embryonic development. The anomalous structure persists, and the lingual papillae are not differentiated in that area.

Diagnosis. Visual inspection reveals a circumscribed, spindle-shaped area around the foramen cecum.

Treatment. Nystatin. Laser resection may be appropriate in patients with carcinophobia.

Allergic Glossitis
Clinical Features. The signs are similar to those of nonspecific glossitis, except that the disease begins suddenly with swelling and redness of the tongue,

with swelling and pain progressing to itching. There is a danger of respiratory obstruction if the reaction progresses to edema.

Pathogenesis. This is an allergic reaction localized to the tongue. Many substances are possible allergens, including serum injections, antibiotics, drugs such as phenothiazine, barbiturates, sulfonamide, aspirin, local anesthetics, and foods such as fruits, fish, protein, or nuts.

Diagnosis. This is based on the clinical picture of a sudden onset with marked symptoms, and on demonstration of the allergen.

Differential diagnosis. Acute infectious enanthema, mycosis, intoxication, local chemical damage, and nonspecific glossitis must be considered.

Treatment. This is both symptomatic and antiallergic. Allergen tests can be done and an allergen-free diet prescribed.

The tongue is also affected by the following specific or chronic inflammations: tuberculosis, syphilis, mycoses, actinomycosis, dermatomyositis, Sjögren disease, and progressive scleroderma.

Surface lesions of the tongue that encourage infection include:

1. *Geographic tongue:* The dorsum of the tongue is covered with smooth red patches, which resemble a map and may gradually change position. The cause is unknown, but this is a harmless condition that does not require treatment.

2. *Fissured tongue:* In this disease, there are clefts and folds of varying depth forming islands on the mucosa of the dorsal surface of the tongue. This appears to be a simple autosomal-dominant hereditary disease. It is one of the aspects of the Melkersson–Rosenthal syndrome of facial paralysis, edema of the face and lips, and fissured tongue. Fissured tongue occurs frequently in trisomy 21 (Down syndrome). Harmless inflammation may occur due to penetration of foreign material into the clefts. The treatment is symptomatic.

The common causes of a coated, red, or fissured tongue are summarized in **Table 3.6**, and the causes of burning of the tongue in **Table 3.7**.

Abscess of the Floor of the Mouth

Clinical Features. These include swelling and limitation of movement of the tongue, increasing pain, difficulty in articulation progressing to complete loss of speech, protrusion and induration of the floor of the mouth with marked sensitivity to pressure, severe difficulty in swallowing, and finally complete inability to eat, limitation of movement of the temporomandibular joint with trismus, fever, severe generalized symptoms, and occasionally stridor.

Pathogenesis. Infected material enters via rhagades of the tongue or the oral mucosa. The infection advances into the loose musculature of the tongue and into the numerous connective-tissue spaces (**Fig. 3.30b**). The base of the tongue, the lingual tonsil, or a carious tooth are also possible portals of infection (see **Fig. 3.30a**). The causal organism is usually common pathogenic bacteria. Penetration of small foreign bodies such as fish bones, bone splinters, kernels of corn, etc. are also possible causes. The infection may arise primarily in the sublingual or submandibular glands lying in the floor of the mouth. An abscess on the floor of the mouth is known as a *Ludwig angina.*

Diagnosis. This is made on the basis of the clinical picture of an inflammatory swelling of the floor of the mouth, severe pain, and a progressive course.

Differential diagnosis. Hematoma, gumma, tuberculosis, and malignancy.

Treatment. Therapy should be started at the onset of symptoms, with high doses of intravenous broad-spectrum antibiotics. If this does not induce remission, the antibiotic must be changed depending on the resistogram. If there is evidence of liquefaction, the abscess is opened widely and drained externally. Adequate diet and fluid intake must be ensured, if necessary with a nasogastric tube or parenteral feeding. A tracheotomy is indicated for respiratory obstruction. If *Ludwig angina* develops, the infected area is opened widely to prevent infection spreading to the larynx or mediastinum.

Course and prognosis. These are favorable provided that suppuration occurs quickly so that the abscess can be drained. Extension of the abscess to the deeper soft tissues of the neck (see **Fig. 3.45a, b**) and to the mediastinum is a life-threatening situation.

Actinomycosis. This is also a possible differential diagnosis, but it is now becoming very rare. This

Table 3.6 Surface lesions of the tongue

Type of lesion	Basic disease	Clinical symptoms	Details
Red tongue	Pernicious anemia	Initially dark red, later caramel-colored spots and striae on the dorsum of the tongue. The surface of the tongue is red, smooth, and shiny	Dysgeusia, paresthesia, xerostomia; the oral mucosa is also affected
	Scarlet fever	Strawberry tongue	Protrusion of papillae
	Hepatic cirrhosis	Glazed, shiny smooth red dry tongue with blue spots, "liver tongue"	Generalized symptoms prominent, glazed lips, yellow staining of the oral mucosa, brownish pallid face
	Sjögren syndrome	Dry, smooth, red glazed tongue	Swelling of the salivary glands, and salivary stones
	Median rhomboid glossitis	A raised or slightly sunken red area free of papillae in the center of the middle third of the tongue in the midline	A harmless lesion confined to the tongue causing no symptoms
	Vascular congestion	Red-violet swollen tongue	Right heart failure, hepatic cirrhosis and malignant tumors
	Hypertension	Pink to carmine red	Hypertension, myocardial insufficiency, left heart failure, valvular heart disease, local allergic reaction and shock
	Allergy	Strawberry or raspberry red, edema	Occurs in local allergic reaction and also in shock
Gray smooth tongue	Vitamin A deficiency	Bluish matt epithelial protrusions and bluish staining of the lips	Xerostomia, dysphagia
	Radiotherapy	Oral mucosal is sensitive to heat, circumscribed mucosal atrophy, mucosal induration	Ageusia, xerostomia
	Lichen planus	Milky bluish striae, spider web leukoplakia, papillae are retained and there is no membrane	Also affects the oral mucosa
	Progressive scleroderma	Dry tongue, limited mobility, initially edema of the tongue, later atrophy of the tongue and increasing rigidity	Dysphagia, interference with speech, mouth is too small, salivary deficiency
Black hairy tongue	Antibiotics, idiopathic, smoking, niacin shortage, liver disease	Hairy, greenish-black membrane, long black cornified papillae	Also occurs in mycosis
Fissured tongue	Lingua plicata	Surface of the tongue is furrowed and fissured	A benign normal hereditary variant
	Melkersson–Rosenthal syndrome	Folded tongue	Periodic swellings of the lips, tongue, and parotid glands, and intermittent facial paralysis
Coated tongue	Nonspecific oral infection	Whitish coat (horny scales)	Connected with reduced food intake in gastritis and enteritis and in feverish infections
	Oral thrush	Whitish, membranous adherent plaques with red edges	*Candida albicans* demonstrated on culture

Table 3.6   Surface lesions of the tongue (continued)

Type of lesion	Basic disease	Clinical symptoms	Details
Coated tongue	AIDS	Commonly associated with oral candidiasis and hairy leukoplakia of the tongue	Multifocal symptoms are typical. Diagnosis, see p. 251
	Scarlet fever	Dirty-white coating with reddened tip and edges to tongue	Pharyngitis, exanthemas; β-hemolytic streptococci found on culture
	Diphtheria	Grayish-white membranous coat, smells sweet and nasty	Adherent membrane, the underlying bed bleeds slightly, generalized symptoms
	Typhus	Grayish-white tongue with very red edges	Infection with *Salmonella typhi,* generalized symptoms
	Uremia	Brownish plaques	Renal insufficiency

AIDS, acquired immune deficiency syndrome.

Table 3.7   Burning of the tongue

Basic disease	Clinical symptoms	Details
Geographic tongue	Burning of the tongue, with red-spotted tongue, absence of filiform papillae	
Toxic stomatitis	Burning of the tongue and grayish-blue discoloration of the gingiva by bismuth and lead, reddened edematous mucosa in mercury poisoning	
Stomach and intestinal disorders of various causes	Manifest or latent symptoms, depending on the site of the cause	
Plummer–Vinson (Paterson–Kelly) syndrome (see p. 275)	Dry tongue, considerable dysphagia. Rhagades of the commissures, atrophic mucosa	Almost exclusively in women, dry pale skin, koilonychia, dry mucous membranes
Sjögren disease	Xerostomia, tough sticky saliva, papillary atrophy, smooth glazed tongue, dysphagia	Dryness affecting the mucosa of the oral cavity, the pharynx, larynx, and trachea; swelling of the major salivary glands
Glossitis in megaloblastic anemia	Burning of the tongue, dysgeusia, paresthesia, dryness, spotted tongue with purple-red areas in striae alternating with bluish areas, smooth surface but not papillary atrophy, partially swollen papillae	May involve the entire oral mucosa
Diabetes mellitus	Intermittent marked burning of the tongue with dry surface	Tendency to oral infections and mycoses
Food allergy and contact allergy	Begins suddenly; marked swelling and redness; burning of the tongue increasing to cause pain and feeling of tension	Typical history or evidence of allergic cause, involvement of the rest of the oral mucosa
Pellagra, niacin deficiency	Hypoesthesia of the tongue, salty taste, feeling of a "chapped" tongue, red swollen and occasionally coated tongue, later chessboard tongue with marked fissuring, and finally atrophy	Inflammation of the remaining oral mucosa, sialorrhea is more common than salivary deficiency
Mucoviscidosis	Dry, burning tongue, tough glutinous secretion	Increased sodium and chloride ions in mucus and saliva
Psychogenic glossodynia	Burning of the tongue without any demonstrable organic cause	Frequent in latent depression

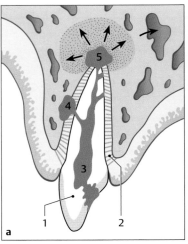 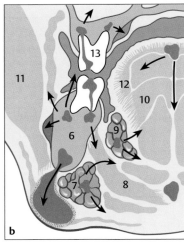

Fig. 3.30a, b Dental infections and infections in the floor of the mouth.
a Infections in and around the teeth. **1**, Carious incisor tooth; **2**, alveolar periosteum; **3**, pulpitis; **4**, periapical abscess; **5**, apical granuloma.
b Sites of origin of inflammations of the floor of the mouth. **6**, Mandibular, arising from the teeth or osteomyelitis; **7**, submandibular gland, due to inflammation or a stone; **8**, musculature of the floor of the mouth; **9**, sublingual gland, inflammation or retention; **10**, tongue musculature; **11**, muscles of the cheek; **12**, abscess of the body of the tongue; **13**, apical granuloma of one of the upper teeth, extending to the antrum.

disease has an indolent course and causes relatively slight pain, but leads to the formation of multiple hard infiltrates with formation of abscesses and fistulas. It is mainly localized to the head and neck (98 % of cases). The organisms are usually *Actinomyces israelii* and accompanying bacteria. *Actinomyces* agglomerations (sulfur granules) can be demonstrated in the pus from the abscess and in tissue specimens. A needle biopsy can be taken, with a specimen of pus being sent for bacteriologic identification. Serologic tests include agglutination and complement fixation. Precipitation tests and intracutaneous tests are not reliable. Treatment is with penicillin in the early phases, sulfonamides in the long term, and incision of any abscesses.

■ **Pharyngeal Lymphatic Ring (Waldeyer Ring)**

Acute Tonsillitis
Clinical Features. Acute tonsillitis usually begins with high temperature and possibly chills, especially in children. The patient complains of a burning sensation in the throat, persistent pain in the oropharynx, pain on swallowing, and pain radiating to the ear on swallowing. Opening the mouth is often difficult and painful, the tongue is coated, and there is oral fetor. The patient also complains of headaches, thick speech, a marked feeling of malaise, and swelling and tenderness of the re-

gional lymph nodes. Both tonsils and the surrounding area, including the posterior pharyngeal wall, are deep red and swollen, but in catarrhal tonsillitis there is no exudate on the tonsil. Later, yellow spots corresponding to the lymphatic follicles form on the tonsils—hence the term *follicular tonsillitis.* Alternatively, yellow spots occur over the openings of the crypts, a condition known as *lacunar tonsillitis.* A membrane occurs in *pneumococcal tonsillitis,* but it is seldom confluent and rarely spreads beyond the tonsil. There is also swelling of neighboring organs such as the faucial pillars, uvula, and base of the tongue. The patient also reports sialorrhea and difficulty in eating (**Figs. 3.31, 3.32**).

Pathogenesis. The most common organism is β-hemolytic streptococci. Staphylococci, pneumococci, mixed flora, *Haemophilus influenzae,* and *E. coli* are much less common. If the symptoms worsen and multifocal symptoms occur, a generalized disorder expressing itself particularly in the lymphoepithelial organs should be suspected. On the other hand, there are also tonsillar infections in which the generalized symptoms are minimal and only the local changes can be recognized. Virus infections are particularly important in this respect—e. g., herpangina (see p. 263). The tonsillar parenchyma is infiltrated with leukocytes in tonsillitis, causing small abscesses in the parenchyma and in the crypts. In addition, a fibrinous exudate is formed and there are marked changes in the parenchyma and the epithelium.

Diagnosis. The diagnosis is based on the clinical presentation of an acute onset with high fever, a sore throat, painful swallowing, redness and exudate on the tonsils, general blood tests, the erythrocyte sedimentation rate (ESR), C-reactive protein (CRP), cardiovascular tests, and urinalysis. Rapid immunoassay testing can identify streptococcus bacteria in 10 min. Appropriate tests or even cultures are performed if diphtheria is suspected, and blood tests are done for mononucleosis (see below)

Differential diagnosis. This includes scarlet fever, diphtheria, infectious mononucleosis, agranulocytosis, leukemia, hyperkeratosis of the tonsils, stage 2 syphilis, and in unilateral disease, ulceromembranous tonsillitis, peritonsillar cellulitis or abscess, tuberculosis, and tonsillar tumors (see below).

Treatment. The standard treatment in patients with streptococcal tonsillitis is penicillin V for 10–14 days (**Table 3.8**). Oral cephalosporins or macrolides can be used in patients allergic to penicillin. As acute tonsillitis is a systemic rather than local disease, treatment should include bed rest, analgesics, a bland liquid diet, and ice packs. The patient should be observed for complications. Local care should include oral and dental hygiene. Local antibiotics should not be given, but antiseptic and analgesic mouthwashes can be used. Moist neck dressings and a sweat pack may be used in the early phases.

Course. Tonsillitis usually resolves within 1 week. However, complications such as respiratory obstruction due to laryngeal edema, otitis media, or rhinosinusitis may occur; sequelae may also develop.

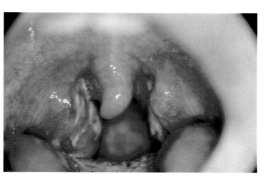

Fig. 3.31 Lacunar tonsillitis. The palatine tonsils are bright red, swollen, and coated.

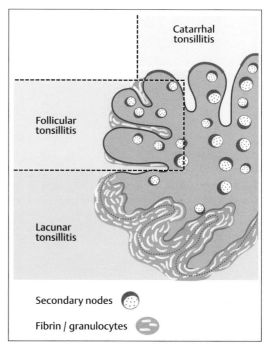

Catarrhal tonsillitis

Follicular tonsillitis

Lacunar tonsillitis

Secondary nodes

Fibrin / granulocytes

Fig. 3.32 The grades of severity and pathomorphology of catarrhal, follicular, and lacunar tonsillitis.

Table 3.8 Initial empirical treatment of acute tonsillitis

Most common pathogens	Initial treatment	Duration
Streptococcus pyogenes	Phenoxymethylpenicillin (penicillin V)	10 days
Haemophilus influenzae	Cefuroxime axetil, loracarbef	5 days
	Amoxicillin	
	Clarithromycin, azithromycin	
	Telithromycin	

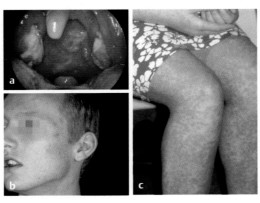

Fig. 3.33a–c a Typical appearance of the mucosa and tonsils in a patient with infectious mononucleosis; the tonsils are swollen and red, with fibrin coatings.
b The nuchal and neck lymph nodes are visibly enlarged.
c A patient with a pseudoallergic rash following treatment with ampicillin.

Nasopharyngitis. The symptoms are as described above but are localized mainly or exclusively to the adenoid. Differential diagnosis includes viral nasopharyngitis.

Infection of the lingual tonsil. This is similar, with symptoms localized to the base of the tongue. Ipsilateral involvement of the larynx or abscess formation in the tongue are possible.

Other types of tonsillitis

1. Simple tonsillitis caused by nonspecific organisms.
2. Tonsillitis in infectious diseases.
3. Tonsillitis in hematologic diseases.
4. Ulceromembranous tonsillitis.

Infectious Mononucleosis (Glandular Fever, Benign Lymphadenosis)

Clinical Features. Salient features include fever in the range of 38–39°C and marked lymphadenopathy of the jugulodigastric group and the deep cervical chain, later becoming generalized (**Fig. 3.33b**). The lymph nodes are moderately tender. The tonsil is very swollen and covered with a fibrinous exudate or membrane (**Fig. 3.33a**). The patient has rhinopharyngitis, hepatosplenomegaly, pain in the neck on swallowing, and a marked feeling of being unwell. There is pain in the head and limbs. The blood picture initially shows leukopenia, and then leukocytosis with a white blood cell count to 20 000–30 000 or more, 80–90% of which are mononuclear cells and atypical lymphocytes.

Two types of disease are distinguished:

1. The *pharyngeal type* is characterized by a very severe sore throat and painful swallowing. The tonsils have a heavy fibronectin coating, and the lymph nodes are enlarged. The virus is located mainly in the mucosa-associated lymphoid tissue (MALT).
2. The *hematogenic type* is characterized by a high fever, severe malaise, abdominal pain, and circulation of the causative virus in lymphocytes (liver, spleen).

Microbiology. The causative organism is the Epstein–Barr virus, which chiefly affects children and adolescents. The disease is probably spread by droplet infection. The incubation period is 7–9 days.

Diagnosis. This is made from the picture of generalized lymphadenopathy and tonsillitis, the characteristic blood picture, a monospot test, and the Paul–Bunnell test (demonstration of heterophile antibodies in the serum; a positive titer is > 1 : 28).

Differential diagnosis. This includes diphtheria (by culture), Vincent angina, scarlet fever, syphilis, rubella, acute leukemia, toxoplasma, listeriosis, and tularemia.

Treatment. Symptomatic treatment includes oral hygiene and measures to reduce fever. Antibiotics may be given against secondary bacterial infection if there is marked ulceration. Cephalosporin or clindamycin is advisable. An allergy-like rash may occur in response to ampicillin (**Fig. 3.33c**). Tonsillectomy may be indicated for severe local symptoms such as respiratory obstruction and dysphagia, and persistent fever.

Complications. The course may be protracted, with paralyses affecting cranial nerves VII and X, serous meningitis and encephalitis, myocarditis (cardiologic supervision), hemolytic anemia, hemorrhagic complications in the gastrointestinal tract, the pharynx, and the skin, hematuria, obstruction of the airway, and a danger of asphyxia. An associated bleeding disorder may also occur in severe disease. Tracheotomy should only be performed in extreme emergencies.

> **Note:** If penicillin does not induce a rapid fall in fever in patients thought to have tonsillitis, they are probably suffering from infectious mononucleosis.

Course. Resolution is marked by a long convalescence (months), during which liver values should be monitored. The patient should refrain from competitive sports during this time, especially if there is any evidence of splenomegaly.

Infection of the Lateral Bands
This is a specific form of infection of the lateral, tubopharyngeal bands, especially in patients who have had their tonsils removed. It may be a "substitute" infection in the absence of tonsils. There is swelling, redness, and yellow spots around the lateral bands, and also in the solitary follicles on the posterior pharyngeal wall (**Fig. 3.34**).

Treatment. Penicillin is administered as in tonsillitis, as complications may also occur in this disease. If the disease recurs frequently, the area should be cauterized with a 2–5 % silver nitrate solution; careful use of a cryoprobe is also possible.

Herpangina
This disease causes marked generalized symptoms such as high fever, headache, pains in the neck, and loss of appetite and mainly affects children up to the age of 15 years. Vesicles form initially, particularly on the anterior faucial pillar, but are very fleeting and are therefore not often seen. The tonsils are often only slightly red and swollen. Occasionally, they are covered in milky white vesicles up to the size of a lentil, arranged like a chain of pearls, or

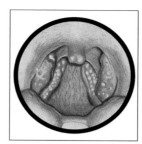

Fig. 3.34 Lateral pharyngitis. Inflammation of the lateral pharynx. Both salpingopharyngeal folds are markedly swollen and reddened, and their surface dotted with numerous small, yellowish-white spots. There is very severe pain, radiating to the ears, and the complaints and generalized symptoms are as in acute tonsillitis.

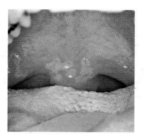

Fig. 3.35 Herpetic angina is usually caused by group A coxsackieviruses, less often by those of group B, retroviruses, or echoviruses.

there are small flat ulcerations of the tonsil. Similar eruptions may occur on the palate or buccal mucosa (**Fig. 3.35**).

Microbiology. The organism is coxsackievirus A, which has an incubation period of 4–6 days.

Diagnosis. This is based on the presence of vesicles, minimal lesions in the tonsils, and the benign rapid course over several days.

Treatment. Symptomatic, including oral hygiene and mouth rinses with chamomile and antiseptic solutions.

Scarlet Fever
The tonsils and pharyngeal mucosa are deep red; there is pain on swallowing, severe malaise, progression to lacunar tonsillitis, and regional lymphadenopathy. After ≈ 24 h, a typical exanthema appears, beginning on the upper part of the body. At the same time, a definite reddening of the tip and edges of the tongue appears, extending later to the entire tongue—strawberry tongue. Facial reddening does not include the perioral skin. It should be noted that the exanthema may not appear. Desquamation of the skin begins on about the eighth day (**Fig. 3.36**).

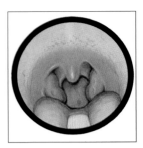

Fig. 3.36   Scarlet fever (scarlatina). Scarlet fever pharyngitis on the first day of the illness. The tonsils and palatal arches are swollen and dusky red. The erythema of the palatal arch is sharply demarcated. A vascular network is frequently visible on the soft palate. The tonsils may have a transient, whitish-gray coating. Necrosis may occur in severe cases.

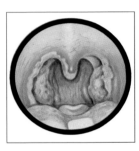

Fig. 3.37   Diphtheria. The tonsils, palatal arches, and uvula are coated with dirty gray–whitish membranes. The tissue is already ulcerated. On forceful depression of the tongue, the epiglottis is visualized. It is not coated.

Microbiology. The type A hemolytic streptococcus is responsible.

Diagnosis. This is made on the basis of the clinical appearances of redness and swelling of the tonsil, strawberry tongue, small erythematous spots on the soft palate, and the Rumpel–Leede phenomenon (petechiae distal to an inflated sphygmomanometer cuff). The blood picture shows leukocytosis and a left shift, and eosinophilia from the fifth day.

Differential diagnosis. This includes diphtheria, which is excluded by smear and/or culture.

Treatment. This is based on penicillin, oral hygiene, and analgesics.

Diphtheria

Two clinical forms are distinguished:
1. Local, benign pharyngeal diphtheria.
2. Primary toxic, malignant diphtheria.

Clinical Features. Patients experience a mild prodromal phase, usually with a temperature of ≈ 38°C and no more than 39°C. There is slight pain on swallowing and often a very high pulse rate. The tonsils are moderately reddened and swollen, with a white or gray velvety membrane that becomes confluent, extends beyond the boundaries of the tonsil to the faucial pillars and soft palate, and is fixed firmly to its base. The membrane can only be wiped off with difficulty and it then leaves a bleeding surface behind. The jugulodigastric lymph nodes are very swollen, tender, and often hard. There is a characteristic smell of acetone on the breath. Sixty percent of cases are localized to the pharynx including the tonsils, and in 8 % the larynx is involved in addition. Albuminuria is common (**Fig. 3.37**).

Microbiology. The infection is due to the diphtheria bacillus, *Corynebacterium diphtheriae*. The disease is transmitted by contact, droplets, or contamination by oral or nasal secretions. The incubation period is 3–5 days. In localized forms, the disease is restricted to the tonsil, the nose, the larynx, or a wound. The generalized form is progressive and toxic.

Diagnosis. This is based on: (1) a bacteriologic smear from the tonsils and pharynx—Gram staining of a smear from the pseudomembrane provides the result within 1 h; (2) culture provides the answer at the earliest after 10 h; (3) isolation of the organism confirms the diagnosis in 2–8 days; (4) there is a membrane that is firmly adherent and extends beyond the tonsil. This is a notifiable disease.

Differential diagnosis. This includes nonspecific tonsillitis, infectious mononucleosis, Vincent angina, candidiasis, agranulocytosis, leukemia, and syphilis.

Treatment. On the earliest reasonable suspicion of diphtheria (possibly *before* bacteriologic confirmation), the patient should be isolated and treated with antiserum administered intramuscularly at a dosage of 200–500 IU/kg. A skin test should be given to exclude allergy to the antitoxin before it is administered. In severe cases, a high dose of 1000 IU/kg may be given, accompanied by antibiotic coverage. In addition, penicillin G should be given, initially 3 × 2 million IU i. v., or alternatively erythromycin for 14 days.

Treatment also includes bed rest, oral hygiene, neck dressings changed several times a day, and steam inhalation. Diphtheria immunization with diphtheria toxoid is protective but does not become effective for several weeks.

Complications. These include general toxicity, failure of the heart and circulation, hemorrhagic nephritis or nephrosis, palatal paralysis due to polyneuritis, airway obstruction, and danger of asphyxia. A proportion of the population are silent carriers of the disease.

Normally, excretion of virulent diphtheria bacteria ceases after several weeks. However, carriers may continue to be a source of infection for months or even years. Cultures are therefore necessary until three cultures at weekly intervals are negative.

Long-term carriers should be treated with local and parenteral antibiotics and local disinfection. If this does not eradicate the organism, it may be necessary to carry out tonsillectomy, accompanied by adenoidectomy in children, to remove the source.

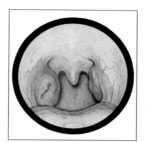

Fig. 3.38 Primary complex on the right tonsil. Among the rare extragenital sites of syphilitic infection, the tonsils are second only to the lips in frequency of involvement. Sharply demarcated ulcerations on the thickened, firm, reddened right tonsil. Painless, hard swelling of the regional lymph nodes, which are readily displaceable. Definitive diagnosis is possible only if spirochetes are found on dark-field microscopy.

Syphilitic Tonsillitis

Clinical Features. All stages of syphilis may be encountered in the oropharynx. After 3 weeks, the primary lesion appears on the lips, buccal mucosa, tonsils, and tongue. Typically, the primary chancre is painless, consisting initially of a papular lesion that develops into an ulcer. Palpable regional lymph nodes are present. Approximately 6 weeks after the primary infection, white, hazy mucosal enanthemas (*plaques opalines*) appear on the tonsils, faucial pillars, and soft palate. The hard palate is usually spared. Later, they progress to dark-red papules. Signs of stage 2 infection are usually present in other parts of the body. The tertiary stage appears after 20–30 years.

Diagnosis. Any ulcer in the oropharynx, especially involving the soft palate and uvula, is suspicious. The diagnosis is confirmed by dark-field examination of organisms from the primary lesion and by serologic testing (**Fig. 3.38**).

Serologic tests. *Treponema pallidum* hemagglutination assay (TPHA), fluorescent treponemal antibody absorption (FTA-ABS) test, 3 weeks after infection, follow-up test of the patient's response to therapy.

Treatment. Penicillin G (600 000 IU daily for 2 weeks). Erythromycin should be used in patients allergic to penicillin.

Tonsillar Tuberculosis

This disease causes a superficial erosive ulcer with a necrotic slough (see p. 389).

Agranulocytosis

Clinical Features. The generalized symptoms are prominent and include high fever and chills. The patient feels very sick and has a typical blood picture. The disease occurs mainly in older individuals. There is ulceration and necrosis of the tonsils and pharynx, with a blackish exudate, severe pain in the neck and on swallowing, sialorrhea, and oral fetor. There is no regional lymphadenopathy.

Pathogenesis. Severe injury to the leukopoietic system may be caused by drugs or by occupational or other toxins.

Differential diagnosis. This includes diphtheria, infectious mononucleosis, Vincent angina, and acute leukemia.

Treatment. This consists of elimination of all possible leukotoxic drugs, avoidance of other sources of injury, and prevention of secondary infection by high-dose penicillin, blood transfusion, and careful oral hygiene. The patient should be in the care of a hematologist.

Vincent Angina (Ulceromembranous Pharyngitis, Trench Mouth)

Clinical Features. The patient usually describes unilateral pain on swallowing, and there is ipsilateral swelling of the jugulodigastric nodes. There is an ulcer, which is often deep, on *one* tonsil, with a

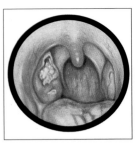

Fig. 3.39 Vincent angina (ulceromembranous pharyngitis, trench mouth). The right tonsil is enlarged and reddened. On its upper end, there is an irregular, crater-like ulcer, the bottom of which is coated with a dirty grayish layer of mucus.

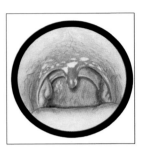

Fig. 3.40 Fungal (*Candida*) pharyngitis. On the soft palate, small, irregularly shaped, slightly prominent, white spots are seen that can be removed easily with a cotton swab. The diagnosis is easy and is based on microscopic findings.

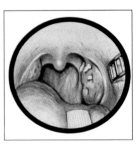

Fig. 3.41 Chronic tonsillitis. When pressure is applied with a spatula to the swollen tonsil, crumbly, fetid cores of pus and liquid pus emerge from the crypts. Taken alone, demonstration of cores of pus is insufficient for diagnosis of chronic tonsillitis, as they may also occur in completely normal tonsils lacking any signs of irritation.

whitish exudate, and the site of predilection for this is the upper pole. The local findings are often impressive in contrast to the symptoms, which are often slight. There may only be a feeling of a foreign body in the throat, and the patient also has a characteristic oral fetor. There is usually no fever. The exudate, which can be easily wiped off, may extend to the palate, buccal mucosa, and gingiva.

Microbiology. Fusiform and spirochetal organisms are always both present.

Diagnosis. This is made on the basis of the clinical picture of a typical infection usually of *one* tonsil, with unilateral lymphadenopathy, and on the results of bacterial culture (**Fig. 3.39**).

Differential diagnosis. This includes diphtheria, tuberculosis, syphilis, tonsillar neoplasms, acute leukemia, agranulocytosis, and infectious mononucleosis.

Treatment. Penicillin is given for 3–6 days. Local treatment with 2–5 % silver nitrate is applied topically.

Course. Usually short, with a good prognosis.

Fungal (*Candida*) Pharyngitis
Clinical Features. A white superficial punctate exudate forms, which can be wiped off and later becomes confluent. There is usually only slight redness in the surrounding mucosa. The tonsils, palate, posterior pharyngeal wall, and buccal mucosa may be affected. Subjective symptoms are few (**Fig. 3.40**).

Treatment. Antimycotic agents. Nystatin and imidazole are given in the form of a suspension or gel. Ketoconazole and fluconazole may be used for longer-term therapy. Systemic treatment with fluconazole is often required and essential in patients with HIV/AIDS.

Hyperkeratosis of the Tonsil (Differential Diagnosis of Interest)
This is a typical yellowish-brown or white, flat, or somewhat nodular prominent hyperkeratotic process on the tonsillar surface which *cannot* be wiped off.
Caution: This condition is frequently misdiagnosed as tonsillitis.
The cause is a benign circumscribed keratinization of the tonsil, especially of the epithelium of the crypt. No treatment is necessary.

Chronic Tonsillitis
Chronic tonsillitis requires particular attention on diagnostic grounds, as it is difficult to differentiate from a normal tonsil. It may also be a focus of infection, with effects on the entire body (**Fig. 3.41**).

Clinical Features. The history usually shows recurrent attacks of tonsillitis, but this is not always the case. There is often little or no pain in the neck and little or no difficulty in swallowing. There is halitosis and a bad taste in the mouth. The jugulodigastric lymph nodes are often enlarged. Chronic tonsillitis often remains more or less symptom-free. The systemic effect may become evident through reduced resistance, fatigue, a tendency to catch colds, unexplained high temperature, and loss of appetite.

Pathogenesis. The organisms are usually a mixed flora of aerobic and anaerobic bacteria in which streptococci predominate. Group A β-hemolytic streptococci are especially likely to cause focal symptoms. Poor drainage of the branching crypts leads to retention of cell debris, which forms a good culture medium for bacteria (see p. 260). From crypt abscesses of this type, the infection extends via epithelial defects in the reticular epithelium into the tonsillar parenchyma to produce a cryptic parenchymatous tonsillitis. Alternatively, it can penetrate into the capillaries surrounding the crypts, allowing toxins and organisms to enter the general circulation intermittently or continuously. In the long term, the tonsillar parenchyma undergoes fibrosis and atrophy.

Diagnosis

- The history shows recurrent acute or subacute attacks of tonsillitis.
- *Local findings:*
  - The tonsils are more or less fixed to their base, as shown by the depressor test (see **Fig. 3.13e**).
  - The tonsillar surface is fissured or scarred.
  - *Watery* pus and grayish-yellow material can be pressed out of the opening of the crypts by a tongue depressor (see **Fig. 3.13e**).
  - Reddening of the anterior faucial pillar is present.
  - Peritonsillar tenderness is present.
  - Lymphadenopathy of the jugulodigastric group is found.
- *General findings:*
  - The history includes recurrent tonsillitis, unexplained high temperature, lowering of resistance, etc.
  - Blood picture: the ESR and antistreptolysin titer are raised (see below).

Note: Fixed yellow concrements observed when pressure is exerted on the crypts with a tongue depressor do *not* signify chronic tonsillitis, but are a physiologic phenomenon (tonsillar plugs).
The size of the tonsil is also *not a* criterion for the presence of chronic tonsillitis. This disease can occur in large hyperplastic tonsils, but is more common in small and medium-sized tonsils. It is not always possible to make the diagnosis of chronic tonsillitis on the basis of the local findings. The history and general findings also need to be assessed critically. The examiner's judgment and experience are often decisive. Immunology has so far not proved to be of any practical diagnostic value.

Focal infection. A "focus" is any local change in the body that is capable of producing remote pathologic effects beyond its immediate surroundings. Poststreptococcal infections after tonsillitis are of special interest.

In clinical experience, diseases that may be based on a focal process include the following:
- Rheumatic fever (acute, febrile joint, and muscle disease).
- Glomerulonephritis and focal nephritis.
- Localized pustular psoriasis.
- Eruptive psoriasis (in children).
- Chronic urticaria.
- Endocarditis, myocarditis, and pericarditis.
- Polyserositis.
- Inflammatory disorders of the nerves and eyes (iridocyclitis).
- Vascular diseases (e. g., recurrent thromboangiitis, nodular vasculitis).

Treatment. Chronic tonsillitis requires treatment whenever it fulfils the criteria for a local pathologic process outlined above (see p. 247). Conservative measures such as gargling, painting, and suctioning are of no benefit. Even antibiotics can at best favorably influence the local process and risk of dissemination during the course of treatment. When the antibiotic is withdrawn, the pathogenic mechanism becomes reactivated, as the anatomic situation has not changed.

Tonsillectomy thus appears to be the only definitive treatment that can be considered for chronic tonsillitis. This applies even to patients with a coexisting coagulation disorder that will require appropriate replacement measures before surgery, special surgical techniques (e. g., "sealing" of the wound surface with fibrin glue and collagen fleece), and meticulous local supervision for a period of several days.

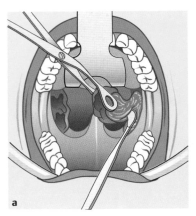 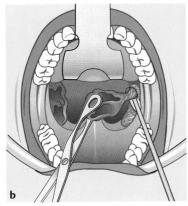

Fig. 3.42a, b Tonsillectomy with the head extended. The tongue is above, the upper incisors are below.
a Incision.
b Dissection and removal of the tonsil.

Tonsillectomy is indicated for the following diseases:

- Chronic tonsillitis.
- Recurrent tonsillitis.
- Peritonsillar abscess.
- Tonsillogenic septicemia.
- Tonsillogenic or posttonsillitis focal symptoms.
- Marked hypertrophy of the tonsil causing mechanical obstruction.
- If a tonsillar tumor is suspected.

Relative indications include:

- Resistant carriers of diphtheria bacilli.
- Stubborn oral fetor as a result of excess production of tonsillar plugs.
- Cervical lymph nodes that are tuberculous (bovine type), in which the tonsil is a possible portal of entry (see p. 389).

Contraindications include pharyngitis sicca, leukemia, agranulocytosis, serious generalized disorders such as tuberculosis or diabetes, and ulcerative or destructive processes extending beyond the tonsil if the diagnosis has not been confirmed. In some cases, cleft palate also represents a contraindication.

The patient's age is not a contraindication in doubtful cases.

The balance between immunobiologic considerations and the local pathologic findings needs to be weighed up carefully before tonsillectomy is recommended, particularly in children.

Principles of tonsillectomy. The operation can be performed under either local or general intubation anesthesia.

Tonsillectomy is usually performed with the patient under intubation anesthesia, with the head extended (**Fig. 3.42a, b**). An incision is made into the anterior faucial pillar, and the connective-tissue layer between the tonsillar parenchyma and the pharyngeal constrictor muscles is demonstrated. The tonsil is then freed by combined blunt and sharp dissection, proceeding from the upper pole to the base of the tongue, preserving the faucial pillars. The *entire* tonsillar tissue has to be removed. Hemostasis is secured by pressure, ligatures, or electrocautery. The same procedure is then performed on the opposite side.

Complications include hemorrhage, which may occur up to the 14th postoperative day. See also page 269.

As tonsillectomy is the most common surgical procedure in otolaryngology, there has been a desire to reduce the risk of hemorrhage through innovative surgical techniques and equipment. The National Prospective Tonsillectomy Audit, conducted in England and Northern Ireland in 2003–04, compared the overall risk of hemorrhage in relation to different surgical techniques (**Table 3.9**).

The following questions are often asked about tonsillectomy:

1. *The tonsils are apparently protective organs. Is it not bad for the body as a whole if they are removed?* The tonsils ought to be removed only if they are a source of irreversible inflammatory disease, if they are acting as a focus of infection, or if they are impeding breathing or swallowing due to their size. In these cases, it is the tonsils' pathologic characteristics that predominate, and their original protective function is reduced or has been lost. There is no doubt that this protective immunologic

function can be taken over satisfactorily by the remaining lymphoepithelial organs and structures in the pharynx. Removing irreversibly diseased or very enlarged tonsils, and those suspected of harboring a focus of infection, is therefore not a disadvantage, but a prerequisite for good health.

2. *Is there a tendency to catch upper respiratory infections more often after tonsillectomy?* A distinction needs to be made between pharyngitis and tonsillitis. Susceptibility to pharyngitis is not reduced by tonsillectomy itself, but it may be reduced if the tonsillectomy restores the airway to normal (e. g., in tonsillar hypertrophy) and if the flora in the mouth and pharynx are restored to normal (e. g., in chronic tonsillitis). Simple pharyngitis can therefore occur just as often after tonsillectomy as before, but tonsillitis can no longer occur, and intratonsillar abscess (a dangerous condition), focal symptoms, and tonsillogenic complications are also eliminated.

3. *What are the best age and the best time of year for tonsillectomy?* The operation can be performed at any age and at any time of year, but in patients under the age of 4 or over the age of 60 it should only be done with the strictest indications.

4. *Does tonsillectomy have any deleterious effects on the voice and speech?* If it is performed with a careful, conservative technique, tonsillectomy usually does not have any deleterious effects on the voice and speech. However, considerable caution is needed before recommending the operation in a patient who has an open, corrected, or occult cleft palate. Reinforcement of palatal insufficiency is described on page 281. In singers, the resonating space may be changed, although this is usually only temporary, and care is advised in these patients.

Tonsillotomy. There has been renewed interest in the traditional procedure of tonsillotomy, which was previously abandoned due to the risk of scarring of the crypts and follicles, with postoperative debris creating a nidus for abscess formation. A major reason for this renaissance is that there is a reduced risk of infection and abscess formation after tonsillotomy. The procedure can be performed using various types of laser (CO_2, diode), radiofrequency surgery, or the Coblation technique. It maintains open crypts (**Fig. 3.43**) and may preserve the immunological function of the tonsils in children younger than 4 years of age.

Indications: Tonsillotomy is only indicated in children or adults who have hyperplasia of the palatine tonsils. It is contraindicated if there is a history of recurrent infections or abscess.

Table 3.9   Results with five commonly used tonsillectomy techniques, based on the findings of the National Prospective Tonsillectomy Audit (Royal College of Surgeons of England, London, 2005)

Cold steel tonsillectomy using ties and /or packs	Technique with by far the lowest risk of postoperative hemorrhage (1.3 %) and return to theater (1.0 %)
Cold steel dissection with (bipolar or monopolar) diathermy hemostasis	Hemorrhage rate of 2.9 %; 1.7 % of the patients returned to theater
Bipolar (forceps or scissors) diathermy for dissection and hemostasis	Hemorrhage rate of 3.9 %; 2.4 % of the patients returned to theater
Monopolar diathermy for dissection and hemostasis	Hemorrhage rate of 6.1 %; 4.0 % of the patients returned to theater
Coblation for dissection and hemostasis	Hemorrhage rate of 4.4 %; 3.1 % of the patients returned to theater

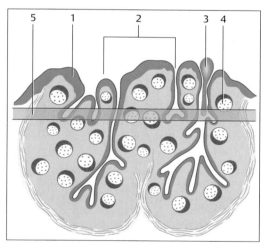

Fig. 3.43   The principle of laser tonsillotomy. **1**, Squamous epithelium; **2**, tonsillar crypts; **3**, cryptic content; **4**, secondary nodes; **5**, dissection level.

Local and General Complications During and After Tonsillitis

Post-tonsillitis complications include rheumatic fever, often with a symptom-free interval of 4–6 weeks, and endocarditis, myocarditis, or pericarditis. Acute glomerulonephritis and focal nephritis, which require urinalysis after the tonsillitis has

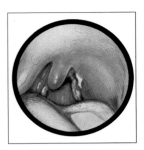

Fig. 3.44 Peritonsillar abscess. There is a rounded, firm protrusion of the left anterior palatal arch, with displacement of the uvula toward the right. The visible parts of the tonsils show patches of pus. Yellow, creamy pus is extruded from the region of the left upper pole.

resolved, are diseases secondary to streptococcal infection (see p. 267).

Peritonsillar Abscess (Supratonsillar or Retrotonsillar Abscess)

Unlike recurrent acute tonsillitis, this usually presents in young adults.

Clinical Features. Rapidly increasing difficulty in swallowing occurs after a symptom-free interval of a few days after tonsillitis. The pain usually radiates to the ear, and opening of the mouth is difficult due to trismus. The speech is thick and indistinct. The pain is so severe that the patient often refuses to eat, the head is held over to the diseased side, and rapid head movements are avoided. The patient has sialorrhea and oral fetor, swelling of the regional lymph nodes, increased fever with high temperatures of 39–40°C, and the general condition deteriorates rapidly. Patients also have an intolerable feeling of pressure in the neck, obstruction of the laryngeal inlet, and increasing respiratory obstruction. However, the symptoms may sometimes only be mild. Simultaneous bilateral abscesses may occur occasionally.

Pathogenesis. Inflammation spreads from the tonsillar parenchyma to the surrounding tissue, producing peritonsillitis, and an abscess forms within a few days (**Fig. 3.44**). This may follow acute tonsillitis or occur spontaneously. In the latter case, it has been suggested that the focus of infection is mucous salivary gland tissue in the supratonsillar space. The pharyngeal constrictor muscle is usually an effective barrier against further spread (**Fig. 3.45a, b**).

Diagnosis. This is made on the basis of the clinical picture of swelling, redness, and protrusion of the tonsil, faucial arch, palate, and uvula. The uvula is pushed towards the healthy side, and there is marked tenderness of the tonsillar area. Inspection of the pharynx may be difficult due to severe trismus. The jugulodigastric nodes are tender. There is an exudate on the tongue, and rarely on the tonsils and palate. The blood count and ESR are typical of an acute infection. When the swelling is fluctuant, it may be possible to aspirate the contents for diagnosis.

Differential diagnosis. This includes peritonsillar cellulitis, tonsillogenic sepsis (see below), allergic swelling of the pharynx without fever (angioneurotic edema), malignant diphtheria, agranulocyto-

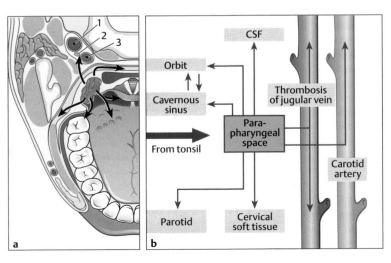

Fig. 3.45a, b Tonsillogenic complications.
a Extension to the immediately surrounding tissues. **1,** Internal jugular vein; **2,** vagus nerve; **3,** internal carotid artery.
b Further possible directions of spread of a tonsillogenic infection.

sis, specific tonsillar infections (tuberculosis and syphilis), and nonulcerating tumors of the tonsil or neighboring tissues (malignant lymphoma, lymphoepithelial tumor, anaplastic carcinoma, or leukemia).

The differential diagnosis also includes dental infections such as peritonsillar abscess due to impacted wisdom teeth and aneurysms of the internal carotid artery (pulsation). An absence of acute local signs of infection and of fever, and a prolonged course, suggest that a diagnosis of peritonsillar abscess is wrong.

Treatment. *Conservative:* High doses of antibiotics—e.g., penicillin or cephalosporin, etc.—for 1 week at least are only able to prevent the formation of an abscess in the early stages of infiltration of the peritonsillar tissues. Analgesics, a fluid diet, cold foods, an ice pack to the neck, and mouthwashes are prescribed.

Surgical treatment:

1. *Abscess tonsillectomy,* which is performed with the patient under general endotracheal anesthesia (see p. 268). This procedure can be carried out in all patients who are fit for surgery, particularly those with a recurrent peritonsillar abscess. It prevents further recurrence, the patient only has to undergo one course of treatment, and time is saved.
2. *Drainage of the abscess,* followed by tonsillectomy 3–4 days later with general anesthesia.

Principles of abscess drainage: Local anesthesia is induced carefully with 1 % topical lidocaine (Xylocaine), and infiltration anesthesia with 1 % lidocaine plus 1 : 200 000 epinephrine is used at the site of the intended incision. Pus often drains from the puncture site when the anesthetic is introduced. The anesthetic has to be allowed ≈ 5 min to act before the incision is made. Endotracheal anesthesia is usually more acceptable to patients.

Site of the incision: The incision is made at the point of maximum protrusion, usually between the uvula and the second upper molar tooth (**Fig. 3.46**). A test aspiration can sometimes be carried out before the incision. A long-handled pointed scalpel is used for the incision. All but 1.5–2.0 cm of the point is wrapped in sterile adhesive tape (**Fig. 3.46**) to prevent the point of the scalpel from penetrating too deeply and injuring the major vessels of the neck. The incision is made parallel to the ascending ramus of the mandible and must not pass externally, as the internal carotid artery and internal jugular vein are in the immediate

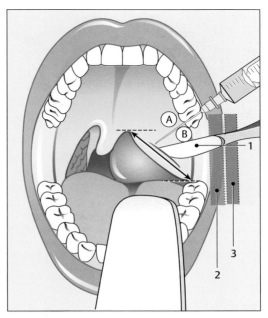

Fig. 3.46 Peritonsillar abscess. **1**, Guarded scalpel; **2**, internal carotid artery; **3**, internal jugular vein. Before the incision into the abscess is made (**B**), it is punctured and aspirated (**A**). The abscess is incised along a line connecting the last molar and the uvula.

vicinity (see **Fig. 3.45a**). If the diagnosis is correct, pus gushes out and must be removed with a powerful aspirator to prevent aspiration into the trachea. After the abscess has drained, a hemostat is introduced into the abscess cavity and opened widely, usually producing a further gush of pus. The abscess cavity must be opened up daily until there is no more pus draining from it.

Note: An incision should not be made until the abscess is "ripe"—i. e., fluctuation can be demonstrated or is probable.
Interval tonsillectomy can be performed after a delay of a few months to prevent recurrence of the abscess.

Course and prognosis. Regression of the inflammation and prevention of an abscess is possible with timely administration of antibiotics. An abscess may also drain spontaneously and heal. However, distressing pain and difficulty in eating usually make active drainage necessary. If tonsillectomy is not performed, there is a high risk of recurrent abscess in the paratonsillar scar tissue.

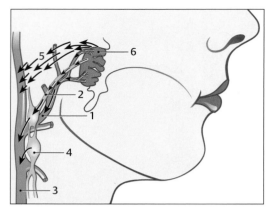

Fig. 3.47 Genesis of tonsillogenic sepsis. **1**, Extension via veins; **2**, extension via lymph vessels; **3**, internal jugular vein; **4**, regional lymph nodes around the internal jugular vein; **5**, extension in continuity via the cervical soft tissues to the internal jugular vein; **6**, palatine tonsil.

Complications and risks. These include extension of the inflammatory swelling and edema to the laryngeal inlet, with increasing respiratory obstruction and a possible risk of asphyxia. The abscess may also rupture into the parapharyngeal space (see **Fig. 3.45a**). From there, it may extend as:

- A descending internal cervical abscess.
- A parapharyngeal abscess.
- Ascending involvement of the orbit or the cranial cavity, causing meningitis, cavernous sinus thrombosis, and brain abscess.
- Thrombosis of the internal jugular vein.
- Erosion of the carotid artery or its branches (rarely).
- Invasion of the parotid (purulent parotitis).

Septicemia During or After Tonsillitis, Tonsillogenic Sepsis

Clinical Features. These include chills with a septic temperature chart, tenderness along the internal jugular vein, which appears as a tender, firm cord under the anterior edge of the sternocleidomastoid muscle, or tenderness of the jugulodigastric lymph nodes. There is often simultaneous reddening of the tonsillar area, but this is not essential. The patient has a severe constitutional upset, a left shift in the blood count with leukocytosis, splenomegaly, possible spread to the lung, skin, or liver, a dry tongue, and a weak rapid pulse.

Pathogenesis. Bacteria enter the bloodstream from the tonsil, or from a neighboring focus of pus. Three different pathways are possible (**Fig. 3.47**):

1. *Hematogenous,* via the tonsillar veins and the facial vein to the internal jugular vein. Thrombophlebitis develops in the vein, and infected thrombi enter the pulmonary or general circulation.
2. *Lymphogenous,* via efferent lymphatics of the tonsil to the regional lymph nodes of the jugulodigastric group and along the internal jugular vein. From there, the internal jugular vein becomes infected, and the disease then progresses as in (1).
3. *Direct spread* of the abscess in or around the tonsil, with rupture into the parapharyngeal space or into the cervical soft tissue, with involvement of the internal jugular vein.

Many organisms may be responsible for tonsillogenic septicemia; they can often be demonstrated in the blood if a specimen is taken during a rigor. Mixed infections are also frequent.

Diagnosis. This is based on the picture of chills and symptoms of septicemia due to continuous or intermittent bacteremia. There is a history of tonsillitis and symptoms of chronic tonsillitis (see p. 266); the ESR increases rapidly, and there is a rapidly rising leukocytosis. There is tenderness in the jugulodigastric lymph nodes or the internal jugular vein. Defensive spasm of the cervical soft tissues occurs, with a relieving posture in the head and neck. The organism can be demonstrated in the blood.

Treatment. If severe sepsis is suspected, high-dose penicillin or broad-spectrum antibiotics are started immediately to protect the body from metastases. Specific, selective antibiotic therapy can be given on the basis of laboratory tests.

Other obligatory measures include:

1. *Tonsillectomy* to eliminate the focus.
2. *Ligature of the internal jugular vein* inferior to the thrombus and resection of the diseased segment, if the internal jugular vein is involved.
3. *Wide opening and drainage* of an abscess of the cervical soft tissues.

Course and prognosis. This is a life-threatening disease, but the prognosis is good if treatment with antibiotics and surgery are instituted promptly.

The following conditions are rare:

Tonsillogenic cavernous sinus thrombosis. This is transmitted via the pterygoid venous plexus or the internal jugular vein to the inferior ophthalmic vein. Symptoms are described on page 272.

Bleeding due to erosion, secondary to tonsillitis. The external and internal carotid artery may be involved, in a similar manner to the cervical veins, by an abscess in the parapharyngeal space. Symptoms include severe hemorrhage from the tonsil, usually after a small prodromal bleed.

> **Note:** An immediate tonsillectomy has to be performed, with massive antibiotic cover, at the first suspicion of tonsillogenic septicemia with recurrent chills. If this unusual clinical scenario is seen, consideration should be given to the possibility of immune deficiency.

■ **Other Pharyngeal Inflammations**

Rare Abscesses in the Pharyngeal Area

Retropharyngeal Abscess in Children
Abscesses can form due to breakdown of lymphadenitis of the retropharyngeal lymph nodes following pharyngeal infection in children, especially during the first 2 years of life.

Clinical Features. These include swelling of the posterior pharyngeal wall, difficulty in swallowing, thick speech, difficulty in eating, elevated temperature, a relieving posture of the neck (differential diagnosis: torticollis), leakage of food through the nose, possibly nasal obstruction, croup, and laryngeal edema (**Fig. 3.48**).

Differential diagnosis. Benign and malignant prevertebral tumors must be considered.

Treatment. This is by paramedian incision and drainage under general anesthesia, with the head hanging if fluctuation occurs. The airway must be protected from aspiration by an endotracheal tube, and antibiotic cover is given.

> **Caution:** Magnetic resonance images should be obtained whenever a retropharyngeal abscess is suspected, due to the risk of extension to the mediastinum between the superficial and deep neck fascia.

Retropharyngeal Abscess in Adults
This is usually a descending prevertebral cold abscess originating from tuberculous caries of a cervical vertebra, or

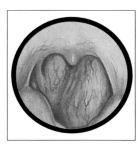

Fig. 3.48 Retropharyngeal abscess. Hypostatic abscess. Rounded, resilient protrusion of the left epipharynx, mesopharynx, and hypopharynx. There is an insidious disease course, as in tuberculosis or syphilis.

suppuration in osteomyelitis of the temporal bone (e. g., petrositis) and in mastoiditis.

Clinical Features. These include pressure in the neck, attacks of coughing, difficulty in swallowing, mild dysphagia, stiffness of the neck, and typical lesions of the cervical spine on radiographs.

Differential diagnosis. Benign and malignant tumors and spondylosis of the cervical spine.

Treatment. A test aspiration is made. If a cold abscess is present, it is drained if possible to the lateral part of the neck and not into the oropharynx. Antituberculous treatment is given, and the patient is referred to a spinal surgeon.

Acute Pharyngitis
Clinical Features. These include pain on swallowing, possibly radiating to the ear, a feeling of dryness, heat, and soreness in the pharynx, itching, scratching, burning, clearing the throat, and attacks of coughing. The patient usually feels sick. The entire pharynx (nasopharynx, oropharynx, and hypopharynx) is usually involved in the infection. Fever occurs, especially in children. In viral infections, the course is often intermittent over several weeks.

Pathogenesis. This is usually a primary virus infection, often with later secondary bacterial infection. Less often, it is a primary bacterial infection due to streptococci, *Haemophilus influenzae*, or pneumococci. There are prodromal symptoms on acute infection, such as measles, scarlet fever, and rubella. Acute pharyngitis may also be rhinogenic and/ or sinogenic, or it may be caused by physical or chemical injury, scalds, caustics, etc.

Diagnosis. The mucosa appears red and thickened. The palatal and pharyngeal mucosa are dry, with a glazed surface. Mucus is produced, which is initially colorless but later tenacious and yellow. Deep-red,

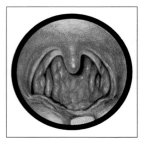

Fig. 3.49 Acute pharyngitis. This is usually a concomitant condition or a prodromal sign of an infectious disease. The mucous membranes of the pharynx, palate, and uvula are diffusely or spottily reddened. The salpingopharyngeal folds and lymph follicles show cushion-like swelling.

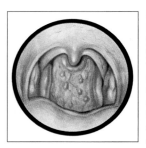

Fig. 3.50 Chronic granular (glandular) lateral pharyngitis. The salpingopharyngeal folds and the scattered or grouped lymphatic follicles are brilliant red and swollen. There is a sensation of burning, itching, and a foreign-body sensation, especially on empty swallowing.

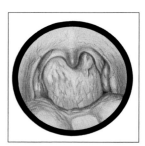

Fig. 3.51 Atrophic pharyngitis (pharyngitis sicca). The mucous membranes of the pharynx are thinned, atrophic, and dry, or covered with a thin layer of mucous, giving them a varnished appearance. Viscous, purulent mucus coming from the nasopharyngeal space or adherent grayish-green crusts are frequently seen. There is a sensation of marked dryness, with painful swallowing due to the adherent crusts, and halitosis.

solitary follicles are usually prominent, and there is regional lymphadenopathy with swelling and tenderness, especially in children. Tonsillitis often occurs, or if the tonsils have been removed there is infection of the lateral bands (**Fig. 3.49**).

Treatment. Symptomatic treatment includes hot milk and honey, cold or warm neck dressings, pharyngeal irrigation, and inhalations with isotonic saline solution to liquefy thick secretions. A mild oil

(applied transnasally) may be helpful in relieving mucosal inflammation.

Smoking is forbidden, and anesthetic and disinfectant lozenges are given. Local antibiotics must *not* be given, and parenteral antibiotics are only given for severe bacterial infections. Bed rest is advised for fever.

Chronic Pharyngitis

This is a comprehensive term for several chronic irritative or inflammatory conditions of the pharyngeal mucosa.

Clinical Features. There are several forms:
1. *Simple chronic pharyngitis:* This causes a globus sensation, constant throat-clearing, bouts of coughing, a feeling of dryness or phlegm in the throat, pain of varying degrees in the neck and on swallowing, and tenacious secretion. The course is intermittent, and there is no generalized upset and no fever.
2. *Chronic hyperplastic pharyngitis:* The mucosa of the posterior pharyngeal wall is thickened and granular, with prominent solitary follicles. It is a smooth red to grayish-red in color, possibly with venous telangiectasis and secretion of stringy, colorless mucus. There is usually a very disturbing, strange sensation in the pharynx with compulsive throat-clearing and swallowing, gagging, and even vomiting (**Fig. 3.50**).
3. *Chronic atrophic pharyngitis:* The posterior pharyngeal wall is dry and glazed, often with dry, tough crusts of secretion. The mucosa is smooth, pink, often very tender and transparent, but may also be red and thickened. Simultaneous atrophic rhinitis and laryngitis sicca may occur. The patient is constantly obliged to spit out the stringy secretion. At night, there is a feeling of choking and disturbance of sleep. Continuous clearing of the throat may produce slight mucosal hemorrhage. The disease depends on climatic or temperature conditions, and the symptoms resolve at the seaside but are worse in hot dry air. Older people are more often affected (**Fig. 3.51**).

Pathogenesis. A functional, constitutional weakness of the pharyngeal mucosa is often present. The disease may be due to chronic exogenous damage from dust, chemicals, or heat (e. g., at work). Common contributing factors are marked temperature changes, working in a drafty or smoky environment (e. g., butchers and restaurant workers), work-ing in a dry or improperly air-conditioned atmosphere, heavy smoking and drinking, oral breathing, chronic nasal airway obstruction, abuse of nose drops and sprays, chronic sinus-itis, and hypertrophic adenoids.

Other causes include endocrine disorders (e. g., meno-pause, hypothyroidism), avitaminosis A, and general disor-ders (e. g., heart and kidney malfunction, diabetes, pulmo-nary insufficiency, chronic bronchial diseases). Finally, mu-cosal allergy and incorrect use of the voice among profes-sional speakers such as teachers, politicians, and singers may be responsible.

Diagnosis. The local findings are typical. The dis-ease lasts for years, with an intermittent course. There is often a discrepancy between the unre-markable local findings and the marked symptoms.

In patients with atrophic pharyngitis, it is im-portant to exclude a nasopharyngeal tumor and a chronic infectious focus in the paranasal sinuses. Nasal function should be tested using rhinoman-ometry.

Differential diagnosis. This includes Sjögren syn-drome (see p. 423), Plummer–Vinson (Paterson–Kelly) syndrome (see p. 275), and malignancy of any part of the pharynx or esophagus. The latter requires careful endoscopy. The disease has to be distinguished from chronic tonsillitis and sinusitis, specific pharyngitis, tuberculosis or syphilis, cervi-cal spondylosis and deficient antibody syndrome (diagnosed by serum electrophoresis), Thornwaldt bursa (see below), elongated styloid process syn-drome (see p. 276), enlarged posterior ends of the nasal turbinates, choanal polyp, and psychoneuro-sis.

Treatment. The examiner should look for the local or distant causes listed above and should eliminate them.

Chronic hyperplastic pharyngitis: Local treatment includes the reduction of hyperplastic mucosal areas with 2–4 % silver nitrate applied under micro-scopic vision. Dry and atrophic areas should be stimulated with Lugol iodine solution, for example. Afterwards, a mild aromatic oil can be used to cover the raw mucosa (applied transnasally).

Chronic atrophic pharyngitis: Iodine solution can be used in an effort to stimulate the remaining secretory elements in the atrophic mucosa. This cannot be done when metaplasia is present.

Symptomatic treatment includes moisturizing the pharyngeal mucosa with steam inhalations. Nicotine and alcohol must be avoided. Local mea-sures are described on p. 277, and include oily prep-arations to provide a protective film for the dry mucosa. A change of climate is advised, and the air humidity at work is tested. Patients may even have to change their job or place of residence.

Thornwaldt Disease, Pharyngeal Bursitis

Clinical Features. These include foul-smelling drainage from the nasopharynx, particularly in the mornings.

Pathogenesis. The cause of this disease lies in persistence of the central groove of the adenoid or formation of a pouch in the roof of the pharynx as an anatomic variant (see **Fig. 3.6**), or on the posterior wall of the nasopharynx, which retains a yellowish-brown secretion and debris, with or with-out accompanying inflammation. Gradual closure and for-mation of a cyst is possible. The symptoms are then inter-mittent. This is a rare disorder.

Diagnosis. This is made by careful endoscopic ex-amination of the entire nasopharynx.

Differential diagnosis. Sinusitis, especially sphe-noid or ethmoidal, or early neoplasm in the naso-pharynx must be considered.

Treatment. Surgical obliteration of the cyst is car-ried out.

Ulceromembranous Pharyngitis
See page 265.

Plummer–Vinson Syndrome, Paterson–Kelly Syndrome

Clinical Features. This disease occurs almost exclusively in women from 40 to 70 years of age and may occasionally cause marked, painful dysphagia. The mucosa of the tongue and of the pharynx is atrophic; the skin is dry, pale, and flaccid; the mucous membranes are dry; the patient also has koilonychia and complains of burning of the tongue, and a loss of teeth is possible.

Pathogenesis. The basic cause is probably an iron defi-ciency. Promoting factors include achlorhydria and avitami-nosis, and chronic atrophic mucosal inflammation with sub-epithelial fibrosis. There is a risk of postcricoid carcinoma in 10–30 % of cases. Tumors may occur many years later even though iron deficiency has been corrected.

Diagnosis. The dysphagia due to stricture of the cervical esophagus and development of webs worsens, so that ultimately only small amounts can be swallowed. The fingernails are curved, and there are rhagades at the corners of the mouth, weight loss, hypochromic anemia, extremely low values for serum iron, anisocytosis and microcytosis, radiologic evidence of spasm of the esophageal opening with a notch at the level of the cricoid, and possibly also a web within the esophageal lumen at that level. Endoscopy should be performed.

Differential diagnosis. This includes postcricoid carcinoma, hypopharyngeal carcinoma, and functional dysphagia.

Treatment. Therapy consists of iron and vitamin B, a bland diet, and possibly endoscopic dilation of the esophageal stenosis.

Pharyngeal Diphtheria
See page 264.

Tuberculosis, Syphilis
See pages 252, 265, respectively.

Other Lesions of the Pharyngeal Mucosa
Lesions of the pharyngeal mucosa occur in blood disorders such as agranulocytosis, panmyelophthisis, acute leukemia, and chronic lymphatic and chronic myeloid leukemia.

■ Other Pharyngeal Diseases

Styloid Process Syndrome (Eagle Syndrome)
Clinical Features. These include dysphagia or neuralgia, usually on one side, and severest in the tonsillar region or behind the angle of the jaw. Pain may radiate to the ear or the temporal region. Pain may occur on swallowing, or on certain movements of the cervical spine. The symptoms can be reproduced by palpating the tonsillar cleft.

Pathogenesis (see Fig. 3.20). Mechanical irritation of the nerves and vessels close to the styloid process when it is excessively long (the normal length is ≈ 3 cm). The neighboring nerves are cranial nerves IX, X, XI, and XII, and the neighboring vessels are the internal and external carotid artery. An elongated styloid is not common.

Diagnosis. Palpation of the tonsillar cleft, which produces the typical symptoms at this point, and by radiography.

Differential diagnosis. Neuralgias of the cranial nerves IX and X (see below), and spondylosis of the cervical spine.

Treatment. Removal of the styloid process from the mouth via a tonsillectomy or an external approach.

Glossopharyngeal Neuralgia (Cranial Nerve IX)
Clinical Features. This is usually a disease of the older age groups. There is a sudden tearing pain of one side of the tongue or the neck, radiating to the ear, accompanied by discharge of tenacious saliva. Pain is induced by swallowing food, chewing, and also by speaking and yawning. As a result, the patient eats extremely carefully and often with the head in a typical position.

Diagnosis. This is made by inducing local anesthesia of the trigger zones, the base of the tongue, the lower pole of the tonsil, which interrupts the attacks of pain for a brief period.

Differential diagnosis. Neuralgia of the intermediate nerve (Ramsay Hunt neuralgia), neuralgia of the trigeminal or the auriculotemporal nerves, and stylohyoid syndrome (see p. 171).

Treatment. *Conservative:* Carbamazepine should be tried. *Surgical treatment* consists of division of the cranial nerve IX in the posterior cranial fossa.

Neuralgia of the Vagus Nerve (Cranial Nerve X)
Neuralgia of the superior laryngeal nerve: There is intermittent episodic violent pain radiating into the lateral part of the neck from the ear to the thyroid gland, with a pressure point over the greater horn of the hyoid bone and at the point of entry of the nerve into the thyrohyoid membrane.

Neuralgia of the auricular branch of the vagus causes intermittent, very severe pain in the retroauricular and suboccipital areas, and in the shoulder.

Diagnosis. The pressure point is the long process of the hyoid, the thyrohyoid membrane, or the musculature around the mastoid process.

Differential diagnosis. Ramsay Hunt neuralgia of the intermediate nerve and geniculate ganglion, and auriculotemporal neuralgia.

Treatment. *Conservative treatment* should be tried first, including warm local applications, poultices, and exposure to infrared light. *Surgical treatment* includes division of the superior laryngeal nerve or injection of absolute alcohol (0.3–0.5–1.0 mL) at the entrance of the nerve into the thyrohyoid membrane.

Globus Hystericus (Functional Dysphagia)

Globus hystericus is a symptom complex that requires investigation even when accompanying pharyngitis.

Clinical Features. These include an intermittent or continuous feeling of a foreign body being stuck in the throat that cannot be dislodged despite swallowing. Occasionally, there is also pain in the throat or radiating to the ears. Swallowing is not affected. Organic lesions are absent.

Pathogenesis. An incorrect psychosomatic response to stress and possibly a tendency to spasm of the muscles of the esophageal inlet.

Diagnosis. Typical tenderness in the midline at the level of the cricoid arch. Radiography is normal, as is esophagoscopy. Other autonomic disturbances are often also present.

Differential diagnosis (see Table 3.1). A benign or malignant tumor of the mouth, pharynx, or esophagus must be excluded.

Treatment. The patient often has a cancer phobia, and this needs to be dealt with by counseling. Sedatives are given, and the patient is removed from the stressful situation. If organic causes are found, they are eliminated if possible; otherwise, the suspected cause is explained to the patient.

■ Basic Conservative Treatment of the Mucosa

Local applications for mucosal diseases of the mouth and pharynx include sprays, cold and warm inhalations, painting, and lozenges. Mouthwashes may also be very useful. A gargle usually maintains direct contact only with the mucosa of the anterior part of the oral cavity and does not reach the faucial pillars, tonsil, posterior pharyngeal wall, or hypopharynx, as this will stimulate the gag reflex. Occasionally, solutions that have been used for gargling reach these regions via saliva.

The substances used in the mouth and pharynx include in particular anti-inflammatory agents, antiseptics, anesthetics (e. g., 1 % tetracaine or lidocaine), vitamin solutions, iodine glycerin solutions, and steroid preparations. Antibiotics should not be used locally because the concentration is too low, and resistance and allergy can develop. Saline solutions or oily preparations are used for dry mucosa. Chamomile has a drying effect and is not indicated in patients with atrophic mucosa. Mucolytics are used to soften tenacious mucus. Pharmacologic agents can also be given to control saliva formation.

Oils should be mild and adhesive to coat the dry epithelium. Oils with a peanut or sesame-seed base are recommended. Standardized Myrtol has secretolytic, secretomotoric, bacteriostatic, and deodorizing effects on the respiratory mucosa (see p. 159).

Enteric or parenteral medication is indicated in many diseases of the mouth and pharynx. However, it must always be remembered that mucosal disorders may have been caused by drugs in the first place—e. g., by antibiotics.

■ Trauma in the Mouth and Pharynx

Alkali and Acid Burns and Scalds

Scalds occur particularly in children. Alkali and acid burns—due to mistaking the contents of a bottle (lye, vinegar essence, cleaning fluids, etc., kept in empty bottles) or to attempted suicide (hydrochloric acid, caustic soda, vinegar essence, sulfuric acid)—occur principally in adults.

Clinical Features. These are dramatic. There is severe pain in the mouth and pharynx, sialorrhea, difficulty in swallowing, redness and vesicle formation on the affected part of the mucosa. Later, a flat white membrane with deep red edges and mucosal edema appears. Caustic substances are usually swallowed, so that the mucosa of the esophagus, the stomach, and the intestine may also be involved (see p. 365). The patient may be in shock.

Diagnosis. The history and local findings in the mouth, pharynx, and perioral tissues form the basis for the diagnosis. Involvement of the stomach and esophagus must be assessed as rapidly as possible using careful endoscopy, at the latest within 8 days. The type of fluid and the amount must be determined, and if possible the ingested fluid should be tested.

Treatment. This includes drinking large amounts of water or (even better) milk. The acids are neutralized with sodium bicarbonate or magnesium salts. Lyes are neutralized with diluted vinegar or lemon juice. Treatment of shock may be needed. Local treatment of the mouth and pharynx includes lozenges or ice cubes, lukewarm mouthwashes, possibly with lidocaine supplements, analgesics, a cool liquid diet, feeding via a nasogastric tube or with parenteral nutrition in severe cases, antibiotics, and steroids, depending on local findings.

Foreign Bodies

These are less common in the mouth and pharynx than in the esophagus (see p. 367). Small pointed foreign bodies, such as splinters of bone, fish bones, bristles from a toothbrush, needles, nails, or bits of wood and glass, can impact in the tonsil, base of the tongue, vallecula, or lateral wall of the pharynx. Larger foreign bodies such as bits of toys, flat bones, coins, buttons, large fish bones, bits of false teeth, etc. often impact in the piriform sinus or hypopharynx before entering the esophagus.

Clinical Features. There is pain of varying severity, which is worse on swallowing, and swallowing may be completely obstructed.

Diagnosis. This is based on the history. Radiography is performed if it is thought that the material may be radiopaque. Radiographically, a swallow is also performed with a contrast medium using a colorless medium such as Gastrografin (not barium) which will not influence assessment of the mucosa at subsequent endoscopy. Endoscopy is then carried out. Small impacted foreign bodies in the tonsil or base of the tongue can often be felt with the finger. Small foreign bodies in the upper pharynx are best removed without endoscopy, using grasping forceps under direct vision.

Treatment. Instrumental extraction of the foreign body is performed as quickly as possible, due to the danger of pressure necrosis or mucosal injury, causing abscess or mediastinitis.

> **!**
> **Note:** If a foreign body is suspected, endoscopy should be performed as quickly as possible using an open rigid esophagoscope or a Weerda diverticuloscope. The search is continued until the foreign body is found or until it is certain that no foreign body is present. Attempts to dislodge foreign bodies by ingesting foods such as salads, bread, etc. are not justifiable, as this often leads to delay and allows complications to develop.

Mucosal Injuries in the Mouth and Pharynx due to Foreign Bodies and Trauma

Because of the good healing properties of this area, suturing of mucosal injuries is only rarely required, unless they are extensive. However, antibiotic cover may be indicated.

Penetrating soft-tissue injuries in the mouth and pharynx, bullet wounds, stab wounds, and wounds due to traffic accidents have to be assessed immediately from within outward, as well as injuries to the soft and related bony tissues, mandible, maxilla, hyoid, teeth, and cervical spine. The injured structures should be debrided, repositioned, fixed, and sutured in layers. Antibiotic cover is given. Entry of air into the cervical soft tissue causes surgical emphysema.

Impalement injuries to the palate and the posterior of the wall of the pharynx usually occur in children, due to falling onto pointed objects. Immediate expert examination and suture of the wound are usually necessary.

Tongue bites usually heal spontaneously if the damage is slight and superficial. Penetrating bite wounds require exploration and possibly suture because of the danger of infection from carious teeth. If a portion of the tongue is completely divided, it should be reimplanted. The result depends on the speed of the reconstruction, the condition of the wound, and the arterial blood supply.

Tongue piercings are now common. Penetration of the tongue muscle by a stud may be followed by serious complications such as infection and bleeding.

Insect bites caused when a live insect (bees, etc.) is swallowed along with food lead to considerable edema of the pharynx and thus respiratory obstruction. For treatment, high-dose steroids are administered intravenously, ice packs are applied to the neck, calcium, and tracheotomy is performed if necessary.

■ Neurogenic Disorders

Motor Paralyses of the Pharynx

Clinical Features. These include absence of the pharyngeal reflex, choking, rhinolalia aperta due to palatal paralysis, difficulty in swallowing fluids, and escape of fluids through the nose during swallowing. It is impossible to suck, or to blow out the cheeks. The soft palate deviates to the healthy, nonparalyzed side.

Pathogenesis. Causes include cerebrovascular accidents, tumors of the base of the skull, jugular foramen syndrome affecting cranial nerves IX to XI, pseudobulbar palsy, syringobulbia, and herpes zoster. In *bulbar paralysis,* the motor cranial nerve centers in the medulla oblongata degenerate gradually, causing muscle atrophy, fibrillation of the tongue, and inability to swallow. Difficulty in swallowing also occurs in *pseudobulbar palsy* due to bilateral lesions of the supranuclear pathways for the lower motor cranial nerves, but *without* muscle atrophy and fibrillation.

Differential diagnosis. Stenosing lesions in the upper digestive tract must be considered.

Diagnosis. Swallowing disorders can be investigated using video fluoroscopy and functional endoscopy. A speech and language therapist (SALT) is often helpful for analyzing these disorders.

Treatment. Nutrition has to be ensured with a nasogastric tube; a pharyngostomy or a gastrostomy may be needed. Pneumonia must be prevented by frequent aspiration, and a tracheotomy may even be needed.

Prognosis. This depends on the underlying disease and the course.

Pharyngeal Spasm

Patients find it very difficult or impossible to swallow. They have tonic spasms or vomit swallowed food, and also have pain behind the sternum.

Pathogenesis. This may be a prodrome preceding complete paralysis due to any of the neurologic causes named above, but may also be a hysterical phenomenon. See also globus hystericus (p. 277).

The results of paralyses of the posterior cranial nerve are summarized in **Table 3.1**.

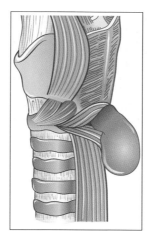

Fig. 3.52 The typical topographical situation in a Zenker diverticulum. It develops in the Killian triangle between the inferior constrictor and the cricopharyngeus muscle.

■ Hypopharyngeal Diverticulum (Zenker Diverticulum)

This is often incorrectly called an esophageal diverticulum, but the pouch lies immediately above the esophageal opening (**Fig. 3.52**). Men are affected three times more frequently than women.

Clinical Features. Small pouches cause a foreign-body sensation or a feeling of pressure in the throat during and after eating, as well as irritation in the neck. Larger pouches cause sticking or regurgitation of food, frothy saliva, a gurgling noise when pressure is applied to the neck, oral fetor, and attacks of coughing—especially at night, when the contents of the pouch may empty into the larynx. There may be associated "heartburn" and reflux esophagitis. The disease mainly affects middle-aged and elderly persons. If the pouch increases in size, swallowing becomes progressively worse until eventually dehydration, electrolyte disturbances, and cachexia develop due to mechanical obstruction of the esophagus.

Pathogenesis. The site of predilection is the Killian triangle (see **Figs. 3.3, 3.7**). Weakness of the wall in the cricopharyngeal area between the cricopharyngeus and the components of the inferior constrictor initially favors temporary bulging, and later persistent and increasing herniation of the mucosa and submucosa of the posterior wall of the pharynx. The pouch passes between the pharynx and the prevertebral fascia. Suspected causes include spasm of the entrance of the esophagus, eating too quickly, or incoordination of the

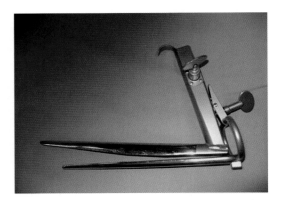

Fig. 3.53   The Weerda diverticuloscope.

pharyngeal phase of swallowing with the opening of the esophagus. Formation of scars at this level may also play a part.

Diagnosis. This is made on the basis of the typical history and symptoms, especially regurgitation of undigested food, and occasionally of food eaten several days earlier. Examination with the mirror often shows frothy secretions in the piriform sinus. A barium swallow (see **Fig. 7.2a–k**) demonstrates the lesion. Esophagoscopy is necessary. It is important to exclude a carcinoma within the pouch.

Differential diagnosis. This includes globus hystericus, malignant tumors of the hypopharynx, esophagus, or stomach, hiatus hernia, achalasia, high esophageal strictures, and congenital vascular rings (see p. 371).

Treatment. There are three management options: conservative, surgery via an external approach, and endoscopic surgery. Conservative treatment aims to advise and reassure the patient (small, frequent meals, last meal no later than 6 PM, sleeping with the head of the bed raised). The principles of surgery are as follows.

Endoscopic surgery: The procedure is performed with the patient under general endotracheal anesthesia, using the Weerda diverticuloscope. The spur is isolated and divided with special endoscopic scissors, or with a laser or stapler (**Figs. 3.53, 3.54**). Endoscopic stapling or laser surgery techniques are the treatment of choice for all pouch surgery.

Complications include damage to large vessels running in the spur and opening of the mediastinum, resulting in mediastinitis. The height of the spur and the size of the diverticulum are therefore the main criteria for selecting this approach.

External removal of the sac is the treatment of choice for large diverticula. General or local anesthesia may be used. Access is gained via an incision along the anterior border of the left sternocleidomastoid muscle. Dissection is continued between the larynx and the carotid sheath at the lateral edge of the cricoid plate. The sac of the pouch is isolated, lying between the esophagus and the prevertebral fascia. The cricopharyngeus muscle, which forms the bar at the entrance to the diverticulum, is identified and divided. The pouch is then resected, and the hypopharynx and cervical soft tissues are closed in several layers. Complications include damage to the recurrent laryngeal nerve.

■ Anomalies of the Mouth and Pharynx

Congenital anomalies of the tongue—such as cleft tongue, microglossia, aglossia, congenital stenosis of the junction between the nasopharynx and the oropharynx, or stenosis at the junction of the hypopharynx and the esophagus—are rare. Macroglossia

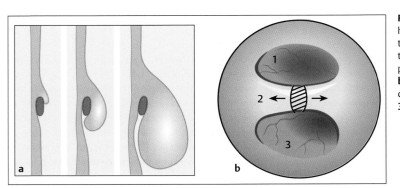

Fig. 3.54a, b   **a** Genesis of a hypopharyngeal pulsion diverticulum. The red area indicates the inferior part of the cricopharyngeus muscle.
b Principle of endoscopic spur division. **1**, Esophagus; **2**, spur; **3**, diverticulum.

is much more common and is treated by surgery. Ankyloglossia is caused by a frenulum that is too short; it is corrected using a Z-plasty. Macroglossia in patients with a pituitary adenoma is a symptom of acromegaly. Pituitary surgery and endocrine therapy may be beneficial in these cases.

Median Cervical Cysts and Fistulas
See page 395.

Clefts of the Lip, Jaw, and Palate
The prevalence of congenital cleft of the lip, upper jaw, or palate is one per thousand among Caucasian ethnic groups. The incidence is considerably lower among Africans and African Americans, but higher among Native Americans and Asians. Clefts of the lip, upper jaw, and palate are more common in boys, whereas pure cleft palates are more common in girls. The following types can be distinguished: cleft lip (harelip), cleft lip and upper jaw, and cleft palate, and the conditions can be unilateral, bilateral, incomplete, or complete (**Fig. 3.55a–c**). Complete clefts of the lip, upper jaw, and palate may occur (total cleft), and if this finding is bilateral it causes the so-called wolf's nose.

Clinical Features. The appearances are typical. In infants, there is considerable difficulty in nursing, as it is not possible to close the lips and shut off the palate. Food escapes through the nose, and the child tends to aspirate milk into the trachea.

Infections of the upper and lower airways occur due to disordered swallowing and respiratory physiology. Abnormal tubal function leads to serous otitis media, chronic otitis media, and conductive deafness. The speech is affected, with rhinolalia aperta, lisping, abnormal articulation, and velopharyngeal insufficiency. There are anomalies of occlusion and position of the teeth. The nose is almost always involved in clefts of the lips and palate.

Pathogenesis. The cause is probably multifactorial. Embryonic damage is caused by hypoxia, embryopathy, virus infections in the mother, toxins, and genetic lesions. There is familial clustering, which is irregularly dominant.

Diagnosis. This is made on the basis of the typical facial appearance and examination with a laryngeal mirror.

Submucous cleft palate is often overlooked. The clue is a slight speech disorder. It is diagnosed by

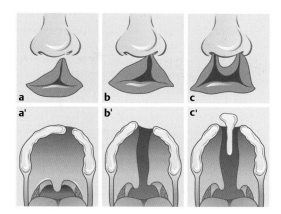

Fig. 3.55a–c Typical cleft formations.
a Cleft lip.
b Cleft lip and upper jaw.
c Bilateral cleft of lip, upper jaw, and palate.
a′ Cleft upper jaw.
b′ Cleft upper jaw and palate.
c′ Bilateral cleft of lip, upper jaw, and palate.

palpation, which shows a bony dehiscence under an intact palatal mucosa.

Complete assessment requires the combined efforts of an ear, nose, and throat surgeon with training in plastic surgery, a phoniatrician, a dentist, an oral surgeon, and an orthodontist, so that all the important aspects and defects can be detected and a common plan of treatment decided on.

Treatment. *Surgical treatment* consists of multilayered closure of the defect to form a solid floor of the nose and to correct the nasal deformity. Often, many corrective operations and orthodontic and phoniatric assessments and treatments are necessary, depending on the type and extent of the defect.

Time schedule for correction of clefts:
- *Cleft lips* are corrected between the fourth and sixth (to eighth) months of life using cheiloplasty, with final correction between age 14 and 16 years if necessary.
- *Cleft lip and maxilla* are corrected between the fourth and sixth (to eighth) months of life by an operation on the lip and nostril. Final correction can be performed between ages 14 and 16 years. Orthodontic measures begin as necessary from age 5.
- *Cleft lip, maxilla, and palate* are corrected between the fourth and sixth (to eighth) months of life using primary

veloplasty and cheiloplasty. The remaining cleft is closed between ages 12 and 14 years, and a final correction of the lip and nose is performed around the age of 16 years. Speech therapy begins at the age of 4 years, and orthodontic management with an obturator for the remaining cleft from the age of 6 years.

- *Cleft palate* is treated between the fifth and eighth months of life with a primary veloplasty. Speech therapy begins at age 4 years, and orthodontic management with an obturator for the remaining cleft from the age of 6 years. The remaining cleft is closed between ages 12 and 14 years.

Plastic procedures to improve speech: Plastic closure of the cleft is intended to improve the speech and articulation and is successful in ≈ 70 % of cases. Tissue available for the repair may be inadequate, so that velopharyngeal insufficiency persists in some cases and further procedures are necessary. Several reconstructive procedures are available for narrowing the pharynx. The principle of pharyngoplasty is to restore the function of the short, immobile, insufficient soft palate to as near normal as possible.

1. Pharyngoplasty is performed with formation of a velopharyngeal flap. The soft palate is brought into contact with the posterior pharyngeal wall using a soft-tissue flap (the Schönborn–Rosenthal or Sanvenero–Rosselli method).
2. Autogenous or synthetic material is implanted to achieve protrusion of the posterior wall of the pharynx, supplementing the Passavant bar by forming a prominence on the posterior pharyngeal wall during contraction of the superior constrictor muscle.
3. The soft palate is displaced posteriorly.

■ Tumors of the Mouth and Pharynx

■ Benign Tumors of the Oral Cavity, Including the Tongue and Oropharynx

In theory, all types of benign tumor can occur in this region, but they are rare. Some arise from the teeth and teeth-bearing organs and are therefore matters for the oral surgeon. The more common *benign connective-tissue tumors* include fibromas, lipomas, myxomas, chondromas, hemangiomas, lymphangiomas, neurinomas, and irritation fibromas—e. g., in malocclusion or absent teeth. The more common *benign epithelial tumors* include papilloma, keratoacanthoma, true adenoma, and pleomorphic adenoma.

The diagnosis is made by biopsy. Treatment is with the appropriate operation if the size of the tumor, its histologic

appearance, its growth tendency, or other properties make this advisable. Biopsy is not necessary for hemangiomas and lymphangiomas.

Specific Tumors

- *Hemangiomas and lymphangiomas* (see also p. 431) are usually congenital, and 90 % affect girls. The sites of predilection are the tongue, cheek, and parotid regions. The tumor may be so large that it becomes life-threatening due to recurrent bleeding, airway obstruction, or obstruction of eating. These tumors often resolve spontaneously within the first 2 years of life, and surgical removal should therefore be delayed if possible until age 3 or 4. Radiotherapy is not indicated, due to the risk that it may inhibit growth of the facial skeleton and later induce carcinoma. If the tumor is growing quickly, embolization of the feeding vessel arising from the external carotid artery may be attempted, or diethylstilbestrol can be given for a limited period.
- *Papillomas* in the mouth usually do not cause any symptoms. Treatment is only necessary if the lesions extend to the pharynx or larynx (see p. 318).
- *Lingual thyroid tumors,* see page 329.
- *Tumors of neighboring organs* may extend into the mouth and oropharynx. The most frequent are tumors of the parotid gland, which penetrate into the oropharynx via the retromandibular space, displacing the lateral pharyngeal wall, tonsil, or soft palate—e. g., pleomorphic adenoma, see page 429. Vascular tumors of the neck—e. g., carotid body tumors—can also cause similar pharyngeal displacement. Intrusion into the oral cavity by benign tumors of neighboring organs—e. g., tumors of the soft tissues of the cheek, nasopharynx, and maxillary sinus—is rare. On the other hand, malignant tumors extend from neighboring organs into the oral cavity more frequently than into the oropharynx.

■ Malignant Tumors of the Oral Cavity, Including Lip, Tongue, and Oropharynx

The great majority of these lesions are keratinizing squamous cell carcinomas. Nonkeratinizing and anaplastic carcinomas, as well as adenoid cystic carcinomas, are unusual, and adenocarcinomas rare. This group forms ≈ 5 % of all malignant tumors. Lymphoepithelioma (Schmincke–Regaud tumor) is a unique tumor, which today is regarded as an anaplastic carcinoma.

Connective-tissue tumors may rarely arise in the oral cavity and on the tongue—especially spindle cell sarcoma, myxosarcoma, malignant lymphoma, Hodgkin disease, plasmacytoma, malignant giant cell tumor, rhabdomyosarcoma, hemangioendothelioma, and malignant melanoma (**Figs. 3.56, 3.57a, b**). The prognosis varies widely even among carcinomas alone, depending on the site, extent, and histologic differentiation of the lesions. The TNM classification is used for documentation, choice of treatment, and prognosis. **Tables 3.10** and **3.11** summarize the staging classification for carcinomas of the lip, oral cavity, and pharynx.

Malignant skin tumors on the upper lip are usually basal cell cancers, and those on the lower lip are mostly squamous cell carcinomas.

Clinical Features. Any ulcer that does not heal rapidly and any hyperkeratotic area should be suspected of being an early malignancy. In the early stages, there is little or no pain.

With increasing size of the tumor, the patient reports pain and there is induration and infiltration of the underlying tissues and regional lymphadenopathy affecting the nodes in the submandibular triangle and the jugulodigastric and deep cervical groups.

Frequency. The lower lip and tongue account for ≈ 50 % of carcinomas in this area, the floor of the mouth for ≈ 10 %, the buccal mucosa for ≈ 10 %, the palate for ≈ 10 %, and the mandible and maxilla for ≈ 10 %. Some 10–15 % of malignant intraoral tumors develop in the tonsils.

The symptoms of carcinoma in the oral cavity affecting the floor of the mouth or the tongue are initially minimal, so that the diagnosis is often delayed. Later symptoms include an ulcer with raised edges, bleeding, and increasing pain radiating to the ear and neck, interference with speaking and swallowing, oral fetor, and sialorrhea. Late symptoms include involvement of the regional lymph nodes and finally loss of weight, due to increasing difficulty in eating. In the tongue, the most frequent site is the lateral margin. Tumors of the floor of the mouth around the opening of the submandibular duct are only slightly less frequent. Often, the first symptom patients notice is that their dentures are not fitting well.

Tumors of the oropharynx (base of the tongue and tonsils) cause symptoms earlier. These include

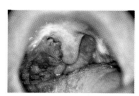

Fig. 3.56 Carcinoma of the right tonsil.

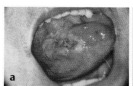
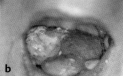

Fig. 3.57a, b Carcinoma of the lateral tongue.

Table 3.10 TNM clinical classification for carcinoma of the lip and oral cavity

T1	≤ 2 cm
T2	> 2 to 4 cm
T3	> 4 cm
T4a	*Lip:* through cortical bone, inferior alveolar nerve, floor of mouth, skin
	Oral cavity: through cortical bone, deep/extrinsic muscle of tongue, maxillary sinus, skin
T4b	Masticator space, pterygoid plates, skull base, internal carotid artery
N1	Ipsilateral single ≤ 3 cm
N2a	Ipsilateral single > 3 to 6 cm
N2b	Ipsilateral multiple ≤ 6 cm
N2c	Bilateral, contralateral ≤ 6 cm
N3	> 6 cm
MX	Distant metastasis cannot be assessed
M0	No distant metastasis
M1	Distant metastasis

From: F.L. Greene et al., *AJCC Cancer Staging Manual*, 6th ed. (New York: Springer, 2002) and UICC, *TNM Classification of Malignant Tumours*, 6th ed. (New York: Wiley-Liss, 2002).

Table 3.11   TNM clinical classification for carcinoma of the pharynx

Nasopharynx

T1	Nasopharynx
T2	Soft tissue
T2a	Oropharynx and/or nasal cavity without parapharyngeal extension
T2b	Tumor with parapharyngeal extension
T3	Bony structures and/or paranasal sinuses
T4	Intracranial, cranial nerves, infratemporal fossa, hypopharynx, orbit, masticator space
N1	Unilateral node(s) ≤ 6 cm, above supraclavicular fossa
N2	Bilateral node(s) ≤ 6 cm, above supraclavicular fossa
N3a	> 6 cm
N3b	In supraclavicular fossa

Oropharynx

T1–T3	See **Table 3.10**
T4a	Larynx, deep/extrinsic muscle of the tongue, medial pterygoid, hard palate, mandible
T4b	Lateral pterygoid muscle, pterygoid plates, lateral nasopharynx, skull base, carotid artery

Hypopharynx

T1	≤ 2 cm and limited to one subsite
T2	> 2 cm to 4 cm or more than one subsite
T3	> 4 cm or with hemilarynx fixation
T4a	Thyroid/cricoid cartilage, hyoid bone, thyroid gland, esophagus, central compartment of soft tissue
T4b	Prevertebral fascia, encases carotid artery, mediastinal structures

Oropharynx and hypopharynx

N1–N3	See **Table 3.10**

Pharynx—distant metastasis (M), see **Table 3.10**

From: F.L. Greene et al., *AJCC Cancer Staging Manual*, 6th ed. (New York: Springer, 2002) and UICC, *TNM Classification of Malignant Tumours*, 6th ed. (New York: Wiley-Liss, 2002).

increasingly severe pain on swallowing, which is often initially unilateral, thick indistinct speech, an ulcer on the tonsil, and increasing size of the tonsil, though this is not essential. Palpation shows induration of the tonsil or base of the tongue. There is oral fetor, bleeding, or bloodstained sputum. The tongue is fixed, and the patient has trismus, thickening of the neck and floor of the mouth, loses weight, and often has a typical pallor.

Note: Assessment of a tumor in this region requires palpation with the finger in addition to examination with the mirror.

Diagnosis. The possibility of a carcinoma must always be borne in mind in any patient with a palpable tissue induration in the oral cavity or on the tongue, or with a mucosal ulcer that does not heal rapidly. A biopsy should always be taken. Palpation of the lymph nodes is described on page 385. If the diagnosis remains uncertain, radiography and direct endoscopy should be undertaken.

Note: Any mucosal lesion persisting for more than 3 weeks with a roughened surface, change in color, ulceration, etc., should be suspected of being an early malignancy and requires biopsy for diagnosis.
The negative biopsy: If the clinical suspicion of malignancy persists, a negative biopsy should not be accepted, as the material may have been sampled from the edge of the tumor or from tumor-free tissue. Biopsy should therefore be repeated until a satisfactory histologic explanation is found for the clinical appearance.

Staging. The purpose of staging is to ascertain the precise extent of tumor spread for topographic diagnosis and to search for regional and distant metastases. For all tumors located in the head and neck region, the presence of local and regional metastases in the lymph nodes of the neck worsens the prognosis exponentially. Distant metastases occur in up to 20 % of cases—most commonly in the lungs, liver, and skeletal system.

CT and MRI make it possible to visualize the deep anatomic structures of the oropharynx and surrounding tissues (e. g., retropharyngeal lymph nodes, deep muscles of the tongue, prevertebral and paravertebral areas, and base of the skull). Ultrasonography can guide fine-needle aspiration for cytologic assessment of suspicious-appearing lymph nodes, the base of the tongue, or the floor of the mouth—e.g., to assess the depth of infiltration.

Searching for distant metastases requires at least a chest radiograph in two planes and ultrasound imaging of the upper abdomen. In view of the serious prognosis for patients with this type of tumor, especially lesions staged as T2–T4, CT or MRI imaging of the neck, chest, and upper abdomen should be carried out if possible. Radioisotope bone scans make it possible to identify skeletal metastases. Positron-emission tomography is the most modern method of detecting unidentified primary tumors in patients with the syndrome of carcinoma with unknown primary (CUP).

Differential diagnosis. This includes tertiary syphilis, tuberculosis, Vincent angina, and agranulocytosis.

Treatment. This is determined by the site and stage of the tumor (the details are described below). The principal goal is radical extirpation of the tumor. When metastasis is present in stage IIa disease, en-bloc tumor resection is the best way to prevent further seeding of tumor cells to the metastasis. The three most important points to consider in malignant tumor surgery are *radicality, functionality*, and *esthetics*.

Neck dissection is the essential surgical procedure to consider in the treatment of all malignant tumors of the head and neck (see Chapter 8, p. 405).

Carcinoma of the Lip

This tumor is much more common in Caucasians than in blacks. The male/female ratio is 30 : 1, and the average age is 60–65 years. The lower lip is affected in the large majority of patients. Exposure to ultraviolet irradiation is an important etiologic factor. Other factors are poor oral hygiene, smoking of cigarettes or pipes, and excessive alcohol consumption. Up to 95 % of tumors of the lower lip are well-differentiated squamous carcinomas. Basal cell carcinomas are more common on the upper lip than squamous cell carcinomas. About 85 % of malignant squamous carcinomas occur on the lower lip, 5 % on the upper lip, and 5 % affect both lips. Carcinoma of the *lower* lip usually grows very slowly to begin with and does not metastasize in the early stages. The prognosis is much less favorable in carcinoma of the *upper*

lip. Ninety-five percent of the tumors are squamous cell carcinomas.

Treatment. Surgery is slightly better than radiotherapy, with a 5-year survival rate of ≈ 85 % compared with ≈ 80 % for radiation. The principle of the operation is wedge excision of the required extent, followed by primary wound closure or reconstruction using various plastic procedures—e.g., an Abbe–Estlander flap. A complete or suprahyoid neck dissection (see p. 405) may also be necessary, depending on the tumor stage.

Results. Most carcinomas of the lip are highly differentiated and are identified in the early stages. With appropriate treatment, the outcome is usually good. Control of local tumor growth is achieved in 78–99 % of cases, depending on the initial tumor stage. Local recurrences are observed in less than 4 % of T1 tumors and in less than 20 % of T2 tumors. Tumor recurrence in regional lymph nodes is observed in 4–27 % of patients.

The tumor-specific survival rate for all patients with cancer of the lip, including those undergoing salvage therapies, is 85 % at 5 years.

Depending on the initial treatment, salvage therapy (e.g., surgery or radiotherapy) is an option that often results in good local and regional control of tumor growth.

Carcinomas of the Oral Cavity and Body of the Tongue

This is a fairly frequent site for carcinoma. The male/female ratio is 70 : 30, but it depends on the site and race. The average age is 50–60 years. There is a statistically significant history of smoking and alcohol abuse in these patients; ≈ 85 % have this history and only 15 % do not. Further suspected etiologic factors include poor dental care and poor oral hygiene. Ninety-five percent are well-differentiated squamous carcinomas. Seventy-five percent are located in the gutter between the lower alveolus and the lateral border of the tongue, the so-called drainage area of the mouth. The lateral border is the part of the tongue most frequently affected (in 50 % of patients), and 90 % of these tumors infiltrate and show superficial ulceration.

Tumors of the oral cavity and the anterior two-thirds of the tongue metastasize to the submandibular, superior subgastric, and middle jugular cervical lymph nodes, or more rarely to the deep cervical lymph nodes. The frequency of lymphatic metastasis increases with the stage of the tumor. With T1

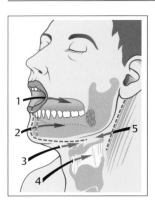

Fig. 3.58 Routes of access for tumors of the mouth and pharynx. **1**, Transoral; **2**, temporary mandibulotomy; **3**, suprahyoid median pharyngotomy; **4**, subhyoid median pharyngotomy; **5**, lateral pharyngotomy.

tumors, it occurs in 10–15% of patients, with T2 tumors in ≈ 30%, with T3 tumors in 35–40%, and with T4 tumors in 55–75%. Gingival tumors and those in the mucosa of the cheek have an even higher rate of regional lymph-node metastasis. There is a very high rate of lymph-node metastases depending on the site of the primary tumor. More than 50% of tongue tumors produce lymph-node metastases, but only 10% of tumors of the hard palate do so. Bilateral lymph-node metastases can occur, especially in tumors of the tongue and the anterior part of the floor of the mouth.

Treatment. In the early stage, T1 (see **Table 3.10**), surgery and radiotherapy are equally effective. Surgery is preferable for larger tumors (T2 and T3) or when lymph-node metastases are present. The prognosis is unfavorable in patients with stage T3 or bone invasion, where combinations of surgery and radiotherapy, possibly combined with chemotherapy, are certain to produce the best results.

T1 tumors: Circumcision or laser surgery of the tumor with a safety margin of 1 cm is usually possible without producing a functional defect. T2 or T3 tumors can be treated with laser surgery or temporary division or partial resection of the mandible, and reconstruction of the defect with a distant flap (pectoralis major flap or microvascular–myofascial radialis flap) is usually required. For T4 tumors, a combination of surgical measures with simultaneous chemoradiotherapy sufficient to permit an acceptable quality of life is indicated.

Principles of surgery: Various routes of access can be used, depending on the site of the tumor (**Fig. 3.58**). The tumor must be removed with a wide margin in three dimensions.

Several techniques are available for a tongue carcinoma depending on its extent, including partial or subtotal glossectomy with partial mandibulectomy. A radical neck dissection is performed. Temporary median division of the lower lip and mandible is often necessary to provide satisfactory access.

The soft-tissue defect resulting from excision of an oropharyngeal malignancy can be closed with regional pedicle flaps from the temporalis muscle, myocutaneous flaps (pectoralis muscle), or free tissue transfer with radialis flaps and microsurgical anastomosis of the blood vessels.

Results. Tumors recur in 10–20% of T1 tumors and ≈ 40% of T2 tumors. The tumor-specific 5-year survival rate for patients with T1 tumors is 95%, and for those with T2 tumors it is 65%. For those with T3 and T4 tumors, the prognosis for survival at 5 years drops to only 40%. These tumors should be treated with a combination of surgery and postoperative radiation or primary simultaneous chemoradiotherapy.

Patients with tumors at this site often require postoperative care for the many attendant problems such as difficulty with speech, mastication, swallowing, tube feeding, and difficulties with false teeth.

Carcinoma of the Tonsil or Base of the Tongue

These are relatively frequent tumors, with a male/female ratio of 4 : 1. The age of predilection is 50–70 years. The history also often shows combined alcohol abuse and smoking. Ninety percent are squamous cell carcinomas, and they are more often well differentiated rather than poorly differentiated. Sixty percent of patients have lymph-node metastases, of which 15% are bilateral. Seven percent have distant metastases affecting the lung, skeleton, and liver. A second carcinoma affecting some other part of the upper aerodigestive tract, either at the same time or later, is relatively frequent. The pathways of spread of this tumor are shown in **Fig. 3.59**.

Treatment. The method of choice is surgery combined with radiotherapy. Surgery is performed either before or immediately after radiotherapy, to a dose of 60–70 Gy, and requires removal of the tonsil, the base of the tongue, the wall of the hypopharynx, the soft palate, and the ascending ramus of the mandible, with a good margin, if these structures are affected or suspicious. Neck dissection is also performed. The soft-tissue defect is repaired with a pedicled regional flap from the temporalis muscle, neck, or chest or with free tissue transfer and microvessel anastomosis (**Fig. 3.60**)

The principles of management described above may apply to all patients, but they will vary according to the size of the tumor and also the individual unit that is administering the treatment. In reality, the therapy for each individual patient is discussed at a multidisciplinary team meeting after MRI of the neck and fine-needle aspiration of any palpable lymph nodes. The following treatment recommendations are observed in the regional head and neck cancer centre at University Hospital Aintree in Liverpool (United Kingdom):

- Small tonsil tumors are treated with local wide excision or laser excision, followed by radiotherapy.
- For a medium-sized carcinoma of the tonsil, good results with minimal functional problems follow extended local excision/laser excision with partial excision of the tongue base after controlling the lingual artery during a neck dissection. The defect is allowed to heal by secondary intention.
- Patients with large tumors (T3, T4) are offered chemoradiotherapy if they are fit enough. Cetuximab, a chimeric monoclonal antibody that inhibits epidermal growth factor receptors (EGFRs), may also be recommended. Salvage surgery is seldom successful. There is currently controversy as to whether all patients with this disorder should be treated with chemoradiotherapy.

- The neck disease is treated with selective neck dissection, followed in some cases by radiotherapy.
- It should be noted some that of these patients may present with a neck mass, and there may well be an occult primary tumor within the tongue base.

Results. The most important prognostic factors are the extent of the tumor and involvement of cervical lymph nodes. Radical tumor surgery followed by radiotherapy alone produces overall 5-year survival

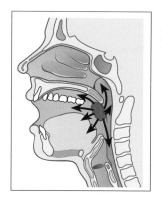

Fig. 3.59 Directions of spread of a malignant tumor of the tonsil.

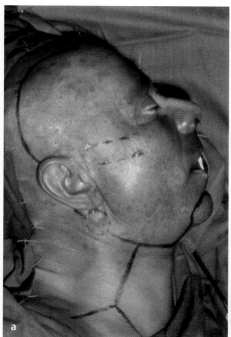
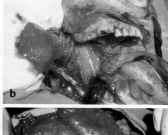
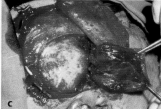
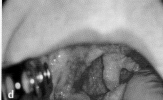

Fig. 3.60a–d Steps in tumor surgery for carcinoma of the right tonsil and reconstruction of the defect using a temporalis muscle flap.
a The incision line is marked for opening the cheek and severing the mandible, right-sided neck dissection, and elevation of the temporal muscle flap.
b The intraoperative field after removal of the tumor and biopsy to examine the cut edges using rapid section diagnosis.
c Elevation of the temporalis muscle flap.
d View of the healed temporal muscle flap 4 months after surgery.

rates of 35–40 %. When bilateral cervical lymph-node metastases are present, the 5-year survival rate falls to 10 %. For T1/T2 N0 M0 tumors, the 5-year survival rate is 75–80 %. Simultaneous chemoradiotherapy improves the prognosis for inoperable patients.

Mesenchymal tumors in this region are usually radiosensitive, as are lymphoepithelial tumors and anaplastic carcinomas. These tumors are therefore not suitable for surgery.

■ Benign Tumors of the Nasopharynx

Benign tumors of the nasopharynx are rare. Nasopharyngeal angiofibroma is the most frequent.

Nasopharyngeal Angiofibroma

This occurs exclusively in males, beginning about the age of 10 years. The tumor is said to resolve spontaneously after the age of 20–25 years, but this is *not* true of all cases.

Clinical Features. These include increasing nasal obstruction, purulent rhinosinusitis due to obstruction of the nasopharynx, severe spontaneous bleeding from the nose or pharynx, rhinolalia clausa, headaches, obstruction of the ostium of the eustachian tube causing conductive deafness, middle ear catarrh, and purulent otitis media. Posterior rhinoscopy shows occlusion of the nasopharynx by a smooth, grayish-red tumor that may be lobulated and have offshoots penetrating the choana or Rosenmüller fossa. The surface of the tumor often shows pronounced vessels. In later stages, there may be deformity of the face and nasal skeleton, protrusion of the cheek, and possibly exophthalmos. Finally, the patient has difficulty in eating. The tumor is firm to palpation.

Pathogenesis. The typical nasopharyngeal angiofibroma is histologically benign but clinically destructive because of its expansive and invasive growth. It is a very coarse angiofibroma rich in fibrous tissue that arises from the roof of the nasopharynx or within the pterygoid fossa. The tumor usually arises from the pterygomaxillary fissure and gains attachment to the soft tissues of the nasopharynx. It grows relatively quickly. After filling the nasopharynx, the tumor sends offshoots into the nasal sinuses, upper jaw, sphenoid sinus, pterygopalatine fossa, cheek, ethmoid sinuses, and orbit. Finally, it may extend into the cranial cavity after eroding the base of the skull.

Diagnosis. This is made by transnasal endoscopy, examination with the mirror or nasopharyngoscope loupe, and CT or MRI. Angiography of the carotid and internal carotid artery is indicated for an extensive tumor. Superselective angiography of the branches of the carotid is performed to allow therapeutic embolization (**Fig. 3.61a–d**).

Differential diagnosis. The differential diagnosis should include hypertrophied adenoids, choanal polyp (which is soft and does not bleed), lymphoma, chordoma, and teratoma.

> **Note:** A biopsy should be done with extreme care, due to the risk of massive bleeding, and probably will not yield accurate information on the hemodynamic activity of the tumor. Only MRI, magnetic resonance angiography, and conventional angiography can supply this information.
> A nasopharyngeal tumor in an individual between the ages of 10 and 25 years for which there is a suspicion that it may be a juvenile nasopharyngeal angiofibroma should only be submitted to biopsy in a hospital, and preparation should be made to proceed immediately to further surgery if massive bleeding occurs. However, angiography provides a characteristic diagnostic picture.

Treatment. The ideal method of treatment is surgery. Different approaches are available: midfacial degloving, transmaxillary access, or transpalatal access. Extensive tumors may need a craniotomy and mandibular osteotomy (**Fig. 3.62a, b**). For smaller tumors, endoscopic techniques are now possible. Preoperative embolization of the feeding vessels may be appropriate in all of these tumors. Embolization should ideally be done within 48 h before surgery (**Fig. 3.61a–d**). Radiotherapy is an effective means of treatment, with a success rate of up to 80 %.

Rare Benign Nasopharyngeal Tumors

Chordoma. This develops from the notochord and occurs mainly in men between 20 and 50 years of age. It grows very slowly and erodes the base of the skull, causing lesions of the cranial nerves, and it may also extend into the sphenoid sinus.

Treatment: Surgery should be performed if possible, but there is a considerable risk of recurrence. Radiotherapy is only palliative. Metastases to the neck are said to occur.

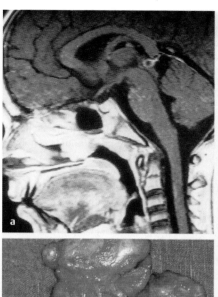

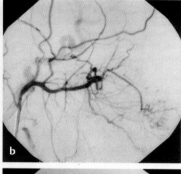

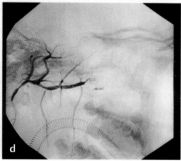

Fig. 3.61a–d
a Nasopharyngeal angiofibroma of the posterior nose in a boy.
b Selective digital subtraction angiography.
c The excised tumor specimen.
d Preoperative embolization of the tumor vessel.

Other types of tumor. Teratoma, dermoid, fibroma, and lipoma.

Treatment: Surgery should be undertaken if the patient has symptoms.

■ Malignant Tumors of the Nasopharynx

The most frequent of these relatively rare tumors is squamous cell carcinoma, together with lymphoepithelial tumor, which is now regarded as an anaplastic tumor. These two together constitute 75 % of tumors in this region. Tumors in children include lymphoma, plasmacytoma, and Burkitt B cell lymphoma in certain parts of Africa. The latter is thought to be due to the Epstein–Barr virus (see p. 262). Nasopharyngeal tumors affect men twice as commonly as women.

Clinical Features. These include nasal obstruction, disorders of tubal aeration causing unilateral conductive deafness, middle ear discharge, middle ear effusion, bloodstained purulent nasal discharge, and headaches felt deep within the skull. Lymphnode metastases are frequent and widespread in 90 % of cases. Enlarged jugulodigastric lymph nodes on one or both sides are often the first symptom that brings the patient to the doctor. Lymph-node metastases may also be retropharyngeal and in the

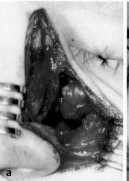

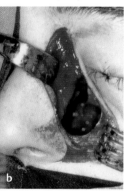

Fig. 3.62 Operation for a large nasopharyngeal angiofibroma via an open approach with lateral rhinotomy, (**a**) before and (**b**) after removal of the tumor.

nuchal area. The primary tumor may remain undiscovered despite careful endoscopic searching, as it grows concealed beneath the mucosa. There is gradual protrusion and loss of mobility of the soft palate and increasing, often unilateral, pain in the head and face (trigeminal nerve). Exophthalmos, oculomotor paralyses of cranial nerves III, IV, and VI, involvement of V, IX, X, XI, and XII as well, oral fetor, and massive nosebleeds occur. Blood-borne metastases to the lung, liver, and skeleton are quite common.

Diagnosis. This is made by rhinoscopy, nasopharyngoscopy, palpation, retraction of the soft palate, and biopsy. Tomograms in the anterior, posterior, and lateral views and CT scans elucidate involvement of the base of the skull. Angiograms may also be needed. The roof of the nasopharynx and Rosenmüller fossa require particular attention, as these are often the site of origin of this tumor. Demonstration of Epstein–Barr viral antigens and antibodies has become extremely important clinically—making early detection of an asymptomatic recurrence possible, for example, and allowing early treatment with afterloading therapy or laser surgery (Ho:YAG laser).

Treatment. Radiotherapy is the method of choice for mesenchymal tumors and anaplastic carcinomas, as they are very radiosensitive. It may be combined with chemotherapy. Surgery should only be considered for very small circumscribed nasopharyngeal tumors, combined with electrocoagulation, if it can be shown that the tumor does not extend into the eustachian tube or the base of the skull. Postoperative radiotherapy should be administered. Advanced carcinomas are treated solely with radiotherapy, at times combined with chemotherapy for the primary tumor. Regional lymphnode metastases may be treated with therapeutic neck dissection, provided that the primary tumor has been destroyed.

Prognosis. This depends on the tumor stage, histologic diagnosis, tumor extension, and presence of metastases. Lymphoepitheliomas (Schmincke–Regaud tumors) have a 5-year survival rate of 40 %; for other malignant tumors in this region the figure is ≈ 20 %.

■ **Tumors of the Hypopharynx**

See p. 328.

■ **Obstructive Sleep-related Breathing Disorders**

Thomas Versey

In the achievement-oriented societies of industrialized countries, nonrestorative sleep constitutes a socioeconomic problem of considerable magnitude. The problem is complex. The International Classification of Sleep Disorders, Revised (ICSD-R) distinguishes more than 80 kinds of sleep disorder. As only a few of these are caused by otorhinolaryngology disorders, the present discussion focuses only on obstructive sleep-related breathing disorders (SRBD) that have their pathophysiologic roots in the upper airways.

Clinically, three types of obstructive SRBD can be distinguished:

1. *Primary snoring (benign snoring, snoring without sleep apnea)*: At worst, the noisy breathing may lead to tension in the patient's social environment, without physically compromising the patient.
2. *Obstructive sleep apnea syndrome (OSAS)*: At least four percent of males and 2 % of females are affected. OSAS is characterized by repeated episodes of obstruction of the upper airways during sleep, with repetitive pauses in breathing, usually associated with oxygen desaturation of the peripheral blood. This results in an elevated risk of cardiovascular disease (stroke, heart attack, arterial hypertension, atherosclerosis) and increased mortality. Snoring, excessive daytime somnolence, and drop in functional performance capacity are the cardinal symptoms of OSAS.
3. *Upper airway resistance syndrome (UARS)*: This is a form of SRBD in which repetitive increases in resistance to airflow in the upper airway lead to brief arousals and daytime somnolence. As UARS is difficult to diagnose, the new version of the ICSD-R does not include UARS any longer and subsumes it under OSAS.

Pathogenesis. The main sites of obstruction are the segments between the choanae and larynx. This region is held open only by voluntary muscles. As sleep deepens, the muscle tone decreases, which in sleep apnea patients leads to an imbalance between the vacuum during inspiration (suction effect) and muscle tone. The resulting collapse of the airways is compounded by pressure exerted by the tissues surrounding the airways. This third factor is determined in large part by fatty deposits associated with obesity or by anatomical peculiarities—e. g., hyperplasia of the tonsils, soft palate, or root of the tongue. As it is so widespread, obesity is the main cofactor in the pathogenesis of OSAS.

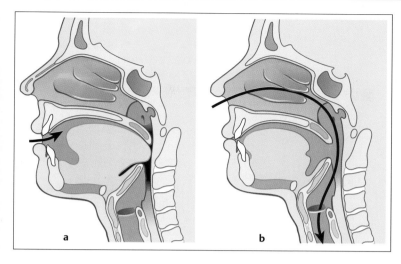

Fig. 3.63a, b   The principle of intermittent nasal respiratory therapy with continuous positive airway pressure (CPAP).

Definition. The definition of OSAS depends on the number of episodes of disordered breathing per hour of sleep. A distinction is made between complete absence of breathing, known as apnea, and phases of shallow and/or slowed breathing, known as hypopnea.

The symptoms of UARS, are identical to those of OSAS, but without obstructive apnea or hypopnea. The leading symptom consists of arousals from sleep caused by disordered respiration.

Diagnosis. Currently, the diagnosis is based on a typical case history, including quantitative assessment of daytime sleepiness, clinical findings, and sleep laboratory findings (indexes of apnea, hypopnea, and arousal).

- *Step 1:* Case history, including a standardized sleep laboratory questionnaire.
- *Step 2:* Physical examination (electrocardiography, blood pressure, pulmonary function, and otorhinolaryngology parameters).
- *Step 3:* Assessment of nocturnal cardiorespiratory parameters without measurements of sleep (sleep apnea screening).
- *Step 4:* Polysomnography (nocturnal measurement of respiratory and sleep parameters).

Treatment. Only since the early 1980s has treatment of OSAS using conservative approaches, technical apparatus, and surgery been used on a large scale. The purpose is to reduce the number of inspiratory standstills, snoring, daytime somnolence,

and cardiovascular risk factors, in order to improve the patient's quality of life. Treatment is individualized, depending on sleep laboratory assessment (severity of the condition) and otorhinolaryngology findings.

Conservative treatment: There is no effective pharmacological treatment for either OSAS or primary snoring. Muscular relaxants and sedative agents are sometimes employed. Avoidance of alcoholic beverages and smoking prior to going to bed and weight normalization are important supportive measures in OSAS.

Technical aids:
- Nocturnal respiratory therapy with positive pressure (continuous positive airway pressure, CPAP). The principle is to provide pneumatic support for the upper airways (**Fig. 3.63**). Although the initial success rate approaches 100 %, 30–40 % of the patients later discontinue respiratory therapy because of side effects.
- Oral appliances. Tongue-restraining devices push the tongue forward. Success rates of 50–70 % have been reported for mild OSAS.

Surgical treatment: The classification of surgical treatment approaches is based on the definition of three levels in the upper airways (**Fig. 3.64**). Level 1 is the nose, level 2 the soft palate, and level 3 the base of the tongue and the hypopharynx.

Surgery of the nose (level 1): Improvement of nasal breathing leads to a better quality of sleep. A reduction in

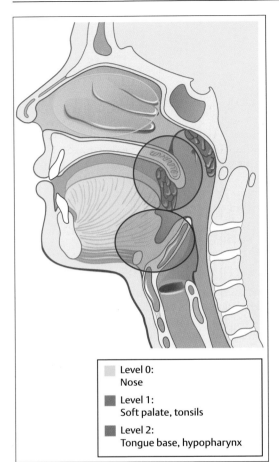

Level 0:
Nose

Level 1:
Soft palate, tonsils

Level 2:
Tongue base, hypopharynx

Fig. 3.64 Classification of upper airway obstruction at various levels.

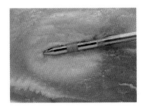

Fig. 3.65 The effects of radiofrequency (RF) therapy on tissue (reproduced with permission of Olympus Celon).

primary snoring is achieved in only ≈ 40 % of patients, and OSAS is not permanently healed in any.

Surgery of the nasopharyngeal region: In children, 85–90 % of OSAS cases can be cured by combined palatine tonsillectomy and adenoidectomy.

Surgery of the palatine tonsils (level 2): In children, hypertrophy of the palatine tonsils and the adenoids is the most common cause of OSAS. Hypertrophy of the palatine tonsils occurs much more rarely in adults. Tonsillectomy is an operation at the level of the soft palate that clearly achieves more space in the upper airway. For this reason, it is often used to treat OSAS.

Surgery of the soft palate (level 2): A uvulopalatopharyngoplasty (UPPP) is often performed in combination with tonsillectomy. The principle of the operation consists of muscle-sparing excision of excess mucosa (by conventional surgery) and forward displacement of the palatopharyngeal arch by appropriate suturing. This results in a tendency toward improvement in 50 % of OSAS patients and long-term improvement in 70 % of patients with primary snoring. An alternative option only for primary snoring or mild OSAS is radiofrequency (RF) surgery, in which adjustable current is applied using needle electrodes (**Fig. 3.65**), resulting in shrinking and stiffening of the soft palate.

Surgery of the tongue (level 3):
- Application of RF to the base of the tongue (cure rate ≈ 33 %) in mild to moderate OSAS.
- Hyoid suspension—i. e., fixation of the hyoid to the thyroid cartilage or the mandible, resulting in forward displacement of the hyoid and subsequent enlargement of the retrolingual air passage.
- Laser-assisted resection of the lingual tonsil.

Oral surgery: Maxillomandibular transposition osteotomy has a success rate of more than 90 %. It consists of forward displacement of the maxilla and mandible, resulting in enlargement of the air passages, particularly in patients with dysgnathias.

4   Larynx and Hypopharynx

Larynx—Applied Anatomy and Physiology

■ Basic Anatomy and Physiology

■ Embryology

The larynx develops from a two-part anlage: the supraglottis develops from a buccopharyngeal bud, and the glottis and subglottis from a tracheobronchial bud. This is clinically significant in the postnatal period. The nerves of the pharyngeal arches are branches of the vagus nerve.

During the course of life, the larynx descends from about the level of the second vertebra at birth, depending on the sex, to about the level of the fifth cervical vertebra in the adult.

■ Anatomy

The laryngeal skeleton consists of the *thyroid, cricoid,* and *arytenoid* cartilages, which are hyaline cartilage; the *epiglottis,* which is fibrous cartilage; and the fibroelastic accessory cartilages of Santorini (corniculate cartilage) and Wrisberg (cuneiform cartilage), which have no function.

Calcification and ossification of the thyroid cartilage begin at the time of puberty. Ossification of the cricoid and arytenoid cartilage follows somewhat later. The female larynx calcifies later than that of the male. On radiography, it is often difficult to distinguish the calcified parts of the laryngeal framework from bony foreign bodies.

Internal and external ligaments and membranes connect the cartilages and stabilize the covering soft tissue.

For clinical purposes, the laryngeal cavity is divided into three compartments (**Fig. 4.1, Table 4.1**):

- Supraglottis.
- Glottis.
- Subglottis.

The *vocal fold* has a cartilaginous part, which is the arytenoid cartilage, and a membranous part. The latter includes the vocalis muscle, the lamina propria, and the epithelium (**Fig. 4.2a, b**). The length of the membranous part of the vocal fold is 0.3 cm in the newborn, 1.0–1.4 cm in women, and 1.5–2.0 cm in men. The *glottis* is the space between the free edges of the vocal folds. The *transglottic space* is illustrated in **Fig. 4.1** and described in **Table 4.1** (see **Fig. 4.13**).

> **Note:** Carcinoma occurs almost exclusively in the intermembranous part of the glottis, whereas intubation granuloma and contact granuloma caused by vocal overuse mainly affect the intercartilaginous part (see pp. 309–311, and **Figs. 4.19, 4.20**).

Superiorly, the larynx is limited by the free edge of the epiglottis, the aryepiglottic fold, and the interarytenoid notch. *Inferiorly,* the lower edge of the cricoid cartilage marks the junction with the trachea (see **Fig. 4.1**).

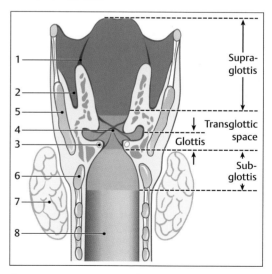

Fig. 4.1 Compartments and individual structures in the larynx. **1**, The aryepiglottic fold, forming the boundary between the larynx and the hypopharynx; **2**, the piriform sinus, which belongs to the hypopharynx; **3**, vocal ligament; **4**, anterior commissure; **5**, thyroid cartilage; **6**, cricoid cartilage; **7**, thyroid gland; **8**, trachea.

Table 4.1 Classification and terminology of the laryngeal cavity

Supraglottic space	Epilarynx	Laryngeal surface of the epiglottis + aryepiglottic fold + arytenoid
	Vestibule	Between the epiglottis and the rima glottidis
	Aditus	Epilarynx + vestibule
Glottal space	Vocal folds and 1 cm inferiorly	
Subglottic space	Down to the lower border of the cricoid cartilage	
"Transglottic space"	Glottis + ventricle + vestibular folds	

The *thyroid cartilage* is united by a joint with the *cricoid cartilage.* Rocking and slight gliding movements occur at this joint. The muscles, ligaments, and membranes between the cartilages allow functionally important movements between different parts of the larynx.

External ligaments and connective-tissue membranes anchor the larynx to the surrounding structures. The most important membranes include the following.

- The thyrohyoid membrane holds the opening for the superior laryngeal artery and vein and for the internal branch of the superior laryngeal nerve, which provides the sensory supply to the larynx above the vocal folds.
- The cricothyroid membrane is the point where the airway comes closest to the skin; this is the site for laryngotomy (see p. 355).
- The cricotracheal ligament provides attachment to the trachea.

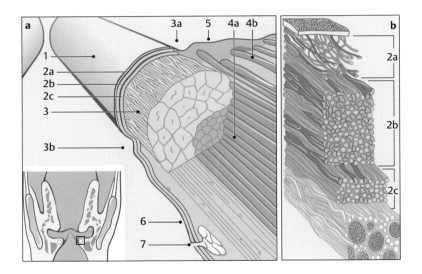

Fig. 4.2a, b **a** A three-dimensional section through the membranous part of the vocal fold, magnified from the frontal section through the larynx as shown in the inset in the lower left corner. **1**, Stratified squamous epithelium; **2a**, superficial layer of the lamina propria; **2b**, intermediate layer of the lamina propria; **2c**, deep layer of the lamina propria, **2b** and **2c** forming the vocal ligament; **3**, vocal ligament enveloping the vocalis muscle; **3a**, superior arcuate line; **3b**, inferior arcuate line; **4a**, medial part of the thyroarytenoid muscle—i. e., the vocalis muscle; **4b**, lateral part of the thyroarytenoid muscle; **5**, epithelium of the laryngeal ventricle (Morgagni ventricle), consisting of cylindrical ciliated epithelium and islets of squamous epithelial cells; **6**, subglottic respiratory cylindrical ciliated epithelial zone; **7**, mucous gland. (Adapted from T. von Lanz and W. Wachsmuth, *Praktische Anatomie. Ein Lehr- und Hilfsbuch der Anatomischen Grundlagen ärztlichen Handelns*, 2nd ed., Berlin: Springer, 1950.) **b** Enlarged schematic drawing of the lamina propria. The numbers correspond with those in **a**. (Adapted from M. Hirano and K. Sato, *Histological color atlas of the human larynx*, San Diego: Singular, 1993.)

The internal ligaments and connective-tissue membranes—e. g., the conus elasticus and thyroepiglottic ligament—connect the cartilaginous parts of the larynx to each other.

The internal muscles and the one external muscle act synergistically and antagonistically to control the functions of the larynx. They open and close the glottis and place the vocal folds under tension (**Fig. 4.3**). This interplay explains the different positions of the vocal folds in paralysis of the recurrent laryngeal nerve or of the external branch of the superior laryngeal nerve (**Table 4.2**).

!

Note: There is only *one* muscle that opens the glottis, the posterior cricoarytenoid. The muscles that close it are clearly in the majority. The ratio of their relative power is 1 : 3. Only the interarytenoid muscle, with a pars obliqua and a pars transversa, is unpaired; all other muscles are paired.

Nerve supply. The nerve supply of the larynx is bilateral, from the superior laryngeal and recurrent laryngeal nerves, which both arise from the vagus nerve (see **Fig. 4.11**).

The *superior laryngeal nerve* divides into a sensory internal branch, which supplies the interior of the larynx down into the glottis, and an external branch, which provides the motor supply to the external cricothyroid muscle.

The *recurrent laryngeal nerve* provides motor supply to the rest of the ipsilateral internal laryngeal musculature and to the contralateral interarytenoid muscle. In addition, it provides sensation to the laryngeal mucosa inferior to the glottic cleft.

The left recurrent laryngeal nerve loops around the aortic arch to reach the larynx in the groove between the trachea and the esophagus. The right recurrent laryngeal nerve passes around the subclavian artery and then runs upward between the trachea and the esophagus.

Both recurrent laryngeal nerves enter the larynx at the inferior horn of the thyroid cartilage. The relations of this nerve to the inferior thyroid artery and thyroid gland are important in surgical anatomy (see p. 303).

When one is diagnosing paralysis of the recurrent laryngeal nerve, pathology should be sought from the skull base around the jugular foramen, along the cervical course of the nerve, and within the chest and mediastinum. Causes of recurrent

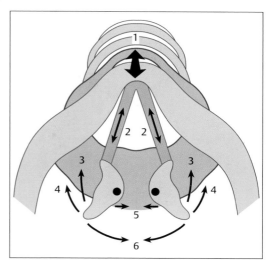

Fig. 4.3 Directions of pull in the laryngeal musculature. **1**, Cricothyroid muscle (the anticus muscle); **2**, medial part of the thyroarytenoid muscle (the vocalis muscle); **3**, lateral part of the thyroarytenoid muscle; **4**, lateral cricoarytenoid muscle (lateralis muscle); **5**, interarytenoid or transverse muscle; **6**, posterior cricoarytenoid muscle (posticus muscle).

Table 4.2 Functions of the laryngeal musculature

Function	Muscle
Opening of the glottis, abduction of the vocal folds	Posterior cricoarytenoid muscle (posticus muscle)
Closure of the glottis, adduction of the vocal folds	Lateral cricoarytenoid muscle
	Transverse and oblique arytenoid muscle
	Thyroarytenoid muscle, lateral part
Tension of the vocal folds	(Anterior) cricothyroid muscle
	Thyroarytenoid muscle, medial part (vocalis muscle)

paralysis include metastases, malignant lymphoma, malignant goiter, esophageal carcinoma, tuberculous lymphadenopathy, aortic and carotid aneurysms, and pulmonary hypertension.

Blood supply. The blood supply to the larynx is divided by the glottis into two areas.

The supraglottic blood supply from the superior laryngeal artery originates from the external caro-

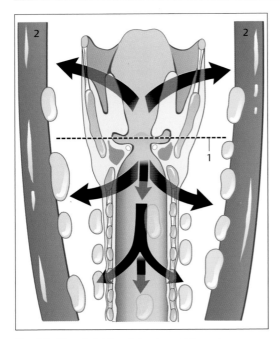

Fig. 4.4 The glottal lymph barrier, which produces supraglottic and subglottic lymph flow. The first supraglottic lymph-node stations are the inconstant prelaryngeal node and the upper deep cervical nodes. The first subglottic node stations are the pretracheal and paratracheal and lower deep jugular lymph nodes. **1**, Glottal lymph barrier; **2**, internal jugular vein.

tid artery, whereas the subglottic supply from the inferior laryngeal artery derives from the thyrocervical trunk of the subclavian artery.

Venous drainage passes superiorly via the superior thyroid vein to the internal jugular vein and inferiorly via the inferior thyroid vein to the left brachiocephalic vein.

Lymphatic drainage. The lymphatic drainage of the larynx (**Fig. 4.4**) is very important clinically.

The free margin of the vocal fold has no lymphatic capillaries. The superior surface of the vocal fold and the floor of the ventricle have several lymphatic vessels running parallel to the free margin of the vocal fold.

On the other hand, the supraglottic space has a rich lymphatic network. A very dense and partly multilayered capillary network is found in the ventricular fold and ventricle. The supraglottic lymphatic pathway converges on the anterior insertion of the aryepiglottic fold and leaves in smaller collections of vessels along the neurovascular bundle

of the larynx. Submucous and preepiglottic horizontal anastomoses are found in the midline of the larynx and are responsible for bilateral and contralateral metastases in carcinoma.

Between the free margin of the vocal fold and the upper border of the cricoid cartilage, the cranial margin of the subglottic region, lies the inferior surface of the vocal fold. It carries lymphatic capillaries. The posterior commissure serves as an important interconnection site for lymphatic capillaries between the various regions of the larynx.

The subglottic capillary network is not as dense as the supraglottic network. Bilateral and contralateral invasion of the lymph nodes is possible via the pretracheal and paratracheal lymph nodes. The additional drainage to the peritracheal and mediastinal lymph nodes is clinically important.

The laryngeal lymph is ultimately collected into the superior and inferior deep cervical lymph nodes.

Mucosal lining. The mucosal lining of the larynx is adapted to its special position at the junction of the respiratory and digestive tracts. Stratified squamous epithelium, partly keratinized, covers the laryngeal surface of the epiglottis, the vestibular folds, the vestibule of the larynx, and the vocal folds. Ciliated columnar epithelium covers the remaining parts of the mucosal surface.

The lamina propria has three layers. The deep and intermediate layers form the vocal ligament, and the superficial layer is also known as the *Reinke space*. This is a closed cleft beneath the epithelium of the vocal fold, with no glands or lymphatic capillaries. It is clinically important in relation to Reinke edema (see p. 319).

■ Physiology

Phonation. The larynx can only form a sound when the vocal folds vibrate. Together with the covering epithelium, the lamina propria is essential for voice production. The sound is modified by the movements of the pharynx, palate, tongue, and lips to form speech.

Vocal function, vocal range, tone amplification, timbre, and resonance are described on pp. 332–334.

Hoarseness is the result of noise formed by endolaryngeal turbulence in the airstream and irregularities in the normally periodic vibrations of the vocal folds.

Respiration. The vocal folds are in the respiratory position; the glottis is open and is under reflex control, which depends on gas exchange and acid–base balance.

The sphincter function is the oldest phylogenetic function of the larynx (**Table 4.3**).

Protection of the lower respiratory tract. The base of the tongue, posterior pharyngeal wall, and faucial pillars are involved in swallowing. The swallowing reflex, transmitted in the glossopharyngeal nerve, ensures cessation of respiration and contraction of the aryepiglottic folds, vocal folds, and vestibular folds, and tilting of the epiglottis by the thyroepiglottic muscle. Simultaneously, the suprahyoid musculature contracts, drawing the larynx anteriorly and superiorly by 2–3 cm.

Experience with surgical removal of the epiglottis shows that this structure is only of limited significance for protecting the larynx. An intact sensory nerve supply to the mucosa of the laryngeal aditus from the internal branch of the superior laryngeal nerve is much more important. It controls reflex muscular contraction.

The cough reflex is stimulated by particles of food touching the vestibular folds or penetrating through the larynx. It consists of a deep reflex inspiration with the larynx open. The glottis closes with rising intrathoracic pressure and then opens suddenly with an explosive expiratory stream, and the foreign body is coughed out.

!

Note: The larynx is a receptor field for other vasovagal reflexes. Mechanical irritation of the internal surface of the larynx can induce arrhythmia, bradycardia, and cardiac arrest. Satisfactory mucosal anesthesia must be ensured during endolaryngeal procedures. Particular care is necessary during repeated attempts at intubation, prolonged laryngoscopy, and laryngotracheal obstruction by foreign bodies, etc. The vagal reflex can be blocked by atropine and increased by opiates. Reflex irritability is increased in smokers.

Thoracic fixation. The respiratory system is closed off by the glottis to provide mechanical assistance during several bodily functions—notably coughing, defecation, micturition, vomiting, and parturition. In addition, the pectoral muscles are supplemented during chin-ups, while digging, and in breathing during asthma attacks.

Table 4.3   Functions of the larynx

Phonation	
Respiration	
Protection of the lower airway	Closure of the aditus on swallowing
	Closure of the glottis
	Reflex respiratory arrest
	Cough reflex
Glottal closure with thoracic fixation and Valsalva maneuver, as occurs when lifting heavy loads	

Methods of Examination

Examinations provide information about:
- The position of the larynx and its relation to neighboring anatomic structures in the neck.
- The external and internal shape of the larynx.
- The type, site, and extent of lesions inside and outside of the larynx.
- Functional disorders.

■ Inspection

Normally, the thyroid prominence can only be seen in men. It moves upward on swallowing; absence of this movement indicates fixation of the larynx by infection or tumor.

Indrawing of the suprasternal notch on inspiration, combined with inspiratory stridor, suggests laryngotracheal obstruction by a foreign body, tumor, edema, etc.

■ Palpation

The laryngeal skeleton and neighboring structures are palpated during respiration and swallowing, with attention being paid to the following:
- The thyroid cartilage.
- The cricothyroid membrane and cricoid cartilage.
- The carotid artery with the carotid bulb, which must not be confused with neighboring cervical

lymph nodes; the palpating finger picks up pulsations.

- The thyroid gland, lying inferior and lateral to the thyroid and cricoid cartilages.
- Simultaneous movement of the larynx and thyroid gland on swallowing.

■ Laryngoscopy

The two ways of examining the larynx are indirect and direct laryngoscopy. The larynx is inspected with the aid of a mirror and the unaided eye, with a flexible or rigid endoscope, or with a laryngoscope and a microscope (**Table 4.4**).

Table 4.4 Summary of areas to be examined in laryngoscopy

Oropharynx	Base of tongue, both valleculae epiglotticae, lingual surface of the epiglottis
Hypopharynx	Piriform sinus
Boundaries between the hypopharynx and larynx	Glossoepiglottic and aryepiglottic folds
Larynx	Epiglottis, arytenoid cartilages, vestibular folds, vocal folds and ventricles
Subglottis	

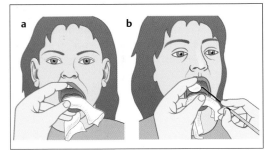

Fig. 4.5a, b   Indirect laryngoscopy with the laryngeal mirror. This technique has become rare since the introduction of endoscopes. The mirror is heated with a hot-air warmer to prevent it from steaming up.

■ Indirect Laryngoscopy

The examination technique is illustrated in **Fig. 4.5a,b**. The tongue is grasped with the thumb and middle finger of the left hand, so that the thumb lies on the tongue. The index finger is used to push back the upper lip. The tongue must be drawn forward carefully to prevent damage to the frenulum by the lower teeth. The light from the mirror is directed toward the uvula. The glass surface of the laryngeal mirror is warmed, and its temperature is tested with the examiner's own hand. It is then introduced along the palate until it reaches the uvula.

Stimulation of the base of the tongue and posterior pharyngeal wall should be avoided, as it can provoke the gag reflex. The posterior surface of the mirror is used to lift the uvula and push it upward and backward. The posterior part of the tongue, the pharynx, and part of the larynx are now visible in the mirror. The patient is asked to say "e" to bring the epiglottis into a more upright position and thus provide a better view of the larynx. The view of the larynx can be considerably improved by using LumiView lenses (Welch Allyn, Skaneateles Falls, New York, USA). In a patient with a sensitive gag reflex, it may be necessary to spray the pharynx first with a topical anesthetic such as lignocaine before the examination can be performed (**Fig. 4.6**).

■ Flexible Nasendoscopy

The most commonly used method for diagnostic assessment of the larynx is flexible nasendoscopy with a nasopharyngoscope (nasopharyngoscopy). The endoscope is introduced through the nose without anesthesia. During endoscopy, the nasopharynx, the movement of the velum, and the motor function of the vocal folds can be observed. The flexible endoscope makes it possible to assess the hypopharynx, as well as laryngeal closure during swallowing, and to identify disorders of vocal fold movement. Endoscopes with charge-coupled device (CCD) chips at the tip provide sharp images and are useful for examining the vocal folds for organic diseases and phonatory movement using stroboscopy.

Rigid Endoscopy of the Larynx

Rigid endoscopes have become very useful in everyday practice. They are light, have wide-angle lenses, and can supplement or replace indirect laryngoscopy with the mirror. Two types with angles of 70° or 90° are commonly used (see also section on nasal endoscopy, p. 133, and **Fig. 2.21**).

The advantages of this procedure are that it provides a good view of otherwise hidden areas, variable magnification, good illumination, and video documentation. Surgical procedures can be performed using rigid videostrobolaryngoscopy (**Fig. 4.7**).

> **Note:** Biopsies can be taken and polyps removed during indirect laryngoscopy using topical anesthesia administered with cotton swabs or a spray (see **Fig. 4.6**). Although most laryngologists prefer microlaryngoscopy, procedures using local anesthesia are still performed for phonosurgery, for taking biopsies, and to remove foreign bodies.

Microlaryngoscopy

The larynx and hypopharynx can be examined directly with a rigid laryngoscope resting via a lever arm on a chest support (**Figs. 4.8a, b**). A binocular operating microscope is added for microlaryngoscopy. A micromanipulator is attached for laser surgery (**Fig. 4.8c**), and suitable instruments have been designed for this (**Fig. 4.9**). Anesthesia is administered intravenously and respiration is secured by endotracheal intubation or jet ventilation. This procedure has represented a considerable advance in diagnostic and endolaryngeal microsurgery. Microlaryngoscopy provides excellent illumination of the larynx, upper trachea, and hypopharynx, making hidden areas accessible. Endolaryngeal surgical procedures can be performed.

The following features are looked for during the examination: the color of the mucosa, abnormal tissue, the appearance of local or diffuse lesions (smooth, rough, ulcerated, exophytic, etc.), the lumen of the trachea, and the shape of the hypopharynx. If the patient is under general anesthesia and relaxed, it is not possible to observe the respiratory movement of the vocal folds properly. For obvious reasons (intubation and an unconscious patient), it is also not possible to see phonatory movement either.

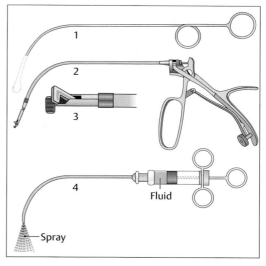

Fig. 4.6 Instruments for administering mucosal anesthesia in the larynx and for small interventions at the vocal folds. **1,** Curved metal cotton applicator; **2,** curved double-cupped forceps with handle; **3,** curved needle holder for intralaryngeal injections; **4,** spray, which can also be used with compressed air.

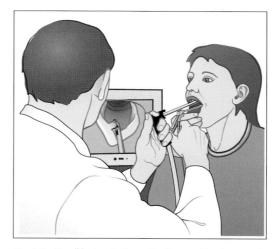

Fig. 4.7 Small lesions in the epithelium and lamina propria can be removed using topical anesthesia. The larynx is observed with a rigid endoscope held in one hand, and the lesion is grasped using the instrument held in the other hand. The patient holds the tongue. The procedure is monitored on a video screen.

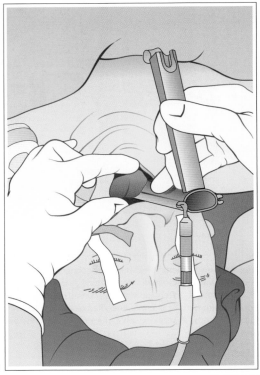

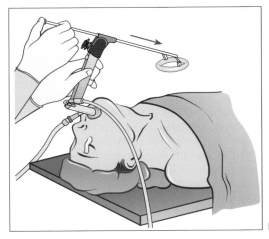

Fig. 4.8a–c   a The first step in microlaryngoscopy. Introduction of the laryngoscope. The patient is in a supine position, with the upper teeth are protected by a tooth guard.
b The suspension arm is used to hold the laryngoscope in position.
c Microlaryngoscopy with an attached laser micromanipulator. The laser beam is directed into the axis of the surgeon's view. The endotracheal tube has to be a specialized laser tube.

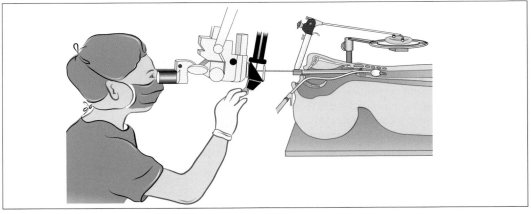

■ Diagnostic Imaging

High-resolution computed tomography (CT) allows accurate assessment of the site and extent of stenoses and tumors, and of any damage to local, laryngeal, and neighboring structures.

Magnetic resonance imaging (MRI) has broadened the range of diagnostic imaging in the larynx and adjacent regions. Soft-tissue findings such as the extent of a tumor and any lymph-node metastases can be displayed.

■ Stroboscopy

See Chapter 5, **Fig. 5.1** and p. 334.

◼ Other Special Techniques

High-speed Glottography

A rigid endoscope is connected to a high-speed camera that can record 2000–4000 frames per second. Observations for short periods during the onset of phonation and during steady-state phonation can then be stored on a computer. This allows scientific analysis of laryngeal function, and of the movement of the vocal folds during sound production in particular.

Electromyography

Electromyography (EMG) is the electrical recording of muscle activity. It aids in the diagnosis of diseases affecting muscle and peripheral nerves. EMG results can help determine whether symptoms are due to a muscle disease or a neurological disorder. In the larynx, EMG is used to examine immobile vocal folds and differentiate between ankylosis or paralysis, for example.

Clinical Aspects

◼ Congenital Anomalies (Table 4.5)

Congenital laryngeal anomalies have three cardinal clinical symptoms: *dyspnea, dysphonia,* and *dysphagia.*

Laryngomalacia

Clinical Features. Inspiratory stridor begins immediately or during the first few weeks postpartum, in severe cases accompanied by cyanosis. The symptoms worsen during feeding.

Pathogenesis. Abnormal calcium metabolism causes weakness in the supraglottic laryngeal skeleton, particularly in the epiglottis.

Diagnosis. Direct laryngoscopy and bronchoscopy. The epiglottis is usually omega-shaped and soft, and covers the laryngeal entrance on inspiration. The arytenoid prominences or aryepiglottic folds may be sucked in during inspiration. The shape and function of the vocal folds is normal.

Treatment. The neonate is observed carefully and the parents are given reassurance. The cartilage becomes stiffer during the course of weeks or months, and the symptoms

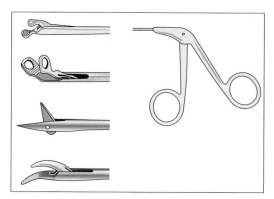

Fig. 4.9 Instruments for endolaryngeal microsurgery. *From top left:* cutting forceps, forceps with fenestrated jaws, scissors, alligator forceps. *Right:* hand piece.

Table 4.5 Frequency of congenital laryngeal anomalies

Frequency	Congenital anomaly
≈ 75 %	Laryngomalacia
≈ 10 %	Neurological disorders (unilateral or bilateral recurrent nerve paralysis)
Rare	Atresia and webs
	Cysts and laryngoceles
	Subglottic stenoses
	Hemangioma
Very rare	Clefts

gradually disappear. Feeding should be interrupted with pauses after every two or three swallows. In cases of respiratory distress, tube feeding is indicated. Severe temporary dyspnea should be managed in a neonatology intensive-care unit (NICU) with continuous positive airway pressure (CPAP) or intubation. Tracheotomy is only required exceptionally.

Neurogenic Disorders

Clinical Features. If the symptoms are unilateral, there is squealing and a weak cry. Bilateral lesions cause inspiratory stridor.

Pathogenesis. Some cases are idiopathic, while some are due to congenital or cardiovascular anomalies or stretching of the neck during birth.

Diagnosis. Fiberoptic laryngopharyngoscopy or direct laryngoscopy, showing one or both vocal folds in the paramedian position. An intermediate position of the folds is considerably rarer.

Treatment. Unilateral lesions do not require treatment. A large proportion of congenital recurrent paralyses recover spontaneously. Bilateral lesions may require intubation initially, and tracheotomy later if obstruction persists.

Atresias and Webs

Clinical Features. Atresias cause powerful, fruitless attempts at respiration, cyanosis, and inability to cry immediately after birth, leading rapidly to death. Webs cause respiratory obstruction of variable degrees.

Diagnosis. Direct laryngoscopy reveals atresia or a (subtotal) web at the glottis.

Treatment. In severe cases of dyspnea, asphyxia can only be prevented by endoscopic division of the web or tracheotomy in the immediate postpartum period. This can be done by incision or endolaryngeal laser surgery and may be repeated if necessary.

Laryngoceles

Internal laryngoceles lie within the larynx in the vestibular fold (**Fig. 4.10**).

External laryngoceles are a prolongation of the ventricle through the thyrohyoid membrane to form a palpable cystic mass in the neck.

Combinations of the two forms and bilateral laryngoceles are rare.

Clinical Features. Dyspnea and dysphonia are accompanied by a foreign-body sensation in the throat.

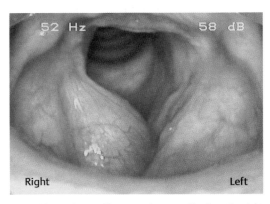

Right   Left

Fig. 4.10 An internal laryngocele protruding into the right vocal fold.

Pathogenesis. This is a congenital or acquired expansion of the laryngeal saccule; a blind sac of the laryngeal ventricle (Morgagni ventricle), filled with air or mucus.

Diagnosis. This is established by laryngoscopy, palpation, and CT. The smooth swelling increases in size on puffing, straining, and on playing wind instruments.

Treatment. If patients have no dyspnea, observation is sufficient as long as the swelling does not increase. External laryngoceles are exposed and removed via an external incision. Small internal laryngoceles are removed using a CO_2 laser during microlaryngoscopy.

Subglottic Stenoses

Clinical Features. Inspiratory *and* expiratory stridor are present. The voice is usually normal. Recurrent pseudocroup may also occur.

Pathogenesis. The cause is usually an anomaly of the cricoid cartilage.

Diagnosis. This is established by direct laryngoscopy, tracheoscopy, and CT.

Treatment. Tracheotomy may be necessary in severe respiratory obstruction. The child is then observed until surgery is possible at the age of 5 years. The procedures used are laryngotracheoplasty, anterior cricoid split, posterior cricoid split, and interposition of costal cartilage.

Hemangioma

Clinical Features. These tumors may cause hoarseness or respiratory obstruction, depending on their location. Spontaneous bleeding with blood aspiration can lead to a dangerous emergency.

Diagnosis. Direct microlaryngoscopy.

Treatment. Spontaneous regression of the hemangioma should be awaited. Occasionally, when respiratory obstruction increases or the hemangioma bleeds spontaneously, laser surgery (with Nd:YAG or CO_2 laser) is indicated. Tracheotomy is not usually necessary.

■ Organic Functional Disorders

These can have neurological, myogenic, or articular causes. They are characterized by voice disorders such as dysphonia and aphonia, or by dyspnea, e. g., laryngospasm.

Dysphonia. Atypical vibrations of the vocal folds or abnormally increased or decreased passage of air through the glottis causes increased hoarseness rather than a clear tone. It is analyzed using endoscopy, stroboscopy, high-speed cinematography, and phoniatry.

Dyspnea. Audible stridor (shortness of breath, at times accompanied by cyanosis) occurs when the diameter of the respiratory tract is reduced by at least one-third. The anoxia can increase dramatically during physical exercise.

> **Note:** A 1-mm mucosal swelling in an infant narrows the lumen by more than 50 %. Edema must be 3 mm thick in the adult to produce the same effect.

Neurogenic functional disorders due to causes in the cortical or subcortical areas mainly cause bilateral abnormalities of vocal fold movement. Bilateral, but more often unilateral, disorders of vocal fold function—usually combined with lesions of the vagus, glossopharyngeal, and hypoglossal nerves—are localized in the medulla oblongata. Cerebral ischemia or bleeding in the area of the brain stem leads to sudden combined paralyses of the superior and inferior laryngeal nerves in older people. Ninety percent of isolated defects of the vagus nerve or its branches are located in the region of the nucleus ambiguus, the inferior ganglion, and down to the peripheral laryngeal musculature. Typical vocal fold palsies result from damage to the vagus nerve inferior to the inferior ganglion (**Fig. 4.11**).

The vocal folds are observed in different positions during function, or when paralyzed in relation to an imaginary reference line provided by the sagittal glottic axis (**Fig. 4.12**).

Physiological positions during function. During phonation, the vocal folds are in the median position (**Fig. 4.13a**) (in adduction), and during inspiration (**Fig. 4.13b**) they are in the lateral position (in abduction).

Vocal fold positions in the most common pareses (see Fig. 4.12)

- The paramedian position is seen in recurrent nerve paralysis with posterior cricoarytenoid paralysis.

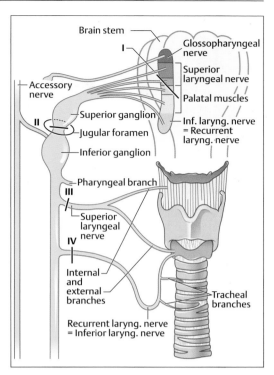

Fig. 4.11 The vagus nerve and its branches, with sites of possible lesions (I–VI) and effects on the larynx. There is no rule for the position of the paralyzed vocal fold, only a trend. **I**, A lesion in the nucleus ambiguus (hemorrhage, neoplasm) produces paralysis in the intermediate or paramedian position. **II**, Loss of continuity in the jugular foramen (skull base tumors, aneurysms of the internal carotid artery) of the inferior ganglion causes paralysis of the superior laryngeal nerve and recurrent laryngeal nerve. The vocal fold is in the intermediate position, and the soft palate is paralyzed. Lesions in and around the jugular foramen may be accompanied by paralysis of the glossopharyngeal, accessory, and hypoglossal nerves. **III**, Interruption of the vagus nerve at the superior laryngeal nerve (carotid surgery) causes a loss of tone of the cricothyroid muscle and loss of tension in the vocal fold. **IV**, Division of the recurrent nerve (bronchial carcinoma, aortic aneurysm, thyroid surgery) causes vocal fold paralysis in the paramedian position.

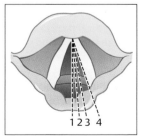

Fig. 4.12 Positions of the vocal fold. **1**, Median, or phonatory position; **2**, paramedian position; **3**, intermediate position; **4**, lateral or respiratory position.

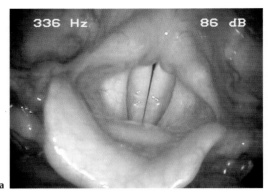

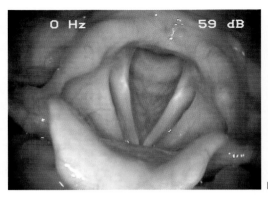

Fig. 4.13a, b   a Normal larynx during phonation.   **b** Normal appearance of the larynx during respiration.

- The intermediate position of the vocal fold is most often seen when the vagus nerve, including the superior and inferior laryngeal nerves, is completely paralyzed, thus affecting all of the internal and external laryngeal muscles.
- "Cadaveric position" is an incorrect term. This should be described as "intermediate position," similar to the position of the vocal folds in flaccid paralysis or in the end stage of a vocal fold paralysis. The vocal folds show bowing due to atrophy of the vocalis muscle. The arytenoid cartilage is tilted anteriorly when the posticus muscle is paralyzed.

Other anomalies of position combined with hyperkinetic or hypokinetic dysphonia include:
- *Vocal fold bowing:* The glottal chink is elliptical during phonation, due to reduced tension in the vocalis muscle as a result of atrophy, as occurs in senile dysphonia.
- *Transversus (interarytenoid muscle) weakness:* A triangular gap remains open between the arytenoid cartilages and the posterior part of the vocal folds during phonation.
- *Combinations of the two forms of inadequate closure* may occur.

It is not possible to predict the final position of the vocal folds after damage to the superior and recurrent laryngeal nerves, as the nerves may recover or partially preserve function (**Fig. 4.14**). Vice versa, the extent of neural injury cannot be deduced from the position of the paralyzed vocal fold. In addition, atypical positions may be adopted due to fibrosis of the muscle or ankylosis of the arytenoid joint.

Recurrent Laryngeal Nerve Paralysis (Table 4.6)
All internal laryngeal muscles are paralyzed on the affected side. If the external cricothyroid muscle, supplied by the external branch of the superior laryngeal nerve, is still active, it stretches the paralyzed vocal fold and forces it into the paramedian position. In incomplete paralysis of the adductors, the paresis of the single abductor of the vocal folds (the posterior cricoarytenoid muscle) is functionally predominant. This unilateral or bilateral form of paresis is known as posticus paresis. Stroboscopy is useful in the long-term follow-up of vocal fold paralyses. If the mucosal wave can be observed in the course of paresis, it is a sign that neural function is recovering, suggesting a positive prognosis.

Unilateral Recurrent Nerve Paralysis
Clinical Features. Often noted incidentally, the symptoms include moderate to severe dysphonia in the acute phase. The voice improves later. There is no appreciable respiratory obstruction except during severe physical activity. The patient cannot sing high notes or raise his voice.

Diagnosis. Laryngoscopy shows an immobile vocal fold in the paramedian, intermediate, or lateral position on one side. Thorough laryngologic, phoniatric, neurologic, and radiologic examinations are indicated in order to identify the cause (see **Table 4.6,** p. 306).

Treatment. If treatment of the causal disease does not restore vocal fold mobility, the patient is given voice therapy to achieve glottal closure by activating the remaining neuromuscular units on the paralytic side and stimulating the mobile vocal fold on the other side.

Bilateral Recurrent Nerve Paralysis

Symptoms

- Dyspnea and a danger of asphyxia due to narrowing of the glottal chink. Inspiratory stridor is noted during physical activity, sleep, or when talking.
- Initially, there is dysphonia, which lasts for a variable period—between 4 and 8 weeks, depending on the cause—and with a weak and hoarse voice thereafter. Speech is interrupted by long inspiratory phases.
- Feeble coughing is also symptomatic.

Pathogenesis. See **Table 4.6**.

Diagnosis. This is based on laryngoscopy. In bilateral paralysis, the vocal folds are usually in the paramedian position.

Treatment

- Relief of the airway takes first priority. Tracheotomy and a cannula with a speaking valve are required only if dyspnea is severe—i.e., if peak expiratory flow goes below 40% of the normal value for the patient. Many patients manage to stay without tracheotomy by avoiding exertion, as the dyspnea is tolerable as long as they are at rest.
- If spontaneous remission does not occur, surgery to widen the glottis is indicated 10–12 months after the onset of the paresis if the patient is suffering from permanent dyspnea and physical activity limitation or, in case of tracheostomy, if the patient wishes to be free of the speaking valve. The recommended procedure is partial arytenoidectomy and posterior cordectomy.

Principles of surgery: The operation is carried out endoscopically with a CO_2 laser (**Fig. 4.15a–e**). The part of the vocal process of the less mobile arytenoid cartilage that is obstructing the lumen of the cricoid ring below is removed (partial arytenoidectomy), and the elastic cone is opened all the way down to the cricoid. The posterior part of the vocal fold is incised and part of the vocalis muscle is removed (posterior cordectomy). The inferior part of the subglottic mucosa is sutured laterally to the floor of the Morgagni ventricle and ventricular fold.

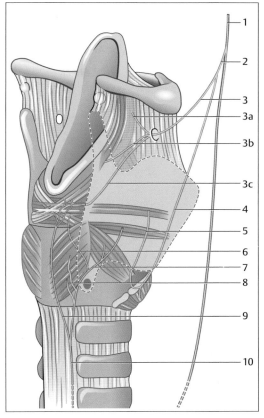

Fig. 4.14 Innervation of the larynx. **1**, Vagus nerve; **2**, superior laryngeal nerve (SLN); **3**, internal branch of the SLN; **3a**, superior branch of the internal SLN; **3b**, middle branch of the internal SLN; **3c**, inferior branch of the internal SLN; **4**, external branch of the superior laryngeal nerve; **5**, ventricular branch of the external SLN; **6**, posterior branch of the recurrent laryngeal nerve; **7**, anterior branch of the recurrent laryngeal nerve; **8**, branches to the posterior cricoarytenoid muscle; **9**, ansa galeni to the inferior branch of the internal SLN and branches to the interarytenoid muscle; **10**, recurrent laryngeal nerve.

Creating a posterior gap for respiration and preserving the anterior part of the vocal fold means that contact for phonation is still possible.

Note: The wider the glottal gap after the operation, the less satisfactory is the voice.

Table 4.6 Unilateral or bilateral recurrent nerve paralysis

Causes	Details
Intracranial portion of the vagus nerve, including nuclei	
Neurological diseases	Wallenberg syndrome (posterior inferior cerebellar artery syndrome). Occlusion of the vertebral or posterior inferior cerebellar artery of the brain stem, in which the lateral part of the medulla oblongata infarcts. Symptoms include difficulties with swallowing, hoarseness, dizziness, nausea and vomiting, rapid involuntary movements of the eyes (nystagmus), and problems with balance and gait coordination
	Poliomyelitis, bulbar paralysis, multiple sclerosis, cerebral tumors
Cervical portion of the vagus nerve	
Thyroidectomy	Most frequent cause of vocal fold immobility
Malignant goiter	
Blunt or sharp cervical trauma	
Cervical metastases near the skull base	Commonly associated with other cranial neuropathies
Intubation anesthesia	Stretching of the recurrent nerve due to incorrect patient positioning; pressure of the tube against the anterior branch inside the larynx; pressing of the larynx against the vertebral column
Thoracic portion (mediastinum) of the vagus nerve	
Operations on the hypopharynx or esophagus	Failure to display the course of the nerve during resection of the hypopharyngeal diverticulum
Esophageal carcinoma	Particularly of the upper third
Mediastinal diseases	Lymphogranulomas, non-Hodgkin lymphoma, metastases, mediastinitis
Aneurysms of the aorta or subclavian artery	Congenital or syphilitic
Duct operations	
Cardiomegaly of various causes	May also occur in Ortner syndrome (a rare cardiovocal syndrome in which there is recurrent laryngeal nerve palsy secondary to cardiovascular disease)
Bronchial carcinoma	Particularly common in tumors arising from the left upper and middle lobes and with involvement of the mediastinal lymph node metastases
Pulmonary tuberculosis	
Pleural plaques	
No specific location	
Infectious and toxic	Influenza; herpes zoster; rheumatism; syphilis; tissue toxins such as lead, arsenic, or organic solvents; streptomycin; quinine
Idiopathic	It should be noted that a diagnosis of idiopathic recurrent nerve paralysis should only be made after all other causes have been excluded. In the great majority of these patients, spontaneous recovery occurs within 2–3 months. After a longer period, the chances of recovery are lower

Speech therapy is used to supplement the operation by restoring the voice either at the level of the glottis or with ventricular fold phonation.

Unilateral or Bilateral Paralysis of the Superior Laryngeal Nerve

Clinical Features. These include aspiration of food and drink, loss of power of the voice, and inability to sing in the head or falsetto register, particularly when bilateral. Breathing is normal.

Pathogenesis. The superior laryngeal nerve has an internal branch that carries afferent fibers from the mucosa of the laryngeal aditus and motor fibers for the quadrangular muscle of the ventricular fold. It is connected with the inferior laryngeal nerve by the ansa galeni in most patients. The external branch of the superior laryngeal nerve supplies motor innervation to the cricothyroid muscle. Paralysis affects the function of the cricothyroid muscle, as well as the sensory innervation of the supraglottic part of the larynx, and is due to mechanical lesions of the nerve, particularly after thyroid gland operations, tumor surgery, and viral infections.

Diagnosis. Laryngoscopy shows that the tension of the vocal folds is reduced so that the glottis does not close completely during phonation. In unilateral paralysis, the ipsilateral vocal fold is often shortened and lies lower than the nonparalyzed side. Respiratory movement of the vocal folds appears to be unimpaired.

Treatment. Corticosteroids and voice therapy should be tried.

Combined Lesions of the Laryngeal Nerves

These include lesions of the superior laryngeal and recurrent laryngeal nerves (see **Fig. 4.11**).

Clinical Features. Unilateral paralysis causes dysphonia with a breathy or rough voice. The patients run out of air when talking. The healthy vocal fold compensates later. Aspiration occurs due to an absence of sensory protection. In bilateral paralysis, there is dysphonia or aphonia. Respiration at rest is generally good. There is also aspiration and a marked feeling of shortage of breath during physical exertion.

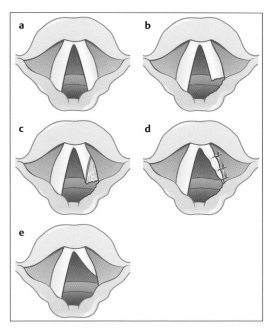

Fig. 4.15a–e   The principle of partial arytenoidectomy and posterior cordectomy with intralaryngeal sutures.
a, b The intraluminal part of the vocal process of the arytenoid cartilage is resected with laser surgery, and the incision through the conus elasticus is extended laterally to the cricoid cartilage.
c The posterior part of the vocal fold is opened with a triangular incision, and the underlying vocalis muscle is resected.
d, e The inferiorly based flap from the posterior part of the vocal fold is sutured laterally to the ventricular fold. This creates optimal conditions for wound healing (**e**), with minimal fibrin and granulation tissue formation. If the anterior part of the vocal fold can still be adducted, it can be used for phonation.

Pathogenesis. The main cause is central or peripheral damage to the vagus nerve, causing flaccid paralysis with immobility of the affected vocal fold in the intermediate position. There is bilateral flaccid paralysis with bilateral lesions (see **Fig. 4.11**).

Diagnosis. Laryngoscopy shows one or both of the vocal folds bowed and paralyzed in the intermediate position (**Fig. 4.16a, b**).

Treatment. It is rarely possible to treat the cause of this form of paralysis, and the mainstay of treatment is speech therapy.

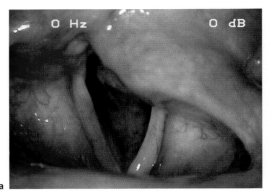

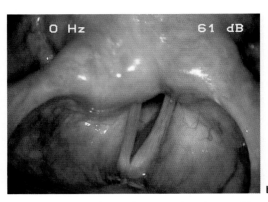

a

b

Fig. 4.16a, b a Palsy of the left vocal fold during respiration, with atrophy of the muscle in the intermediate position. The arytenoid cartilage is tilted anteriorly, as there is no pull from the posterior cricoarytenoid muscle.

b The same patient during phonation. There is a considerable gap between the vocal folds, causing phonatory dyspnea.

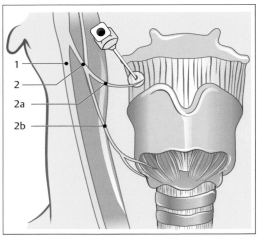

Fig. 4.17 Infiltration anesthesia of the superior laryngeal nerve. **1**, Vagus nerve; **2**, superior laryngeal nerve; **2a**, internal branch; **2b**, external branch.

Note: If speech therapy for a unilateral atrophic vocal fold paralysis does not succeed in closing the glottal gap and normalizing the voice, the immobile vocal fold can be medialized using laryngoplasty or injection techniques.

Neuralgia of the Superior Laryngeal Nerve

This is one of the localized or mononeural pain syndromes of the head and neck, such as trigeminal neuralgia or occipital neuralgia.

Clinical Features. Episodic stabbing pain, usually on one side, radiating to the upper part of the thyroid cartilage, the angle of the jaw, or the lower part of the ear. Pain on pressure is experienced at the level of the greater horn of the hyoid or in the region of the thyrohyoid membrane.

Pathogenesis. The cause is unknown but may relate to viral infection, previous trauma (or surgery), or mechanical-morphologic factors (e.g., hyoid bone variations). The disease occurs between the 40th and 60th years of life. The trigger zone lies in the piriform sinus and is set off by swallowing, speaking, and coughing.

Treatment. Repeated anesthetic block of the superior laryngeal nerve should be tried. The site of injection lies between the greater horn of the hyoid and the superior horn of the thyroid cartilage (**Fig. 4.17**). Medical treatment with carbamazepine may also be helpful.

■ Trauma

Laryngeal function may be affected by vocal overuse, intubation injury, external trauma, chemical toxins, and foreign bodies. Symptoms caused by abnormal laryngeal function include voice disorders, respiratory obstruction, coughing, and surgical emphysema of the neck. Appropriate endo-

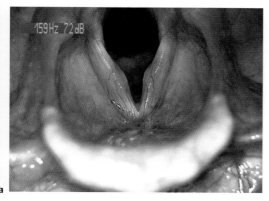

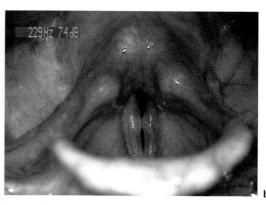

Fig. 4.18a, b   **a** Vocal fold nodules during respiration. They are bilateral but often of different sizes, located in the middle of the membranous part of the vocal fold.

b Vocal fold nodules during phonation. The glottis has a typical hourglass shape. The narrowing is caused by the vocal fold nodules touching.

scopic and radiographic procedures are used to diagnose and localize the lesion (see pp. 297-301).

Acute Vocal Trauma

Clinical Features. These include dysphonia or even aphonia, and pain on speaking.

Pathogenesis. The condition is caused by extreme overuse of the voice among spectators at sports events, politicians, market traders, and regular visitors to discos or clubs with loud music.

Diagnosis. Indirect or direct laryngoscopy, which shows hyperemia or swelling of the vocal folds and subepithelial bleeding.

Treatment. Strict voice rest and inhalations are required. If polyps form, they are removed under local anesthesia or with direct microlaryngoscopy under general anesthesia.

Chronic Vocal Trauma

Clinical Features. The voice is hoarse and croaking, or ceases during stress. Singing is difficult or impossible.

Pathogenesis. Vocal nodules develop due to chronic vocal strain or misuse of the voice. In children, vocal nodules occur predominantly in boys, while among adults mainly women are affected. Nodules have been observed in mothers of large families and among schoolteachers. When singers develop vocal nodules, it may be due to unsatisfac-

tory singing technique or excessive vocal strain. A wide angle between the vocal folds at the anterior commissure as an anatomical precondition fosters the development of vocal nodules.

Diagnosis. Direct or indirect laryngoscopy demonstrates the nodules at the typical site in the middle of the vocal folds, which is the point of maximum amplitude of the vibrations and of tearing/shearing and colliding forces of the vocal folds. The nodules are usually bilateral (**Fig. 4.18a, b**).

Treatment. When the nodules progress beyond a certain size, they become fibrotic, and voice rest and speech therapy are no longer successful. Most patients then require endolaryngeal microsurgery, with postoperative speech therapy.

Contact Granuloma

Clinical Features. These include dysphonia and shooting pain in the larynx when speaking.

Pathogenesis. Almost all patients have a history of psychological stress. Vocal overuse causes the arytenoid cartilages to impinge sharply against each other. Gastroesophageal reflux is another likely cause.

Diagnosis. Indirect or direct laryngoscopy typically shows a swelling at the vocal process on one side (**Fig. 4.19a, b**). A reactive pachydermia (thickened epithelium) on the other side may sometimes occur.

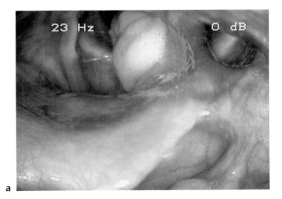

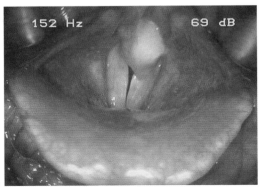

Fig. 4.19a, b **a** Contact granuloma during respiration. **b** Contact granuloma during phonation.

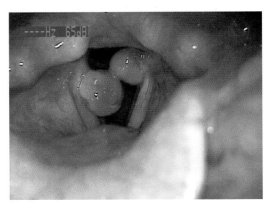

Fig. 4.20 Bilateral intubation granulomas in the cartilaginous part of the glottis.

Differential diagnosis. This includes ulceration or granulation due to intubation, tumors, and tuberculosis.

Treatment. The patients are usually hyperactive and do not persist with voice rest or speech therapy. Treatment centers on psychosomatic exploration and counseling. Excision is only useful in order to exclude a malignancy histologically.

Acute Intubation Injury

Clinical Features. Immediately or shortly after removal of the tube, patients develop dysphonia, attacks of coughing, and hemoptysis. They also have pain in the larynx and neck.

Pathogenesis. The injury is caused by repeated or incorrect intubation, intermittent positive pressure respiration, a protruding guide wire, use of a tube of the wrong size, insufficient relaxation, overextension, and pressure from the tube cuff. These factors lead to myogenic or neurologic paralysis. Drying of the mucosa by the premedication can exacerbate the mucosal injury. Laryngeal complications can be expected after less than 48 h of intubation in adults and after 3–7 days in young children, who tend to develop subglottic mucosal injuries.

Diagnosis. Laryngoscopy shows a subepithelial hematoma, superficial and deep mucosal injuries, and rarely torn epithelium at the vocal fold or subluxation of the arytenoid cartilage. Intubation granulomas are usually bilateral and located on the vocal process (**Fig. 4.20**).

Treatment. A hematoma or superficial mucosal or epithelial lesion can heal spontaneously within 2 weeks. Pressure-induced paralysis of the recurrent laryngeal nerve may also resolve spontaneously. Subluxation of the arytenoid cartilage, which is usually connected with paresis of the inferior laryngeal nerve, may require surgery.

Chronic Intubation Injury

Clinical Features. Dysphonia or laryngeal dyspnea develop 2–8 weeks after intubation anesthesia or prolonged intubation.

Pathogenesis. Incorrect intubation, a tube that is too large or too rigid, incorrect (endolaryngeal or subglottic) positioning of the cuff, or prolonged intubation can cause damage. Additional pathogenetic factors include general conditions that the patient may have, such as shock, retching, and vomiting.

> **Note:** Early lesions—including endolaryngeal or subglottic hyperemia, edema, ischemic mucosal defects with fibrinous membrane, necrosis, and ulceration—lead to late injuries such as ulceration, granulation, perichondritis, cartilaginous necrosis, synechiae, and strictures.

Diagnosis. Laryngoscopy, CT scan, measurement of ventilatory function, and spirometry.

Treatment. Granulomas are removed with endolaryngeal microsurgery or laser treatment. Postoperative speech therapy may reduce the tendency for recurrences to develop (see below).

Laryngotracheal Stenoses and Synechiae

These often require several surgical procedures over a long period. The operations include excision or splitting of the scar tissue and of the cricoid cartilage if necessary, with mucosal or cartilaginous grafts. A stent has to be worn in the reconstructed larynx for at least 6 weeks until the patent lumen stays open without narrowing again (see p. 352; **Figs. 6.9, 6.10, 6.11 b, d**).

External Trauma

Blunt and penetrating injuries, open and closed, have to be examined and diagnosed.

Clinical Features. Immediate or increasing dyspnea up to complete obstruction of the airway due to hematoma, edema, and dislocation of cartilage fragments; bleeding; and dysphonia. Dysphagia and pain occur when the esophagus is affected.

Pathogenesis. Causes include athletic injuries, karate blows, fighting, and attempted strangulation. In addition to direct trauma resulting in subluxation and disruption of the laryngeal framework, a blow may force the larynx against the vertebral column, causing vertical, horizontal, or combined fractures and endolaryngeal mucosal tearing. Subluxation of the larynx from the trachea can occur. Perforations or contusions in the neighboring hypopharynx and upper esophagus lead to tracheoesophageal or laryngoesophageal fistulas. The neighboring nerves and vessels may also be injured (**Figs. 4.21a–e, 4.22**).

Diagnosis. Inspection, palpation, and laryngoscopy demonstrate fractures, crepitation, or displacement of laryngeal fragments and surgical emphysema of the neck. CT scans and measurement of ventilatory function should also be performed.

Treatment. Preservation of the airway is the most important measure, if necessary using bronchoscopy, tracheotomy, or intubation (see **Table 6.3**). Emergency bronchoscopy can be carried out with bronchoscopes of the appropriate size. Distressing coughing attacks are suppressed with antitussive medication. Some patients may require admission to an intensive-care unit. Further procedures are listed in **Table 4.7**.

Table 4.7 Types of laryngeal trauma and treatment. The basic principle of treatment is to secure a patent airway

Type of injury	Treatment
Hematoma and edema, small mucosal tears	Voice rest, steroids; tracheotomy if necessary
Extensive soft-tissue injuries of the neck, exposed cartilage with otherwise intact or easily reconstructible laryngeal skeleton	Open exploration and reconstruction; a silicone stent or keel can be used in the anterior commissure or glottis to prevent webbing
Loss of thyroid cartilage and mucosa	Mucosal grafts and stenting of the inside of the larynx
Laryngeal fractures, vertical or horizontal	Suturing of the fragments with or without stenting
Laryngotracheal subluxation	End-to-end anastomosis of the cricoid cartilage and tracheal rings
Late stenosis	Open exploration, excision of scar, mucosal and cartilaginous grafts and stenting with Montgomery T-tube
	Endoscopic stenting via tracheoscopy with a silicone stent (Dumont)

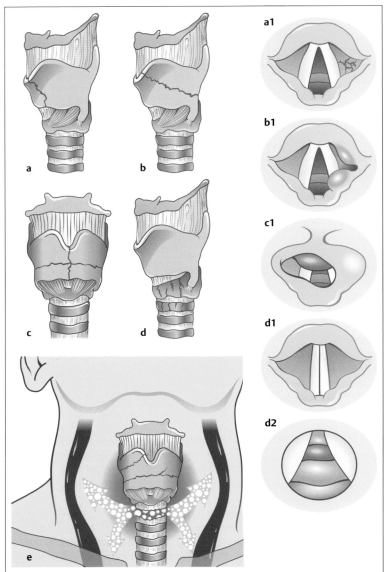

Fig. 4.21a–e Laryngeal trauma, showing fractures of the thyroid cartilage.
a Vertical, with laryngoscopic signs of supraglottic hematoma and swelling (**a1**).
b Oblique, with hematoma of the aryepiglottic fold and arytenoid region (**b1**).
c Crushed, with supraglottic narrowing due to a torn-off epiglottic petiole (**c1**).
d, e Fracture of the cricoid cartilage, with bilateral immobility of the vocal folds (**d1**), subglottic hematoma or granulation (**d2**), tearing of the trachea, with air escape into the surrounding tissues and congestion due to compression of the large cervical veins caused by hematoma, edema, and surgical emphysema (**e**).

Inhalational Trauma Due to Chemical Toxins

Clinical Features. *Acute:* severe attacks of coughing, a feeling of burning and asphyxia, and epiphora. *Chronic:* hoarseness, a feeling of dryness, lump in the throat, throat clearing, and coughing attacks.

Pathogenesis. The trauma is caused by gases or steam escaping after industrial explosions and the effect of smoke during fires. The most common chronic toxin is inhalation of tobacco smoke.

Diagnosis. Laryngoscopy shows redness, mucosal maceration, and edema.

Treatment. Voice rest, cessation of smoking, humidification of the air, corticosteroids for edema, inhalation therapy, and laryngoscopic follow-up

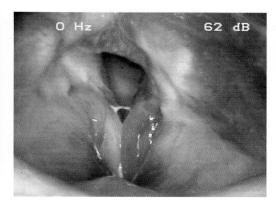

Fig. 4.22 Laryngeal trauma, with a hematoma on the inner larynx.

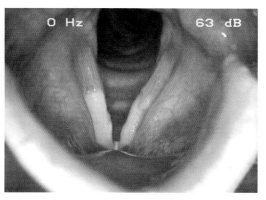

Fig. 4.23 Acute laryngitis, with a fibrinous exudation in the anterior half of the membranous part.

are indicated. Antibiotics are given as required. Intubation can be carried out if there is acute respiratory insufficiency (p. 355).

Foreign Bodies

Clinical Features. The initial symptoms are attacks of coughing, stabbing pain in the larynx, and dysphagia when eating. Dyspnea may occur, particularly in infants, due to the tendency of the infant's mucosa to produce edema. Large foreign bodies, especially vegetables, may cause asphyxia due to mucosal swelling.

Pathogenesis. Laryngeal foreign bodies are rarer than tracheal or bronchial foreign bodies. Sharp-edged, pointed, or large foreign bodies may become trapped in the larynx. The danger of foreign-body aspiration is particularly severe during sudden fright, laughing, or when there is a lack of sensory innervation of the larynx.

Diagnosis. Indirect laryngoscopy, rigid video-laryngoscopy. Laryngotracheobronchoscopy should be performed in all doubtful cases. There may be edema overlying a foreign body that has been trapped. Radiography can only detect foreign bodies that are radiopaque, especially metallic ones.

Treatment. The foreign body is removed carefully using a rigid endoscope, with care being taken to preserve the mucosa. A tracheotomy may be neces-

sary in order to remove large foreign bodies in the larynx with associated edema.

A laryngeal foreign body may occasionally be coughed out, but it is more often aspirated into the tracheobronchial tree.

Course. The mucosa tends to produce reactive edema, particularly in children. Steroids are indicated in these cases. The physician should be prepared to carry out intubation if severe dyspnea develops after a foreign body has been removed.

■ Inflammation

Acute Laryngitis

Clinical Features. Hoarseness, aphonia, pain in the larynx, and coughing attacks. In children, there is a danger of airway obstruction. Acute laryngitis is usually due to ascending or descending viral infections from other parts of the airway.

Pathogenesis. The cause is viral or, rarely, bacterial infection.

Diagnosis. Laryngoscopy shows red and swollen vocal folds. Depending on the underlying disease, the neighboring pharyngeal or tracheal mucosa may also be inflamed (**Fig. 4.23**).

Treatment. General measures include steam inhalation, aspirin, and fluids by mouth. Steroids are indicated for marked edema. As acute laryngitis is

Table 4.8 Treatment of acute subglottic laryngitis. The basic principle is to relieve both obstruction and a distressing cough that impedes circulation

Sedation in children (drug-mediated respiratory depression should be avoided)
Steroids
Antibiotics to prevent secondary infection
Administration of fluids
Croup tent (moist cloth over the bed)

mainly due to viral infections, antibiotics should not be given unless bacterial infection is confirmed by a smear test with microbiological culture and susceptibility testing.

!
> **Note:** Oil-containing inhalations should not be used. Only aerosols with a particle size of 30 ± 20 µm precipitate in the larynx.

Voice rest is indicated, and smoking should be forbidden. Chemicals such as certain dyestuffs or artificial products and allergic toxins such as hair sprays, shellfish, and crustaceans should be eliminated.

!
> **Note:** If the symptoms do not improve considerably or resolve within 3 weeks, rigid endoscopy and stroboscopy should be used to identify suspicious findings. Ulceration, proliferation, and exudate are not typical of uncomplicated nonspecific laryngitis. Specific diseases, premalignant lesions, and tumors must be excluded by biopsy via microlaryngoscopy.

Croup Syndromes

Diphtheritic croup, beginning with laryngeal membranes and obstruction, is rare. However, sparse endemic foci still persist in western Europe. Diphtheritic laryngitis with grayish-white membranes, occurring as an isolated condition, is also rare. It is usually combined with oropharyngeal lesions. Tracheotomy is required for increasing dyspnea.

The term "pseudocroup" includes a group of acute laryngotracheal diseases mainly affecting children.

Acute Subglottic Laryngitis

Clinical Features. A dry barking cough following a head cold that rapidly becomes worse; hoarseness; inspiratory, expiratory, or mixed stridor; retraction of the suprasternal notch and of the intercostal spaces during inspiration; cyanosis; perioral pallor. The severity of respiratory obstruction depends on the degree of mucosal swelling in the subglottis. Worsening symptoms in children lead to concern due to the impending threat of airway obstruction.

Pathogenesis. This is a very serious acute disease of early infancy, most common between the ages of 1 and 5 years. Within a short time, life-threatening narrowing of the child's airway can develop due to inflammatory mucosal swelling of the elastic cone in the subglottic space. The disease is basically caused by viral infection with accompanying secondary bacterial infection. Cool, damp, and foggy weather in fall and winter appear to increase the morbidity. However, recurrent infections in the nasopharynx and nasal obstruction due to chronically inflamed hypertrophied adenoids and tonsils are important etiological factors. The role of air pollution in the pathogenesis of this disease is still unclear.

Diagnosis. The clinical picture is usually very typical. Laryngoscopy reveals glottal mucosal edema and redness, potentially with crust formation.

Treatment. See **Table 4.8**. Mild cases, assessed by the degree of respiratory obstruction, can be managed by the family practitioner or pediatrician. The efficacy of the treatment needs to be closely monitored.

If treatment fails and dyspnea increases, the child must be admitted to hospital urgently on an emergency basis for treatment with oxygen therapy and standby for an endotracheal intubation, depending on the degree of dyspnea and the results of blood gas analysis (oxygen saturation, partial pressure of carbon dioxide). Tracheotomy is carried out when there is severe obstruction and progressive sicca-type crust formation.

Acute Epiglottitis

Clinical Features. There is a classic presentation with the clinical triad of drooling, dysphagia, and distress. Severe pain during swallowing and refusal of food and liquid intake may lead to dehydration and potential circulatory collapse. Inspiratory stridor usually forces the patient to sit upright in bed with the nose pointing upward in a "sniffing position." Speech is muffled ("hot potato speech") and temperature is raised.

Pathogenesis. Acute epiglottitis is essentially laryngeal supraglottitis. The main cause is infection with *Haemophilus influenzae.* Since the introduction of vaccination against this, however, infection may be caused by several other upper respiratory tract organisms. The disease is sometimes caused by mucosal damage resulting from swallowing sharp-edged food, allowing pathogenic organisms to enter. The disease is life-threatening for children between 2 and 8 years of age, with a mortality of up to 20 % if not treated. Adults are also affected.

Diagnosis. The diagnosis is "epiglottitis acutissima" if the course is particularly fulminant. Laryngoscopy or examination with a tongue depressor shows a thick, swollen, red epiglottic rim (**Fig. 4.24**). Epiglottic swelling is visible on a lateral radiograph.

Differential diagnosis. Pseudocroup may also be caused by congenital anomalies, foreign bodies, angioneurotic edema of the larynx, hypocalcemic laryngospasm, tumors, infected epiglottic cysts, and laryngoceles.

Treatment. Immediate transfer to the nearest appropriate facility (an emergency department approved for pediatrics). Ventilation is supported with a bag valve mask. If respiratory arrest occurs, the airway is secured by nasotracheal intubation. Tracheotomy is rarely required nowadays, due to the usually short course of the disease. An intravenous line is required for administration of broad-spectrum antibiotics (with second-generation or third-generation cephalosporins) at high doses and steroids.

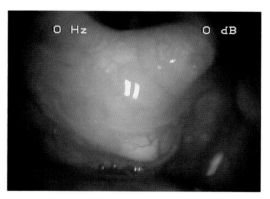

Fig. 4.24   Epiglottitis with abscess formation.

Note: In patients with respiratory obstruction, particularly children, diagnostic procedures may lead to complete obstruction. Preparations must therefore be made for intubation or tracheotomy *before* the examination. The patient should be referred to hospital if a diagnosis of epiglottitis is suspected.

Prognosis and course. The disease usually improves rapidly within a few days. Possible complications include epiglottic abscess and perichondritis.

Chronic Laryngitis

Chronic nonspecific laryngitis needs to be distinguished from the group of specific forms such as tuberculosis, Wegener granulomatosis, amyloidosis, etc. Chronic nonspecific laryngitis requires assessment and treatment by an otolaryngologist.

Chronic Nonspecific Laryngitis

Clinical Features. These persist for weeks or months, in contrast to those of acute laryngitis. They include hoarseness, a deeper voice, and sometimes a dry cough. The voice is less robust and there is a globus sensation in the larynx and a feeling of needing to clear the throat, but little or no pain.

Pathogenesis. This disease is mainly due to exogenous toxins such as cigarette smoking, occupational air pollution, and climatic influences. Another cause is vocal overuse in bartenders, construction workers, call center agents and other professional speak-

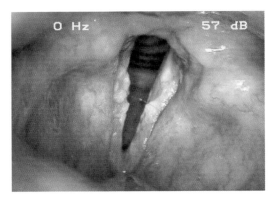

Fig. 4.25   Chronic laryngitis, with epithelial keratosis.

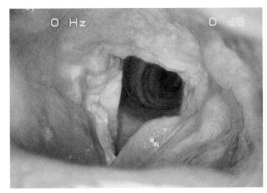

Fig. 4.26   Laryngeal tuberculosis.

ers. Nasal obstruction may also be a factor in the pathogenesis.

> **Note:** Laryngopathia gravidarum, due to vocal fold edema with dysphonia and deepening of the voice, is sometimes observed in the second half of pregnancy. The hoarseness almost always resolves spontaneously after delivery.
> Administration of male sex hormones and anabolic steroids causes voice changes in women, including deepening of vocal pitch, disorders of the singing voice, and a reduction in the ability of the speaking voice to carry. These disorders persist as a result of virilization of the laryngeal structures.

Diagnosis. Laryngoscopy shows thick and red vocal folds with rough edges (**Fig. 4.25**). There is tenacious mucus, and the rest of the laryngeal mucosa often looks similar. Microlaryngoscopy should always be performed, and malignancy should be excluded by biopsy.

Treatment. The treatment is protracted. Eliminating exogenous toxins such as tobacco is the mainstay of treatment. Voice rest can be useful for a few days in case of acute exacerbations, and if necessary, a deviated nasal septum can be corrected to restore normal nasal respiration. Antibiotics are not administered unless pathogenic bacteria are identified in a smear test with microbiological culture and susceptibility testing. Steroids, saline inhalations, and mucolytic agents are given for a period of ≈ 4 weeks (see pp. 313-314). If the epithelial

changes do not resolve, a biopsy should be taken to exclude malignant transformation. The epithelium must not be completely removed, as in cases of cancer. As long as there is no malignancy, the patient must be observed closely with stroboscopic examinations.

> **Note:** Regular laryngoscopic follow-up examinations are advisable in patients with chronic laryngitis, because of the possibility of dysplasia. Microlaryngoscopy and biopsy should be performed in all doubtful cases. This is the only way to detect malignancy early.

Specific Forms of Chronic Laryngitis
Laryngeal Tuberculosis
Clinical Features. Hoarseness and coughing persisting for several months and pain, radiating to the ear, on swallowing.

Pathogenesis. Laryngeal tuberculosis is almost always secondary to active pulmonary tuberculosis. The infection is transmitted to the larynx by bacilli contained in the sputum. The posterior part of the larynx, interarytenoid area, and epiglottis are most commonly affected. There is a danger of perichondritis. Monocorditis can be caused by a miliary tuberculous deposit.

Diagnosis. In fresh cases, microlaryngoscopy initially shows reddish-brown submucous nodules, which are partly confluent. Later, ulcerations or granulations develop (**Fig. 4.26**). Monocorditis is characterized by redness and thickening, occasionally with small ulcerations of one vocal fold. Other investigations include histology, culture, radiography, and examination by an internist.

Differential diagnosis. This includes vasomotor mono-corditis, nonspecific chronic laryngitis, and carcinoma.

Treatment. Antituberculous treatment is given in cooperation with an internist (rifampicin and isoniazid). Pain is treated by blocking the superior laryngeal nerve (see **Fig. 4.17**). Isolation of the patient is rarely necessary owing to the chemotherapeutic options available, but contacts with other persons should be investigated. This is a notifiable disease.

Course and prognosis. Laryngeal tuberculosis is infectious. Mucosal lesions often heal with no permanent effects on laryngeal function, but if the tuberculosis has affected the laryngeal cartilaginous framework, defects arise during healing. The prognosis is good nowadays, with potent antibiotics given for 6–12 months.

Laryngeal Sarcoid

Laryngeal sarcoid is nowadays rare as an extrapulmonary manifestation. Dysphonia and a globus sensation are caused by sarcoid deposits in the larynx.

Biopsy, if necessary combined with prescalene lymph-node biopsy, is necessary to establish the diagnosis.

In contrast to tuberculosis, the epithelioid cell nodules do not caseate or ulcerate. Radiography is a supplementary examination. The disease is treated by an internist.

Laryngeal Syphilis

Isolated laryngeal syphilis is unusual, and it is much more often a manifestation of oropharyngeal syphilis in the secondary generalized stage of the disease.

Mucous plaques or hazy, smoke-colored mucosal lesions occur in the larynx, similar to those of syphilitic pharyngitis (see p. 253). The patient is also hoarse. This is a notifiable disease.

Respiratory obstruction only occurs in the presence of marked mucosal swelling. The cartilage is destroyed in a gumma in the tertiary stage. Differential diagnosis from carcinoma is difficult.

Scleroma of the Larynx

Pale red swellings and granulations with crusts develop, mainly in the subglottic space. Subglottic, laryngeal, and intratracheal stenoses occur in stage III of the disease, causing hoarseness, cough, and increasing stridor.

Diagnosis. Microlaryngoscopy, histopathology, and culture (*Klebsiella rhinoscleromatis*).

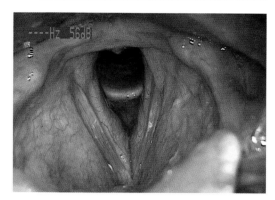

Fig. 4.27 Amyloidosis of the larynx.

Treatment. Tracheotomy, followed by appropriate surgical treatment of laryngotracheal stenosis, is necessary for respiratory stridor.

Pemphigus Vulgaris and Pemphigoid Vesicles

These conditions preferentially affect the epiglottis and are often incidental findings. The vesicles are usually painless, but may occasionally cause a globus sensation and lead to stenosis due to extensive scarring (this may also affect the adjacent pharynx). Paraneoplastic symptoms may be present. Treatment is directed toward the underlying disease.

Generalized Rheumatoid Arthritis

The cricoarytenoid joint is often affected, causing hoarseness, stridor, and pain, radiating to the ear, on swallowing.

Laryngeal Amyloid

Amyloid in the head and neck most often causes macroglossia. Laryngotracheal amyloid is next most common finding. It is usually isolated and is very rarely associated with other systemic diseases. Tumorous, polypoid lesions covered with smooth mucosa, with a pale waxy appearance, may develop in the larynx in this form of dysproteinemia. The sites of predilection are the vocal folds and the subglottic space (**Fig. 4.27**). Surgical removal is required for severe hoarseness and respiratory obstruction.

Laryngeal Perichondritis

Clinical Features. Pain in the larynx that increases on swallowing or with external pressure, hoarseness, and dyspnea.

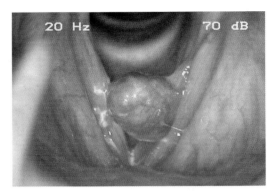

Fig. 4.28   A large polyp on the left vocal fold.

Pathogenesis. Surgical and accidental trauma, infiltration of cartilage by tumor, infection—e. g., tuberculosis—and irradiation can all be causes. If the cartilage is not invaded by tumor, it usually tolerates radiation up to 60 Gy. The usual clinical problem is chondroradioneurosis, with inflammation of the overlying mucosa.

Diagnosis and findings. A laryngoscopic picture of radiogenic pallid mucosal edema, particularly on the epiglottis and the arytenoid cartilages, is very typical along with the history. Intralaryngeal and extralaryngeal swelling, fistulas, and sequestration of necrotic pieces of cartilage are seen.

Treatment. Sequestrated or exposed cartilage must be removed. Broad-spectrum antibiotics are given in high doses, combined with steroids.

Note: Radiation edema is very difficult to treat and often disguises persistent or recurrent tumor.

■ **Tumors**

■ **Benign Tumors**

Vocal Fold Polyps
Clinical Features. These include hoarseness, aphonia, and attacks of coughing. If the polyp has a pedicle and is floating between the folds, the voice may return to normal for short intervals.

Pathogenesis. This is the most common benign tumor of the vocal folds, mainly affecting men between 30 and 50 years of age. It is often initiated by agents that cause laryngeal inflammation. Hyper-

kinetic voice disorders and vocal overuse are important factors.

Diagnosis. Laryngoscopy (**Fig. 4.28**) shows the polyp usually lying on the free edge of the vocal fold, either on a pedicle or sessile. It is edematous and occasionally hemorrhagic. Older polyps appear firm, due to fibrosis and thickening of the overlying epithelium.

Treatment. The polyp is removed by endolaryngeal microsurgery, with preservation of the lamina propria. The patient is advised to rest the voice for ≈ 3 days. The defect epithelializes faster when the voice is resting.

Note: The polyp should always be examined histologically to confirm the diagnosis.

Reinke Edema
Clinical Features. These include hoarseness and deepening of the voice. Stridor may occur, particularly on exertion, if the edema is marked.

Pathogenesis. The edema is almost always bilateral and broad-based. It develops in the Reinke space. The edema usually affects women over the age of 40 years who are smokers and frequent professional speakers.

Diagnosis. Laryngoscopy shows a bilateral broad-based edematous mass on the vocal folds (**Fig. 4.29**).

Treatment. The epithelium covering the edema has no definite border separating it from the surrounding normal epithelium. On the cranial surface, the incision, or a narrow excision of epithelium, follows the arcuate line laterally. The myxoid acellular substance of the lamina propria is suctioned or pressed out. Redundant epithelium is trimmed and the epithelium is redraped so that the edges are adjacent (**Fig. 4.30a–g**). The epithelium must not be excised or stripped as was advocated formerly.

Recurrent Respiratory Papillomatosis
Clinical Features. Hoarseness, often severe, and respiratory obstruction, depending on the site and extent of the lesions.

Pathogenesis. The benign tumor is caused by human papillomavirus (HPV). During normal vaginal delivery, infants may be infected through exposure of the aerodigestive tract to the cervix and vagina of a mother with genital HPV infection. Papillomas in adults may have persisted since early childhood. The course of the disease is unpredictable.

Diagnosis. This is established by direct laryngoscopy and histologic examination. Papillomas may be pedicled, solitary, or widespread. Their surface is pale-yellow to red, granular, villous, and often has a raspberry appearance.

Other areas of papillomatosis may lie in the oropharynx and subglottic space (**Fig. 4.31**).

Treatment. Spontaneous regression rarely occurs. The effects of immunologic and antiviral treatment and vaccines have not been reproducible. There is currently no alternative to surgery. Removal of papillomas during microlaryngoscopy can be achieved with microlaryngeal dissection and CO_2 laser. Suction diathermy, and more recently microdebrider treatment, are also used to remove papillomas, but these techniques have to be handled with extreme caution, as the glottis forms bad scars as a result of overtreatment. In severe cases, local injection of an antiviral agent such as cidofovir is used to try and prevent recurrence. Children often require surgical excision as often as every 2–4 weeks. Tracheotomy has to be avoided, as it may lead to the disease progressing at sites from laryngeal to tracheal to pulmonary.

Note: Progression of papilloma to squamous cell carcinoma can occur, but this is rare (< 5 % of cases).

Retention Cysts

These are glazed, white, or occasionally blue cysts derived from mucosal glands. They are localized to the vestibular fold, ventricle, epiglottis (**Fig. 4.32**), aryepiglottic folds, and valleculae.

Small cysts are sometimes found incidentally; larger cysts can cause a globus sensation, dysphonia, and dyspnea.

Treatment. Removal using microsurgery with the CO_2 laser.

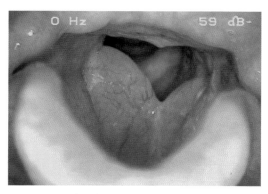

Fig. 4.29 Reinke edema.

Chondromas

Clinical Features. Hoarseness, dyspnea, dysphagia, or globus sensation, depending on the site.

Pathogenesis. The tumors grow slowly and often arise from the cricoid cartilage.

Diagnosis. Laryngoscopy usually shows a subglottic tumor covered with smooth mucosa. The tumor is sometimes palpable externally. CT demonstrates the site and extent of the tumor.

Treatment. Surgical. Chondromas are radioresistant.

Leukoplakia, Dysplasia, and Carcinoma in Situ of the Laryngeal Mucosa

Leukoplakia is a clinical term that covers lesions of different histologic grades. A leukoplakic lesion may signify a premalignant or malignant process and therefore requires histologic examination. Histomorphologic definitions of the grades of dysplasia help eliminate ambiguous terminology and facilitate prognostic assessment:

Grade I: *Simple dysplasia*—i. e., epithelial hyperplasia without nuclear atypia, without disturbances of maturation or stratification of the squamous epithelium. This is a clinically benign disease.

Grade II: *Middle-grade epithelial dysplasia* with basal cell hyperplasia, loss of basal cell polarity, moderate cell polymorphism, a slightly increased mitotic rate, and occasional dyskeratosis. This should be regarded clinically as a premalignant lesion.

Grade III: *High-grade dysplasia* with basal cell hyperplasia, loss of basal cell polarity, cell polymor-

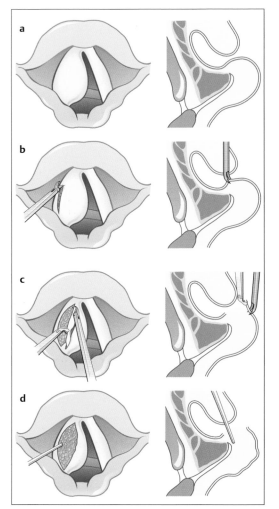

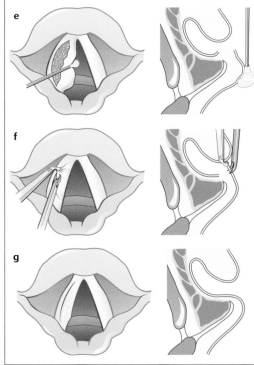

Fig. 4.30a–g The principle of surgery for Reinke edema.
a The epithelium over the edematous area is not sharply demarcated from the surrounding epithelium.
b, c An incision or very small excision is made into the epithelium as far laterally as possible on the upper surface of the bulging vocal fold (**b, c**).
d, e The liquid or gelatinous intercellular material is suctioned (**d**) or extruded (**e**) from the lamina propria.
f, g Finally, the redundant, stretched epithelium is resected (**f**) until the wound margins are smoothly apposed (**g**).

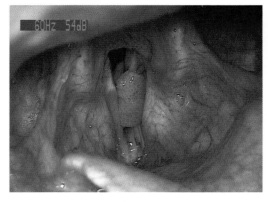

Fig. 4.31 Laryngeal papilloma.

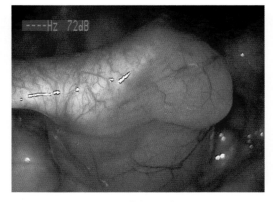

Fig. 4.32 Retention cyst of the epiglottis.

phism, increased mitotic rate, numerous dyskeratoses, and abnormalities of epithelial stratification. Transition to carcinoma in situ is shown by intensification of high-grade dysplasia, loss of epithelial stratification, but no invasion of the stroma. Carcinoma in situ may be a forerunner of a carcinoma, an intraepithelial offshoot, or an isolated satellite focus.

!

> **Note:** Squamous cell carcinomas of the larynx arise on the basis of precancerous changes lasting various periods of time. They can be diagnosed at this stage using microsurgery. Excisional biopsy with complete removal at the preinvasive stage not only establishes the diagnosis, but also provides definitive treatment.

Clinical Features. Hoarseness, a foreign-body sensation in the throat, and a desire to clear the throat.

Pathogenesis. Exogenous toxins—e.g., smoking and irradiation.

Diagnosis. Microlaryngoscopy shows rough, thickened mucosa in the larynx or vocal folds, occasionally deepened by scar tissue and altered in color.

Treatment. The histologic classification determines the type and extent of treatment. Lesions confined to the vocal folds are treated with subepithelial cordectomy via microlaryngoscopy (see **Fig. 4.35a–f**). Obvious etiologic agents should be eliminated. These procedures are usually performed with the laser. The underlying structures are protected by subepithelial infusion.

■ **Malignant Tumors**

Laryngeal Carcinoma

Laryngeal carcinoma accounts for ≈ 40 % of carcinomas of the head and neck. It is most common between the ages of 45 and 75 years. Men are affected ten times more frequently than women. There has been a trend since 1990 for the cancer death rate to decrease, although the absolute number of deaths has increased owing to increasing life spans.

Clinical Features. Hoarseness is the first and main symptom when the tumor affects the glottis. Further symptoms, which may occur alone or in combination depending on site and extent, include a foreign-body sensation, clearing the throat, pain in the throat or referred elsewhere, dyspnea, dysphagia, cough, and hemoptysis. Regional lymph-node metastases may also occur.

!

> **Note:** Hoarseness persisting for more than 2–3 weeks must always be investigated by a laryngologist, and this step must not be omitted.

Pathogenesis. Invasive carcinoma may develop from epithelial dysplasia, particularly carcinoma in situ. More than 90 % of laryngeal carcinomas are keratinizing or nonkeratinizing squamous cell carcinomas. Rare malignant forms include verrucous carcinoma, adenocarcinoma, carcinosarcoma, fibrosarcoma, and chondrosarcoma.

Most patients with squamous carcinoma of the larynx were or are heavy cigarette smokers and, in addition, often heavy drinkers. Chronic exposure to irritation with heavy metals such as chromium, nickel, and uranium, or asbestos exposure and radiation exposure, are rarer causes.

There are regional and ethnic variations in the frequency of site distributions within the larynx. For example, supraglottic carcinoma is more common in Spain and in parts of South America than it is in Germany.

Laryngeal carcinoma infiltrates locally into the mucosa and underneath the mucosa and metastasizes via the lymphatics and the bloodstream. The limits of vascular spread are embryologically determined (see p. 293 and **Fig. 4.4**). Supraglottic carcinomas therefore usually remain confined to the supraglottic space and spread anteriorly into the preepiglottic space (**Fig. 4.33**). Glottic carcinomas spread into the subglottic space, rather than into the supraglottic region (**Fig. 4.34a, b**). Transglottic carcinoma is a glottic carcinoma involving the ventricle and the vestibular folds. The site of origin cannot be recognized. The characteristics of the intralaryngeal lymphatics (see p. 296) influence the frequency of regional lymph-node metastases. Other factors influencing the frequency of metastases are the duration of symptoms, histologic differentiation, and the size and site of the tumor. Lymph-node metastases are rare at the time of presentation in patients with carcinomas of the vocal fold, but are found in ≈ 20 % of subglottic carcinomas, ≈ 40 % of supraglottic carcinomas, and ≈ 40 % of transglottic carcinomas.

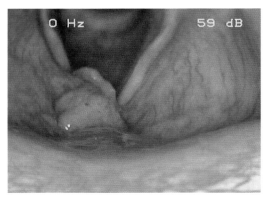

Fig. 4.33 Supraglottic carcinoma at the ventricular fold and stalk or petiole of the epiglottis (T2 N1 M0).

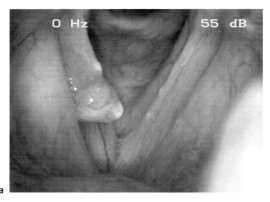

a

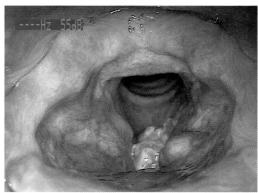

b

Fig. 4.34a, b   a Carcinoma of the right vocal fold (T1 N0 M0).
b Carcinoma of the left vocal fold comprising the anterior commissure (T3 N2 M0).

Contralateral metastases are unusual in unilateral glottic tumors. Bilateral metastases become more common if the carcinoma crosses the midline, at the anterior or posterior commissure or in the trachea, or if the tumor arises primarily in the supraglottic space.

Distant hematogenous metastases are relatively unusual in laryngeal carcinoma when the patient is seen for the first time. Second primary carcinomas of the respiratory and digestive tracts (synchronous or metachronous) also occur.

Diagnosis. The clinical diagnosis is initially based on the findings of indirect laryngoscopy, video laryngoscopy, and stroboscopy. The site and extent of the tumor and the mobility of the vocal fold have to be assessed (**Table 4.9**). Microlaryngoscopy (see **Figs. 4.8, 4.9**) allows accurate evaluation of the site and extent of the tumor, provides a view of hidden angles such as the ventricle and the piriform sinus, and facilitates assessment of superficial characteristics of the tumor, such as nodular, exophytic, granulomatous, or ulcerating (see **Figs. 4.33, 4.34**). CT and MRI are used to assess the depth of involvement.

Differential diagnosis. Chronic laryngitis and its specific forms, and benign laryngeal tumors.

Treatment. If untreated, laryngeal carcinoma leads to death within an average of 12 months due to asphyxia, bleeding, metastases, infection, or cachexia. The existence of cardiovascular or pulmonary diseases and diabetes mellitus determines the course of treatment and the course of the disease. Patients are treated on an individual basis following presentation and discussion at a multidisciplinary team meeting. The indications for radiotherapy, chemotherapy, or surgery for laryngeal carcinoma vary depending on the site and stage of the tumor, as well as the patient's geographical location. They are often used in combination. Chemotherapy alone has so far proved to be ineffective with this type of tumor, but it is often combined with postoperative radiotherapy and leads to an absolute benefit of ≈ 10 % in the 5-year survival rate. Radiotherapy is mainly administered in the form of telecobalt megavoltage radiation. With the exception of T1 N0 glottal tumors and some T2 N0 tumors, and especially if lymph-node metastases are present, surgery is clearly superior to radiotherapy.

Table 4.9   TNM classification and involvement of laryngeal carcinomas (see Figs. 4.33, 4.34 a, b)

Glottis		*Supraglottis*	
T1	Limited to vocal fold(s), normal mobility	T1	One subsite, normal vocal cord mobility
T1a	One vocal fold	T2	Mucosa of more than one adjacent subsite of supraglottis or glottis or adjacent region outside the supraglottis; without fixation
T1b	Both vocal folds		
T2	Supraglottis, subglottis, impaired vocal fold mobility	T3	Vocal cord fixation or invades postcricoid area, pre-epiglottic tissues, paraglottic space, thyroid cartilage erosion
T3	Vocal fold fixation, paraglottic space, thyroid cartilage erosion		
T4a	Through thyroid cartilage; trachea, soft tissues of neck: deep/extrinsic muscle of tongue, strap muscles, thyroid, esophagus	T4a	Through thyroid cartilage; trachea, soft tissues of neck: deep/extrinsic muscle of tongue, strap muscles, thyroid, esophagus
T4b	Prevertebral space, mediastinal structures, carotid artery	T4b	Tumor invades prevertebral space, mediastinal structures, or encases carotid artery
Subglottis		*All sites*	
T1	Limited to subglottis	N1	Ipsilateral single ≤ 3 cm
T2	Extends to vocal fold(s) with normal/impaired mobility	N2a	Ipsilateral single > 3 to 6 cm
		N2b	Ipsilateral multiple ≤ 6 cm
T3	Vocal fold fixation	N2c	Bilateral, contralateral ≤ 6 cm
T4a	Through cricoid or thyroid cartilage; trachea, deep/extrinsic muscle of tongue, strap muscles, thyroid, esophagus	N3	> 6 cm
		Distant metastases	
T4b	Prevertebral space, mediastinal structures, carotid artery	MX	Distant metastasis cannot be assessed
		M0	No distant metastasis
		M1	Distant metastasis

Chemoradiotherapy is appropriate for patients with inoperable tumors, patients who decline cancer surgery, and laryngeal tumor manifestations that are not amenable to surgical palliation. Extension of laryngeal carcinoma to the hypopharynx is another possible indication for chemoradiotherapy.

Multimodal treatment with surgery and postoperative chemoradiotherapy appears to yield the best results for selected patients in advanced stages.

Complications after radiotherapy include persistent edema, which makes it difficult to assess the local appearance and detect a recurrence. The edema is usually due to chondroradionecrosis, leading to cartilaginous necrosis, which may require laryngectomy. Other complications include dysphagia, ageusia, xerostomia, and sicca syndrome. In patients who undergo surgery after a full course of radiotherapy, wound healing and the prognosis are considerably poorer.

Surgical procedures for laryngeal carcinoma. In selected cases, decortication and cordectomy can be carried out using endoscopic laser surgery, with good oncological and functional (voice) outcomes. The European Laryngological Society has published a proposed classification of endoscopic cordectomies:

Type I: Subepithelial cordectomy of the vocal fold is indicated for severe dysplasia and some carcinomas in situ (**Fig. 4.35a**).

Type II: Subligamental cordectomy is indicated for a vocal fold carcinoma with a mobile vocal fold (T1 N0) (**Fig. 4.35b**).

Type III: Transmuscular cordectomy is indicated for cases of small superficial cancer of the mobile vocal fold, or where cancer reaches the vocalis muscle without deeply infiltrating it (T2 N0) (**Fig. 4.35c**).

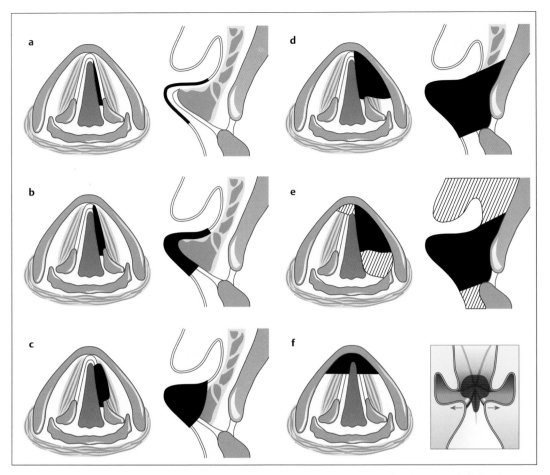

Fig. 4.35a–f   The classification of cordectomies.

a Subepithelial cordectomy (type I): resection of the vocal fold epithelium, passing through the superficial layer of the lamina propria.

b Subligamental cordectomy (type II): resection of the epithelium, Reinke space, and vocal ligament.

c Transmuscular cordectomy (type III): through the vocalis muscle.

d Total cordectomy (type IV) extends from the vocal process to the anterior commissure. The depth of the surgical margins reaches the internal perichondrium of the thyroid ala,
and sometimes the perichondrium is included in the resection.

e Extended cordectomy: Type Va encompasses the contralateral vocal fold and the anterior commissure; type Vb includes the arytenoids; type Vc encompasses the subglottis; and type Vd includes the ventricle.

f Anterior commissurectomy (type VI): a bilateral anterior cordectomy for cancer originating in the anterior commissure without infiltration into the thyroid cartilage, either extending or not extending to one or both vocal folds.

Type IV: Total or complete cordectomy is indicated for cases of T1a cancer, where cancer is infiltrating the vocal fold and is diagnosed before surgery (**Fig. 4.35 d**).

Type Va–d: Extended cordectomy can encompass the contralateral vocal fold, the (still mobile) arytenoid cartilage, the ventricular fold, or the subglottis as deep as 1 cm under the glottis. This may be suitable for selected cases of T2 carcinoma (**Fig. 4.35e**).

Type VI: Cordectomy of the anterior commissure is an anterior commissurectomy with bilateral anterior cordectomy (**Fig. 4.35 f**).

Vertical or horizontal partial laryngectomies are used for carcinomas for which a cordectomy is not suitable because of the extent or site of the tumor, but for which total laryngectomy is not necessary. Partial laryngectomies preserve vocal function and a normal airway. The prerequisites for success are careful assessment and good surgical judgment to ensure that the tumor is removed completely.

- *Vertical partial laryngectomy:* Principle of the operation (**Fig. 4.36a, b**). Several methods are available, but the principle common to all of them is that a wide vertical segment of the thyroid cartilage, and occasionally the cricoid cartilage, is removed together with the laryngeal soft tissues and the tumor. A *hemilaryngectomy,* removal of half of the larynx, can be performed for a tumor limited strictly to one side.
- *Horizontal partial laryngectomy:* Principle of the operation (**Fig. 4.37a, b**). The supraglottic space is completely removed, with retention of the vocal folds and the arytenoid cartilage.

After a partial resection, the functional results are good and the airway is normal, as is vocal function, but the latter depends on the type of resection, the results of which are variable. The patient may have temporary difficulty in swallowing, which may persist in elderly patients. There is a danger of recurrence at the excisional margins if the tumor was incorrectly evaluated preoperatively or if the technique is inadequate.

Total laryngectomy may sometimes be combined with removal of the hypopharynx. This technique is indicated for tumors that cannot be removed using cordectomy or partial laryngectomy and for tumors that have spread to neighboring structures such as the tongue, hypopharynx, thyroid gland, and trachea. Total laryngectomy is also indicated for tumors that have recurred after radiotherapy or partial procedures.

Surgical technique (**Figs. 4.38–4.41**): The entire larynx is removed from the base of the tongue to the trachea, if necessary with removal of parts of the tongue, pharynx, trachea, and thyroid gland. If part of the tongue or pharynx is removed, the defects are reconstructed with flaps—e. g., a platysma flap, pectoralis musculocutaneous flap, or radial forearm flap. After this operation, the patient can only breathe via the tracheostomy. Swallowing is almost normal once the wound has healed, and the voice is produced either at the pharyngoesophageal

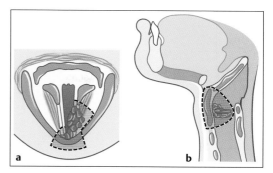

Fig. 4.36a, b Vertical frontolateral partial resection. The dashed line marks the area of resection.

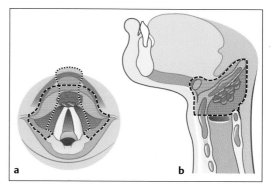

Fig. 4.37a, b Horizontal supraglottic partial resection. The limits of the resection are shown by the dashed line. The dotted line indicates the area to be resected that is not clinically visible on laryngoscopy.

segment by vibrations in the esophageal mucosa driven by a voice prosthesis (**Fig. 4.41**), by ructus (esophageal speech; see under rehabilitation, below), or using an external electronic larynx.

Complications after laryngectomy include pharyngocutaneous fistula and recurrent tracheobronchitis.

!

Note: Removal of the primary tumor using partial or total laryngectomy should be combined with curative en bloc neck dissection if lymph-node metastases are present (**Fig. 4.42**). If there is a known high risk of lymphatic metastases for a tumor at a particular site, many surgeons carry out a selective neck dissection even if lymph-node metastases cannot be palpated. The results of treatment are summarized in **Table 4.10**.

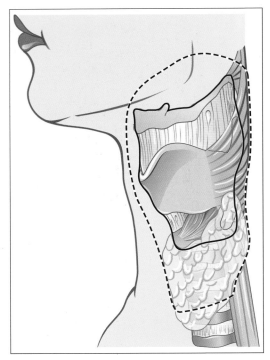

Fig. 4.38 The area resected in laryngectomy. The boundaries of the resection area can be extended for involvement of the tongue, hypopharynx, upper trachea, and thyroid gland (shown by the dashed line).

Table 4.10 Five-year survival in patients with laryngeal carcinoma*

Type of tumor	Survival rate (%)	Treatment
Glottal carcinoma		
T1N0	95	Endoscopic surgery
T2N0	90	Endoscopic surgery (or radiotherapy)
T3	60–70	Surgery (or combined surgery and radiotherapy)
T4	< 60	Surgery or combined surgery and radiochemotherapy
Supraglottic carcinoma		
T1	80, 90 †	Surgery
T2	60, 90 †	Surgery, or combined surgery and chemoradiotherapy
T3 and T4	50, 80 †	Surgery, or combined surgery and chemoradiotherapy
Subglottic carcinoma	40, 50 †	Surgery, or combined surgery and chemoradiotherapy

* The survival rate is considerably reduced when regional lymph-node metastases are present, and is reduced even more if the nodes are fixed (see pp. 321–322).

† The first figure is the disease-free survival, the second is the overall survival.

Rehabilitation of the laryngectomee

1. Voice and speech
   - Approximately 20 % of laryngectomees can learn esophageal speech, or use nonvocal speech. The upper esophageal sphincter vibrates when air is released by eructation. Learning the technique is guided by a speech therapist.
   - Tracheoesophageal puncture is promoted by clinicians as a better method. About 20 % of patients are successfully rehabilitated in the long term.
   - The most widely used (55 %) form of voice rehabilitation after total laryngectomy and postoperative radiotherapy is the artificial larynx. This electronic device produces sound by conducting externally produced vibrations via the skin and tissue of the neck to the pharyngeal wall or the floor of the mouth. Speech in the vocal tract is articulated in the usual manner. Voiced parts can be heard at a conversational volume.

2. Tracheostomy
   - As breathing is only possible via the tracheostomy, aspiration of water during showering, bathing, and swimming should be prevented by special accessories such as a stoma cover or a snorkel.
   - Once the tracheostomy has stabilized, it is usually unnecessary to use a tracheostomy tube. If the tracheostomy tends to shrink, a short individually fitted stoma button can be used, or it may be necessary to widen the stoma surgically.

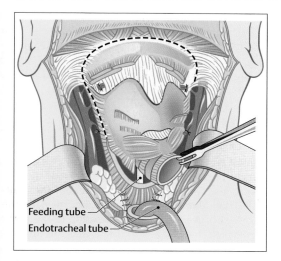

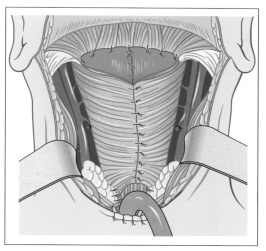

Fig. 4.39 Laryngectomy. A U-shaped incision is made, and the skin–platysma flap is turned superiorly over the chin. The larynx together with the hyoid bone (dashed line above) is freed from its connection with the surrounding soft tissue and from the trachea and is divided from the trachea inferiorly. It is also divided from the esophagus below and from the hypopharynx. The excision may also proceed from above downward. The feeding tube is usually replaced with a tube positioned via percutaneous endoscopic gastrostomy (PEG). The thyroid gland, which is divided and sutured laterally, is visible in the lower part of the drawing.

Fig. 4.40   The situation after removal of the larynx and closure of the pharyngeal mucosa in layers.

- There is a tendency for tracheitis with crusts to develop, particularly in the spring and fall, because of the absence of the air-conditioning mechanism provided by the nose.

3. Social reintegration
   - Patients and their relatives need thorough instruction before the operation about future functional deficits. Medical and psychological training is necessary after the operation. The patient is encouraged to join a laryngectomee club.

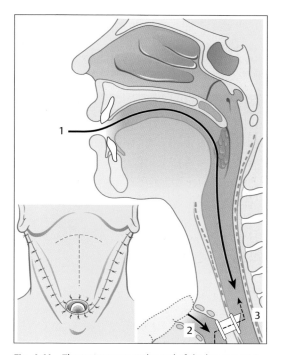

Fig. 4.41   The appearance at the end of the laryngectomy. The replaced U-shaped skin flap covers the newly repaired pharynx. The T-shaped pharyngeal suture line is shown by the dotted line in the inset on the left. **1**, The food passage has been reconstructed. Normal swallowing can be resumed after healing. **2**, Tracheostomy for a new airway. **3**, Closing the tracheostomy with a finger or a valve enables the patient to talk over a voice prosthesis, which is inserted via a tracheoesophageal puncture.

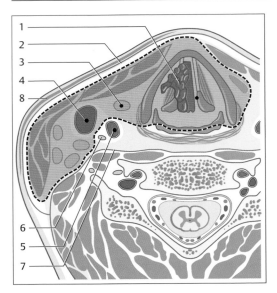

Fig. 4.42 Laryngectomy with radical neck dissection. The area to be resected is shown by the dashed line. **1**, Larynx with the tumor; **2**, superficial cervical fascia, which coincides with the limits of radical neck dissection; **3**, cervical lymph nodes; **4**, internal jugular vein; **5**, carotid artery; **6**, vagus nerve; **7**, deep cervical fascia; **8**, platysma.

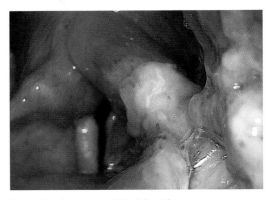

Fig. 4.43 Carcinoma of the left piriform recess.

Hypopharynx

Anatomy. See pp. 232 and 233.

The most important diseases in this region are foreign bodies, pulsion diverticulum (see p. 362), and carcinoma (**Fig. 4.43**).

■ **Hypopharyngeal Carcinoma**

The TNM classification distinguishes three regions (**Fig. 4.44**):

- Pharyngoesophageal junction (postcricoid area).
- Piriform recess.
- Posterior pharyngeal wall.

The T staging is shown in **Table 3.11**.

Clinical Features. In more than 40% of cases, the patient presents as a result of lymph-node metastases. The typical site is at the angle of the jaw under the sternocleidomastoid muscle. The patient also has dysphagia and pain radiating to the ear. Hoarseness and dyspnea indicate that the tumor has extended to the larynx or paralyzed the recurrent laryngeal nerve. Oral fetor (degenerating tumor) and bloodstained sputum may also occur.

Pathogenesis. Alcohol and nicotine abuse are predisposing factors in the development of hypopharyngeal squamous cell carcinoma. The ratio of men to women is estimated at 3 : 1. Postcricoid carcinoma occurs more frequently in women. The disease may be related to Plummer–Vinson (Paterson–Kelly) syndrome. About 50% of patients have T3 N1–2 tumors when first seen. Carcinomas of the posterolateral pharyngeal wall and of the postcricoid region have a particularly high rate of metastases, often bilateral in postcricoid lesions. Distant metastases in the lung, liver, and skeleton are found at the time of diagnosis in 10% of cases, and at autopsy in as many as 80% of patients. Virtually all of the tumors are poorly differentiated squamous cell carcinomas.

With regard to the order of frequency of various sites of hypopharyngeal carcinoma, tumors in the piriform recess are the most common, followed by lesions in the posterior pharyngeal wall. Postcricoid tumors are rare (**Fig. 4.45**).

Diagnosis. Early symptoms involving swallowing difficulties and cervical lymph-node metastases are often neglected, so that the diagnosis is delayed. The time elapsing between the early symptoms and the first examination by a specialist is often too long. Endoscopic examination should always be carried out when a hypopharyngeal carcinoma is suspected. The tumor may be ulcerating or exophytic in type, and it is often surrounded by edema and covered with retained saliva and food remnants.

> **Note:** Cervical lymph-node metastases with an unknown primary tumor require thorough examination of the hypopharynx.

Treatment. Surgery depends on the site and extent of the tumor and the presence of lymphatic or blood-borne metastases. For T1 tumors, partial resection of the hypopharynx with endoscopic access or via open surgery is appropriate. T2 tumors require partial resection of the hypopharynx, which may involve parts of the larynx and thyroid gland. Transoral resection with CO_2 laser is an alternative. T3 tumors require hypopharyngectomy and laryngectomy, including the thyroid gland and reconstruction of the hypopharyngeal walls. T4 tumors usually cannot be treated surgically.

The pharynx and upper esophagus can be reconstructed with a forearm free flap, jejunal free flap, gastric pull-up, platysma flap, or myocutaneous flap from the chest wall.

A neck dissection is indicated on one or both sides, due to the very high rate of metastases to the cervical lymph nodes. Selective neck dissection is carried out in patients with N0 and N1; modified radical neck dissection in patients with N2; and radical neck dissection in patients with N3.

Postoperative radiotherapy is indicated when there are positive resection margins, multiple pathologic lymph nodes, or in patients with an advanced tumor stage.

In patients with advanced stages of the disease who are in poor general condition, chemoradiotherapy is indicated instead of surgery. This can lead to 5-year survival rates of 25–50 %.

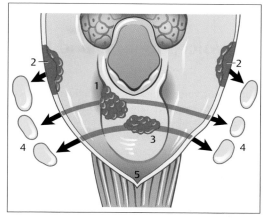

Fig. 4.44 The sites of carcinomas in the hypopharynx (**1–3**) and pathways of lymphatic metastasis. The hypopharynx has been opened posteriorly. The esophageal inlet (**5**) lies inferiorly. **1**, Piriform sinus; **2**, posterior pharyngeal wall; **3**, postcricoid region; **4**, chain of deep cervical nodes along the internal jugular vein.

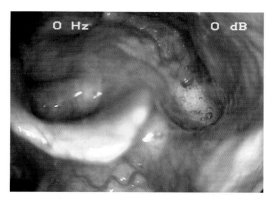

Fig. 4.45 Carcinoma of the postcricoid region at the esophageal inlet.

5 Voice, Speech, and Language

Nonorganic voice disorders, speech fluency, articulation, and language are a field for specialized physicians, known as phoniatricians. The training provided for these specialists is not standardized across Europe. Some start as otolaryngologists for 2 years and then focus on the diagnosis and treatment of communication disorders. Others are otolaryngologists who specialize later during their career. Phoniatrics is not a commonly known subspecialty, but phoniatric centers are scattered all over Europe. In the U.S., otolaryngologists with a special interest in laryngology provide care for voice patients. Communication disorders that are not treated medically are subject to treatment by speech and language therapists or speech-language pathologists. In the Scandinavian countries and in central and eastern Europe, these therapists are also called logopedists.

Voice

■ Voice Production

Voice involves interaction between the respiratory system, larynx, vocal tract, articulatory organs, and cerebral coordination. *Vocalization* means producing sound, preferably on an emotional level; *phonation* is sound production with the aim of communicating by speech or singing. The two terms are interchangeable. The coordination of phonation originates in two centers in the brain—the limbic system and the primary motor area of articulatory organs in the cortex.

■ Glottal Sound Generation

Modulation of the air stream during phonation is controlled through the interaction of the vocal folds with the air stream, which results in passive vibration of the vocal folds. The configuration of the glottal aperture and its elasticity during phonation is adjusted by the neuromuscular system. The vocal folds adduct, contract, and tense. According to the myoelastic–aerodynamic theory in voice initiation, the vocal folds adduct, forming a slightly closed or narrow channel between the subglottic and supraglottic airways. During expiration, air pressure builds up at the level of the glottis and pushes against the vocal folds. Sufficient air pressure pushes air through the glottal aperture. The following forces close the glottis:

- Bernoulli's effect of airflow through the glottis generates a negative force that pulls the vocal folds medially.
- The elasticity of the vocal folds (passive recoiling) returns the vocal fold tissue to the shape it had before it was deformed by transglottic pressure.
- Air passing through the glottis from the subglottic reservoir causes a fall in subglottic pressure. The driving force pushing the vocal folds apart decreases.

When the vocal folds close and obstruct airflow, subglottic pressure builds up to deform the vocal fold tissue and start another cycle of the opening phase. This process as a whole is called the *glottic cycle*. Characteristic phases of glottal deformation during vibration are shown in **Fig. 5.1**.

The fundamental frequency determines the perceived pitch of the voice, which is related to the number of vibrations of the vocal folds per second (Hz). The recurrent laryngeal nerve sends neural signals to the laryngeal musculature, which varies the tension of the folds and their configuration. This leads to tones at different frequencies and loudness levels.

■ Body-cover Model

The *body-cover model* is an attempt to classify the connective-tissue structures of the vocal fold into functional units (**Table 5.1**). It groups the five anatomical tissue layers of the vocal fold (see **Fig. 4.2a, b**) into three functional layers: The first layer, called the *cover*, consists of the epithelium and superficial lamina propria. The cover is pliable, elastic, and nonmuscular. The second layer, called the *transi-*

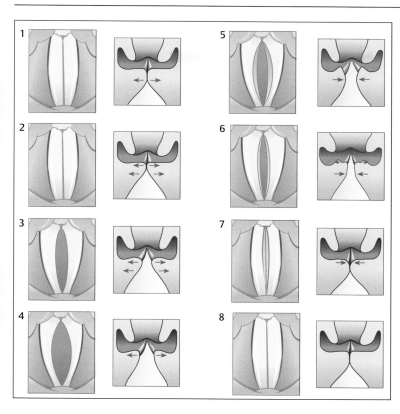

Fig. 5.1 Characteristic features of normal vocal fold vibration as seen in stroboscopy. **1**, The lower part of the glottis starts to open; **2**, the upper part of the glottis starts to open; **3**, the lower and upper part of the glottis open; **4**, the lower part of two glottis is maximally open, and the upper part of glottis is still opening; **5**, the lower part of the glottis closes and is visible; **6**, the lower and upper part of the glottis close, and a mucosal wave propagates on the surface; **7**, the lower part of the glottis is closed; **8**, the upper part of the glottis is closed.

tion, is the vocal ligament, consisting of the elastic and collagen fibers of the intermediate and deep layers of the lamina propria. The third layer, called the *body*, consists of the medial thyroarytenoid or vocalis muscle. It is stiff. The effective tension of the vocal folds depends on the interaction between the cover and the body, which is adjusted by muscle contraction.

■ **Source-filter Theory**

Vocalization is sound production in the larynx. It does not necessarily involve articulation. However, all human voice productions are altered when they pass the vocal tract. The configuration of the tract determines the sound that emerges from the lips. The acoustic properties of the vocal tract shape the spectrum of the primary glottal source, as explained by the *source-filter theory*. This is based on the notion that the spectrum of the laryngeal voice source and the vocal tract resonator are clearly separable and independent. Sound produced in

Table 5.1 Layers of the vocal folds: anatomical tissue layers compared with functional layers in the body-cover model

Five tissue layers		Body-cover model	
Epithelium		Mucosa	Cover
Lamina propria	Superficial layer		
	Intermediate layer	Vocal ligament	Transition
	Deep layer		
Thyroarytenoid muscle (vocalis)		Muscle	Body

the glottis travels through the air-filled supraglottic space, the throat, and the oral and nasal cavities before being emitted into the environment (**Fig. 5.2**). The air in this vocal tract resonator has multiple resonance frequencies at which it enhances existing spectral components (*harmonics*). These vocal tract resonances (*formants*) act as filters that shape the spectrum of the sound generated by

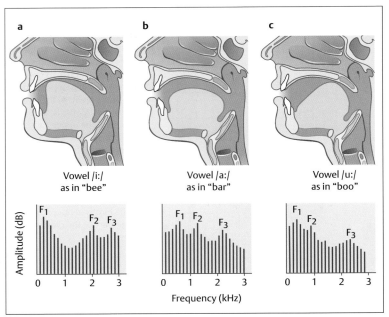

Fig. 5.2a–c A sagittal section through the vocal tract for three different vowels, /i:/ as in bee, /a:/ as in bar, and /u:/ as in boo, showing the tongue position and the power spectra of the emitted sound with the first (F₁), second (F₂), and third (F₃) formants.

the source (larynx) to produce an output signal that is a combination of source and filter (**Fig. 5.3**). The different sounds of human speech (*phonemes*) depend strongly on formants. In all human languages, vowels are distinguished by the frequencies of the two lowest formants (**Fig. 5.4**). The third, fourth, and fifth formants are of greater significance to personal voice timbre.

■ Voice Diagnosis

The following aspects need to be taken into account when assessing common forms of dysphonia.

History. The patient's history should reveal causes of the disturbed voice function—beginning with the age, the voice problem, whether it is acute or chronic, and whether it is related to vocal load or environmental irritants. What is the patient's overall physical condition? Are there any allergies or breathing problems, or is the patient a smoker? Is food affecting the voice? Reflux may cause voice problems. Sex hormones can alter the voice. Hearing loss is a source of vocal problems. Surgery in the throat, larynx, or neck, or intubation, as well as medications and drugs, can alter the voice.

Is the voice abused during speaking or during singing? Does the patient have pain when talking or singing? Laryngologists should ask about the amount of vocal exercises and their duration, the time of day, and activities that have adverse effects on the vocal folds such as weightlifting, aerobics, and playing of some wind instruments. Information about voice training may reveal technical deficiencies. Pressing commitments to events requiring public speaking or singing may cause physical and emotional stress.

Voice registration. Audio recording is the most valuable basic tool for voice assessment, for blind perceptual evaluation by a panel, or for sophisticated acoustic analyses. It is essential for all recordings of voice patients to be filed as an archive from which it is easy to retrieve an earlier sample. A digital recording system should be used to store signals, unless analogue–digital conversion and storage can be done directly by the computer. A sampling frequency of at least 20,000 Hz is recommended. For the recordings, a quiet room with ambient noise < 50 dB is acceptable. The mouth-to-microphone distance needs to be kept constant at 10 cm.

Perception. The rating is based on the patient's speech while reading a text. Two main components of hoarseness have been identified:

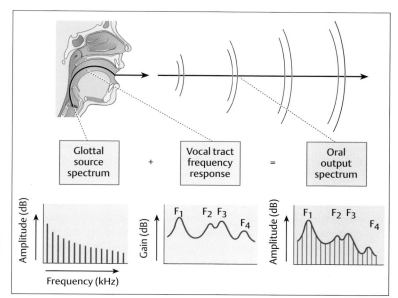

Fig. 5.3 The source-filter model. The spectrum of the sound produced at the level of the glottis (left) is altered by the shape, and thus by the acoustic properties, of the vocal tract (middle), which leads to a characteristic spectrum in the emitted sound (right).

Breathiness (B): an audible impression of turbulent air leakage through an insufficient glottic closure may include short aphonic moments (unvoiced segments).

Roughness (R) or harshness: an audible impression of irregular glottic pulses, abnormal fluctuations in fundamental frequency (F_0), and separately perceived acoustic impulses (as in vocal fry), including diplophonia and register breaks.

The severity of hoarseness is quantified using the parameter G (grade). This represents the overall voice quality, integrating all deviant components. The term "hoarseness" (H) may also be used for this overall perceptual parameter.

A more extended rating known as GRBAS—including G (grade), R (roughness), B (breathiness), A (asthenia), and S (strain)—is sometimes used for assessing the voice, and this may be encountered in the literature. However, there are no clear pathophysiologic explanations for "asthenia," which may sound breathy, or "strain," which also may include roughness.

A scale known as RBH has therefore been developed from the above components of auditory perceptual analyses. For reporting purposes, each component is graded on four points (0, normal or absence of deviance; 1, slight deviance; 2, moderate deviance; 3, severe deviance). The highest score becomes the grade. This is a very simple but reliable way of documenting voice quality. It is subjective, and is best evaluated by speech and language therapy practitioners and phoniatricians.

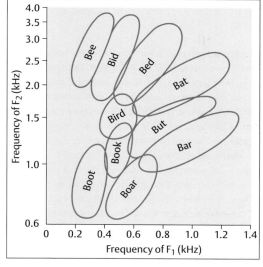

Fig. 5.4 Vowels are mainly determined by their first (F_1) and second (F_2) formants. Formants are resonances of the vocal tract altered by tongue motion, jaw opening, and widening or narrowing of the pharynx. Their frequency changes due to the preceding and following phonemes, a phenomenon known as coarticulation.

It is also possible to score RBH on a visual analogue scale (VAS), which is a line 100 mm long. Marking a distance on this line reflects the perceived severity. The left end indicates an absence (0 mm) and the right end indicates full expression (100 mm) of any of the deviations. For easier rating, anchoring points indicating mild, moderate, and severe may be provided along the line.

Video stroboscopy. Video laryngostroboscopy is the main clinical tool for the etiological diagnosis of voice disorders. It can also be used to assess the quality of vocal fold vibration and thus the effectiveness of medical or surgical treatments. The basic parameters involved are:

Glottal closure: Insufficient closure can be longitudinal (over the whole length of the glottis and without sufficient adduction), dorsal (posterior triangular chink—occurs in ≈ 60 % of middle-aged healthy women during normal voice effort), ventral, irregular, oval (over the whole length of the glottis, but with a dorsal closure), or hourglass-shaped.

Regularity. *Mucosal wave*: accounts for the physiology of the layered structure of the vocal folds; see **Table 5.1** and **Fig. 5.1**.

Symmetry: The "mirror" motion of the two vocal folds. Usually, asymmetry is caused by limited vibratory quality due to a lesion—e. g., diffuse scar, localized cyst, or leukoplakia.

Acoustics. Acoustic parameters provide objective and noninvasive measures of vocal function. Perturbation measures (in period and amplitude) and harmonics-to-noise computations have emerged as the most robust measures, and these appear to capable of determining the basic perceptual elements of voice quality—*grade, roughness,* and *breathiness*. Percentage jitter and percentage shimmer are currently used as the basic acoustic measures, computed using a voice sample of a sustained /a:/ at a comfortable frequency and intensity. *Jitter* is computed as the mean difference between the periods of adjacent cycles divided by the mean period. It is a measurement that is therefore related to the fundamental frequency (F_0). *Shimmer* is computed as the mean difference between peak-to-peak amplitudes divided by the mean amplitude. Obviously, comparisons of voice quality before and after treatment require the use of similar techniques and materials in both tests.

Aerodynamics. The simplest aerodynamic parameter in voicing is the maximum phonation time (MPT) in seconds. This consists of a prolongation of the vowel /a:/ for as long as possible after maximum inspiration and at a spontaneous, comfortable pitch and loudness. A prior demonstration is necessary, and three trials are required, the longest time being selected.

Voice range profile (VRP). This determines the upper and lower limits of both the pitch range and loudness. The VRP is recorded using specialized software on a computer equipped with a microphone. The patient sits in front of the computer (ideally, in a soundproof room) and says "/a:/" at various pitches and loudness levels. On the monitor, the computer draws a graph of the sounds of the patient's voice. Pitch (frequency) is measured from left to right, with the lowest-pitched notes at the far left. Loudness (intensity) is measured from bottom to top, with the softest sounds near the bottom. When pitch and loudness are displayed together, the shape of the whole voice recording is often like a football. The range of loud and soft sounds is wide in the comfortable middle of the pitch range and more limited near the higher and lower pitches. The basic acoustic measures include three critical points of the VRP. The *highest frequency* and the *softest intensity*—dB(A) at 30 cm—appear to be the most sensitive for changes in voice quality, the latter being related to the phonation threshold pressure. The additional measurement of the *lowest frequency* makes it possible to compute the pitch range.

Subjective rating by patient. This evaluation of voice is becoming increasingly important in everyday clinical practice. It is the patient who has to live with his/her voice. A voice handicap index can be computed on the basis of a patient's responses to a carefully selected list of questions that investigates the severity of disability/handicap in everyday social and/or professional life and the possible emotional repercussions of the dysphonia. An easy subjective evaluation can be provided by patient themselves on a double visual analogue scale of 100 mm (see above). On the first scale, the impression of the voice quality in the strict sense is marked; on the second scale, the impression of what impact the voice problem has on everyday social and, if relevant, professional life and activities is marked.

A score of "0" (at the extreme left) means a normal voice and no voice-related disability or handicap in everyday life, whereas "100" (at the extreme right) means extreme voice deviance and extreme voice-related disability or handicap in everyday social (and professional) activities, as rated by patients themselves.

■ Functional Voice Disorders

Vocal Misuse and Musculoskeletal Tension Dysphonia

Signs and symptoms. The main symptom is vocal fatigue. The voice is loaded but unable to be heard in a given environment (e. g., a classroom). Patients feel a sore throat, pain in the neck, or a lump in the throat. The voice presents with mild to moderate hoarseness.

Pathogenesis. Voice generation with disrupted balance of the respiration, phonation, and resonation that are necessary for efficient voice production. Overuse or abusive voice behaviors may lead to organic changes such as vocal nodules, vocal polyps, vocal fold cysts, or contact granulomas. Misuse of extrinsic and intrinsic laryngeal muscles causes tension or pain at the larynx and vocal fatigue.

Diagnosis. Organic changes are described in Chapter 4. In nonorganic disorders, video stroboscopy shows no specific findings, with the exception of a posterior gap in the closed phase of the glottal cycle in most patients. Voice diagnosis generally reveals a breathy voice with mild hoarseness, a reduced MPT, reduced vocal intensity in the VRP, normal jitter, and mild to moderate handicap on subjective assessment.

Treatment. In accordance with the history, it has to be decided whether treatment should be conservative in order to achieve the long-term goals desired in the patient's career.

If a nonorganic voice disorder is obviously due to vocal misuse and muscle tension, a more symptom-orientated voice therapy should be favored. Organic changes should be treated by combining surgery and voice therapy.

Psychogenic Voice Disorder
Signs and symptoms. Total inability to speak; whispered speech in cases of conversion aphonia; strained or strangled speech in cases of conversion dysphonia.

Pathogenesis. The voice disorder is a manifestation of psychological disequilibrium—such as anxiety, depression, conversion reaction, or a personality disorder—that is interfering with volitional control over phonation. This may lead to musculoskeletal tension disorders or vocal abuse, which can be observed or retrieved from the patient's history.

Diagnosis. During video laryngoscopy, organic changes may be visible such as vocal nodules, contact ulcers, or ventricular phonation. Voice diagnosis is difficult, as the patient is often unwilling or unable to comply with the tasks it involves.

Treatment. This is carried out by a speech and language therapist or psychotherapist. A patient with psychogenic or conversion aphonia should be treated immediately during the first visit to a voice clinic. Treatments for conversion dysphonia may require 10–20 sessions, and with further sessions depending on the progress the patient makes. Psychotherapy may also be required.

Spasmodic Dysphonia
Clinical Features. Adductor spasmodic dysphonia comes with a tight voice quality, abrupt initiation and termination of voicing, a broken speech pattern, and short breaks in speech. In very rare cases of abductor spasmodic dysphonia, the glottis opens when the patient attempts to speak and only whispering is possible.

Pathogenesis. Spasmodic dysphonia is a focal form of dystonia. Dystonia disorders are thought to be due to abnormal functioning in the basal ganglia of the brain. Involuntary excessive contraction of the muscles that bring the vocal folds together affects the flow of air through the vocal folds. The air is pressed through the glottis with strong effort.

Diagnosis. An interdisciplinary approach is required. The otolaryngologist or phoniatrician can exclude any structural abnormality of the larynx such as nodules, polyps, neoplasms, or inflammation. The speech and language therapist evaluates the patient's voice production and voice quality. The neurologist evaluates the patient for other signs of dystonia, other muscle movement disorders, or other neurological conditions.

Treatment. The most frequent treatment today is local injection of botulinum toxin into the vocal fold muscles. There is not enough evidence regarding surgery, but attempts are being made to develop reliable procedures. Complementary speech therapy is often terminated by the patients themselves when they receive repeated botulinum toxin injections.

Paradoxical Vocal Fold Movement

Clinical Features. Wheezing or inspiratory stridor due to inappropriate closure of the true vocal folds during respiration.

Pathogenesis. The nature of this disease is not well understood, and its incidence is still unknown. It may occur in patients with asthma; focal laryngeal dystonia; Gerhardt syndrome (congenital laryngeal abductor paralysis); psychogenic, drug-induced laryngeal dystonia; gastroesophageal reflux; or it may be exercise-induced.

Diagnosis. This is made by exclusion. Transnasal fiberoptic endoscopy during an acute attack reveals a pattern of vocal fold adductory and abductory movement consistent with paradoxical movement during repeated tasks such as phonating the vowel / ee/ and sniffing, coughing, panting, or throat-clearing. Spirometry (assessment of pulmonary flow volume loops), arterial blood gases, bronchial challenge testing, and chest radiography are carried out.

Treatment. This consists of psychotherapy, pharmacologic management (to relieve the symptoms), and behavioral management (speech therapy). Botulinum toxin can sometimes be effective.

Speech

Functional Speech Disorders (Dyslalia, Articulation Disorder)

Clinical Features. Functional speech disorder is one of several speech sound disorders that can occur in children and persist to adulthood. A child with a functional speech disorder has difficulty in learning to make a specific speech sound (e. g., /r/), or a few specific speech sounds, which may include some or all of these: /s/, /z/, /r/, /l/ and /th/. The most common disorder is lisp (stigmatism).

Causes. Unknown.

Diagnosis. This is made by a speech and language therapist.

Therapy. Treatment is given by a speech and language therapist. In general, the prognosis for the successful treatment of functional speech disorders in children is good.

Developmental Phonological Disorders

Clinical Features. By the age of 4 years, children with this disorder will show an impaired ability to produce sounds as expected for their developmental level. These children have poor phonological awareness (the ability to recognize and manipulate the sounds and syllables used to compose words) in particular, and poor metalinguistic ability (the capacity to think about and talk about language) generally.

Affected children do not pronounce sounds clearly, or replace one sound with another, e. g., / k/ is replaced by /t/, or /g/ is replaced by /d/: "I'm a dood dirl." The child has difficulty in learning and organizing all the sounds needed for clear speech, reading, and spelling. Difficulties in speech sound production interfere with academic or occupational achievement, or with social communication.

Pathogenesis. The disorder is more common in boys and affects ≈ 10 % of children under the age of 8 years. Five percent of those above 8 years of age have this disorder. By the age of 17 years, the incidence of phonological disorder is reduced to 0.5 % (an estimate, as there are no reliable data). A phonological disorder will occur if the sound is stored wrongly in the child's mind, or if the sound is actually said incorrectly by the child, or the cognitive processes that correlate storage and articulation are absent or incorrect.

Diagnosis. Assessment by a speech and language therapist helps determine what the particular needs of an individual child are. The child may have:

- A problem with speech clarity during preschool years, with no subsequent reading and spelling problems.
- A problem with speech clarity during preschool years and in early school years, difficulty in learning to read and difficulties with reading comprehension.
- Speech and reading problems as described above, plus difficulty with spelling.
- Speech and spelling problems (i. e., no reading difficulties).

- Speech clarity problems during preschool years, and difficulties with written expression in elementary school (primary school).

Differential diagnosis. Hearing impairment, delayed speech, mental retardation, and learning disability also lead to language use that is not easily understood.

Treatment. Most children with dyslalia or phonological disorders need speech and language therapy for a long period.

Stuttering

Stuttering is a disorder in which speech is interrupted by repeated movements and fixed postures of the speech mechanism. These interruptions may be accompanied by signs of struggle and tension. The speech disruptions involved in stuttering range from mild to severe. Stuttering may also be quite variable within individuals.

The impact of stuttering on everyday life. Someone who stutters may experience extreme frustration and anxiety about speaking. Stuttering interferes with communication and with people's social interactions, causes embarrassment, prevents attainment of the vocational potential, and may lead to social anxiety or social phobia.

Causes. Stuttering is most likely due to a problem with neural processing (brain activity) that underlies speech production. It appears to be almost entirely confined to speech production. People who stutter are not as a group less intelligent or less well coordinated than those who do not stutter. Adults who stutter are more prone to social anxiety than others. Stuttering is thought to be a physical disorder and is not thought to be caused by psychological factors such as nervousness or stress, or parenting practices, or the way parents communicate with their children when they are young. The learning theory assumes that stuttering results from an effort not to stutter. The breakdown theory claims that the coordination of the anatomical structures involved in speech is affected. The demands and capacities model regards stuttering as a result of high demands on fluent speech with inadequate motor, cognitive, and linguistic abilities on the part the speaker. There is a genetic element in the etiology, but the precise nature of the inheritance is at present unknown.

Developmental stuttering. About 5% of children start to stutter, usually during the third and fourth years of life. The onset typically occurs as children are starting to put words together into short sentences. The onset of stuttering can be gradual or sudden, and at onset the severity of stuttering ranges from mild to severe. In a few cases, the onset can be so sudden and severe that parents think their child has a serious illness.

Symptoms

- Repeating syllables or part-word repetition: "I … I … I … wanna …" or "Where … where … where is …?" or "W – W – W – Where are you going?"
- Stoppage of speech: holding the lips and tongue in one position for brief periods (when attempting to start a word, as in "………………… can I have a drink?")
- Sound prolongation, as in "*Wwwwwww*here is my drink?"
- Interjections: the speaker produces several interjections in order to say the word "around" smoothly ("I'll meet you – *um um you know like* – around six o'clock"), because he or she expects to have difficulty in smoothly joining the word "you" with the word "around."
- Unusual facial and body movements associated with the effort to speak.

Natural recovery. Many children recover from stuttering naturally, although the exact rate of recovery and the average time taken to recover is not known. It seems that more girls recover naturally than boys, and that having a family history of recovery from stuttering may increase a child's chances of recovering naturally. The chances of recovery seem to be best shortly after the onset of the condition. However, at present, it is not possible to say whether an individual child will recover naturally or will require treatment.

Therapy. Developmental stuttering is often treated by providing parents with information about how to restructure the child's speaking environment in order to reduce episodes of stuttering. Parents are often urged to:

- Provide a relaxed home environment that provides ample opportunities for the child to speak. Setting aside specific times when the child and parent can speak free of distractions is often helpful.
- Refrain from criticizing the child's speech or reacting negatively to the child's disfluencies. Parents should avoid punishing the child for any disfluency or asking the child to repeat stuttered words until they are spoken fluently.
- Resist the urge to encourage the child to perform verbally for people.
- Listen attentively to the child when he or she speaks.
- Speak slowly and in a relaxed manner. If a parent speaks this way, the child will often speak in the same slow, relaxed manner.
- Wait for the child to say the intended word. Do not try to complete the child's thoughts.
- Talk openly to the child about stuttering if he or she brings up the subject.

A speech evaluation is recommended for children who stutter for more than 6 months or for those whose stuttering is accompanied by struggle behaviors.

Two main therapeutic strategies have been developed. *Fluency shaping* focuses on relearning how to speak or unlearning faulty ways of speaking. Following the *nonavoidance strategy,* the stutterer (1) identifies the symptoms, (2) reduces anxiety, (3) releases blocks by modification, and (4) stabilizes speech by applying these methods. The psychological side effects of stuttering should also be addressed. Any of a variety of treatments may improve stuttering to some degree, but there is at present no cure for stuttering. Stuttering therapy, however, may help prevent developmental stuttering from becoming a lifelong problem.

Medications or drugs which affect brain function often have side effects that make them difficult to use for long-term treatment. Electronic devices that help an individual to control fluency may be troublesome in most speaking situations and are therefore often abandoned by individuals who stutter.

Unconventional methods of stuttering therapy also exist. It is a good policy to check the credentials, experience, and goals of the person offering treatment and to avoid working with anyone who promises a "cure" for stuttering.

Language

Normal Language Development
Milestones for normal language development are provided in **Table 5.2**. These are helpful for comparing a child's developmental stage with what can be expected at various ages.

Table 5.2 Normal language development

Age of child	Typical language development
0–2 months	Phonation stage. The baby should produce comfort sounds and coo with normal-sounding vocalizations. A few utterances may sound "vowel-like"
2–3 months	Cooing stage. The baby should produce "vowel-like" sounds and "consonant-like" sounds made in the back of the mouth
4–6 months	Expansion stage. The baby produces a variety of sounds, including raspberries (labial trills), squeals, growls, yells, whispers, and isolated vowel-like syllables
7–10 months	Canonical stage. The baby will say /bababa/, /dadada/, /mamama/ or other reduplicated syllabic sequences. Vocalization with intonation. Responds to name, to human voices without visual cues by turning the head and eyes, and to friendly and angry tones
11–12 months	Variegated babbling. The baby will produce gibberish speech with a wide variety of sounds and sequences. Uses one or more words with meaning (this may be a fragment of a word). Understands simple instructions, especially if vocal or physical cues are given. Practices inflection. Is aware of the social value of speech
18 months	Has vocabulary of around 5–20 words, made up chiefly of nouns. Some echolalia (repeating a word or phrase over and over). Much jargon with emotional content. Child's speech is 25 % intelligible. Is able to follow simple commands

Table 5.2 Normal language development (continued)

Age of child	Typical language development
2 years	Can name several objects common to the surroundings. Is able to use at least two prepositions, usually chosen from the following: in, on, under. (Mean) length of sentences is given as one or two words, largely noun–verb combinations. Vocabulary of around 150–300 words. Child's speech is 50–75 % intelligible. Can use the pronouns "I/me" and "you" correctly, although "me" and "I" are often confused. "My" and "mine" are beginning to emerge. Responds to commands such as "show me your eyes (nose, mouth, hair)"
3 years	Uses the pronouns "I," "you," and "me" correctly, and some plurals and past tenses. Knows at least three prepositions, usually "in," "on," and "under." Knows the main parts of the body and should be able to indicate these if not name them. Handles three-word sentences easily. Has 900–1000 words. The child's speech is 75–100 % intelligible. Verbs begin to predominate. Understands most simple questions dealing with the environment and activities. Relates experiences so that they can be understood. Able to reason out questions such as "What should you do when you are sleepy, hungry, cold, or thirsty?" Children this age should be able to state their own sex, name, and age. They should not be expected to answer all questions, although they understand what is expected
4 years	Knows names of familiar animals. Can use at least four prepositions or can demonstrate understanding of what they mean when given commands. Names common objects in picture books or magazines. Knows one or more colors. Can repeat four numbers when they are given slowly. Can usually repeat words of four syllables. Demonstrates understanding of "over" and "under." Has most vowels and diphthongs and the consonants /p/, /b/, /m/, /w/, and /n/ well established. Often indulges in make-believe. Extensive verbalization when carrying out activities. Understands concepts such as longer and larger, when a contrast is presented. Readily follows simple commands even if the stimulus objects are not in sight. Much repetition of words, phrases, syllables, and even sounds
5 years	Can use many descriptive words spontaneously—both adjectives and adverbs. Knows common opposites: big–small, hard–soft, heavy–light, etc. Has number concepts of four or more. Can count to ten. Speech should be completely intelligible, in spite of articulation problems. Should have all vowels and the consonants /m/, /p/, /b/, /h/, /w/, /k/, /g/, /t/, /d/, /n/, /ng/, /y/ (yellow). Should be able to repeat sentences as long as nine words. Should be able to define common objects in terms of their use (hat, shoe, chair). Should be able to follow three commands given without interruption. Should know his or her age. Should have simple time concepts: morning, afternoon, night, day, later, after, while, tomorrow, yesterday, today. Should be using fairly long sentences and should use some compound and some complex sentences. Speech on the whole should be grammatically correct
6 years	In addition to the above consonants, these should also be mastered: /f/, /v/, /sh/, /zh/, voiced /th/ (this). Speech should be completely intelligible and socially useful. Should be able to tell a fairly connected story about a picture, seeing relationships between objects and events
7 years	Should have mastered the consonants /s/ and /z/, /r/, voiceless /th/ (thing), /ch/, /wh/, and the soft /g/ as in George. Should handle opposite analogies easily: girl–boy, man–woman, flies–swims, blunt–sharp, short–long, sweet–sour, etc. Understands terms such as alike, different, beginning, end, etc. Should be able to tell time to quarter hour. Should be able to do simple reading and to write or print many words
8 years	Can give quite involved accounts of events, many of which occurred at some time in the past. Complex and compound sentences should be used easily. There should be few mistakes in grammatical constructions—tense, pronouns, plurals. All speech sounds, including consonant blends, should be established. Should be reading with considerable ease and now writing simple compositions. Social amenities should be present in his speech in appropriate situations. Control of rate, pitch, and volume are generally good and appropriately established. Can carry on conversation at rather adult level. Follows fairly complex directions with little repetition. Has well-developed time and number concepts

If a baby is not babbling or imitating any sounds by the age of 7 months, it may mean there is a problem with hearing or speech development. Babies with partial hearing loss still can be startled by loud noises or will turn the head toward them, and babies may even respond to their parents' voices. But they will have difficulty in imitating speech. A newborn's hearing should be checked by hearing screening. Later on, observations by parents are an early warning system. A baby should be referred to a children's hearing specialist (pediatric audiologist) if there is any suspicion.

Specific Language Impairment

Language acquisition is the primary area of concern as the child grows and develops. There are no obvious related causes such as hearing loss or low intelligence quotient (IQ) for the condition known as *specific language impairment* (SLI; this is a precise name for terms also used, such as developmental language disorder, language delay, or developmental dysphasia). The condition may be genetic. The incidence of SLI in children of kindergarten age may be as high as 7–8 %, and SLI is known to persist into adulthood.

Clinical Features. SLI is a language disorder. This means that the child has difficulty in understanding and using words in sentences. Both receptive and expressive skills are typically affected. Late talking may be a sign of disability. Five-year old children with SLI sound approximately 2 years younger than their age. Children who do not ask questions or tell adults what they want may have a communication disorder. Children with SLI may not produce any words until they are nearly 2 years old. At the age of 3 years, they may talk, but cannot be understood. As they grow, they struggle to learn new words, make conversation, and sound coherent. An incomplete understanding of verbs is a sign of SLI. Typical errors include dropping the -s off present-tense verbs and asking questions without the usual "be" or "do" verbs, or dropping the past tense ending from verbs. SLI affects a child's academic achievement, and 40–75 % of these children have problems in learning to read.

IQ, hearing, emerging motor skills, social–emotional development, and the child's neurological profile are all normal.

Diagnosis. The signs of SLI are present by the age of 3 years. The Rice–Wexler Test of Early Grammatical Impairment can identify specific gaps in a child's language abilities. It can be used with children aged 3–8 years.

Treatment. Early identification and intervention during preschool years is time well spent to minimize possible academic risks. Children with SLI need extra opportunities to talk and listen. Interactions with other children are especially difficult, as they are less supportive and patient than adults. The focus of class activities may be role-playing, sharing time, or hands-on lessons with new, interesting vocabulary. This kind of preschool will encourage interaction between children, and will build rich layers of language experience. Equipping a child for success at ages 3 and 4 years will lead to positive experiences in the kindergarten. Parents can also send their preschool child to a speech and language therapist.

Differential diagnosis. Several other disabilities, such as mental retardation, autism, hearing loss, or cerebral palsy also involve difficulties communicating, but are not SLI. Speech impediments are different from language disorders. A child with a speech impediment makes errors in pronouncing words, or may stutter.

Aphasia

Aphasia is a communication disorder that occurs after language has been developed, usually in adulthood. Not simply a speech disorder, aphasia can affect the ability to comprehend the speech of others, as well as the ability to read and write. In most instances, intelligence per se is not affected.

Clinical Features. To a variable degree, symptoms include deficiencies in speech production, auditory language comprehension, and phonemic, morphological, and semantic paraphasias. Most experts in aphasia recognize that aphasia varies along two major dimensions, auditory comprehension ability and fluency of speech output, leading to the concept of *nonfluent* and *fluent types* of aphasia.

Nonfluent aphasia (Broca aphasia): Disordered fluency of speech output is characterized by slow, labored speech with limited output and prosody. Individuals have difficulty in using the substantive words of their native language and in producing grammatical sentences. Verbs and prepositions

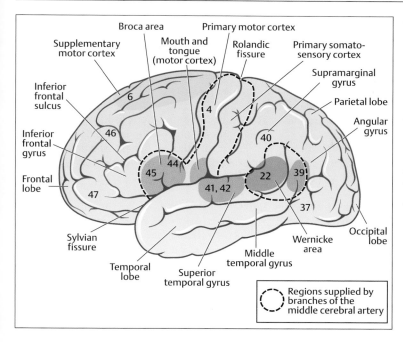

Fig. 5.5 The lateral surface of the left cerebral hemisphere. Brodmann areas 44 and 45 correspond to the Broca area, and area 22 to the Wernicke area. Areas 41 and 42 correspond to the primary auditory cortex; these areas are deep in the sylvian fissure and cannot be visualized in a lateral view of the brain. Area 40 is the supramarginal gyrus, and area 39 is the angular gyrus. The names of gyri and corresponding Brodmann numbers mentioned in **Table 5.3** are also listed.

are disproportionately affected. Speech errors occur mostly at the level of speech sounds, producing sound transpositions and inconsistencies. Auditory comprehension is only minimally affected. Reading abilities parallel comprehension. There is an inability to repeat what someone else says. Broca's aphasia is quite likely to co-occur with motor problems. Hemiplegia on the side of the body opposite the side of brain damage affects walking and writing. Writing problems parallel speech output, but there are diminished abilities if the arm used for writing is paralyzed.

Fluent aphasia (Wernicke aphasia): Individuals with fluent aphasia have problems in comprehending and monitoring their own speech. They are verbose and use inappropriate and jargon words. There is a disproportionate difficulty in understanding spoken and written language. Reading and writing are impaired in similar ways to auditory comprehension and speech output. The patients' comprehension difficulties make them unable to repeat words spoken by others. Individuals with fluent aphasia seldom have coexisting difficulty with the mechanics of speech, arm use, or walking.

In *anomic aphasia,* individuals have problems with naming.

Conduction aphasia is due to damage to the neural links between the posterior and anterior speech areas, which makes it quite difficult for these individuals to correct the errors they hear themselves making and affects their ability to repeat the speech of others.

Pathogenesis. The language zone in the brain includes the portion of the frontal, temporal, and parietal lobes surrounding the sylvian fissure and structures deep to these areas (**Fig. 5.5**). Aphasia is most frequently caused by damage to the cerebral cortex of the left hemisphere of the brain, which is dominant in language processing and language skills. Hemispheric laterality is reversed in a small minority of patients: this feature is seen in about half of left-handed individuals and in a few right-handed persons. In these cases, right-hemisphere damage is the cause of aphasia. Aphasia occasionally results from damage to subcortical structures such as the basal ganglia or thalamus, which has rich interconnections with the cerebral cortex.

Stroke is the most common cause of aphasia. Twenty percent of individuals who suffer strokes develop some form of aphasia. Other causes include head injuries, brain tumors, and infection.

Diagnosis. Information about the location of the damage is obtained with magnetic resonance imaging (MRI) and computed tomography (CT). Language function tests (naming, comprehension, reading, writing, and repetition) and tests of other cognitive functions should be performed immediately after a stroke. Language is the medium through which most cognitive functions are observed. It should therefore be assessed first. If extensive aphasia is present, only cautious interpretations of other cognitive functions may be given.

The examination involves listening to spontaneous speech and evaluating the individual's ability to recognize and name objects, comprehend what is heard, and repeat sample words and phrases. The individual may also be asked to read text aloud and explain what the passage means. In addition, writing ability is evaluated by having the individual copy text, transcribe dictated text, and write something without prompting.

Standardized measures provide an inventory of aphasic symptoms (e. g., the Aachen Aphasia Test and the Boston Diagnostic Aphasia Examination). These tests provide baseline and follow-up assessments to measure progress in treatment, and guide the treatment itself. Assessment of aphasia should comprise the following linguistic levels:

- *Communication abilities:* conversation, comprehension, and passing of information
- *Articulation and prosody:* precision, fluency, speech velocity, rhythm, and vocalization
- *Automated speech*: repeated, invariable, unintended utterances such as verbal automatisms, stereotypes, and echolalia
- *Semantic structure:* retrieving words, combining words, differentiating the meaning of words, sidestepping to meaningless set phrases

- *Phonemic structure*: appearance and order of sounds in words (mix-up, elision, addition, alteration, etc.)
- *Syntactic structure:* completeness and complexity of sentences, number and position of parts of sentences, inflections and linking elements, diagnosis of agrammatism and paragrammatism

The major symptoms used in identifying aphasia syndromes are provided in **Table 5.3**.

Individuals without aphasia should perform on aphasia tests (such as the Token Test) with almost no errors.

Differential diagnosis
- Dysarthria caused by paralysis affecting the many muscles involved in speaking, such as the muscles of the tongue. Dysarthria often co-occurs with aphasia.
- Traumatic brain injury (TBI). Physical trauma to the head, causing damage to the brain, which may be focal or restricted to a single area of the brain, or diffuse and affecting more than one region of the brain.
- Dementias such as Alzheimer disease. In these cases, general cognitive disturbances lead to the linguistic consequences of language disturbances.

Treatment. Medical treatment in stroke units and neurological wards in the early phase is necessary for reducing the long-term effects of stroke. Language therapy and cognitive rehabilitation by speech and language therapists are aimed at modifying language and communication skills and training the aphasic patient to communicate with relatively intact language skills such as reading and writing. Aphasia treatment includes restitutive and compensatory exercises and psychosocial support.

Table 5.3   Lesion location and clinical manifestations in the classic aphasia syndromes

Aphasia syndrome	Classical lesion location	Clinical manifestation
Broca aphasia	Posterior aspects of left inferior frontal convolution known as the Broca area (Brodmann areas 44 and 45), adjacent premotor and motor regions, with extension into underlying white matter, basal ganglia, and insula	Major deficit of speech production, nonfluent, sparse, halting, hesitating, effortful, slow speech, often misarticulated, frequently missing function words
Wernicke aphasia	Posterior region of left superior temporal gyrus and possible adjacent parietal cortex (lower segment of supramarginal and angular gyri)	Major deficit of auditory comprehension, with fluent paraphasic output (phonemic, morphological, and semantic paraphasias)
Anomic aphasia	Inferior parietal lobe (angular gyrus) or the connections between parietal and temporal lobes; damage to left anterior temporal cortex	Deficit of single word production, typically for common nouns, with variable auditory comprehension problems, fluent
Global aphasia	Large left perisylvian region, extending deep into underlying white matter, lenticular and caudate nuclei	Major deficits affecting both language comprehension and production, nonfluent
Conduction aphasia	Left perisylvian damage to primary auditory cortex (areas 41 and 42), surrounding association cortex (area 22), and variable damage to the insula, its subcortical white matter, and the supramarginal gyrus (area 40); sparing of superior temporal gyrus (Wernicke area)	Deficits of repetition and spontaneous speech (phonemic paraphasias), fluent
Transcortical motor aphasia	Anterior and superior to Broca area (watershed zone); or white matter tracts deep to Broca area	Deficit of speech production similar to Broca aphasia with relatively spared repetition, nonfluent
Transcortical sensory aphasia	Posterior parietotemporal lesions; posterior section of middle temporal gyrus (area 37) or in underlying white matter, with relative sparing of Wernicke area (area 22 in the superior temporal gyrus—watershed zone)	Deficit of auditory comprehension, with relatively spared repetition, fluent

From: A.F. Johnson and B.H. Jacobson, *Medical speech-language pathology: a practitioner's guide* (New York: Thieme, 2007).

6   Tracheobronchial Tree

The trachea is located predominantly in the neck and is a continuation of the larynx, so that diseases of one organ can often affect the other. This makes the tracheobronchial system of particular interest to the otolaryngologist. In fact, endoscopic diagnosis and treatment (laryngotracheobronchoscopy) were developed by ear, nose, and throat surgeons and are still practiced by them, although other specialists in bronchial diseases such as pulmonologists and thoracic surgeons also practice diagnostic tracheobronchoscopy (common term: bronchoscopy). The following overview is presented from the otolaryngologist's point of view and illustrates relationships with associated disciplines.

Applied Anatomy and Physiology

■ Basic Anatomy

The *trachea* is attached to the cricoid cartilage, which is the narrowest rigid element of the airway and moves in response to movements of the floor of the mouth and cervical muscles. It is 10–13 cm long in adults, and its lumen is held open by 16–20 horseshoe-shaped *cartilaginous rings*. Posteriorly, the tracheal tube is formed by the *membranous part,* which lies in contact with the anterior esophageal wall.

The *carina*—i. e., the origin of the two main bronchi—lies at the level of the sixth thoracic vertebra. It has an inferiorly open angle of 55°. The right main bronchus lies at an angle of ≈17° to the midline and the left bronchus at an angle of ≈ 35° (**Fig. 6.1a, b**).

The *bronchial tree* has an extrapulmonary and an intrapulmonary course. The horseshoe-shaped cartilaginous rings of the bronchial wall gradually become complete rings, fully encircling the bronchus in its more peripheral parts. The bronchioles do not have cartilaginous elements in their walls, but only a spiral muscle. Changes in the lumen are produced by the bronchial musculature and additionally, in the middle and small bronchi, by the bronchial veins.

The trachea and bronchi are lined by respiratory mucosa, which becomes flatter toward the periphery and passes into a single layer of cuboidal epithelium in the bronchioles.

Vascular supply. The blood supply to the trachea is mainly from the inferior thyroid arteries, but there are also connections with the superior thyroid arteries. The bronchi and carina derive their blood supply directly from the aorta via bronchial arteries. Numerous anastomoses with the pulmonary arteries supply the lung tissue.

Lymphatic drainage. The trachea mainly drains to the lymphatic network of the neck, but it also connects with the thoracic lymph system, which is important for the spread of metastases.

Nerve supply. This is provided by the vagus nerve and sympathetic trunks. **Figure 6.1a–c** shows the anatomy of the central parts of the bronchial tree.

■ Basic Physiology

The self-cleaning mechanism and secretions, etc. are described on pages 124–127. The mucociliary apparatus works in the direction of the larynx. The process of warming, humidifying, and cleaning inspired air begins in the nose and is completed in the lower airway, so that in normal anatomic conditions, the intratracheal air temperature is maintained at ≈ 36°C when the external temperature is above 0°C. These temperatures are considerably lower during mouth breathing. The relative humidity of the intratracheal air is also considerably lower during mouth breathing; during normal nasal breathing, intratracheal humidity is 99%.

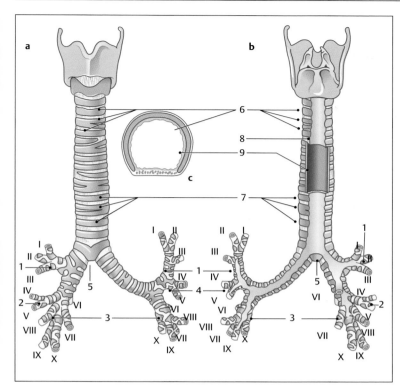

Fig. 6.1a–c The tracheobronchial tree. Nomenclature of the segmental bronchi. *Right.* 1, Superior lobar bronchus: I, apical; II, posterior; III, anterior. 2, Middle lobar bronchus: IV, lateral; V, medial. 3, Inferior lobar bronchus: VI, superior segmental; VII, medial basal; VIII, anterior basal; IX, lateral basal; X, posterior basal. *Left.* 1, Superior lobar bronchus: I, apical; II, posterior; III, anterior. 4, Lingular bronchus: IV, superior; V, inferior. 3, Inferior lobar bronchus: VI, superior segmental; VII, medial basal; VIII, anterior basal; IX, lateral basal; X, posterior basal. 5, Tracheal bifurcation; 6, tracheal cartilage; 7, annular ligaments; 8, membranous wall, with tracheal glands and trachealis muscle; 9, mucosa. **a** Anterior view. **b** Posterior view, with the posterior wall partly fenestrated. **c** Cross-section of the trachea.

Methods of Investigation

■ Tracheobronchoscopy

Two tracheobronchoscopy methods are available:
- *Rigid endoscopy* (**Fig. 6.2a–c**)
- *Flexible endoscopy* (**Fig. 6.3**)

Rigid tracheobronchoscopes (common term: bronchoscope) are tubes of various calibers with a proximal cold-light source (**Fig. 6.2**). As tracheobronchoscopy is usually performed with the patient under general anesthesia, the bronchoscope is directly connected to the anesthetic apparatus (*respiration bronchoscope*) so that it acts like an elongated rigid anesthetic tube. These bronchoscopes can be combined with instruments for aspiration, lavage for cytologic diagnosis, swabs for culture, aspiration biopsy, peribronchial needle biopsy, injection, curettage, biopsy, and foreign-body extraction. They can also be used in combination with catheters for bronchography or catheter aspiration

biopsy, and with telescopes of various angles. Simultaneous bronchoscopy and radiographic screening is especially useful for aspiration biopsy, catheter manipulation, and foreign-body extraction, which is a common indication for bronchoscopy, especially in children.

The rigid bronchoscope can also be used for photographic and video documentation in combination with rigid telescopes. A laser beam can be guided via a rigid endoscope for relatively bloodless removal of benign tumors, but laser beams transmitted through flexible fibers in combination with flexible endoscopy are more suitable.

Indications for the use of the rigid bronchoscope are listed in **Table 6.1**.

With diameters of 2.5–5.0 mm, *flexible bronchoscopes* (**Fig. 6.3**) are thinner than rigid ones. The movement of the distal end can be controlled externally to allow introduction into lobar bronchi, segmental bronchi, and even into the subsegmental bronchi. The instrument can be introduced via the nose or mouth, or through a tracheostomy if one is present. Fine flexible instruments can be used,

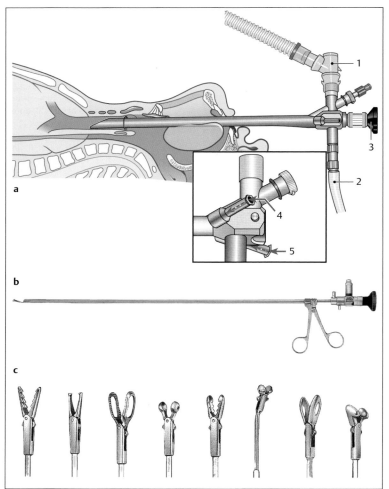

Fig. 6.2a–c   Rigid bronchos-copy.
a Bronchoscope with **1**, anes-thetic attachment; **2**, light car-rier; **3**, interchangeable window; **4**, special side tubes for jet-ven-tilation attachment; **5**, CO_2 measurement device.
b Long forceps with an attached telescope (optic forceps).
c Specially designed microfor-ceps for bronchoscopy.

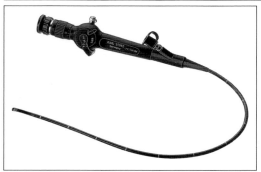

Fig. 6.3   A flexible fiberoptic bronchoscope.

guided via a working channel in the flexible bron-choscope, so that procedures such as cytologic di-agnosis, curettage, biopsy, and foreign-body extrac-tion are also possible in limited cases. Simultaneous fluoroscopic monitoring and laser treatments are also possible.

Flexible bronchoscopy can be performed with the patient under local or general anesthesia. In the latter case, the endoscope is introduced through the endotracheal tube or laryngeal mask. Indica-tions for the diagnostic and therapeutic use of flex-ible tracheobronchoscopy are listed in **Table 6.1**.

Mediastinoscopy is described on page 404.

Table 6.1　Indications for bronchoscopy with a rigid tube or flexible endoscope

Indication	Rigid bronchoscopy	Flexible bronchoscopy
Emergency bronchoscopy as a temporary measure in sudden obstructive respiratory failure	+++	+
When intubation is difficult or impossible	+	+++
To remove tracheal or bronchial foreign bodies	++	++
To arrest bleeding in the trachea or bronchi	+++	+
To remove retained secretions in obstructive disease of the lung or trachea (tracheobronchial lavage)	+	+++
To aspirate tuberculous lymph nodes at the carina, and lung abscesses	++	++
To allow the use of laser to remove a benign endotracheal or endobronchial tumor or a cicatricial membrane	+	+++
To diagnose tracheal and bronchial stenoses	++	++
Suspected tracheal tumor or a tumor in the surrounding tissue. The elasticity of the tracheal wall and its mobility should be assessed	+++	+
Suspected peripheral bronchial tumors—i. e., distal to the segmental ostia	+	+++
Unexplained persistent attacks of coughing and wheezing	++	++
Hemoptysis of uncertain origin	++	++
Suspected tracheal or bronchial trauma	+++	+
Transtracheal or transbronchial aspiration of a lymph node or a central tumor	+	+++
To control percutaneous tracheotomy	+	+++
Tracheobronchial stent implantation	++	++
Undiagnosed disorders of the lung parenchyma, unresolved pneumonia, interstitial pneumopathy, pleural effusion of uncertain origin, middle lobe syndrome	+	+++

+++ Method of choice; ++ method of similar value; + alternative method.

Clinical Aspects

■ Stenoses

Acute and chronic stenosis may occur in the trachea or bronchi. In addition, stenoses can be classified as intramural (arising within the tracheal wall), extramural (compression from outside of the tracheal wall), and endoluminal (arising from the mucosal lining). Finally, there are those that affect the mucosa and the supporting elements of the wall (compression stenosis and tracheomalacia) (**Fig. 6.4a–c**).

A classification according to the site of the stenosis is shown in **Fig. 6.5a–c**.

Tracheal stenoses usually require urgent treatment due to the risk of asphyxia, as compensation is not possible.

Acute Stenoses

Clinical Features. The main symptom is inspiratory stridor, which may be accompanied by restlessness, coughing attacks, fear of imminent death, cyanosis, and choking.

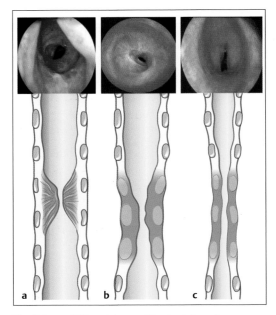

Fig. 6.4a–c   Different types of tracheal stenosis.
a Scars forming webs and sails on the internal lining alone. There is a web-like scar in the subglottic space.
b Cicatricial changes affecting all of the elements of the tracheal wall. The endoscopic view shows a stenosis in the middle part of the trachea.
c Compression of the trachea and loss of stability lead to tracheomalacial stenosis.

> **!**
> **Note:** Inspiratory stridor is an important sign of *obstructive respiratory failure*. Retraction of the suprasternal notch and the supraclavicular and intercostal areas on inspiration is a typical sign of high resistance in the airways.

Pathogenesis. The cause is sudden narrowing of the tracheal lumen by more than 50 % secondary to blunt trauma, aspiration of a foreign body, edema, swelling, bleeding, infection, crusts, etc.

Diagnosis. The severity of inspiratory, and often expiratory, stridor also indicates the urgency of the situation. The history usually indicates the cause. The level of the obstruction can be localized by auscultation. Bronchoscopy is performed using the rigid bronchoscope, with preparations being made for immediate tracheostomy. Radiographs are taken only when a delay does not involve any risk.

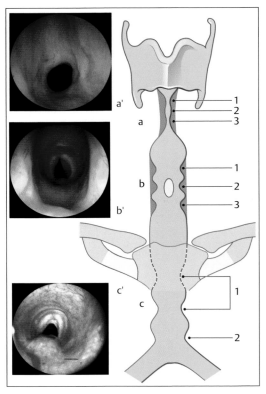

Fig. 6.5a–c   Typical locations of laryngotracheal stenosis.
a Glottis/subglottic area: **1**, laryngeal stenosis; **2**, laryngotracheal stenosis; **3**, subglottic stenosis. Stenoses are caused by damage to the laryngeal and subglottic mucosa, the cricoid cartilage or first tracheal rings secondary to prolonged or incorrect intubation, incorrect tracheostomy, or trauma. The endoscopic image shows scars inferior to the vocal cords, narrowing the subglottic space.
b In the area of the tracheostomy: **1**, suprastomal; **2**, stomal; **3**, infrastomal. Stenoses can occur as a result of a tracheostomy, an incorrectly performed tracheotomy, tracheomalacia, or scar tissue. The endoscopic image shows stenosis at the level of the tracheostomy.
c Retrosternal area: **1**, high retrosternal stenoses are caused by prolonged intubation or excessive cuff pressure of the intubation tube; **2**, low retrosternal stenoses are caused by the end of an intubation tube or tracheal cannula. The endoscopic image shows stenosis in the retrosternal area of the trachea.

Differential diagnosis. This includes laryngeal stenosis, bronchial stenosis located near the carina, pulmonary emboli and edema, and an asthmatic attack that does not cause inspiratory stridor (see

Table 6.2). Other causes of dyspnea include:
- Restrictive respiratory failure.
- Cardiac respiratory failure.
- Extrathoracic respiratory failure (decreased respiratory drive due to central respiratory paralysis, diabetes, uremic coma, conditions of increased oxygen requirement, etc.).
- Psychogenic respiratory distress.

Treatment. Rigid bronchoscopy is undertaken. A tracheotomy may be necessary in cases of nonacute and high-lying stenosis. The bronchoscope is left in place to ensure respiration during this procedure. Foreign bodies, if present, are extracted. Otherwise, the patient is intubated.

Chronic Stenoses

Clinical Features. The typical history will be of a long period of increasing dyspnea, occasionally previous attacks of dyspnea, and a weak voice. The degree of severity of the respiratory obstruction often depends on the position of the head. Previous diagnostic measures during acute exacerbations will already have indicated the cause of the respiratory obstruction. The head is held forward with the chin downward. The patient prefers to have the body upright. The differential diagnosis of dyspnea originating from the oropharynx or the upper respiratory tract is listed in **Table 6.2.**

Pathogenesis. This includes trauma presenting as scar formation secondary to tracheal injury or after incorrect or prolonged intubation, which also

Table 6.2   Differential diagnosis of dyspnea

Site of stenosis	Type of disease	Details
Oropharynx and hypopharynx	Inflammation	Peritonsillar or retropharyngeal abscess, infectious mononucleosis, abscess of the base of the tongue, diphtheria
	Functional disturbance	Obstructive sleep apnea, foreign body, posterior displacement of the tongue in unconscious patients, allergic reaction, angioneurotic edema
	Tumor	Benign tumors (e. g., hyperplastic tonsils, lingual thyroid, lymphangioma, hemangioma)
		Malignant tumors (oropharyngeal/hypopharyngeal carcinomas)
Larynx	Congenital stridor	Laryngomalacia, congenital webs
	Inflammation	Epiglottitis, epiglottic abscess, laryngitis, pseudocroup (subglottic laryngitis), laryngeal diphtheria
	Functional disturbance	Vocal cord paralysis, laryngeal spasm, glottic edema, foreign body, scars secondary to trauma or surgery
	Posttraumatic disturbance	Larynx fracture, glottic edema or hematoma
	Tumor	Benign tumors (e. g., cysts, polyps, granulomas)
		Malignant tumors (laryngeal carcinoma)
Trachea and bronchial tree	Inflammation	Tracheitis and/or bronchitis
	Stenoses	Cicatricial stenosis due to long-term intubation or after tracheotomy, tracheomalacia due to compression of the trachea (e. g., goiter) or after tracheotomy or trauma
	Functional disturbance	Foreign body, allergic reaction, asthma
	Trauma	Tracheal subluxation, tracheal rupture, intratracheal bleeding
	Tumor	Benign or malignant tracheal or bronchial tumors

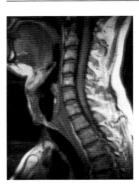

Fig. 6.6 Magnetic resonance image showing a lateral view of a suprastomal stenosis.

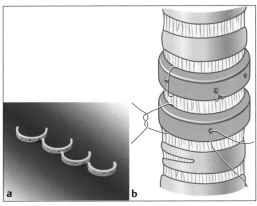

Fig. 6.7a, b Tracheopexy using extratracheal synthetic rings.
a Ceramic rings of different sizes.
b Two rings in position. The rings are secured to the tracheal wall with sutures.

causes injury to the tracheal wall, incorrect tracheotomy (see p. 353 and **Fig. 6.5a**), intratracheal tumors, goiter, malignant thyroid conditions, bronchial and esophageal tumors, and lymphadenopathies. Other possible causes are tracheomalacia, chondro-osteoplastic tracheopathy, or specific infections such as tuberculosis, syphilis, and scleroma, which can gradually destroy the structures of the tracheal wall. In addition, nonspecific infection in the neck, radiotherapy, and mediastinal causes such as dermoid cysts, emphysema, tumors, abscess, and aortic aneurysm can cause destructive local pressure on the structures of the tracheal wall.

Diagnosis
- Rigid or flexible endoscopy (bronchoscopy).
- Chest radiography.
- Magnetic resonance imaging (MRI) of the neck (**Fig. 6.6**).
- Lung function tests.
- Ultrasound and scintigraphy of the thyroid.

Differential diagnosis. See **Table 6.2** and **Fig. 6.5**.

Treatment. This is always surgical, but varies depending on the cause.
1. *Tracheopexy* consists of holding open the tracheal lumen using retaining loop sutures—e. g., in tracheomalacia due to goiter (see **Fig. 6.4c**).
   Principle of the operation: Several techniques are used:
   - Introduction of loop sutures—e. g., after thyroidectomy, into the weakened wall of the trachea and anchoring the loop to structures close to the trachea, such as the muscles and the clavicle.
   - Stiffening of the collapsed trachea with titanium or ceramic rings (**Fig. 6.7a, b**).

2. *Tracheal resection,* with end-to-end anastomosis for scars, strictures, and tracheal trauma, is used for severe destruction of *all* elements of the tracheal wall (**Fig. 6.8a–f**).
   Principle of the operation: The stenosed or scarred segment is resected and the stumps are anastomosed end-to-end. Resection of more than 4 cm requires release of the attachments of the strap muscles above or below the hyoid (suprahyoid or infrahyoid mobilization of the larynx). In addition, the hyoid is transected from the cornua of the thyroid cartilage on each side. Stenosis in the laryngotracheal connection can be treated with *cricotracheal resection.* In this procedure, the stenosed part of the larynx is resected together with one part of the cricoid plate and anastomosed with the remaining part of the larynx (**Fig. 6.9a–d**).

3. *Tracheoplasty,* with or without a previous open gutter, is used for long-segment stenoses.
   The trachea is incised in the midline and the stenosed scarred segment is removed. An autologous cartilage graft harvested from the rib is interposed between the edges of the incision. Depending on the enlargement required for the tracheal lumen, the procedure can be performed in the anterior as well as the posterior wall of the trachea (**Fig. 6.10a–d**). Large defects of the tracheal wall are covered with pedicled or free grafts of mucosa, cartilage, and skin. Healing is achieved by forming an

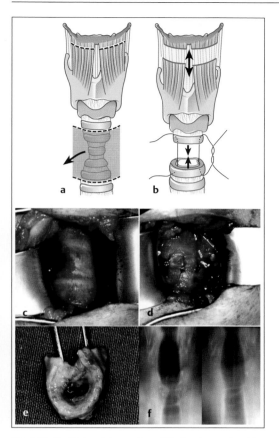

Fig. 6.8a–f Horizontal resection of the trachea and end-to-end anastomosis.

a Resection of the stenosed area and incision for infrahyoid laryngeal mobilization.

b End-to-end anastomosis of the tracheal stumps by laryngeal mobilization.

c, d Intraoperative views. The stenotic area before (**c**) and after (**d**) resection.

e The resected stenotic par.

f Preoperative and postoperative tomograms of the trachea.

open gutter, which is closed secondarily. Temporary synthetic tubes are placed to maintain the lumen and secure ventilation (**Fig. 6.11a–d**).

4. *Endoscopic removal* is used for stenoses, webs, diaphragms, and small benign tumors. The technique involves using a rigid bronchoscope. The stenosed area is divided. The scars are incised

using fine instruments or laser. A tracheotomy is not performed, provided that the stenosis is not too extensive and does not affect the cartilaginous rings.

■ **Tracheotomy, Cricothyrotomy, and Intubation**

Tracheotomy, cricothyrotomy, and intubation are life-saving measures that are often performed as emergency procedures.

Tracheotomy

Depending on the site of tracheal entry (**Fig. 6.12a**), tracheotomy can be divided into a *superior* approach, above the thyroid isthmus; a *middle* approach, after division of the isthmus; and an *inferior* approach, below the isthmus. In urgent cases, a superior tracheotomy is usually performed, although an inferior tracheotomy is usually undertaken in children. If the isthmus is in the normal position and there is enough time, a middle tracheotomy is preferred, due to the lower complication rate. Particularly in prolonged mechanical ventilation, a tracheostomy lowers the complication rate by reducing the dead space by 70–100 mL.

Principle of the operation. *Elective tracheotomy:* **Table 6.3** summarizes the indications for elective tracheotomy. The operation can be performed with the patient under intubation anesthesia using an endotracheal tube or rigid bronchoscope (see p. 345 and **Fig. 6.2a**), or under local anesthesia. A collar incision is made halfway between the suprasternal notch and the superior border of the thyroid cartilage (**Fig. 6.12a**). A median vertical incision can also be used. The trachea is dissected out in the midline and a flap incision is created, spanning across two to four tracheal rings (**Fig. 6.12b**). Hemostasis must be secured, due to the danger of valve-like aspiration of blood from disrupted vessels. A suitably sized tracheotomy tube (see **Figs. 6.11c, 6.13**) is introduced, suturing the neck skin to the tracheal mucosa to create a mucocutaneous anastomosis.

Emergency tracheotomy: In patients with acute respiratory distress, the procedure is indicated when intubation is unsuccessful and rapid surgical conditions are available. The neck is fully extended, so that the laryngeal and tracheal structures are palpable. The most important step is the swift pro-

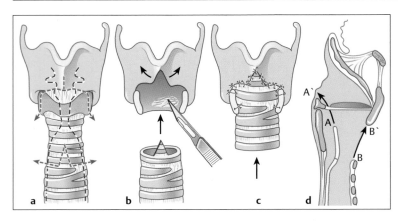

Fig. 6.9a–d Cricotracheal resection and laryngotracheal anastomosis.
a The anterior part of the cricoid ring and the trachea below the subglottic stenosis are dissected.
b Scars in the mucosa on the cricoid plate are resected.
c, d The stump of the trachea is anastomosed posteriorly with the cricoid plate of the larynx (A–A′) and anteriorly with the inner part of the thyroid cartilage (B–B′).

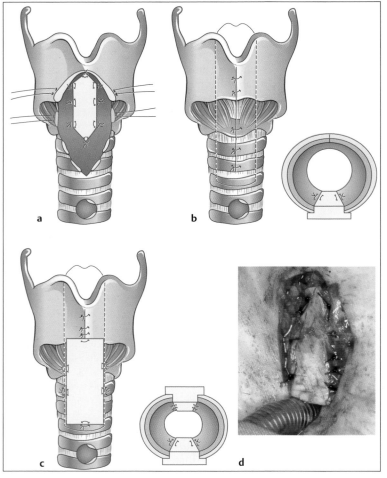

Fig. 6.10a–d Partial tracheoplasty.
a Midline incision in the anterior and posterior wall of the trachea. A rhomboid-shaped piece of cartilage is inserted into the posterior incision between the cut edges of the cricoid plate. The perichondrium is secured to the tracheal mucosa.
b The anterior tracheal wall is closed after insertion of a Silastic tube as a temporary stent.
c Enlargement of the stenotic airway can be achieved by expanding the anterior wall in addition to the posterior wall using the same technique.
d The intraoperative situation. A cartilage graft has been inserted into the anterior tracheal wall.

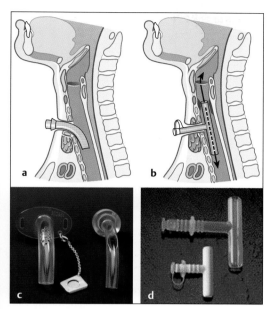

Fig. 6.11a–d   A tracheal tube (cannula) and endoprosthesis secure and stabilize the tracheal lumen.
a Position of a curved synthetic or silver tracheostomy prosthesis.
b A Montgomery silicone T tube. The upper part of the tube bridges the airway across a subglottic stenosis after reconstruction.
c A plastic cannula with a speaking valve. The inner tube (right) is fenestrated, the outer tube (left) is perforated.
d Silastic T tubes.

cedure of opening the tracheal lumen and inserting a respiration tube or tracheotomy tube. A horizontal incision should be made in emergency tracheostomy to avoid accidental damage to laterally positioned vessels. The skin of the neck is secured onto the tracheal cartilage of the opened trachea in the next step. Because of the high risk of bleeding and tissue damage, emergency tracheostomies should be avoided by carrying out an elective tracheostomy before an emergency situation arises.

Complications. Intraoperative complications include massive hemorrhage, especially secondary to venous congestion or from goiters or tumors overlying the trachea. Damage to the cricoid cartilage causes cricoid stenosis. For this reason, the first tracheal ring should not, if at all possible, be included in the tracheostomy. Damage to the pleura may produce a pneumothorax, which is more likely if the pleura lies higher than normal. Other complications include recurrent nerve paralysis, sudden cardiac arrest, and vasovagal collapse.

Postoperative complications include secondary hemorrhage, with aspiration of blood from the wound into the trachea. Serious hemorrhage can occur due to erosion into an aberrant brachiocephalic artery by a displaced tube, usually preceded by less severe warning bleeds. In children, the tube may be coughed out if it is not fixed securely. Other complications include emphysema, tracheitis, cer-

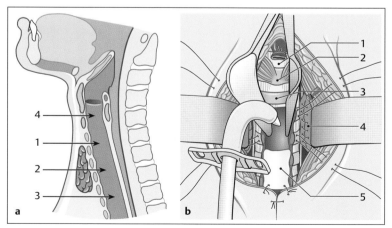

Fig. 6.12a, b   Surgical access routes for tracheotomy or laryngotomy.
a 1, Superior tracheotomy; **2**, middle tracheotomy; **3**, inferior tracheotomy; **4**, cricothyrotomy.
b The intraoperative situation during tracheotomy. **1**, Cricothyroid ligament; **2**, cricoid cartilage. The tracheal wall is incised below the first tracheal ring (**3**), the isthmus of the thyroid gland is divided, and the lateral lobes are held apart. **4**, An anterior tracheal wall flap is reflected downward and fixed to the skin; **5**, a speculum guides the insertion of the tracheal tube.

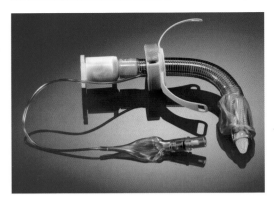

Fig. 6.13 A flexible tracheal cannula with inflatable cuff.

Table 6.3 Indications for elective tracheotomy

Mechanical airway obstruction caused by:

Tumors affecting the pharynx, larynx, trachea, or esophagus

Congenital anomalies of the upper respiratory or digestive tract

Trauma of the larynx or trachea

Bilateral recurrent nerve paralysis

Soft-tissue swelling due to trauma or radiation

Edema due to inflammation of the larynx and oropharynx

Laryngotracheal stenoses

Prophylactic airway management

Improvement of bronchial toilet

Prolonged mechanical ventilation

Postoperative airway management (upper respiratory tract surgery)

vical cellulitis, mediastinitis, pneumonia, lung abscess, esophagotracheal fistula, and difficult decannulation (see p. 356).

Percutaneous Tracheotomy

In today's intensive-care units, surgical tracheotomy is increasingly being replaced by percutaneous tracheotomy, which is most often performed as a percutaneous dilational tracheotomy (PDT).

Principle of the operation. The trachea is punctured with a hollow needle through which a guidewire is passed. Correct positioning of the guidewire

is controlled by flexible bronchoscopy via the ventilation tube. Plastic dilators are then advanced over the guidewire, and the punctured hole is widened until the tracheotomy tube fits. In addition, a special adapter is passed over the guidewire to avoid false positioning outside the trachea. It is very important to check the position of the tracheostomy tube bronchoscopically after insertion. After removal of the tracheotomy tube, the tracheostomy closes spontaneously within a few days. Even within a few hours of the procedure, reintroduction of a tracheotomy tube may prove difficult or impossible.

International PDT techniques include the Ciaglia, Frova, and Fantoni procedures (translaryngeal tracheotomy, TLT), and the Griggs procedure (guidewire dilating forceps, GWDF), which are named after their inventors.

Cricothyrotomy

This is an *emergency procedure.* It has to be revised as soon as possible with a formal tracheotomy, due to the risk of tracheolaryngeal hemorrhage. The area of the cricoid has a dense network of afferent blood vessels that can be damaged. This operation is the method of choice if intubation or emergency bronchoscopy or tracheotomy is not available.

Principle of the operation (Fig. 6.14a). A skin incision is made just superior to the prominent arch of the cricoid cartilage, with the head extended. At this point, the cricothyroid ligament lies superficially under the skin, and there are no large vessels at this site. The membrane is exposed, through which a horizontal incision is made. The incision is held open with a tube or a spreading instrument. A special instrument for the cricothyrotomy connected with a tube is shown in **Fig. 6.14a**. Other single-use sets are available (**Fig. 6.14b**).

!

Note: Cricothyrotomy should not be performed if intubation, emergency bronchoscopy, or tracheotomy is feasible. In life-threatening situations, the incision into the cricothyroid ligament can be held open with a piece of rubber tube or other suitable utensil. A definitive tracheostomy must then be created as soon as possible.

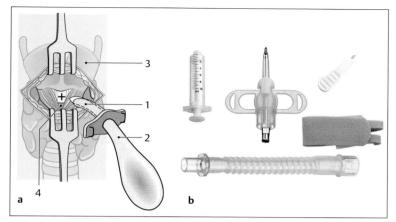

Intubation

Indications. *Short-term intubation* (< 48 h):

- For respiration of patients receiving muscle relaxants—e. g., intubation anesthesia.
- In acute obstructive respiratory insufficiency, the cause of which can probably be relieved within 24–48 h by minor surgical procedures or anti-inflammatory measures such as steroids and antibiotics, or which can be relieved within a short period by assisted respiration as a temporary emergency measure.
- If tracheotomy is impossible or contraindicated.

Long-term intubation (several days or weeks): Long-term intubation should not be undertaken in adults, due to the major risk of subsequent scar tissue stenosis in the larynx or trachea. In addition, modern forms of tubes and cuffed tubes do not reliably prevent the development of stenosis, which may become manifest only several months later. Patients with infections of the airway, those receiving steroids, those suffering from hypotension, and those under the influence of intoxicants are particularly at risk. On the other hand, in small children, prolonged intubation using the correct technique (transnasal–endotracheal) and inert soft materials often produces fewer complications than tracheotomy.

Intubation technique (Fig. 6.15). Intubation can be carried out without anesthesia in patients who are already deeply unconscious. Otherwise, general anesthesia with muscular relaxation is required.

1. The patient must be positioned in such a way that the head and neck are mobile and accessible.
2. The laryngoscope blade is introduced and the glottis exposed.
3. The tube, stiffened with a guidewire, is introduced *under direct vision* into the trachea through the glottis.
4. The tube is secured and the guidewire is withdrawn. Correct positioning of the tube is confirmed by assessing airflow. The tube is connected to a respirator and secured with adhesive tape.

> **Note:** An indwelling tube to provide assisted respiration—e. g., in the intensive-care unit or after cervical injuries—should not be retained for longer than 24–48 h, and certainly for no more than 72 h. Otherwise, there is a danger of endotracheal and peritracheal inflammation, leading to tracheal stenosis. If assisted respiration is needed for longer periods, the tube should be replaced with a tracheostomy.

The Tracheotomy Patient

A tracheostomy can represent a substantial handicap for the patient, and quality of life is reduced. It is therefore important for both patients and carers to be aware of the effects of a tracheostomy and the requirements relating to it.

- Speaking is possible with an intact larynx. The tracheostomy tube can be plugged with a finger or a cap. A speaking tube with a valve suspended in the airflow will support phonation.

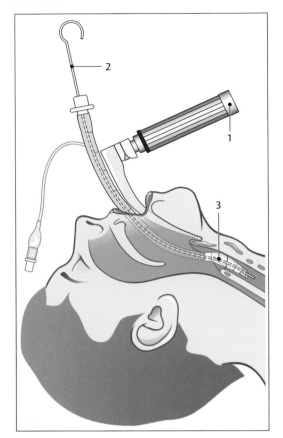

Fig. 6.15 Intubation: the ventilation tube is introduced using the McIntosh laryngoscope (**1**) and guided with a stylet. After introduction (**2**), the cuff (**3**) is inflated with air.

- Patients and their partners and relatives should be taught specific tracheostomy care and measures in emergency situations.
- A kit containing care products such as a special vacuum, a humidifier, replacement tracheal cannulas, and appropriate hygienic articles must be on hand.
- The selection of tracheal cannulas (in terms of size, shape, and material) must be appropriate relative to the original illness and its prognosis.

Practical points for nursing care of a tracheostomy patient

- The tube must be cleaned daily, or even more often when there are profuse secretions or crusts.
- Secretions must be aspirated from the trachea several times a day using a sterile technique.
- The tube must not be left out of the trachea for too long, as the tracheostoma has a tendency to shrink rapidly.
- Crusting is prevented by the use of mucolytic agents, by applying ointment to the stoma, and by instilling a 1–2 % saline solution into the tracheostomy.
- A heat and moisture exchanger ("artificial nose") can be attached to the opening of the tracheostomy.
- The skin surrounding the tracheostomy should be protected by an aluminum-coated gauze stoma dressing and bland fatty ointments or skin oil.

Complications:
- Difficulty in breathing through the tracheostomy may be due to: incorrect placement of the tracheostomy cannula; crusts within the trachea or distal end of the tracheostomy tube; obstruction of the distal end of the tracheostomy tube by tracheal granulations; an incorrectly sized tracheostomy tube; tracheal/bronchial stenosis distal to the tracheostomy.
- Bleeding in a tracheostomy may be due to: tracheitis; granulations in the trachea; erosive hemorrhage from the brachiocephalic trunk or other vessels surrounding the trachea—e. g., due to ulceration/erosion caused by the end of the tube; bleeding from a tumor.

!

Note: Immediate expert advice should be sought and a team approach adopted when there is difficulty in breathing or a bloodstained tracheal secretion is seen.

Difficult decannulation: Decannulation may be impossible due to insufficiency of the tracheal wall, combined with rapid shrinking of the tracheostomy. Factors that lead to instability of the tracheal wall include failures in surgical technique or tracheostomy care. These are:
- Injury to the first tracheal ring or cricoid arch, leading to perichondritis of the cricoid cartilage.
- Infected tracheostoma due to insufficient epithelial covering.
- Inadequate opening in the tracheal wall (too small or too large).

- Granulations around the orifice.
- Tracheomalacia.
- Extratracheal compression by goiter or tumor.

In these cases, the cause of the stenosis must be addressed initially using reconstructive procedures in the trachea or larynx (see pp. 350–351), or by dealing with the extratracheal cause as appropriate—e. g., by thyroidectomy.

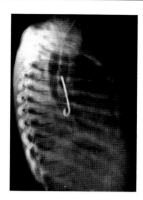

Fig. 6.16 The chest radiograph shows an aspirated needle in the trachea of a 3-year-old child.

■ Foreign Bodies and Trauma

Foreign Bodies
Foreign bodies in the trachea or bronchi usually occur in children, with ≈ 80 % occurring between the first and third years of life. Typical foreign bodies include peanuts, nails, needles, buttons, coins, balls, peas, and pieces of eggshell (**Fig. 6.16**).

Clinical Features. The main symptoms are episodes of coughing or intermittent or continuous dyspnea, with cyanosis, pain, and intermittent hoarseness. Total occlusion of the airway causes sudden death. Apparently symptom-free intervals of days to weeks may also occur.

Site. This depends on the size and shape of the foreign body. The right main bronchus has a straighter angle of origin from the trachea, so that this is the most common site of inhalation. If the foreign body is retained for a longer period, the following may occur: accumulation of secretions; tracheitis or bronchitis with edema, swelling, and granulations; bleeding and bloodstained secretions; inspiratory and expiratory valvular stenoses; partial obstruction of the lower airway or emphysema; atelectasis or overinflation of the poststenotic part of the lung. The type of foreign body is also important.

Pathogenesis. The cause is usually aspiration. Peanuts are notable for causing a severe inflammatory response and obstruction by swelling. Rare causes include broncholiths, due to calcification of retained sputum, rupture of tuberculous lymph nodes into the trachea, and ascarids.

Diagnosis. The history is one of sudden onset, often coinciding with eating.
- *Percussion* shows a dull or hyperresonant note.

- *Auscultation* reveals a hissing stenotic noise at the level of the foreign body and rhonchi. If the bronchus is occluded, there is loss of respiratory sounds and delayed movement of one half of the thorax on respiration.
- *Imaging* includes plain chest radiographs, computed tomography (CT) of the chest, and bronchography.
- *Bronchoscopy* is the most important diagnostic and therapeutic procedure.

Differential diagnosis. This includes diphtheria, pseudocroup, laryngeal spasm, whooping cough, bronchial asthma, intraluminal tumors, pulmonary tuberculosis, pneumonia, and laryngeal stenosis. Marked vertical movements of the larynx are absent in tracheal stenosis.

Treatment. Endoscopy is performed and the foreign body is extracted.

> **Important:** Suspected tracheobronchial foreign body is an absolute indication for endoscopy.

Trauma
Trauma may be caused by stabbing and gunshot injuries, blunt and penetrating injuries from road traffic accidents, and injuries to the neck and thorax.

Clinical Features. These are very variable. The history indicates the cause.

The main symptoms are dyspnea or danger of suffocation, hemoptysis, escape of air from an unusual site, surgical emphysema, pneumothorax, tension pneumothorax, and atelectasis.

Pathologic anatomy includes rupture of the trachea or bronchi, damage to the major vessels, infection of surrounding structures, and mediastinitis.

Diagnosis. This is confirmed by auscultation, chest radiographs, CT, and bronchoscopy.

Treatment. Ruptures or tears in the trachea or main bronchi should be treated as rapidly as possible by exploration and *immediate* repair or anastomosis. Peripheral bronchial rupture is treated using lobectomy (thoracic surgery). Scar tissue stenosis is described on page 347.

Tracheoesophageal fistula is dealt with by separation of the trachea and esophagus and reconstruction (see p. 350). This is usually a technically demanding surgical procedure.

■ Infections

Tracheitis

Acute tracheitis is usually viral and may be primary or secondary to laryngitis or bronchitis. Chronic tracheitis may occur in chronic inflammation of the sinuses, larynx, and bronchi; bronchiectasis; neoplasms; pulmonary cavities; and in unfavorable climatic and occupational environments.

Clinical Features. These include coughing, retrosternal pain, increased purulent or nonpurulent sputum, occasionally mixed with blood, and mild dyspnea. By itself, this disease is not a life-threatening condition and often there is no fever.

Treatment. This is the same as for laryngitis (see p. 313).

Acute Laryngotracheobronchitis in Children, Subglottic Laryngitis, Croup (see p. 314)

This occurs in infants and young children up to about the age of 3 years. It is a life-threatening disease, with barking cough, stridor, retraction of the suprasternal notch and intercostal spaces, cyanosis, and moderate fever.

Pathogenesis. Infection by viruses or bacteria produces severe inflammation of the mucosa of the upper trachea with edema, tenacious secretions, and the formation of crusts. There may be cardiac and circulatory failure and a risk of atelectasis or suffocation.

Differential diagnosis. These include epiglottitis and diphtheria.

Treatment. Therapy consists of oxygen inhalation, steroids, humidification of the air, and antibiotics. If severe respiratory obstruction occurs, the airway must be secured and protected by nasotracheal intubation or occasionally tracheotomy. Sedatives are contraindicated.

Diphtherial Tracheitis

Main symptoms. The typical signs of diphtheria are found in the larynx or the pharynx. Membranous particles, formed from secretions on the mucosal surface, are expectorated, accompanied by coughing and inspiratory stridor. Obstruction of the laryngotracheal airways can occur due to clotted membranes.

Pathogenesis. The infection is caused by *Corynebacterium diphtheriae*, a Gram-positive bacterium that produces an exotoxin. Since the introduction of vaccination in Europe and industrialized countries, the prevalence of the disease has been very low.

Treatment. High-dose penicillin and antitoxic serum (see p. 264) are given and tracheotomy is performed if indicated.

Tracheitis Sicca

This usually accompanies rhinitis or laryngitis sicca. Dry crusts are expectorated, and there is an audible wheeze.

Treatment. This includes removal of the crusts, liquefying the secretions, inhalation, humidification of the air, and antibiotics.

Rare forms of tracheitis include tuberculosis, sarcoidosis, secondary and tertiary syphilis, and scleroma.

■ Congenital and Hereditary Anomalies

These include accessory bronchi opening into the trachea, megatrachea, megabronchi, and congenital stenoses of the trachea and bronchi.

Bronchiectasis

Bronchiectasis may be congenital or acquired, usually affecting the lower lobes on the right more often than the left. *Congenital* forms are due to weakness of the wall of the bronchi or mucoviscidosis. *Acquired* forms are due to bronchitis, emphysema, chronic destructive bronchitis, and secondary bronchial stenosis. Kartagener syndrome is a triad consisting of bronchiectasis, sinusitis and/or nasal polypi, and situs inversus.

Clinical Features. The main symptom is chronic coughing and profuse sputum. Examination demonstrates finger clubbing. CT or MRI of the chest is performed if there is any suspicion of tumor in the mediastinum.

■ Tumors

Neoplasms of the trachea are relatively rare. Malignant tumors occur mainly in the form of carcinomas invading from neighboring anatomical organs and structures (larynx, esophagus, hypopharynx) into the trachea. Adenoid cystic carcinoma is a primary malignant tumor and is the most common form of this generally rare type of neoplasia.

■ Benign Tracheal Tumors

Benign tumors of the trachea are very rare and include adenomas (common in the bronchi), fibromas, lipomas, chondromas, amyloid tumors, neurinomas, hemangiomas, papillomas (usually accompanied by papillomas of the larynx), and pleomorphic adenomas. Another lesion is intratracheal goiter, which involves thyroid tissue growing into the trachea, usually the posterior wall.

Main symptoms. These include coughing attacks, increasing dyspnea, and occasionally hemoptysis. Pain in the chest, wheezing, and expectoration are less common.

Treatment. The tumor is removed endoscopically, using bronchoscopy-guided flexible laser techniques (argon, Nd:YAG laser) if possible. Otherwise, the tracheobronchial tree must be opened using the cervical or thoracic route.

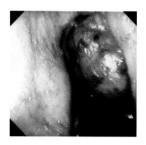

Fig. 6.17 Endotracheal growth of a bronchial carcinoma.

■ Malignant Tracheal Tumors

Adenoid Cystic Carcinoma

This primary tumor of the trachea grows slowly, especially along nerve sheaths. It extends very aggressively and tends to produce hematogenous and lymphatic metastases.

Treatment. Extensive surgery is required.

> **Note:** Adenoid cystic carcinoma must *always* be treated as an extremely aggressive malignancy (see p. 433).

Carcinoma

A tumor arising in the trachea is relatively unusual and is much more likely to occur in the lower half than in the upper section. More often, the tumor extends from a neighboring organ such as the larynx, esophagus, bronchus, mediastinum, or thyroid gland (**Fig. 6.17**).

Morphology. Squamous cell carcinoma and adenocarcinoma are roughly equally frequent, and they both metastasize frequently.

Main symptoms. Bronchial carcinomas frequently arise in major bronchi, and common problems therefore include cough, hemoptysis, breathlessness, wheeze, and stridor. Some patients have diffuse, poorly localized chest pain, and many have chest infections. Of these symptoms, hemoptysis, progressive breathlessness, and persistent respiratory infection are the most important. Dysphonia or aphonia occurs if the recurrent laryngeal nerve is invaded.

Diagnosis. Specific features of note should include the extent and infiltration of the lesion, cervical lymphadenopathy, mediastinal lymphadenopathy, and metastatic disease.

- Diagnostic imaging should include a plain chest radiograph and CT scan of the trachea, neck, and chest, ideally supplemented by MRI as well.
- Bronchoscopy with biopsy.

Treatment. Malignant tumors of the cervical trachea are treated, if possible, by resection and neck dissection. Extended resections require tracheotomy and later reconstruction with pedicled or microvascular flaps. Postoperative radiotherapy is always mandatory, due to the tumor's rapid lymphatic spread. Primary radiotherapy is indicated if surgery is not possible.

Bronchial Carcinoma

The tumor originates from the epithelium of terminal bronchioles, in which the neoplastic tissue extends along the alveolar walls and grows in small masses within the alveoli; involvement may be uniformly diffuse and massive, or nodular or lobular. Metastases to regional lymph nodes, and even to more distant sites, are known to occur, but are infrequent.

Main symptoms. In the early phases, the symptoms may be mild. They include attacks of coughing, pains in the chest, difficulty in breathing, sputum, hemoptysis, a feeling of being unwell, loss of weight, and atypical and recurrent infections of the airway with fever, pneumonia, and dyspnea.

Diagnostic procedures

- Diagnostic imaging is similar to that described above for tracheal neoplasms Bronchoscopy, needle biopsy, and cytology.
- Mediastinoscopy.
- Lung function tests.
- Exploratory thoracotomy is indicated, depending on the individual lesion.

Immediate expert advice and assistance should be sought if there is difficulty in breathing or blood-stained tracheal secretions are seen.

7 Esophagus

Diseases of the esophagus encompass several disciplines. This chapter discusses the otolaryngologic aspects involved, particularly endoscopy and the clinical aspects and treatment of esophageal disorders.

Applied Anatomy

The esophagus begins at the caudal border of the cricoid cartilage, at the level of the sixth cervical vertebra, and ends at the cardia, at the level of the eleventh thoracic vertebra. In adults, the opening of the esophagus lies ≈ 15 cm from the upper incisor teeth and the cardia at ≈ 35–41 cm from the incisors. The full length of the esophagus is thus ≈ 20–26 cm (**Fig. 7.1a**).

The wall of the esophagus is capable of expanding and contracting and is resistant to considerable mechanical stress. The internal lining consists of stratified nonkeratinizing squamous epithelium. The outer longitudinal musculature and inner circular muscle form two separate layers of the wall (**Fig. 7.1b**). There are also muscle fibers running spirally.

The esophageal musculature is striated in the upper third; consists of both mixed smooth-muscle fibers and striated fibers in the middle third; and is almost exclusively smooth muscle in the lower third.

The esophagus has three physiologic sphincters (see **Fig. 7.1a**):

- The *upper* sphincter is the opening of the esophagus formed by the cricopharyngeus muscle.
- The *middle* sphincter is caused by the crossing of the esophagus by the aortic arch and the left main bronchus. This lies ≈ 27 cm from the incisors in the adult.
- The *lower* sphincter is at the level of the esophageal hiatus, the cardia.

The *cervical* and *thoracic* parts of the esophagus are located above the diaphragm. The *abdominal* part is located below it. The blood supply is segmental, as is the lymphatic drainage.

Innervation. The nerves are derived from the vagus nerves and from the sympathetic trunks. Together, they form a plexus between the two layers of the muscular coats, and also a second plexus in the

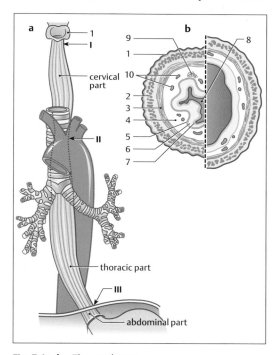

Fig. 7.1a, b The esophagus.
a The esophagus has three physiologic constrictions, caused by neighboring structures: **I**, the upper constriction—the upper entrance to the esophagus, at the level of the cricoid (**1**); **II**, the middle constriction (thoracic constriction of the esophagus), at the level of the aortic arch; and **III**, the lower constriction (diaphragmatic constriction of the esophagus), where the esophagus passes through the diaphragm.
b A cross-section through the esophageal wall, with the left side contracted and the right side relaxed. **1**, Adventitia; **2**, longitudinal muscle layer; **3**, circular muscle layer; **4**, submucosal layer; **5**, muscle layer of the mucosa; **6**, lamina propria of the mucosa; **7**, epithelial mucosal layer; **8**, lumen; **9**, submucosal glands; **10**, submucosal venous vessels.

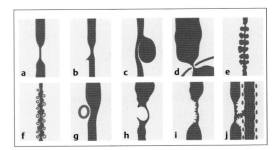

Fig. 7.2a–j   Typical findings on a contrast swallow.
a Stenosis due to caustic injury.
b Traction diverticulum.
c Pulsion diverticulum.
d Achalasia with superimposed megaesophagus.
e Idiopathic esophageal spasm.
f Esophageal varices.
g External compression of the esophagus.
h Benign intraluminal tumor.
i Esophageal carcinoma.
j Tracheoesophageal H-type fistula.

submucous tissue. Striated muscle in the upper third is supplied by somatic fibers from the vagus nerve. Autonomic supply from the vagus to smooth muscle is provided in the middle to lower third. The significance of the segmental sympathetic supply from blood vessels is uncertain.

Physiology and Pathophysiology

The esophagus has its own active mobility, as well as a passive form of mobility produced by respiration and the movements of the neighboring major vessels and the heart. The act of swallowing can be divided into an oral phase, which is under voluntary control, and pharyngeal and esophageal phases. The pharyngeal and esophageal phases are under autonomic control and depend on stimulation of the posterior pharyngeal wall. This is associated with involuntary elevation of the larynx (see p. 235).

The entrance to the esophagus and the gastric cardia are usually closed. The entrance to the esophagus opens during swallowing, and the cardia opens in response to the oncoming peristaltic wave.

The sphincter and transport functions of the esophagus can be investigated using the following procedures: contrast radiography, video fluoroscopy, cineradiography, and manometry (intraluminal measurement of pressure in the esophagus; see p. 364).

Disorders of peristalsis and tone may result from mechanical obstruction and narrowing or from paralysis of the muscles or nerves.

In presbyesophagus, the coordination of the various phases of motility is disturbed, with increased tertiary contractions and atonic phases. This prolongs the transit time of food.

Investigation Methods

■ Clinical Examination

Inspection and palpation of the external part of the neck may demonstrate redness, swelling and tenderness—e. g., over the carotid sheath—as well as venous congestion and lymphadenopathy in cases of inflammatory processes. Indirect mirror examination of the nose and throat should be performed and the pharynx and larynx should be examined. Paralysis of cranial nerves IX, X, and XII should be excluded.

■ Diagnostic Imaging

A contrast swallow with Gastrografin is commonly used to demonstrate the mucosa and lumen. Typical findings are shown in **Fig. 7.2a–j**.

> **Note:** Barium must *not* be used if a perforation or a foreign body is suspected, if there is a risk of aspiration, or in neonates with suspected esophageal atresia. Barium masks foreign bodies, adheres to the mucosa, causes a significant foreign-body reaction, and makes subsequent endoscopy more difficult.

Radiologic investigations include contrast administration, computed tomography (CT; with dual-source and 64-line techniques), and magnetic resonance imaging (MRI) to analyze the composition, distribution, and propulsion of esophageal contents during swallowing. Scintigraphy and video fluoroscopy are noninvasive procedures that have been used to visualize bolus transit. However, the techniques require access to specialized laboratories

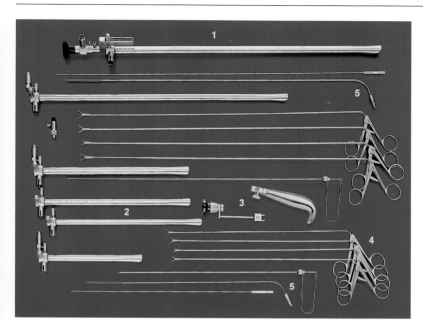

Fig. 7.3 Rigid esophagoscopes. **1**, Standard esophagoscope with telescope;
2, esophagoscopes with
different diameters and
lengths; **3**, interchangeable
eyepiece and handpiece;
4, endoscopic forceps;
5, suction tubes.

and involve radiation exposure. Multichannel intraluminal impedance (MII) is a new technique that
has been used to evaluate bolus transport and gastroesophageal reflux. This method depends on
changes in the resistance to alternating current
between two metal electrodes produced by the
presence of bolus inside the esophageal lumen.

■ Esophagoscopy

Two methods are available for examining the
esophagus. Each method has its own indications,
and the two may need to be combined.

Rigid esophagoscopy (**Fig. 7.3**) is undertaken
under general anesthesia in combination with
muscle relaxant and endotracheal intubation. Light
is transmitted to the distal end of the scope through
glass fibers inside a rigid rod. Telescopes or optical
forceps allow magnification. In addition, continuous lavage and suction can be used. A range of
instruments are available for extraction, excision,
and coagulation, as well as injection. Pneumatic
pressure can be increased in the esophagus to expand a particular part. Rigid esophagoscopy and
endoscopes facilitate photographic and video re-
cords. Laser surgery is also possible for malignant
strictures.

With the patient under general anesthesia with
a muscle relaxant, the rigid esophagoscope is introduced into the esophagus with direct visualization
of the oropharynx, hypopharynx, and postcricoid
area. The instrument is then advanced to the cardia
(**Fig. 7.4**). The diameter of the scope provides ample
space for procedures inside the lumen or on the
walls of the esophagus. The procedure also makes
it possible to assess the elasticity, stiffness, and
mobility of the esophageal wall. The indications
are listed in **Table 7.1**.

Flexible esophagoscopy has specific indications
and can performed with the patient under local
anesthesia with mild sedation. The advantages are
the instrument's narrow caliber, maneuverability, a
working channel allowing the use of miniaturized
instruments, and a fiber for laser treatment.

Gastroscopy and duodenoscopy can also be carried out during the same session (**Table 7.1**). **Figure
7.5** shows a fiberoptic esophagoscope.

Table 7.1   Indications for esophagoscopy

Indication	Rigid esophagoscopy	Flexible fiberoptic esophagoscopy
Removal of foreign bodies and impacted food remnants	++	++
Esophageal perforation	++	++
Endoscopic removal of tumors, postcricoid region	+++	+
Endoscopic removal of tumors, thoracic region	+	+++
Endoscopic division of the spur of a hypopharyngeal diverticulum	+++	–
Dilation of a stenosis or stricture	+++	–
Injection of varices, hemostasis, occasionally combined with laser treatment	–	+++
Intubation of malignant esophageal tumors to maintain food passage	+	+++
Functional evaluation (motility and swallowing disorders)	–	+++
Diagnostic evaluation of diverticula of the hypopharynx and esophagus	++	++
Esophagitis	–	+++
Caustic ingestion	+	+++
Gastroesophageal reflux disease (GERD)	–	+++
Percutaneous endoscopic gastrostomy	–	+++
Panendoscopy	++	++

+++ Method of choice; ++ suitable method; + suitable with qualifications; – not suitable.

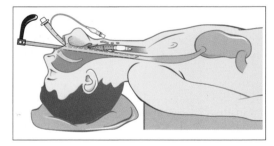

Fig. 7.4   A rigid esophagoscope introduced into the esophagus.

■ Manometry

Intraluminal pressure is measured at various levels in the esophagus. Various methods are used:
- *Three-channel manometry* involves continuous recording of pressure using three measuring catheters at separate measurement points.
- *Pull-through manometry* involves continuous recording of pressure as the end of the catheter is withdrawn continuously from the stomach into the esophagus.
- *Radiomanometry* combines radiography and manometry.
- *Pharmacomanometry* is manometry with the administration of autonomic drugs.

pH-metry is carried out using special pH electrodes, which are connected to a data storage device. Simultaneous pH recording and manometry are possible with a pressure-measuring device. This method helps evaluate reflux and motility disorders, as well as other clinical syndromes such as globus sensation and upper chest pain. It is also important for assessing the efficacy of drug therapy and surgery.

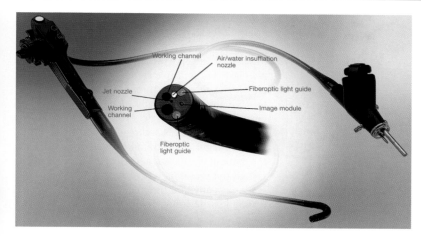

Fig. 7.5 A flexible fiber-optic esophagoscope.

Clinical Aspects

■ Trauma

Caustic Ingestion

Clinical Features. Ingestion of caustic substances causes very severe pain in the mouth, pharynx, behind the sternum, and in the epigastric region, accompanied by gagging, vomiting, sialorrhea, and occasionally glottic edema and dyspnea. White corrosive crusts and burned areas are found in the mouth and the surrounding area. Shock becomes progressive, with falling blood pressure and a rising pulse rate, cyanosis and pallor, cold sweats, and circulatory collapse. After 24–48 h, there are increasing signs of intoxication such as renal damage, hematuria, evidence of liver damage, hemolysis, disturbance of electrolyte and water metabolism, and occasionally involvement of the central nervous system (CNS). There is an increasing risk of perforation or mediastinitis, pleuritis, peritonitis, and tracheoesophageal fistula. Rapid wasting occurs. In the longer term, patients develop a long esophageal stricture, with progressive dysphagia.

Pathogenesis. Coagulation necrosis due to acids and liquefactive necrosis due to alkaline substances penetrate to varying depths. The corrosive scars in the mouth and pharynx may be minimal due to the rapid passage of the agent, but severe damage extending into the esophagus and possibly the stomach and intestine is possible. The esophagus is more severely affected than the stomach in alkaline burns, due to reflex cardiospasm, while acid burns cause more severe damage to the stomach.

Events usually take the following course: 1, primary local necrosis in the mouth, pharynx, esophagus, stomach, and intestine; 2, generalized intoxication; 3, acute, subacute, and chronic corrosive esophagitis; 4, healing of the esophagitis with scarring or stricture; 5, late complications such as late or recurrent stenosis and possibly malignant degeneration. Scar tissue stenosis begins around the third week.

Diagnosis. This is based on the typical history of an accident or attempted suicide and typical local findings. The corrosive substance must be identified. Radiographs are taken of the chest and abdomen. If the corrosive burns appear to be mild, contrast views of the esophagus are taken and careful esophagoscopy can be carried out to assess the esophagus and stomach and insert a feeding tube. *Contraindications* include shock and suspected perforation. Immediate esophagoscopy is only performed if the degree and extent of the corrosive burn are uncertain.

Treatment. If possible, the patient should drink large quantities of fluids (water). Analgesics and sedatives are given, and the patient is admitted to intensive care for intravenous management of shock, fluid administration, parenteral nutrition, broad-spectrum antibiotics, and, if necessary, gastrotomy and tracheotomy. High-dose steroids are

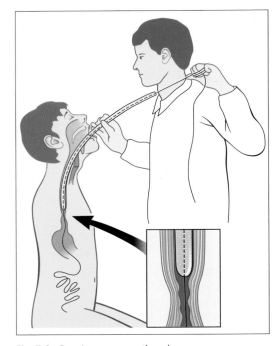

Fig. 7.6   Bougienage over a thread.

given intravenously, and these are continued for at least 4 weeks, with the dosage being adjusted according to the endoscopic findings (granulations).

The first careful esophagoscopy is performed after 6–8 days. Dilation can start at the end of the second week if radiography and endoscopy demonstrate stricture formation. Follow-up esophagoscopies are performed at 10-day intervals until mucosal defects have epithelialized. The patient is then followed up with radiography and esophagoscopy after 1, 3, 6, and 12 months.

Two methods of *bougienage* can be used:

- Early bougienage, approximately 8–12 days after the burn injury, using a thick bougie of ≈ 40 Fr in adults, 20 Fr in children, and 30 Fr in adolescents, with the caliber being increased daily until the patient is able to swallow without difficulty. The intervals are then prolonged until radiography no longer demonstrates a stenosis.
- *Late bougienage* is only used if an organic stenosis develops despite steroid administration. This may only occur several weeks later. Bougienage must *never* be done blindly, but must always be performed using esophagoscopy or over a thread (see below) or stylet.

Bougienage is started with a bougie of the appropriate caliber, with visualization using an esophagoscope. Contrast radiographs should be taken first to localize the stricture and exclude intraluminal neoplasms or multiple stenoses.

Bougienage over a thread (**Fig. 7.6**) can be used to save the patient daily esophagoscopy and to ensure that the bougie is correctly introduced through the stenosis and reaches the distal part of the esophagus. Fenestrated bougies are used. First, the patient swallows a perforated lead shot attached to several meters of silk suture. The thread is let out daily and the metal shot reaches the intestine via the stomach and can be verified by radiography. The thread is then securely anchored. Fenestrated bougies of increasing caliber can now be introduced safely over the thread and through the stricture. Bougienage may take several weeks. When it is no longer needed, the end of the thread is then cut off at the mouth and the sphere and thread are passed normally.

The goal of bougienage treatment is to achieve an esophageal lumen of ≈ 45 Fr (i. e., a diameter of 15 mm) in adults; ≈ 30–35 Fr in children up to 10 years; and 30–40 Fr in adolescents.

The thread can also be brought out via a gastrostomy, with retrograde bougienage performed from the stomach to the mouth.

The risks in bougienage include perforation of the esophageal wall. This does not occur when bougienage is carried out over a thread. Perforations tend to occur particularly in the area of the necrotic stricture—e. g., when there are blind pouches—and cause mediastinitis, pleuritis, or peritonitis, which require external drainage.

If bougienage treatment is unsatisfactory, surgical treatment of the stricture, partial esophageal resection, and replacement with a segment of stomach or bowel must be considered. Due to the tendency for recurrent stenosis and malignant degeneration to develop in the elderly, patients with esophageal strictures must be kept under medical supervision with radiography and endoscopy at increasing intervals.

Blunt Injuries

These traumatic injuries to the esophagus occur especially in road traffic accidents, when the impact of the chest against the steering wheel produces tears in the esophageal wall. Traumatic esophagotracheal fistulas, often delayed, can also occur as a result of localized necrosis of the wall.

The main symptom is coughing on swallowing. Rupture in the lower third of the esophagus is usually the result of blunt trauma to the thorax.

Open Penetrating Injuries

These injuries usually lie in the cervical segment and occur as a result of sharp forces to the neck and upper chest. The main symptoms are the escape of saliva or food from the wound.

Every traumatic injury to the esophagus should be examined using esophagoscopy. Minor damage to the mucosa can be controlled for 4–6 days using a feeding tube, and large open penetrations with injury to the muscle should be treated surgically, with thoracotomy and open exploration.

Foreign Bodies

These mainly involve unintentionally swallowed objects of various types. Children, usually under the age of 3, swallow objects such as coins (**Fig. 7.7**) or toys, whereas adults swallow fish bones, glass splinters, parts of false teeth, nails, needles, large fruit stones, or even cutlery (e.g., among prison inmates).

Clinical Features. These include considerable dysphagia (difficulty in swallowing), odynophagia (pain on swallowing) localized to the neck or retrosternal area and rarely the epigastric region, and attacks of coughing. Life-threatening symptoms include severe pain in the back between the shoulder blades and behind the sternum, and indicate early mediastinitis.

Pathogenesis. Foreign bodies usually become lodged in the upper sphincter, the esophageal orifice, and rarely at the second or third sphincters. Retained or impacted foreign bodies cause necrosis of the esophageal wall, and, depending on the site, lead to mediastinitis, pleuritis, or peritonitis, with paraesophageal abscess formation and, on occasion, surgical emphysema.

Diagnosis. This is based on the history. Initially, pain on swallowing is localized to a specific area, and the neck and cervical spine are held rigid. There may be swelling of the neck or surgical emphysema, or crepitation on palpation of the neck and the supraclavicular fossae. Lateral radiographs of the

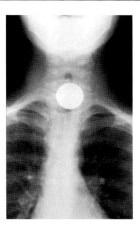

Fig. 7.7 A 3-year-old child with a coin lodged in the upper esophageal constriction.

neck and chest are taken to determine the position of radiopaque foreign bodies. Air shadows in the esophagus above a foreign body are also shown, as is mediastinal emphysema after perforation. Gastrografin is used for foreign bodies that are radiolucent. Esophagoscopy is performed, both to establish the diagnosis and for treatment.

Differential diagnosis. This includes persistent mucosal lesions caused by a foreign body that has already been passed, and early obstructive tumor.

Treatment. If the foreign body is soft and unlikely to perforate, a period of observation is acceptable. These foreign bodies may pass with observation and administration of a sedative that has muscle-relaxant properties (diazepam). Agents that induce esophageal motility such as hyoscine butylbromide (Buscopan) may also be given. Hard and large foreign bodies with sharp edges and hooks are managed using rigid esophagoscopy with the patient under general endotracheal anesthesia. If this is not successful, cervical esophagotomy is performed, or thoracotomy for a more distal foreign body. Perforations are treated by suturing the defect and administering high-dose antibiotic cover. Periesophagitis and abscesses are treated by drainage.

Course and complications. There may be no sequelae if the foreign body is removed rapidly and without complications. If it is retained for a long period, pressure and perforation occurs, leading to mediastinitis with symptoms of rapidly increasing pain behind the sternum or between the shoulder blades. Lateral neck and chest radiographs show gas emphysema (appearing as a "cloudy" prevertebral shadow), widening of the prevertebral stripe, and possible fluid retention. Oral Gastrografin demonstrates the perforation site. Small foreign bodies often reach the stomach initially and have a 95% chance of being passed spontaneously. The feces should be checked for up to 8 days or even longer to ensure that the foreign body has been passed.

> *!*
>
> **Note:** If a foreign body is suspected, the hypopharynx and esophagus must be inspected endoscopically, even if radiographs are negative.

Perforation and Rupture

Iatrogenic esophageal perforation is most likely to occur during esophagoscopy, particularly if there is a stricture that requires dilation. There is also a risk of perforation with feeding tubes, nasogastric tubes, and endotracheal tubes, particularly if they are passed blindly. The sites of predilection are the three sphincters, stenotic areas, and the piriform sinus. It is vitally important for the condition to be explored and repaired as soon as possible using mediastinotomy, thoracotomy, or laparotomy, depending on the site of the perforation.

   Spontaneous rupture of the esophagus (Boerhaave syndrome) is caused by a sudden increase in intraesophageal pressure due to vomiting or cicatricial stenosis, and is relatively common in patients with habitual vomiting or alcohol abuse. The symptoms are dramatic and include blood-stained vomit, hematemesis, severe pain behind the sternum and between the shoulder blades, pain in the left upper quadrant and in the renal area, pallor, a rapid fall in blood pressure, dyspnea, and rapid circulatory collapse.

Diagnosis. This is based on the simultaneous appearance of surgical emphysema of the neck, acute abdominal signs, pneumothorax, and dyspnea.

Differential diagnosis. This includes rupture of the diaphragm, incarcerated hiatus hernia, perforation of a gastric or duodenal ulcer, acute pancreatitis, and myocardial infarction.

Treatment. Open surgical intervention with thoracotomy, primary closure of the defect and pleura, drainage of the pleura and mediastinum, and additional broad-spectrum antibiotic administration are necessary.

Mallory–Weiss syndrome

This consists of severe, painless, and sometimes fatal hemorrhage in the upper gastrointestinal tract due to a tear in the mucosa of the esophagus or esophagogastric junction, usually following severe retching and vomiting. Most cases are associated with chronic alcoholism, but the syndrome can also be caused by malignant tumors, pernicious vomiting during pregnancy, and other diseases. The signs include pallor, tachycardia, and in some patients shock. In most cases, the bleeding stops spontaneously after 24–48 h, but endoscopic or surgical treatment is sometimes required, and rarely the condition is fatal.

■ Esophageal Diverticulum

Hypopharyngeal diverticulum is the most common type of diverticulum in the upper gastrointestinal tract (see p. 279). Diverticula of the esophagus proper are usually acquired and can affect any part of the esophagus (**Fig. 7.8a**).

Clinical Features. Diverticula in the upper esophagus often cause no symptoms at all. Those at the level of the carina cause mild symptoms related to breathing, a retrosternal feeling of pressure, and attacks of coughing. An epiphrenic diverticulum causes pressure at the corresponding site, heartburn, epigastric pain, and dysphagia. Twenty percent of cases are combined with hiatus hernia.

Diagnosis. The diagnosis is based on radiography (**Fig. 7.8b**) and endoscopy.

Differential diagnosis. This includes achalasia, hiatus hernia, and globus hystericus.

Treatment. This involves transthoracic removal, but only if the symptoms are severe or if complications such as ulceration, bleeding, spontaneous perforation, and malignant degeneration are suspected.

Traction Diverticula

Traction diverticula are due to scar tissue contracture caused by inflammatory paraesophageal or paratracheal (bifurcation) lymph nodes. The diverticula are visible on radiographs as an inverted cone arising from the wall, usually located in the middle third of the esophagus.

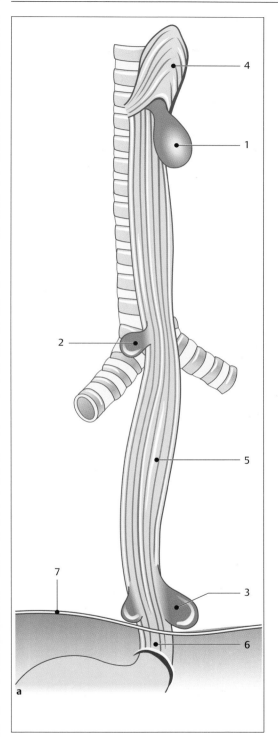

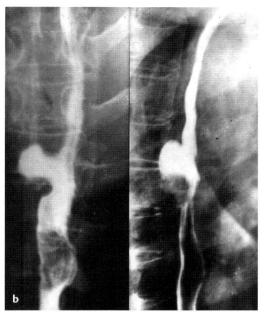

Fig. 7.8a, b   Esophageal diverticula.
a 1, Hypopharyngeal diverticulum; **2**, peribronchial diverticulum; **3**, epiphrenic diverticulum; **4**, lower pharyngeal constrictor muscle; **5**, thoracic part of the esophagus; **6**, abdominal part of the esophagus; **7**, diaphragm.
b Anteroposterior (left side) and lateral (right side) chest projections showing oral contrast studies of the esophagus, with pooling of contrast medium in the diverticulum pouch.

Clinical Features. There are no symptoms. There may be attacks of coughing and a vague retrosternal feeling of pressure and slight dysphagia.

Diagnosis. Radiography is more reliable than endoscopy, but esophagoscopy always has to be carried out to exclude malignancy.

Treatment. Usually no treatment is necessary, but transthoracic removal may be indicated if there are severe symptoms.

■ Inflammations

Nonspecific acute esophagitis accompanies trauma, stenosis, or obstruction due to diverticula, achalasia, presbyesophagus, or retention esophagitis. Esophagitis is uncommon in the absence of any additional etiologic factors.

Ulcerative esophagitis may be due to drugs (tablets or capsules) that are taken without sufficient fluid. Examples include doxycycline, tetracycline, clindamycin, quinidine, iron preparations, aspirin, indomethacin, etc.

Gastroesophageal Reflux

Gastroesophageal reflux disease (GERD) is a gastrointestinal disorder in which stomach contents are regurgitated into the esophagus—reflux. This occurs when the lower esophageal sphincter (LES) muscle is weak, or when it relaxes inappropriately. The retrograde movement of acidic gastric contents causes a burning sensation (heartburn) in the throat or chest.

GERD is extremely common, with 20% of adults reporting at least weekly episodes of heartburn. Up to 10% of adults have daily symptoms. Most patients have mild disease and few develop esophageal mucosal damage (reflux esophagitis) or more severe problems such as esophageal cancer. A hiatal hernia may weaken the LES and cause reflux. Dietary and lifestyle choices may also contribute to GERD. Certain foods and beverages, including chocolate, peppermint, fried or fatty foods, and coffee or alcoholic beverages can also weaken the LES and cause symptoms. Studies have also shown that cigarette smoking, obesity, pregnancy, and asthma may be associated with GERD.

Signs and symptoms. The most common symptom of GERD is heartburn, which most often occurs 30–60 min after meals. It is usually intensified by eating, lying down, bending over, or exercising. Patients often report relief when they take antacids or baking soda. Additional, atypical symptoms may include regurgitation of acidic materials, chest pain, asthma, chronic cough, chronic bronchitis, chronic sore throat, morning hoarseness, swallowing difficulty, bloating, belching, nausea, and weight loss. However, some patients with severe esophagitis may still be almost asymptomatic.

Diagnosis. The medical history is very important, as the physical examination and laboratory tests are often normal in uncomplicated GERD. Flexible esophagogastroscopy is performed if the symptoms do not respond to medication, and 24-h pH monitoring can demonstrate a pathological reflux condition.

Differential diagnosis. This includes carcinoma of the cardia, which may grow beneath the mucosa, achalasia, scleroderma, pregnancy esophagitis, and the changes produced by vagotomy. Angina pectoris has to be ruled out.

Treatment. *Nonsurgical treatment:* For patients with mild GERD, simple lifestyle changes such as quitting smoking, losing weight, dietary changes, and antacids are recommended. Eating smaller meals and avoiding acidic and fatty foods, peppermint, chocolate and alcohol, as well as avoiding eating 3 h before going to bed or before lying down can also help. The upper body should be raised about 15–20° in bed so that gravity reduces the reflux of gastric contents into the esophagus at night. Patients with mild to moderate GERD symptoms that fail to improve with lifestyle changes and antacids can be treated with H_2-receptor antagonists (cimetidine, ranitidine, famotidine, or nizatidine). Another option is to prescribe prokinetic drugs (metoclopramide). In severe cases, proton-pump inhibitors (omeprazole, pantoprazole, and lansoprazole) are indicated.

Surgical treatment: Surgery may be indicated in patients in whom medical therapy has failed, who have experienced complications or side effects with the drug treatment, who have had relapses of GERD, or who have been diagnosed with Barrett's esophagus, esophageal stricture, esophageal ulcers, esophageal bleeding, or hiatal hernia. The most common surgical technique is laparoscopic Nissen fundoplication, in which the upper end of the stomach is modified to serve as a sphincter.

■ Motility Disorders

These may present as atonic or spastic dyskinesias and may be due to a primary disease or may be secondary to other organic disorders.

Idiopathic Esophageal Spasm

Clinical Features. These include dysphagia of varying severity, a feeling of pressure behind the sternum, and prolongation of the act of swallowing.

Pathogenesis. This is a disorder of autonomic innervation ("dyschalasia").

Diagnosis. Radiographic findings are characteristic and show a variable traveling constrictor ring of the esophagus on a contrast swallow (see **Fig. 7.2e**). Manometry is performed with esophagoscopy to exclude organic intraesophageal diseases.

Treatment. Antispasmodic agents are prescribed, and small meals at regular intervals are advised.

Achalasia (Cardiospasm)

This involves an absence of relaxation of the lower esophageal sphincter during swallowing. Normal peristalsis is lost. Material is retained in the esophagus, causing megaesophagus, especially in children. The condition mainly affects those aged 30–50 years, but it also occurs in children.

Clinical Features. The symptoms are prolonged, gradually becoming more severe. There is a feeling of retention of food in the esophagus, and a tendency to wash every mouthful down with fluid. Vomited material does *not* smell acidic, as it is not mixed with gastric acid. In the late stage, there is a severe weight loss or even cachexia.

Pathogenesis. The disease is thought to be due to a neuromuscular disorder, possibly degeneration of the myenteric plexus (Auerbach plexus). Psychogenic or hormonal factors are also possible.

Diagnosis. Contrast radiography shows a dilated, atonic esophagus (see **Fig. 7.2 d**), reduced peristalsis, and smooth walls. Esophagoscopy demonstrates the esophageal lumen, filled with decomposed food, and esophagitis. Endoscopy is also necessary to exclude carcinoma or other organic stenoses of the cardia. Manometry is also performed.

Differential diagnosis. This includes carcinoma of the cardia, scleroderma, and gastric disorders.

Treatment. Long-term medical treatment is ineffective, and the sphincter muscle has to be dilated using a special tube. Recurrences are managed using a Heller extramucosal cardiomyotomy and possibly fundoplication. Malignant degeneration occurs in ≈ 4 % of patients after 15–20 years.

Dilation technique: An expandable dilator is used. Esophagoscopy should be performed first to exclude a tumor as the cause of the stenosis. As soon as the dilating part of the instrument is in the cardia, the sphincter is dilated by rapid closure of the handgrip of the instrument. There is a striking improvement in the dysphagia, which is often permanent. Dilation of the cardia can also be performed using a water-filled or air-filled balloon instead of the dilator. Pressure is controlled with a manometer.

Complications. These include esophageal perforation, especially when intramural carcinoma of the cardia has not been recognized.

Cricopharyngeal Achalasia

Clinical Features. There is a globus sensation, accompanied by a "sticking" feeling when food is being ingested (dysphagia).

Pathogenesis. In primary cricopharyngeal achalasia, the underlying cause may be unknown (idiopathic), or the condition may be caused by intrinsic disorders of the cricopharyngeus muscle (e. g., polymyositis, muscular dystrophy, hypothyroidism, or inclusion body myositis). The basic pathogenic mechanism is neuromyogenic impairment of upper sphincter relaxation, often combined with gastroesophageal reflux. Cricopharyngeal spasm may be secondary to neurologic disorders such as polio, oculopharyngeal dysphagia, stroke, and amyotrophic lateral sclerosis (ALS). Peripheral neurologic disorders such as diabetic neuropathy, myasthenia gravis, and peripheral neuropathies can also cause cricopharyngeal dysfunction.

Diagnosis. An upper gastrointestinal contrast examination, a swallowing study with video fluoroscopy, and manometry are the essential studies for diagnosis.

Differential diagnosis. The condition needs to be differentiated from Zenker diverticulum and malignant disease.

Treatment. Several surgical approaches are available for treating cricopharyngeal dysfunction. The classic approach is external cricopharyngeal myotomy. The current treatment of choice appears to be a transoral approach for endoscopic cricopharyngeal myotomy using laser surgery.

■ Esophageal Involvement in Diseases of Neighboring Organs

The esophagus may be compressed or completely obstructed by goiter, osteophytes of the cervical spine (especially the fifth to the seventh cervical vertebrae), marked kyphoscoliosis, mediastinal tumors, aortic enlargement, and hypertrophy of the left ventricle.

Esophageal Varices

Clinical Features. These include hematemesis, which is often severe, with fresh, clear, red blood; tarry stools; and intermittent, usually mild dysphagia. The patient may bleed to death.

Pathogenesis. The cause is almost always portal hypertension. Blood from the portal venous system is obstructed and drains via collateral vessels. The causes of obstruction include cirrhosis. Among patients with cirrhosis, 50 % have varices, hepatitis, thrombosis of the portal arterial, splenic venous, or vena caval systems, and mediastinal tumors.

Diagnosis. The diagnosis is confirmed by flexible esophagoscopy. The latter is more accurate than radiography.

Differential diagnosis. This includes pulmonary bleeding, bleeding from the nasopharynx, gastric or duodenal ulcer, and erosive gastritis.

Treatment. Emergency measures consist of rapid replacement of blood loss and control of bleeding, including treatment of shock. A Sengstaken–Blakemore tube can be used to achieve immediate hemostasis. Surgical or medical treatment is also necessary. During a symptom-free interval, a portal venous shunt may be appropriate, but alternatives include obliteration of the bleeding vessels using local laser treatment and/or injection of sclerosing agents.

Hiatus Hernia

Part of the cardia and the fundus of the stomach protrude through the esophageal hiatus. There are two main types:
- *Sliding hiatus hernia,* which is clinically silent in 80 % of patients.
- *Paraesophageal, fixed hernia,* which is symptom-free in 50 % of patients.

Clinical Features. These are often absent, but include retrosternal pain or pressure after eating, heartburn, dysphagia, vomiting, and reflux esophagitis.

Diagnosis. Contrast radiography is used. It is sometimes necessary to examine the patient in the Trendelenburg position. Esophagogastroscopy with a fiberoptic endoscope is indicated.

Treatment. This is not necessary for a sliding hiatus hernia if it is not causing symptoms. A transabdominal gastropexy is performed for a paraesophageal hernia, due to the danger of incarceration.

■ Congenital Anomalies and Fistulas

Most congenital anomalies in the esophagus are managed by thoracic or pediatric surgeons. Only those that are of interest during esophagoscopy are discussed here.

Congenital Esophageal Stenosis

Clinical Features. Dysphagia, coughing attacks, and possibly vomiting are symptomatic.

Diagnosis. Radiography and endoscopy.

Treatment. Bougienage or endoscopic laser removal of circumscribed webs is performed.

Short Esophagus

This is a congenital disorder. Reflux symptoms are already present in some 50 % of these infants. The lower esophageal segment is absent.

Clinical Features. As in reflux esophagitis.

Diagnosis. This is provided by contrast radiography and endoscopy, which shows heterotopic gastric mucosa above the diaphragm, thoracic stomach, congenital short esophagus, or Barrett syndrome.

Differential diagnosis. Sliding hiatus hernia must be considered.

Treatment. As in reflux esophagitis.

Tracheoesophageal Fistula

This is a congenital or acquired communication between the lumen of the esophagus and the trachea. It may or may not be accompanied by atresia. **Figure 7.2j** illustrates an H fistula.

Clinical Features. The disease is usually recognized immediately after birth, with choking attacks, dyspnea, and cyanosis. The fistula may remain symptom-free for a long period due to valvular action or the formation of scar tissue. The fistula may occasionally produce symptoms only in later life, including coughing on eating or drinking, expectoration of food, and recurrent aspiration pneumonia.

Diagnosis. This is made by contrast radiography and endoscopy, consisting of combined bronchoscopy and esophagoscopy.

Differential diagnosis. This includes acquired tracheoesophageal fistula due to necrosis of the esophageal wall secondary to trauma, ruptured diverticulum, or breakdown of a malignancy of the esophagus or the trachea.

Treatment. The trachea and esophagus are divided and reconstructed, using a cervical or thoracic approach (depending on the site).

Dysphagia Due to Congenital Double Aortic Arch
Double aortic arch is one of the two most common forms of vascular ring—a group of congenital anomalies of the aortic arch system in which the trachea and esophagus are completely encircled by connected segments of the aortic arch and its branches. Although there are various forms of double aortic arch, the common defining feature is that both a left and right aortic arch are present instead of a single arch. The atypical artery passes between the vertebral column and the esophagus in 80 % of patients, between the trachea and the esophagus in 15 %, and in front of the trachea in 5 %.

Clinical Features. Swallowing difficulties depend on the degree of esophageal compression and typically manifest as vomiting and feeding intolerance in infants and younger children, or as dysphagia later in life. Swallowing dysfunction may contribute to respiratory symptoms as a result of aspiration and/or compression or irritation of the membranous portion of the trachea as a food bolus traverses the area of esophageal obstruction.

Diagnosis. This is made by contrast radiography, arteriography, and esophagoscopy, which shows a pulsating horizontal bar at various levels in the esophageal wall.

Treatment. Surgical division of the vascular ring is indicated in any patient with symptoms of airway or esophageal compression and in patients who need to undergo surgery to repair associated cardiovascular or thoracic anomalies.

■ Tumors of the Esophagus

■ Benign Tumors

These tumors are rare and may demonstrate intraluminal, intramural, or periesophageal growth. The most common are leiomyomas, rhabdomyomas, fibromas, hemangiomas, lipomas, neuromas, and papillomas. They do not often cause symptoms until they reach a considerable size, at which point they produce dysphagia, stenosis, pain, pressure behind the sternum, and bleeding.

Diagnosis. This is made by contrast radiography, esophagoscopy, and biopsy.

Treatment. The tumor is removed either endoscopically or surgically using a transcervical, transthoracic, or transabdominal approach, depending on the type of tumor and its site of origin.

■ Malignant Tumors

The most frequent esophageal malignancy is squamous cell carcinoma, which is often histologically undifferentiated. This tumor represents 40 % of all gastrointestinal malignancies. It almost exclusively affects men over the age of 50. Esophageal carcinoma may develop without previous disease, but may also arise from chronically irritated esophageal mucosa due to corrosion, diverticula, short esophagus of the Barrett syndrome type, reflux esophagitis, hiatus hernia, achalasia, or Plummer–Vinson (Paterson–Kelly) syndrome. In rare cases, it may spread from neighboring organs such as the thyroid, larynx, trachea, bronchi, or stomach. Lymphnode metastases from distant organs are also possible. Rare histological forms include adenocarcinoma, usually affecting the lower segment of the esophagus, and sarcoma.

Clinical Features. These include increasing dysphagia, initially only for solid foods, burning or a feeling of fullness behind the sternum, pain which is late and inconstant and felt behind the sternum or the back, weight loss, hiccups, vomiting, coughing, and hoarseness due to paralysis of the recurrent laryng-

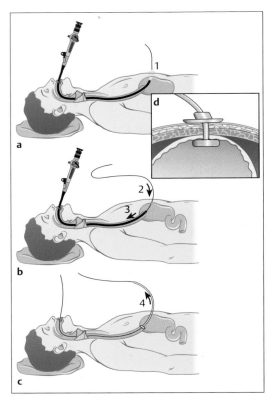

Fig. 7.9a–d Percutaneous endoscopic gastrostomy (PEG).
a A flexible endoscope is used to transilluminate the gastric wall. A sharp needle **(1)** is used to perforate the gastric wall at the illuminated point.
b A guide wire is introduced **(2)** and is retracted with the esophagoscope **(3)** and led out of the mouth.
c The gastrostomy tube is connected to the guide wire. The wire is retracted through the gastric wall together with the tube **(4)**.
d A double-layered plate is used to seal the gastric wall.

eal nerve. On average, the symptoms only become obvious after 4–5 months. Later, there is marked weight loss, inability to eat, vomiting, severe thirst, and severe pain.

Diagnosis. This is often made very late. Radiography shows widening of the mediastinum and lateral displacement of the trachea. Contrast radiography shows a filling defect or delay, an irregular outline in the wall, and narrowing of the esophageal lumen (see **Fig. 7.2i**). Paralysis of the recurrent laryngeal nerve is sometimes the first symptom.

Esophagoscopy with a rigid esophagoscope and biopsy is the most useful diagnostic measure.

Differential diagnosis. This includes achalasia, esophageal stricture, diverticulum, Plummer–Vinson syndrome, benign esophageal tumors, bronchial carcinoma invading the esophagus, and an intraesophageal foreign body.

Treatment. Surgery is only indicated in a third of the cases, usually those arising in the middle and lower thirds of the esophagus. Radiotherapy and chemoradiotherapy are alternative measures, with only limited benefit.

Additional palliative measures include a bypass with an endoprosthesis (intubation) or gastrostomy (for the surgical procedure used in percutaneous endoscopic gastrostomy, see **Fig. 7.9**).

8   Neck (Including the Thyroid Gland)

Applied Anatomy and Physiology

The neck supports the head, allows it to move, and connects it to the trunk. It consists of an *osteomuscular part,* which is adapted to the upright human posture. The *visceral part* of the neck accommodates the upper respiratory and digestive tracts—the larynx, which functions as a sphincter and as the voice organ; the thyroid gland; the carotid sheath and its contents on either side; and the cervical lymphatic system.

The upper border of the neck courses along the inferior border of the mandible, through the apex of the mastoid process to the external occipital protuberance. For clinical and surgical reasons, the suprahyoid triangle is regarded as part of the neck. Inferiorly, the neck ends in a plane formed by the suprasternal notch, the clavicle, and the spinous process of the seventh cervical vertebra. Laterally, the borders of the trapezius muscle form the boundary with the posterior part of the neck (**Fig. 8.1a**). The external shape of the neck depends on factors determined by constitution and sex. In men, the larynx is angular and forms the Adam's apple, and the sternocleidomastoid muscle is well developed. In women, the structures are more slender and delicate.

The sternocleidomastoid muscles and the borders of the trapezius muscle on each side, the hyoid bone, the laminae of the thyroid cartilage, and the cricoid cartilage contribute to the profile and are visible and palpable.

An enlarged thyroid gland (goiter) and tumor masses are readily detected visually and by palpation (see p. 408).

■ Basic Anatomy and Physiology

■ Regions

For clinical purposes, the sternocleidomastoid muscle divides the neck into:

- *The median region of the neck:* inferior to the hyoid are a) the superior carotid triangle (**Figs. 8.1b, 8.2**), which is clinically important, with boundaries formed by the anterior borders of the sternocleidomastoid muscle, the superior belly of the omohyoid muscle, and the posterior belly of the digastric; and b) the small inferior carotid triangle, the boundaries of which are the anterior and posterior borders of the sternocleidomastoid muscle, the medial edge of the omohyoid muscle, and the root of the neck (sternocleidomastoid region). The suprahyoid triangle (see **Fig. 8.1a**) is divided into the submandibular triangle and the submental triangle.
- *The lateral region of the neck* is divided into two triangles by the inferior belly of the omohyoid muscle (**Fig. 8.1b**). The lower of these is the omoclavicular triangle, the boundaries of which are the omohyoid muscle, the clavicle, and the internal jugular vein. It corresponds to the supraclavicular fossa, which is often visible. The upper triangle is the posterior cervical triangle (**Fig. 8.1a**).

■ Fascia

The cervical muscles, viscera, and carotid sheath (**Fig. 8.3**) are enclosed in a fascia which is partly tight, partly loose, and partly incomplete.

- The *superficial cervical fascia* lies beneath the platysma, encloses the sternocleidomastoid and trapezius muscles, inserts into the hyoid bone, and extends superiorly to the border of the mandible and inferiorly to the superior border of the sternum and the clavicle.
- The *medial cervical fascia* is a multilocular system enclosing the entire cervical viscera—the thyroid gland, esophagus, trachea, pharynx, vessels, and nerves. It stretches between the two

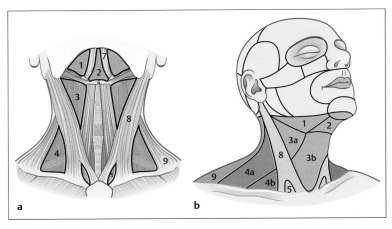

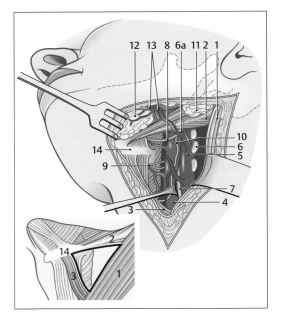

Fig. 8.2   Superior carotid triangle. **1**, Sternocleidomastoid muscle; **2**, posterior belly of the digastric muscle; **3**, superior belly of the omohyoid muscle; **4**, common carotid artery; **5**, internal jugular vein; **6**, deep cervical lymph node; **6a**, lymph node in the jugulofacial venous angle; **7**, vagus nerve; **8**, hypoglossal nerve; **9**, superior laryngeal neurovascular bundle; **10**, ansa cervicalis; **11**, lower pole of the parotid; **12**, submandibular gland; **13**, facial artery and vein; **14**, hyoid bone.

omohyoid muscles, the hyoid, the clavicle, the upper part of the sternum, and the scapula.

- The *deep cervical fascia* forms a tight tube around the deep cervical muscles arising from the spinous processes of the bodies of the cervical spine. The prevertebral layer is part of the fascial system, running continuously from the base of the skull to the inferior end of the spinal column.

The deep cervical fascia is divided into the alar fascia and a prevertebral part lying directly on bone. The prevertebral fascial space is thus divided into two to form the "danger space" (**Fig. 8.4**). Infection can spread directly within it into the posterior mediastinum.

The contents of the carotid sheath—the common carotid artery, external and internal carotid artery, internal jugular vein, vagus nerve, and sympathetic plexus—have their own relatively thick fascial envelope, consisting of parts of all three layers of the cervical fascia.

The interfascial spaces are extremely important functionally and clinically. They can change in shape and move relative to each other, adapting to head movements, vascular pulsation, chewing, swallowing, and respiration.

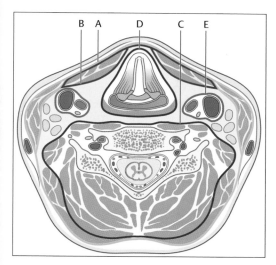

Fig. 8.3 Fascial envelopes. Cross-section at the level of the fifth cervical vertebra. Muscle fascia can be divided into: **A**, superficial cervical fascia; **B**, pretracheal lamina or middle cervical fascia; and **C**, prevertebral fascia or deep cervical fascia. **D**, cervical visceral fascia; **E**, carotid sheath.

Note: The space between the superficial and middle cervical fascia is closed inferiorly as a sac, because of their common insertion onto the sternum and clavicle. This prevents inferior extension of infection. In contrast, the space between the middle and deep cervical fascia communicates freely below with the mediastinum (see **Fig. 8.4**). This allows abscesses to track downward and allows infection secondary to esophageal injuries or surgical emphysema to spread.

■ **Spaces**

The deep spaces of the neck can be divided into spaces that involve the entire length of the neck (including the retropharyngeal space, the danger space, and the prevertebral space); those that are limited to the area above the hyoid bone (the submaxillary, sublingual, and parapharyngeal spaces); and the space limited to the area below the hyoid bone (the anterior visceral space).

- The *anterior visceral space* (see **Fig. 8.4**) lies in the anterior aspect of the neck, is enclosed by the visceral layer and completely surrounds the trachea, esophagus, and thyroid gland. It extends from the thyroid cartilage to the level of the

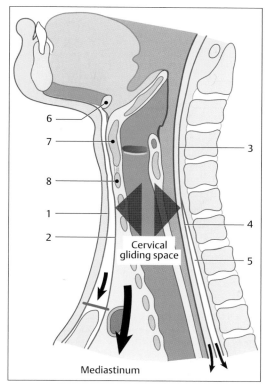

Fig. 8.4 Cervical interfascial spaces. **1**, Superficial cervical fascia; **2**, middle cervical fascia; **3**, deep cervical fascia; **4**, alar layer of the prevertebral fascia; **5**, "danger space"; **6**, hyoid bone; **7**, thyroid cartilage; **8**, cricoid cartilage.

fourth thoracic vertebra in the superior mediastinum.

- The *retropharyngeal space* is the potential space that exists between the posterior aspect of the visceral layer and the alar division of the deep layer. It extends from the base of the skull to the level of the first or second thoracic vertebrae. It contains two lateral chains of lymph nodes separated by a midline raphe. The danger space lies between the alar and prevertebral layers of the deep cervical fascia. It extends from the base of the skull to the posterior mediastinum at the level of the diaphragm and is limited laterally by its fusion with the prevertebral layer and the vertebral transverse process. The prevertebral space lies between the vertebral bodies and the prevertebral layer of the deep cervical fascia. It

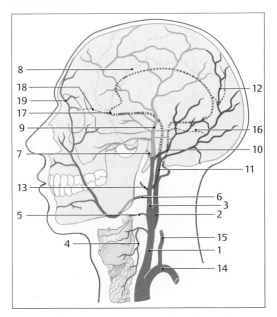

Fig. 8.5   The carotid artery and its branches. **1**, Common carotid artery; **2**, internal carotid artery; **3**, external carotid artery; **4**, superior thyroid artery; **5**, lingual artery; **6**, facial artery; **7**, internal maxillary artery; **8**, middle meningeal artery; **9**, superficial temporal artery; **10**, posterior auricular artery; **11**, occipital artery; **12**, posterior branch of occipital artery; **13**, ascending pharyngeal artery; **14**, subclavian artery; **15**, vertebral artery; **16**, meningeal anastomoses; **17**, carotid siphon; **18**, ophthalmic artery; **19**, angular artery.

extends from the base of the skull to the level of the coccyx.

- The *parapharyngeal space* can be compared with an inverted cone, with its base lying superiorly at the base of the skull and its apex inferiorly at the hyoid bone. It is divided into a prestyloid and a poststyloid component. Its medial border is formed by the lateral pharyngeal wall, and its lateral border is the superficial layer of the deep cervical fascia overlying the mandible, the parotid gland, and the internal pterygoid.
- The *submandibular space* is divided by the mylohyoid muscle into the sublingual space above and the submaxillary space below. These two spaces communicate freely around the posterior edge of the mylohyoid muscle. The entire space is bounded by the mandible anteriorly and laterally. The hyoid bone limits its inferior aspect and the intrinsic muscles of the base of tongue

from its posterior border. The sublingual space contains the sublingual gland, the hypoglossal nerve and Wharton's duct. The submandibular space contains the submandibular gland.

- The *sublingual space* encloses the sublingual gland and is a site for abscesses of the floor of the mouth (see **Fig. 3.1**, p. 229).
- The *submental space* is important in Ludwig angina (see p. 257).
- The *parotid space* encloses the parotid gland and the preauricular lymph nodes.

Note: These boundaries, defined on the basis of individual anatomic structures, are often not respected by nonspecific and specific inflammations, primary tumors of the cervical organs, lymph-node metastases, and primary and malignant lymphomas.

■ **Blood Vessels**

The *common carotid artery* is the main artery of the neck. On the right side, it rises from the brachiocephalic trunk and on the left from the aortic arch. Superiorly, it runs lateral to the trachea and larynx, without giving off any branches, to reach the level of the upper border of the thyroid cartilage, where it divides into the external and internal carotid artery.

The *external carotid artery* is the anterior branch of the common carotid artery. It runs superiorly in the carotid triangle, where it gives off branches, and runs beneath the posterior belly of the digastric muscle and the stylohyoid muscle. It crosses the retromandibular fossa and then courses in front of the external ear to reach the temporal region, where it divides into its final branches.

The branches of the external carotid artery are: the superior thyroid; lingual; facial; ascending pharyngeal; occipital; posterior auricular; internal maxillary, which gives off the middle meningeal artery; and the superficial temporal arteries (**Fig. 8.5**).

The *internal carotid artery* is the posterior branch of the common carotid artery. It supplies the brain and the eyes, and initially runs (as does the external carotid artery) in the carotid triangle before coursing deeper in the retromandibular fossa and through the carotid canal into the skull.

The lower part of the neck receives its important arterial supply from branches of the *thyrocervical trunk:* the suprascapular, inferior thyroid, and ascending and superficial cervical arteries (**Fig. 8.6**).

The *carotid sinus* lies in the bulging part of the carotid bifurcation. It is provided with pressor receptors for blood-pressure regulation.

The *carotid body* is a small structure measuring up to 5 mm in size. It lies in the adventitia of the medial wall of the bifurcation and has chemoreceptor properties that control respiration, blood pressure and heart rate, depending on the blood's O_2 and CO_2 levels and pH. It may undergo malignant degeneration as a chemodectoma (nonchromaffin paraganglioma, carotid body tumor) (see pp. 89–91; 397).

The *vertebral artery* does not participate in the blood supply to the soft tissue of the neck, but it gives off branches for the meninges and the cervical medulla and supplies the circle of Willis. The vertebral arteries transport ≈ 30 % of the cerebral blood supply.

The *internal jugular veins*, together with their main tributaries the anterior and external jugular veins, provide the main venous drainage for the head. The *vertebral veins* and the *venous plexus* in the cervical spinal canal normally carry ≈ 30 % of the cerebral venous drainage. When one or both internal jugular veins are ligated, the vertebral venous plexuses can restore an adequate level of cerebral venous drainage (**Fig. 8.7a, b**) within a few days.

A *central venous catheter* can be introduced via the internal jugular vein or the subclavian vein. Indications include total parenteral nutrition, drug administration, and measurement of central venous pressure. The position of the catheter should be confirmed on radiography before an infusion is started.

> **Note:** The *greater jugulosubclavian venous angle* is situated posterior to the sternoclavicular joint at the root of the neck, and lateral and superior to it lie the supraclavicular or prescalene lymph nodes. The *lesser jugulofacial venous angle* is formed by the opening of the facial vein into the internal jugular vein. There is also a collection of important lymph nodes at this point (see **Fig. 8.7**).

Circulatory disorders of the internal carotid artery. These may cause little or no symptoms, provided there is adequate collateral circulation via the circle of Willis or from the external carotid artery: firstly,

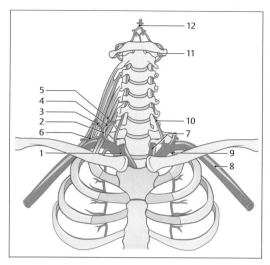

Fig. 8.6 The subclavian artery and its branches. The subclavian artery divides into different arteries, which supply the base of the neck and the upper thoracic aperture. **1**, Brachiocephalic trunk; **2**, thyrocervical trunk; **3**, transverse cervical artery; **4**, inferior thyroid artery; **5**, ascending cervical artery; **6**, suprascapular artery; **7**, common carotid artery; **8**, left subclavian artery; **9**, internal thoracic artery; **10**, vertebral artery; **11**, transverse foramen; **12**, basilar artery.

via the facial, angular, and ophthalmic arteries to the carotid siphon (ophthalmic collaterals; **A** in **Fig. 8.8a**); or secondly, via the occipital, meningeal, and vertebral arteries (occipital anastomosis; **B** in **Fig. 8.8a**).

Acute occlusion of this arterial system and its collaterals causes hemiplegia and unilateral sensory deficits. If the occlusion develops slowly (as in arteriosclerosis, for example), ischemic cerebral attacks initially occur, followed by generalized cerebral insufficiency.

Prior to surgery for head and neck carcinoma with cervical metastases (N3), it is important to test the capacity of the cerebral collateral reserve before proceeding with resection of the internal carotid artery.

Vertebrobasilar insufficiency. One of the sites of predilection for stenosis of the vertebral artery is the segment between its origin from the subclavian artery and its entry into the canal in the transverse process of the sixth cervical vertebra. Stenosis at this site causes temporary, recurrent, or prolonged attacks of dizziness, drop attacks, hearing disor-

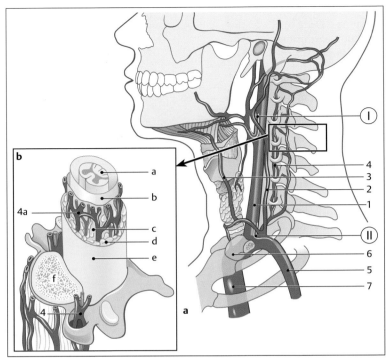

Fig. 8.7a, b Cervical venous system. **1**, Internal jugular vein; **2**, external jugular vein; **3**, anterior jugular vein; **4**, vertebral veins; **4a**, venous plexus in the cervical vertebral canal; **5**, subclavian vein; **6**, brachiocephalic vein; **7**, superior vena cava. **a**, Cervical medulla; **b**, arachnoid; **c**, dura; **d**, epidural space with venous plexus and fat; **e**, periosteal tube; **f**, vertebral body. **I**, Greater jugulosubclavian venous angle; **II**, lesser jugulofacial venous angle.

ders, disorders of vision, and sudden syncope. Chronic vertebral arterial deficiency may present with the medulla oblongata or Wallenberg syndrome.

Wallenberg syndrome. The syndrome is characterized by difficulty in swallowing and hoarseness due to paralysis of the ipsilateral vocal cord. In some cases, taste may also be affected in the ipsilateral half of the tongue. The glossopharyngeal nerve (IX) and vagus nerve (X) are the primary cranial nerves involved in the syndrome. Occlusion of the posterior inferior cerebellar artery (PICA) or branches from it leads to damage to the posterior lateral region of the medulla. The disorder is also known as posterior inferior cerebellar artery syndrome or lateral medullary syndrome.

Subclavian steal syndrome. The resulting cerebral circulatory disorders are due to occlusion of the subclavian artery between its origin in the aorta and the origin of the vertebral artery. Vascular anomalies, trauma, and arteriosclerosis cause a reverse flow in the vertebral artery in favor of the arterial supply to the ipsilateral arm and the thyrocervical trunk at the expense of cerebral circulation (see **Fig. 8.8b**).

■ **Cervical Lymphatic System**

Approximately 300 lymph nodes can be found in the human neck. The cervical lymphatic system is a component of the reticuloendothelial or reticulohistiocytic system. Portals to this system include the lymphoepithelial organs of the nasopharynx and oropharynx (see p. 233).

> **Note:** Up to the age of ≈ 8 or 10 years, hyperplasia of the cervical lymph nodes in the drainage area of the nasopharynx or oropharynx, due to reactive swelling of the tonsils, often results from the close connection between the lymphoepithelial and reticuloendothelial systems. Newly developed lymphadenopathy always requires investigation at any age.

Lymph channels lead from tributary tissue areas to regional lymph nodes or groups. The lymph nodes in the neck are incorporated into a network of lymph capillaries and lymph vessels, which drain on both sides into the large lower deep cervical

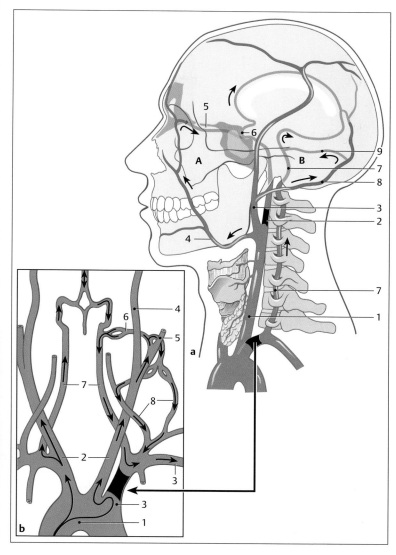

Fig. 8.8a, b **a** Collateral circulation in insufficiency of the internal carotid artery. **A**, Ophthalmic collateral; **B**, occipital anastomoses. **1**, Common carotid artery; **2**, internal carotid artery with stenosis; **3**, external carotid artery; **4**, facial artery; **5**, ophthalmic artery; **6**, carotid siphon; **7**, vertebral artery; **8**, occipital artery; **9**, meningeal anastomoses.

b Bypass circulation in subclavian steal syndrome. **1**, Aortic arch; **2**, common carotid artery; **3**, occluded subclavian artery (black); **4**, internal carotid artery; **5**, external carotid artery; **6**, occipital anastomoses (see also **a**); **7**, vertebral artery; **8**, branches of the thyrocervical trunk.

lymph nodes, from which the lymph finally flows back into the venous system (**Fig. 8.9**).

On the left side, the thoracic duct usually ends in a delta-shaped network. On the right side, the right lymphatic duct sinks into a cervical lymph trunk, 1–2 cm long, in the respective jugulosubclavian angle. These cervical lymph trunks receive afferents on both sides from the cranial area via the jugular trunks, from the axilla via the subclavian trunks, and from the thoracic area via the bronchomediastinal trunks.

The main drainage of the intrathoracic lymph is to the right jugulosubclavian angle, with the exception of the lymph of the left upper lobe of the lung. Lymph from the lower half of the body reaches the left jugulosubclavian angle via the thoracic duct. Lymph from the left superior lung segments also flows into the venous system via the left jugulosubclavian trunk (**A** in **Fig. 8.10**).

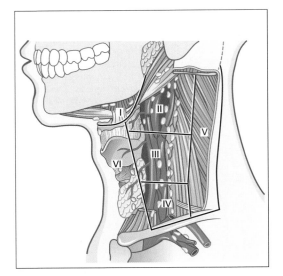

Fig. 8.9 Classification of cervical lymph nodes. The neck is divided into six three-dimensional levels containing lymph-node groups. The superficial border is formed by the superficial cervical fascia below the platysma muscle. The deep plane is formed by the prevertebral fascia and the cervical visceral fascia (see **Fig. 8.3**). **I**, submental and submandibular groups; **II**, upper jugular group; **III**, middle jugular group; **IV**, lower jugular group; **V**, posterior triangle group; **VI**, anterior compartment group.

Note: The lymph-node groups in both jugulosubclavian angles, the supraclavicular lymph nodes, are the last stations for lymph from the entire body (see **Fig. 8.10**). This explains the importance of prescalene lymph-node biopsy in clinical diagnosis (see **Fig. 8.22** and p. 404).

The chains of lymph nodes around the major veins of the neck, especially the internal jugular vein, are embryologically determined. The lymph-node groups of greatest clinical importance lie between the middle and deep cervical fascia. Horizontal and vertical chains anastomose in the carotid triangle. They can be palpated below the angle of the jaw and can be demonstrated surgically in the jugulofacial venous angle in the carotid triangle (see **A** in **Fig. 8.10**).

■ **Nerves**

The motor, sensory, and autonomic nerve supply of the neck is complex.

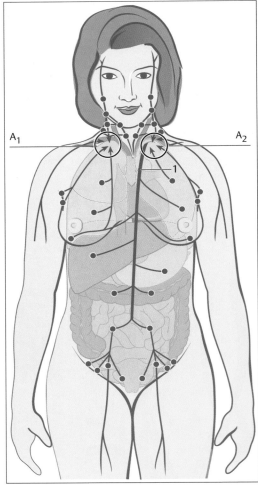

Fig. 8.10 Central lymph spaces of the body at the base of the neck on both sides and their efferents from the cranial lymph nodes, cervical lymph nodes; thoracic (mediastinal and tracheobronchial) lymph nodes; abdominal lymph nodes (mesenteric, lumbar, inguinal, and iliac nodes); and inferior lymph nodes. **A1**, Right central lymphatic space; **A2**, left central lymphatic space with the opening of the thoracic duct. **1**, Thoracic duct.

Motor supply of the cervical musculature and the diaphragm (Fig. 8.11)
- The accessory nerve supplies the sternocleido-mastoid and trapezius muscles.
- The hypoglossal nerve supplies the tongue.
- The ansa cervicalis supplies the infrahyoid muscles.

- Branches of cranial nerves V, VII, and XII innervate the suprahyoid musculature of the floor of the mouth.

The phrenic nerve, arising from C3 to C5, runs inferiorly over the scalenus anterior muscle to supply the diaphragm.

Sensory nerve supply of the external neck. This arises from the cervical plexus, C1 to C4, and consists of the great auricular nerve, the greater and lesser occipital nerves, the transverse nerve of the neck, the supraclavicular nerves, and the dorsal rami over the nape.

The *Erb point* marks the convergence of the anterior branches at the midpoint of the posterior border of the sternocleidomastoid muscle. Infiltration at the Erb point produces local anesthesia in the lateral part of the neck (**Fig. 8.12**).

> **Note:** The nerves of the cervical plexus, especially the great auricular nerve, are often used as grafts for reconstruction of the facial or hypoglossal nerves.

Vagal nerve system—mixed nerves. This system consists of the vagus nerve, glossopharyngeal nerve, and the cranial root of the accessory nerve. These nerves leave the base of the skull through the jugular foramen and have motor, sensory, and parasympathetic functions in the neck, especially for the pharynx and the larynx. The superior ganglion of the vagus nerve lies at the base of the skull, and the inferior ganglion at the level of the hyoid bone (for functions of the vagal nerve system, see **Table 8.1**).

The cranial sympathetics. The sympathetic nervous system is dominant during physical and mental stress. It innervates all of the smooth muscles, the various glands of the body, and the striated muscle of the heart, triggering increases in blood pressure and heart rate, dilation of the pupils, and sweating, in addition to many other somatic reactions.

The cell bodies of the preganglionic neuron are located in the lateral horn of the spinal cord. The nerve fibers leave the spinal cord through the anterior root, and via a communicating branch reach the sympathetic trunk. This consists of several ganglia and nerve fibers and extends from the neck to the sacrum along each side of the vertebral column.

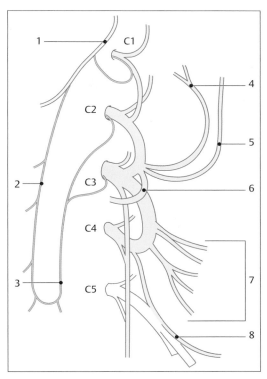

Fig. 8.11 Motor nerves in the neck. **1**, Hypoglossal nerve; **2**, ansa cervicalis superior radix; **3**, ansa cervicalis inferior radix; **4**, minor occipital nerve, **5**, great auricular nerve; **6**, transverse cervical nerve; **7**, supraclavicular nerves; **8**, to the brachial plexus.

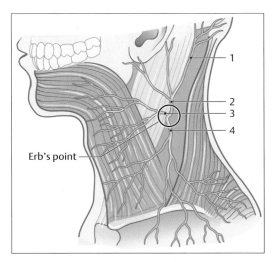

Fig. 8.12 Sensory nerves in the neck. **1**, Occipital nerve; **2**, great auricular nerve; **3**, transverse cervical nerve; **4**, supraclavicular nerves.

Table 8.1   Motor, sensory, and autonomic parts of the vagus nerve system

Motor	*Larynx:* The recurrent laryngeal nerve curves around the subclavian artery on the right side and the aortic arch on the left side. The paired nerves then run superiorly between the trachea and the esophagus on each side. The recurrent nerves supply all the laryngeal muscles, with the exception of the cricothyroid muscle (see **Figs. 4.14; 8.26**)
	Pharynx: Motor vagal impulses reach the pharyngeal musculature via the glossopharyngeal nerve
Sensory	In the neck, these nerve branches are responsible for sensory supply to the base of the tongue, epiglottis, and larynx. The tracheal and bronchial branches of the vagus are involved in the reflex control of respiration. Sensory impulses from the posterior meatal wall and the tympanic membrane run in the auricular branch of the vagus
Parasympathetic	Secretory parasympathetic fibers run from the neck to the organs of the thorax and abdomen. Secretory regulation of the parotid gland is controlled via the glossopharyngeal nerve (see p. 233)
Sympathetic chain	The cervical part of the sympathetic trunk lies in front of the prevertebral fascia and the transverse processes of the cervical spine. The sympathetic trunk supplies the heart, blood vessels, glands, smooth muscular organs, and accessory glands of the skin
	The *superior cervical ganglion* and the inconstant *middle cervical ganglion* arise from several segments
	The *inferior cervical ganglion,* with the upper thoracic ganglia, forms the *stellate ganglion.* It lies between the transverse process of the seventh cervical vertebra and the head of the first rib. Postganglionic fibers from the superior ganglion run to the carotid, middle ear, salivary and lacrimal glands, and the ciliary ganglion via cranial nerves IX, X, and XI and the upper three cervical nerves

The sympathetic nerve fibers supplying the glands (e. g., salivary glands) and smooth muscle of the head (e. g., vessel walls, piloerector muscles, pupilloconstrictor muscle) leave the spinal cord as preganglionic fibers in the first thoracic nerve (T1) and travel by way of the white communicating branches to the cervical portion of the sympathetic trunk. This contains three sympathetic ganglia—the inferior, middle, and superior cervical ganglia. The inferior cervical ganglions fuse with the first thoracic ganglion of the sympathetic trunk to form the stellate ganglion. Postganglionic neurons leave the spinal cord in the first thoracic segment and ascend and enter the sympathetic trunk at the highest sympathetic ganglion in the neck (the superior cervical ganglion). The postganglionic axons reach their effector organs with efferent fibers for the oculomotor, facial, glossopharyngeal, and vagus nerves by winding around arteries on their way to supplying the innervated structures. In this way, the neurons reach and supply the glands and smooth muscles together with the arteries. There are also afferent sympathetic fibers in the facial, glossopharyngeal, and vagus nerves.

Note: Stimulation of the superior cervical ganglion (fright response) produces dilation of the pupil and widening of the palpebral cleft, exophthalmos, sweating, and an increase in vascular tone. Blockage of the stellate ganglion by drugs or tumor leads to the opposite reaction—i. e., enophthalmos, miosis, and ptosis (Horner syndrome).

■ **Basic Physiology**

Coughing. Afferent impulses running in the vagus nerve cause reflex deepening of inspiration, followed by glottic closure. The glottis opens suddenly, with an explosive escape of compressed air after contraction of the expiratory thoracic muscles. High air speeds are obtained during coughing attacks, which can eject mucus, crusts, and foreign bodies (see pp. 313, 357, 367).

Straining. The thoracic and abdominal muscles are strongly contracted with voluntary closure of the glottis. The trunk becomes a mechanically fixed unit, so that the hip and shoulder muscles can respond with a coordinated brief and maximum effort—e. g., when lifting objects or bringing the body into the upright position.

In the Valsalva maneuver (see p. 26), the thoracoabdominal muscle pump develops high-compression pressure on the vascular system with an extrathoracic increase in venous pressure, producing protrusion of the veins of the head and neck and a decrease in arterial pressure due to obstruction of venous return to the heart. The patient may faint.

Methods of Investigation

■ Specific History

The following typical symptoms are reported when the patient's history is taken:
- *Pain:* This can be characterized as constant pain, pain during swallowing, during pressure or palpation, or during neck movement.
- *Signs of local inflammation:* The skin above the suspect area is red and warm or swollen, often in combination with local or diffuse pain.
- *Restricted movement of the cervical vertebrae:* The head and neck show restricted active and passive mobility in the anterior and posterior, and also lateral, directions.
- *Globus feeling:* This includes a foreign-body sensation, a feeling of pressure in the neck area, and a pulsing sensation.
- *Swelling:* The swelling can be characterized by its consistency (hard, smooth, mobile, fixed) and extent (circumscribed, diffuse).

■ Inspection of the Neck Region

Inspection is oriented to the neck structures that contribute to the profile. This includes examination of the color of the overlying skin and of any lesions (e. g., rubor, vascular signs, venous congestion, pigmentation) as well as fistulous openings, swellings, or indurations (lymphadenopathy, tumor, abscess). The position and mobility of the head are examined, with observation for spasm of the neck muscles (e. g., in inflammatory processes) or functional disorders of the cervical spine.

Table 8.2 Differential diagnosis of cervical swelling

Thyroid swelling
Lymphadenopathy
<ul><li>Nonspecific lymphadenopathy</li><li>Specific lymphadenopathy – Mononucleosis – HIV lymphadenopathy – Malignant lymphadenopathy (metastatic carcinoma, Hodgkin and non-Hodgkin lymphoma)</li></ul>
Median and lateral cervical cysts
Inflammation and tumors of the submandibular gland and the cervical part of the parotid gland
Deep inflammation or abscess
Lipoma
Hemangioma, lymphangioma, cystic hygroma
Carotid body tumor
Less common tumors include sebaceous cysts, dermoid cysts, neuroma, vascular aneurysms, infective lymphadenopathy—e. g. rubella, toxoplasmosis

■ Palpation

Palpation is carried out either from the front or behind, and both sides are palpated and compared. The head should be tilted slightly forward to relax the soft tissues. Palpable abnormalities mostly affect the thyroid gland, lymph nodes, salivary glands, tumors, cysts, and abscesses (**Table 8.2**).

Characteristic palpable findings in the neck are tumor, rubor, pain, resistance, fluctuations, pulsations, and indurations.

The evaluation and description note the shape, size, and mobility of the lymph nodes.

Auscultation and palpation are performed for suspected vascular anomalies (carotid body tumors, vascular aneurysms, carotid artery stenosis).

Lymph nodes—palpation technique. It is advisable to palpate the individual lymph node groups bimanually in sequence (**Fig. 8.13**), recording their topographic sites, number, shape, and size. The consistency of the nodes, which may be soft, elastic, fluctuant, firm, or hard, should also be recorded. Other important characteristics are pulsation and mobility. In addition, the neck muscles, shoulder, and thyroid gland should also be evaluated.

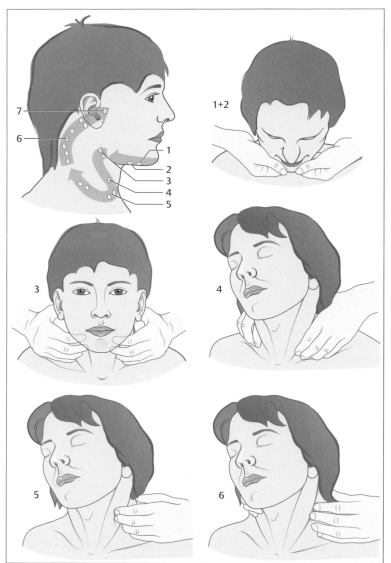

■ Diagnostic Imaging

■ Main Techniques

Two-dimensional B-mode ultrasound. This is regarded as the gold standard for detecting soft-tissue lesions in the neck. Ultrasonography can provide useful information helping to identify specific lesions on the basis of morphological ultrasound criteria.

Note: Ultrasound is not able to distinguish positively between benign and malignant tissue structures.

Computed tomography (CT). Axial CT scans provide detailed views of anatomical structures, differentiating between vascular lesions, inflammatory and tumor-based tissue structures (especially in the lymph nodes), cysts, and destructive cervical mass lesions.

Magnetic resonance imaging (MRI). This provides excellent discrimination of soft tissue, with differentiation between neoplastic, cicatricial, and inflammatory lesions. Contrast administration makes it possible to demonstrate vascular structures. Multiplanar imaging allows precise localization of suspicious tissue.

Positron-emission tomography (PET). This is a specific imaging modality that demonstrates increased metabolic activity in neoplastic tissue after the injection of fluorodeoxyglucose (FDG).

Conventional plain radiography of the neck. In the anteroposterior and lateral projections, conventional plain radiography provides an overview of bony structures (cervical spine), cartilaginous structures (larynx), soft-tissue swellings (prevertebral), cysts, emphysema, foci of tuberculous calcification, sialoliths, radiopaque foreign bodies, and phleboliths.

■ Special Techniques

Plain radiographs of the cervical spine (four views). These show the morphological basis of functional disorders.

Digital subtraction angiography (DSA). This method can detect pathological changes in the vascular structures of the neck (e. g., stenosis, aneurysm, glomus tumor of the carotid body).

Doppler/duplex ultrasound. This is used to assess blood flow in the extracranial vessels (common carotid, external, and internal carotid artery, subclavian and vertebral artery).

Lymphoscintigraphy. This is a method for intraoperative verification of a sentinel lymph node in the head and neck region, as a criterion for selective lymph-node biopsy or neck dissection.

■ Biopsy

Fine-needle aspiration. This method allows sampling of solid tissue masses for cytologic analysis and should usually be performed under ultrasound guidance. The procedure requires considerable experience in cytomorphological evaluation of the sample material.

Core biopsy. Tissue aspiration for histologic evaluation. Only positive results can be used to establish a diagnosis.

Open biopsy. Excision of isolated lymph nodes or wedge excision of a solid tumor mass is the most reliable method for histological assessment.

Clinical Aspects

■ **Inflammation of the Cervical Soft Tissues**

Superficial infections affecting the skin and its appendages have to be distinguished from deep infections affecting the viscera. Superficial infections are usually primary infections of the skin and its appendages, caused by staphylococci. Inflammations of the cervical visceral spaces are usually secondary to necrosis or inflammation of the regional lymph nodes, with or without suppuration, or extend from internal organs such as the airway and the esophagus. The infection is caused by mixed flora of staphylococci, streptococci, Gram-negative organisms, or tuberculous bacilli.

Superficial Infections
Furuncles or *carbuncles* on the neck are most common on the nape in men and are often found in diabetic patients and in patients with alcoholism. Furuncles are treated surgically by deroofing. Carbuncles are treated using parallel incisions and undermining of the subcutaneous septal skin, followed by drainage and concomitant antibiotic therapy.

Infected *sebaceous cysts* and subcutaneous *dermoids* may mimic a cervical abscess. They are excised completely after a course of antibiotics to suppress local inflammation.

Abscesses

Clinical Features. The site of an inflammatory process in the fascial spaces determines the clinical picture. The parapharyngeal and submandibular spaces are most commonly involved. Collections of pus lying deep in the neck often cannot be palpated. The functions of the soft tissue of the neck are restricted, and deep swellings cause pain such as trismus, pain on swallowing, and muscle rigidity. Examination of the blood shows the typical signs of infection. Shivering, respiratory obstruction, or mediastinitis indicate thrombophlebitis or early septicemia.

Pathogenesis. The cause is a soft-tissue infection originating from the head, primary or secondary inflammation of the cervical lymph nodes, a purulent thyroid infection, and/or infected cysts. Descending specific otogenic abscesses (Bezold mastoiditis, see p. 66) are uncommon today.

Diagnosis. This is based on the history, clinical findings, special imaging studies, and microbiology.

Treatment. In severe cases, broad-spectrum antibiotics are given immediately, without waiting for the results of culture and sensitivity tests. The site of the abscess may be determined by aspiration. However, antibiotics and aspiration are no substitute for incision and drainage of the abscess. Definitive surgical treatment often has to be performed in a second stage due to infection of the surrounding soft tissues, veins, arteries, and nerves.

Mediastinitis

Clinical Features. These include severe malaise, fever, retrosternal or intrascapular pain, cutaneous emphysema (gas formation), and venous congestion.

Pathogenesis. The visceral space in the neck is not closed off from the superior mediastinum (see pp. 375–377) so that an inflammation in the former may spread into the area of the latter. A common cause is perforation of the hypopharynx or esophagus, particularly at the beginning of its inlet, during diagnostic endoscopy, removal of a foreign body, or operations on a pharyngeal pouch.

Diagnosis. This is based on the history, clinical findings, chest radiographs—if necessary with contrast films using a watery medium to demonstrate the perforation—and computed tomography.

Treatment. The posterosuperior mediastinum is drained. An incision is made along the anterior border of the sternocleidomastoid muscle, and blunt dissection is carried down to the esophagus. The sternocleidomastoid muscle and thyroid gland are separated by retractors, and a finger is directed along the esophagus into the posterosuperior mediastinum. A drain is introduced once the abscess has been opened. The anterior mediastinum is entered through a horizontal incision above the suprasternal notch. The anterior wall of the trachea is exposed as for an inferior tracheotomy, and a finger is used to open the upper mediastinum. A drain is introduced.

Actinomycosis is a chronic disease causing fistulas. It is relatively painless, with hard infiltrates mainly affecting the neck, but also less commonly the cheek and the floor of the mouth. The skin undergoes livid discoloration. The infection responds to penicillin.

■ Inflammatory Cervical Lymphadenopathy

Acute Cervical Lymphadenitis

Clinical Features. These include acute, painful swellings of the lymph nodes. If the course is subacute, induration and decreasing tenderness occur. The site of the lymphadenitis depends on the primary site of the inflammatory disease. The lymph nodes may fluctuate if treatment is inadequate or the organisms are very virulent. Fluctuation and spontaneous perforation through the skin are possible. In a primary infection with human immunodeficiency virus (HIV), an incubation period of 1–3 weeks is followed by an "acute" stage marked by flu-like symptoms, an itchy skin rash, and generalized lymphadenitis.

Pathogenesis. The first frequency peak is in children up to the age of 10 years and is usually due to nasopharyngeal infection. Streptococcal infections are the most frequent causes. Other potential causes are viruses (rubella, cytomegalovirus, Epstein–Barr, HIV) and mycobacteria.

The second frequency peak is in adults between 50 and 70 years of age. In these older patients, lymphadenitis is often an expression of inflammation accompanying malignancy.

If acute cervical lymphadenitis is found, a careful topographic search of the head and neck region for the primary infection has to be carried out.

Note: The primary focus may have already resolved, but enlarged cervical lymph nodes may still persist.

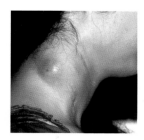

Fig. 8.14 An inflamed cutaneous reaction and lymph-node swelling due to a tuberculous infection.

Diagnosis. The primary focus of infection is looked for in the area of lymph-node drainage. The enlarged and fluctuant lymph nodes may be tender. If there is any doubt, lymph-node incision and drainage accompanied by biopsy are needed.

Differential diagnosis. This includes metastatic carcinoma, Hodgkin and non-Hodgkin lymphoma, inflamed thyroglossal duct of branchial cysts, tuberculous lymphadenopathy, toxoplasmosis, and acquired immune deficiency syndrome (AIDS).

Treatment. Broad-spectrum antibiotics are administered. If there is abscess formation, incision and drainage are necessary. Aspiration of the abscess is not an adequate form of treatment. The wound can be closed, but a drain must be inserted. A specimen of pus is taken for culture and sensitivity testing, and any tissue removed is submitted for histology.

Note: Acute cervical lymphadenitis resolves after treatment of the primary infection. Occasionally, induration of the lymph nodes persists. Central caseous necrosis in the swollen lymph nodes following acute inflammation is suspicious for tuberculosis, infected branchial cyst, lymph-node tumors, fluctuating lymphadenitis in cat-scratch fever, or tularemia. In these cases, a lymph-node biopsy has to be taken for histological examination.

Chronic Cervical Lymphadenitis

Chronic cervical lymph-node enlargement that has been present for more than 4 weeks has to be distinguished from malignant diseases such as malignant lymphoma and cervical lymph-node metastasis.

A diagnostic procedure for cervical lymphadenopathy is mandatory, taking into consideration the presence of risk factors, the patient's age, specific and nonspecific symptoms, and disease history.

Clinical examinations using palpation and B-mode ultrasound allow initial localization and measurement of the lymphadenopathy. Serological screening tests are helpful for differentiating specific lymphadenopathies. Surgical removal of the lymph node will provide the most accurate diagnosis, but must only be done after a full and thorough assessment of the respiratory tract to exclude a primary tumor.

Specific Lymphadenopathy

Tuberculous Lymphadenopathy

Clinical Features. Any group of lymph nodes in the cervical region may be affected; the disease is bilateral in 20% of patients. Nowadays, the upper jugular, supraclavicular, and nuchal lymph nodes are most often involved. This specific lymphadenopathy is painless or only produces slight pain. The lesions may be solitary, multiple, small or large, firm or fluctuant. Often there may be fistulas or old retracted fistulous scars in addition to acute reactivated lymph nodes, possibly with reddening of the skin and fluctuation (**Fig. 8.14**).

Pathogenesis. Tuberculosis lymphadenitis is mainly a secondary hematogenous infection, usually caused by human tuberculous mycobacteria; occasionally, it is due to atypical mycobacteria, particularly in children. The infection spreads from patients with active tuberculosis who may be apparently healthy and tuberculin-positive.

Note: Calcification of tuberculous lymph nodes is often considered to be an indication that they have healed, but this is incorrect. Tubercle bacilli can survive for decades in caseous and calcified centers of lymph nodes.

Diagnosis. Important points to elucidate from the patient's history include country of origin, a family history of tuberculosis, and visits to epidemic areas in Asia, Africa, and south-eastern Europe. Radiographic and CT images of the neck showing calcification of the lymph nodes are almost always pathognomonic. Chest radiography and an intracutaneous tuberculin test complete the diagnostic procedure.

The diagnosis is confirmed by the histological appearance of the excised lymph nodes and by microbiology.

Differential diagnosis. Acute cervical lymphadenitis, branchial cleft cyst, metastatic carcinoma, Hodgkin's disease, sialadenitis, salivary tumor, non-Hodgkin's lymphoma, neurinoma, nodular goiter, dermoid cysts, and salivary stone.

Treatment. Antituberculous treatment is usually a combined triple drug therapy using isoniazid, rifampicin, and ethambutol.

Surgery: The indications for surgery are:
- Lymph nodes 2 cm or more in diameter that show no tendency to resolve.
- Lymph nodes with calcification.
- Fluctuant lymph nodes.
- Fistulas.
- Collar-stud abscess, involvement of the lymph nodes, soft-tissue abscess, and involvement of the overlying skin.

Surgical treatment should include removal of specifically affected lymph nodes, affected soft tissues, and cervical skin. In many cases, particularly with collar-stud abscess, a selective neck dissection (see p. 406) with reconstruction of the skin defect may be necessary. Elimination of a tuberculous primary focus using tonsillectomy is now much less important in the light of present-day knowledge of epidemiology and pathogenesis.

Syphilis (see also p. 253)
- Stage I, primary chancre: an indolent regional lymphadenopathy appears 1–2 weeks after the primary lesion on the lips, mouth, tonsils, or facial area.
- Stage II: multiple cervical lymphadenopathy may occur.
- Stage III: rarely causes lymphadenopathy.

Sarcoidosis (Boeck Disease)

Clinical Features. Lymphadenopathy affects the mediastinal and supraclavicular nodes in 65–75% of cases and the peripheral nodes in 10–20%, and may include the retroperitoneal nodes. The eyes, lacrimal glands, and salivary glands are affected in 5–25% of cases. The skin is affected in 10–40% of cases with erythema nodosum or lupus pernio. The mucous membranes of the nose and sinuses, pharynx, larynx, trachea, mouth, and esophagus demonstrate pale-red granular areas.

Heerfordt syndrome is a rare but distinctive presentation that includes uveoparotitis and facial paralysis; see p. 424.

Pathogenesis. The cause of this condition remains unknown. Affected tissues display a noncaseating epithelioid cell granulomatous reaction, spreading in the reticulohistiocytic system.

Treatment. Systemic steroids are the mainstay of active sarcoidosis. Cytotoxic therapy and anti–tumor necrosis factor-α drugs are used in severe cases.

Catscratch Disease and Tularemia

Clinical Features. A pustulous primary focus occurs in the skin or oral mucosa, and usually ulcerates. This is followed 1–5 weeks later by a regional painless, or almost painless, lymphadenopathy. In more than one-third of cases, the lymph nodes fluctuate and a fistula forms.

Pathogenesis. *Catscratch disease* is caused by *Bartonella henselae*, a small aerobic Gram-negative coccobacillus. In most cases, the infection follows a scratch or a bite from a cat, but dogs, rodents, and hedgehogs may also be carriers.

Tularemia is caused by *Francisella tularensis,* named after the county of Tulare in California. The zoonosis is widespread in rodents, particularly in hares. It is transmitted by ticks and other biting insects.

Diagnosis. History reveals contact with the above animals. Both conditions are confirmed by serology and antibody assay. Histological examination of the affected lymph node in catscratch disease and in tularemia shows reticulocytic lymphadenitis with abscess formation.

Treatment. Both conditions respond to treatment with various antibiotics. However, catscratch disease will often resolve without anitbiotics. In tularemia, the severity and type of lymphadenopathy determine the need for surgical treatment. Lymphadenopathy may resolve spontaneously. Tetracyclines are the treatment of choice.

Toxoplasmosis
Signs and symptoms. Acquired toxoplasmosis causes an acute or subacute influenza-like illness with subfebrile temperatures for 6–8 weeks. An important clinical feature is lymphadenopathy affecting especially the nuchal, periauricular, jugulodigastric, supraclavicular, and rarely axillary and inguinal nodes. The chronic form affects adults and produces few characteristic symptoms, but may cause headache or chronic eye disease.

Pathogenesis. Infection in humans is caused by *Toxoplasma gondii*, which is mainly acquired through consumption of raw beef or pork, but also from contact with feline feces. There is evidence of previous infection in a high proportion of the population, as antibodies are found in up to 70% of clinically healthy people. The great majority of postnatal infections proceed without causing characteristic clinical symptoms.

Diagnosis. *Serological tests:* Sabin–Feldman dye test, indirect immunofluorescence test. The complement-binding reaction is a valuable supplementary method. High titers of immunoglobulins G and M indicate an acute or chronic infection.
   Histological examination of lymph nodes usually reveals Piringer-Kuchinka syndrome—an epithelioid cell lymph-node reaction with no necrosis and argyrophilic granules in the protoplasm of the reticulum cells.

Differential diagnosis. The above serologic findings, particularly in combination with lymph-node biopsy, are very characteristic of toxoplasmosis. Lymphadenopathy with similar lymphocytic changes in the blood picture also occurs in infectious lymphocytosis, rubella roseola infantum, and listeriosis. Similar findings occur in lymphadenopathy in response to antiepileptic drugs—sodium channel blockers, γ-aminobutyric acid (GABA) receptor blockers, and carbamazepine—antitoxins, some antibiotics and serum injections, in the drain-

age area of transplanted tissues, and in mononucleosis.

Treatment. The preferred regimen involves a combination of pyrimethamine and sulfonamides (sulfadiazine).

Lyme Disease
Signs and symptoms. The initial clinical features are erythema migrans and pain at the bite site, with lymphadenitis. Variable organ involvement supervenes at 3–8 weeks. Peripheral facial palsy develops in 60% of cases. The late stage is dominated by neurologic symptoms such as meningopolyradiculitis.

Pathogenesis. The disease is caused by the spirochete *Borrelia burgdorferi*, transmitted mainly by the bite of the tick *Ixodes ricinus* (middle Europe), *Ixodes scapularis* (eastern states of USA), *Ixodes pacificus* (western states of USA), and *Ixales persulcatus* (Russia).

Diagnosis. Serological proof of specific antibodies.

Differential diagnosis. Differentiation is required from spring–summer meningoencephalitis.

Treatment. The antibiotic treatment of choice is doxycycline (in adults), amoxicillin (in children), and ceftriaxone for 3–4 weeks. Alternative choices are cefuroxime and cefotaxime.

Prognosis. The prognosis is favorable with treatment.

■ Cervical Spine Syndrome

Clinical Features. Although cervical spine syndrome is an imprecise term, it is frequently diagnosed by doctors, and simply indicates that the patient has pain in the area of the spine. This does not indicate any causal factors. Possible causes of pain include muscular strain caused by physical stress or incorrect posture. Protrusion or dislocation of an intervertebral disk, or arthrosis and inflammation of the facet joints, can also cause this syndrome. Blockage of a facet joint can cause localized pain, as well as sympathetic nervous system reactions. Clinical symptoms can also be caused by exaggerated motion in single segments of the cervical vertebrae, due to abrasion of stiffened neighboring segments.

Additional clinical symptoms caused by disturbances of the cervical spine are acute cochleovestibular disorders with hearing difficulties, tinnitus, and vertigo. Dysphonia of an undefined origin, chronic pharyngitis, and globus sensation are characteristic signs and symptoms in the pharyngeal and laryngeal sections of the neck area. Other more complex syndromes accompanied by the cervical spine syndrome include acute torticollis, cervical fusion syndrome, and subclavian steal syndrome.

Diagnosis. The history provides preliminary, and often decisive, indications of disorders of the cervical spine. Inspection can identify soft-tissue changes as indications of reflex secondary changes in the area of blocked facet joints. Palpation can detect trigger points, and an analysis of the quality of skin and muscle is carried out. An important examination method is testing the segmental movement of the cervical spine and cervicothoracic junction. This can identify any restricted movement of individual intervertebral joints. This examination method requires chiropractic experience for accurate assessment of alterations.

Treatment. Chiropractic measures and manual therapy form the basis of treatment for disorders of the cervical spine and include soft-tissue techniques to relax the muscles, passive mobilization of individual joints, stretching of muscles, manipulations, and therapeutic use of local anesthesia. All of these can be supplemented with physical measures (application of warmth), physiotherapy, and additional prescription of medications (anti-inflammatory drugs, antirheumatics, muscle relaxants).

■ Trauma

Injuries to the larynx are described on pages 308–313, injuries to the trachea on pages 357–358, and injuries to the esophagus on pages 365–367.

Depending on the force involved, blunt trauma to soft tissues leads to tissue swelling secondary to edema or hematoma, and to surgical emphysema if a defect occurs in the mucosal continuity of the subglottis, trachea, or hypopharynx. The degree of injury is determined by the direction and varying degrees of force. Open injuries to the respiratory or digestive tracts are only slightly less dramatic than a tear in the carotid artery or internal jugular vein. The danger associated with opening one of the major veins is air embolism. If the volume of air aspirated is more than 10–20 mL, the result is fatal. Emergency treatment of air embolism consists of immediate digital compression, flat body posture, and subsequent surgical repair.

Patients with carotid artery hemorrhage usually die at the time of injury due to hemorrhagic shock. Even with immediate digital compression and rapid surgical treatment, a high proportion of the survivors of open injuries to the common and internal carotid arteries have residual cerebral defects. Successful treatment depends on interdisciplinary management involving trauma surgeons, anesthesiologists, and vascular surgeons.

Injuries to the cervical spine can present directly or indirectly. Indirect injuries are often accompanied by other injuries to the head and neck area, and lead to chronic damage to the senses of hearing and balance. There are three typical mechanisms of injury that usually occur during sports and road-traffic accidents:

1. Sprain injury.
2. Torsion injury, often combined with sprain.
3. Whiplash, or injury caused by acceleration/deceleration.

Nausea and vomiting, cochleovestibular reactions (loss of hearing, tinnitus, vertigo) and optical sensations are symptomatic of these injuries. Disturbances of sensation and paralysis can also appear. Diagnosis and therapy of injuries to the cervical spine always require interdisciplinary management involving otolaryngologists, orthopedic and emergency surgeons, neurologists, and neurosurgeons. Patients with suspected injury to the cervical spine should undergo specific investigation starting with plain radiographs of the neck and moving on to CT and MRI. Possible injuries include fractures of C1 (the atlas) or C2 (the dens). These injuries require multidisciplinary expertise from the fields of orthopedics, emergency medicine and possibly neurosurgery.

■ Congenital Anomalies

■ Thyroglossal Duct Cysts and Fistulas

Clinical Features. A firm elastic swelling, the size of a cherry or an apple, is found in the midline of the neck at the level of, above, or below the hyoid bone (**Fig. 8.15**). The patient may have a globus sensation and a visible lump. If a fistula is present, its external opening is often inflamed.

Pathogenesis. *Thyroglossal cysts* are remnants of the thyroglossal duct.

Median cervical fistulas may be caused by perforation of the thyroglossal duct through the skin, by spontaneous perforation of median thyroglossal cysts due to infection, or by surgery (**Fig. 8.16a,b**).

Diagnosis. This is based on the typical site. The cyst or fistula moves up and down when the patient swallows. A probe can be introduced into a fistula as far as the body of the hyoid bone. The lesion can be delineated with ultrasonography.

Differential diagnosis. This includes tumors of the pyramidal lobe of the thyroid gland, ectopic thyroid tissue, inflammatory or malignant lymphadenopathy, epidermoid cyst, and submental dermoid cyst.

Treatment. The cyst or fistula is removed. It is essential to remove the body of the hyoid bone to prevent recurrence, as it contains epithelial remnants. Careful hemostasis and drainage are particularly important, since oozing of blood and postoperative swelling can lead to acute laryngeal obstruction and suffocation.

■ Branchial Cysts and Fistulas

Embryology. Between the third and fourth weeks of embryonic life, five entodermal pharyngeal pouches develop in the lateral part of the foregut. Four ectodermal branchial grooves develop at corresponding sites on the external surface of the embryo. Five mesodermal branchial arches develop in humans between these external and internal grooves. Each contains one cartilaginous bar, one branchial arch artery, one branchial arch nerve, and branchial arch musculature (**Table 8.3**). In the sixth week, the second arch grows over the third and fourth arches and fuses with the neighboring cau-

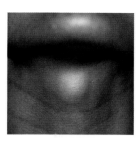

Fig. 8.15 A thyroglossal duct cyst typically forms an elastic swelling in the midline of the neck at the level of the hyoid bone.

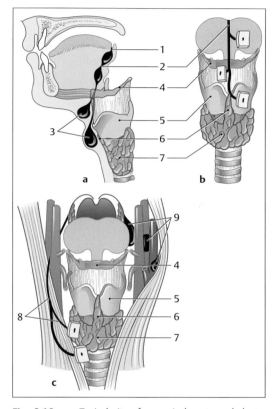

Fig. 8.16a–c Typical sites for cervical cysts and ducts. **1**, Foramen cecum; **2**, thyroglossal duct; **3**, submental and prelaryngeal cysts; **4**, hyoid bone; **5**, thyroid cartilage; **6**, thyroid gland isthmus; **7**, thyroid gland.
a Thyroglossal duct cysts.
b Fistulas.
c Branchial cleft cysts and fistulas. **8**, Fistular tube; **9**, lateral cervical cysts.

Table 8.3 Embryologic development of the branchial arches

First branchial arch, mandibular arch

Ectodermal: Skin of the cheek, mandible, anterior half of the auricle, external meatus, trigeminal nerve, parenchyma of the salivary glands, tooth enamel, epithelial covering of the lip, the tongue as far back as the foramen cecum, tympanic membrane

Mesodermal: Masticatory muscles, anterior belly of the digastric muscle, tensor tympani muscle, articular process of the mandible, malleus, incus, tragus, helical crus, stratum fibrosum of the tympanic membrane

Entodermal: Epithelium of the floor and lateral surfaces of the mouth, eustachian tube, and mucosa of the tympanic membrane, middle ear cavity, and mastoid

Second branchial arch, hyoid bone

Ectodermal: Skin of the posterior surface of the auricle and of the upper part of the neck, parts of cranial nerves VII and VIII

Mesodermal: Stapedius muscle, helix–anthelix, body of the hyoid bone

Entodermal: Epithelium of the base of the tongue, foramen cecum, central part of the thyroid gland, palatine tonsil

Third branchial arch

Ectodermal: Skin of the central part of the neck, parts of cranial nerve IX

Mesodermal: Superior part of the pharyngeal constrictor muscle, common and internal carotid artery

Entodermal: Epithelium of the pharynx, base of the tongue, epiglottis, and piriform sinus

Fourth branchial arch

Ectodermal: Cranial nerve X

Mesodermal: Inferior part of the pharyngeal constrictor muscle, laryngeal musculature, thyroid cartilage, parts of the epiglottis, right subclavian artery, aortic arch

Entodermal: Epithelium of the base of the tongue, pharyngeal epithelium, epiglottic epithelium, parts of the thyroid gland

Fifth branchial arch

Ectodermal: Skin of the lower part of the neck, cranial nerve XI

Mesodermal: Laryngeal musculature, arytenoid and cricoid cartilages

Entodermal: Submucosal lymphoid tissue, lungs

dal precardial swelling. The cervical sinus is thus formed from the disappearing second, third, and fourth branchial grooves. At the same time, the internal third, fourth, and fifth pharyngeal pouches disappear and form the branchiogenic organs, the parathyroids, and the thymus. Normally, the cervical sinus disappears completely. Lateral branchial cervical fistulas are caused by persistence of the external opening of the sinus. Persistent parts of the cervical sinus with obliteration of the external opening are said to cause lateral branchial cervical cysts (**Fig. 8.16c**).

Branchial Fistulas
Branchial fistulas are distinct from the obliterated sinus of branchial clefts.

Clinical Features. Periodically, the cutaneous fistulous opening may become red and swollen. In some cases, there is a noninflamed skin pit. The opening of the fistula is always at the anterior border of the sternocleidomastoid muscle, either at the level of the carotid triangle if it arises from the second branchial arch, at the level of the cricoid cartilage if it arises from the third branchial arch, or close to the suprasternal notch if it arises from the fourth arch (**Fig. 8.16c**). The discharge may be milky or purulent, recurrent, or persistent. The fistula is bilateral in 5 % of patients.

Pathogenesis. The causes are genetic or external toxic factors during pregnancy, such as hypoxemia, hypercarbia, smoking, alcohol, aspirin, urethane, thalidomide, lead, mercury, metabolic disturbances, or irradiation leading to incomplete obliteration of the branchial groove or to persistence of the cervical sinus.

Diagnosis. A subcutaneous cord running superiorly is often palpable and originates from the fistulous opening at the anterior border of the sternocleidomastoid muscle. Secretion can usually be expressed from the fistula by stroking in a downward direction. Introduction of a contrast medium through the fistula shows its course and branches. If the fistula is complete, with a pharyngeal ostium, then the contrast medium flows into the pharynx and the patient can taste it.

Treatment. Recurrence as a result of epithelial remnants can only be prevented by complete excision of the fistula. Complete dissection is facilitated by using a binocular loupe or microscope and by injecting dye into the fistula.

> **Note:** Lateral cervical fistulas may have variable courses. The most common fistulas from the second branchial arch run through the carotid bifurcation (the tonsillopharyngeal duct), whereas inferior fistulas run superiorly behind the common carotid artery (the thymopharyngeal duct).

Branchial Cysts

Clinical Features. Although the origin is congenital, these cysts are mainly noticed during childhood or early adulthood. The cyst is firm, elastic, and fluctuant, but may also be fixed as a result of infection. It is usually oval, with a diameter of ≈ 5 cm. Over the course of years, very large cystic sacs can form in patients who are not concerned with their health (**Fig. 8.17a**). Epipleural or mediastinal branchial cysts arising from the fifth branchial arch system may also be found on rare occasions. Secondary infection may cause severe pain with inflammation of the overlying skin. Bilateral branchial cysts are very uncommon.

Pathogenesis. The assumption that these cysts are branchial arch rudiments is still regarded as likely, although a lymph-node origin has also been proposed (cystic structures formed by epithelial debris).

> **Note:** Epithelial cysts rarely undergo malignant degeneration. A diagnosis of branchiogenic carcinoma should not delay the search for an occult primary tumor; cystic metastases from an occult primary tumor may be interpreted as a branchiogenic carcinoma.

Diagnosis. This is based on the history, palpable findings, ultrasound, CT, and MRI findings. The main risk at diagnosis is missing a cystic malignant squamous cell carcinoma (**Fig. 8.17b, c**).

Treatment. The cyst requires complete excision.

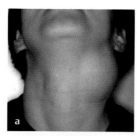
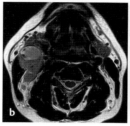
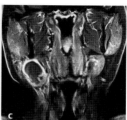

Fig. 8.17a–c a A large branchial cyst. **b, c** Magnetic resonance images show a cystic formation inside an area of inflamed tissue, which is a sign of acute inflammation of the branchial cyst associated with lymphadenitis.

■ **Musculoskeletal Defects**

Klippel–Feil Syndrome

This is a congenital synostosis of the cervical spine, often accompanied by a high spina bifida. The ears are set low on the head, and the patient may have a hearing defect or be totally deaf.

Oculoauriculovertebral Dysplasia (Goldenhar Syndrome)

This involves fusion or absence of a cervical vertebra, auricular tags, and middle ear anomalies, occasional unilateral hypoplasia or aplasia of the ascending ramus of the mandible, a coloboma of the iris, and an epibulbar dermoid.

Cervical Rib, Costoclavicular Compression Syndrome, and Scalenus Syndrome (Naffziger Syndrome)

About 1 % of the general population have a cervical rib, usually arising from the seventh vertebra. Only ≈ 10 % of these cause symptoms, mainly compression of the brachial plexus or of the subclavian artery and vein: the thoracic outlet compression syndrome. Other manifestations include circulatory disorders of the forearm and hand, brachialgia, paralysis of the brachial plexus, intermittent cerebral ischemia with attacks of vertigo, occipital headache, and double vision. Surgery is only carried out when conservative measures have failed, and in particular when there are severe neurologic signs or intermittent venous thrombosis. Treatment consists of division of the scalenus anterior muscle or resection of the cervical rib.

Torticollis

Clinical Features. Typically, the head and neck are held to the affected side and the chin is turned to the healthy side. It is almost always unilateral.

Pathogenesis. Muscular torticollis is the most common form. In congenital torticollis, it is assumed that there was intrauterine damage or birth trauma causing a muscle tear or hematoma, so that the sternocleidomastoid muscle is shortened by fibrosis of the muscle.

All forms of torticollis in early childhood, if untreated, cause damage to the growth of the face and the base of the skull, or scoliosis of the cervical spine. Congenital bony anomalies of the cervical spine can also cause torticollis.

Diagnosis. In muscular torticollis, the sternocleidomastoid muscle is thickened, usually in its lower third, and is hard and tender. It is noticed several days or weeks after birth by the increasingly obvious incorrect position of the head.

Differential diagnosis. See **Table 8.4.**

Treatment. Congenital muscular torticollis should be treated before the beginning of the second year of life at the latest if there has not been spontaneous remission or if conservative orthopedic measures have proved unsuccessful. Several forms of tenotomy and plastic elongation of the sternocleidomastoid muscle are possible.

■ **Vascular Malformations**

Hemangiomas

Clinical Features. The most common site is the face and the nape of the neck. A symmetrical median nevus flammeus (capillary hemangioma) sometimes gives rise to cosmetic problems. Asymmetrical hemangiomas are often combined with other anomalies, such as Sturge–Weber syndrome (a neurocutaneous disorder with angiomas involving the leptomeninges and skin of the face; the cutaneous angioma is called port-wine stain), Klippel–Trénaunay–Parkes–Weber syndrome (a disorder of blood vessels with a classic symptom triad of unilateral

Table 8.4   Causes of torticollis

Muscular	Inflammatory or cicatricial lesions, neoplastic infiltration of the sternocleidomastoid muscle and the overlying skin
	Removal of the sternocleidomastoid muscle, in radical neck dissection
	Paralysis of the accessory nerve
	Rheumatic torticollis, fibromyalgia (area of abnormal hardening in a muscle)
	Progressive myositis ossificans
	Neuralgic–neurovascular symptom complex in the scalene syndrome
Osseous	Torticollis due to nontraumatic atlantoaxial joint subluxation, radiotherapy, or nasopharyngeal surgery (Grisel syndrome)
	Subluxation of a vertebra due to trauma
Symptomatic	Ocular and reflex torticollis in compensation for unilateral lesions of the ocular muscles
	Stiffness of the neck in peritonsillar, retrotonsillar, or parapharyngeal abscesses
	Acute and subacute cervical inflammatory lymphadenopathy
	Otitis externa and media, particularly Bezold mastoiditis (see p. 66)
	Unilateral labyrinthine disorders
Psychogenetic and neurotic	

nevus flammeus, excessive growth of connective tissue and bones, as well as primary varicosis.). The lesions tend to bleed spontaneously and in response to mild trauma.

Pathogenesis. Two-thirds are cutaneous hemangiomas, which are evident at birth. The remainder lie subcutaneously or deeper, with a particular tendency to penetrate the masseter muscle. They are mainly flat hemangiomas that grow rapidly in the first months of life but tend to atrophy spontaneously. If they do not atrophy, they are dealt with surgically in one or more stages.

Lymphangioma (Cystic Hygroma)

Clinical Features. Cystic hygromas usually lie on the lateral part of the neck. They may be large enough to occupy the entire lateral part of the neck and cause stridor, cyanosis, and dysphagia due to displacement of cervical viscera. They may also cause difficulty at birth due to their size. Large hygromas cause torticollis. They may also cause parotid swelling; lymphangioma is the second most common parotid tumor in neonates and infants after hemangioma.

Pathogenesis. Capillary, cavernous, and cystic lymphangiomas are sequestrated parts of the embryonic lymphatic vascular system.

Diagnosis. This is based on the presence of a compressible swelling containing lymph fluid, usually in the lateral cervical area but also in the parotid area.

Differential diagnosis. This includes hemangioma, branchial cyst, and solid or cystic congenital teratoma (dermoid cyst).

Treatment. Spontaneous remission is very uncommon. Aspiration is helpful if the patient is at risk of suffocation. Cystic hygromas are usually multilocular and radiopaque. The treatment of choice is removal in one or more stages, with preservation of vital structures and nerves.

Aneurysms

Clinical Features. A pulsating cervical swelling ("pseudotumor"), causing a hissing noise on auscultation, usually lies anterior to the sternocleidomastoid muscle. It may also be visible and palpable in the parapharyngeal area, depending on its site and growth propensity.

Pathogenesis. In rare cases, the cause is birth trauma or congenital anomalies. Acquired aneurysms are usually due to trauma or syphilis.

Diagnosis. This depends on palpation and auscultation of the neck and oropharynx. The diagnosis can be established using angiography and ultrasonography.

Treatment. Vascular surgery is performed when indicated.

Malignant vascular tumors in the neck include angiosarcoma, which is very uncommon, and hemangiopericytoma (a soft-tissue sarcoma arising from capillary pericytes),

which is more frequent. The prognosis is poor, as the lesions are not usually resectable, tend to recur, and metastasize. They are resistant to radiotherapy and chemotherapy.

Carotid Body Tumor (Chemodectoma)

Clinical Features. The tumor is usually a painless and well-defined swelling located in the carotid triangle. It grows slowly and causes no symptoms in ≈ 70 % of cases. It may cause a feeling of globus or dysphagia. About 20 % of patients have Horner syndrome. The carotid sinus syndrome includes vertigo, tinnitus, and attacks of sweating in ≈ 2 % of cases, particularly on turning the head. It is bilateral in 2–5 % of patients.

Pathogenesis. The tumor of the carotid body consists of precapillary arteriovenous anastomoses, and contains a collection of chemoreceptor non-chromaffin paraganglion cells. These cells belong to a group with a similar appearance in the area of distribution of the vagus and glossopharyngeal nerves: tympanic, jugular (see pp. 89–91), vagal, or periaortic glomus. The tumor may grow around the external or internal carotid artery and narrow it. Hypertrophy of the carotid body is observed significantly more often in persons living in conditions of chronic oxygen deficiency. Malignant changes or metastases develop in 1–10 % of patients.

Diagnosis. Auscultation reveals a vascular bruit. Carotid angiography and Doppler ultrasonography are definitive. On MRI or CT, a typical egg-shaped splaying of the carotid bifurcation, caused by a displacement of the internal and external carotid arteries, may be visible with large tumors.

!
> **Note:** Biopsy is contraindicated, due to the severe danger of bleeding.

Differential diagnosis. This includes aneurysms, branchial cysts, neurogenic cervical tumors, lymph-node metastases, and Hodgkin and non-Hodgkin lymphoma.

Treatment. The carotid body tumor is radiopaque and should be treated surgically, as its future growth is unpredictable. Advances in vascular surgery have reduced the incidence of neurologic deficits and death. Embolization significantly reduces intraoperative bleeding and is routinely advised before surgery.

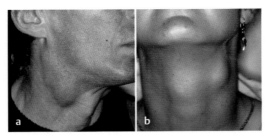

Fig. 8.18a, b **a** A cervical lipoma forms a smooth, soft tumor with no clinical symptoms.
b A schwannoma of the vagus nerve can occur as a solid nonmobile tumor along the course of the nerve.

■ Tumors

■ Benign Tumors

Cervical Lipoma
Clinical Features. Simple lipomas may arise in all parts of the neck and may be solitary or multiple. They are subcutaneous, grow slowly, and are clinically and histologically benign, causing few symptoms. They are often removed for cosmetic reasons (**Fig. 8.18a**).

Lipomatosis of the neck mainly affects the nuchal region. The fatty deposits may become so large that the patient has to hold the head forward. On the neck, the tumors are typically occipital and notched in the midline, and there may be coexisting lipomas on the trunk.

Anterior lipomatosis often begins as a double chin, grows slowly downward in the neck, and tends to infiltrate the muscles. Removal in one or more stages is indicated, as patients are unable to hold the head in the correct position and the condition interferes with function.

Neurinoma
Neurogenic tumors occur relatively often in the neck. They arise either from the autonomic nervous system or from the sheaths of peripheral nerves. Neurofibromas and schwannomas arise from the Schwann cells of the peripheral nerves (**Fig. 8.18b**).

Von Recklinghausen disease is a generalized neurofibromatosis. Solitary tumors are unusual. Twenty-five percent of schwannomas occur in the head (vestibular neurinoma) and in the neck. The lesions in the neck arise from the sheaths of the glossopharyngeal, accessory, and hypoglossal

nerves. The most frequent site of origin is the vagus nerve, and these lesions are known as parapharyngeal neurilemomas.

Schwannomas are firm to palpation, which usually causes fairly severe pain. Their size varies from several millimeters to 20 cm. They are solitary tumors that are mobile only in the horizontal plane when they arise from the vagus nerve. They grow slowly and only rarely cause neurologic deficits.

Definitive diagnosis is provided by histology of tissue removed at surgery, if necessary. The differential diagnosis includes paraganglioma, lymphoma, and metastases.

> **Note:** An amputation neuroma has to be excised in order to exclude persistent or recurrent tumor at the edge of the surgical field.

■ Malignant Tumors of the Cervical Lymph Nodes

In cervical lymph-node malignancies, a distinction needs to be made between lymphomas and metastatic tumors.

Malignant Lymphomas
The number of new cases of malignant lymphoma diagnosed each year is around 20 per 100,000 population. Currently, malignant lymphoma is the fifth most common malignant disease, after lung, breast, colon, and prostate cancer. Lymphomas are classified according to the World Health Organization (WHO) system, which applies to all tumors originating from lymphatic cells. All nodal and extranodal manifestations are included. The nodal subtypes, which include Hodgkin and non-Hodgkin lymphomas, appear as lymph-node tumors. Extranodal lymphomas, which include mucosa-associated lymphoid tissue (MALT) lymphomas, appear in the mucous membranes of the aerodigestive tracts and saliva glands, as well as in the internal organs (liver, spleen, lung, skeleton). **Table 8.5** presents a summary of the WHO classification of lymphomas.

Malignant lymphomas typical for the neck area are:
- Hodgkin disease.
- Non-Hodgkin lymphoma.

Clinical Features. The generalized symptoms are often not very typical and consist of fatigue and

Table 8.5 Summary of the World Health Organization lymphoma classification (2008)

B cell neoplasm

Precursor B cell neoplasm

Mature B cell neoplasm

Chronic lymphocytic leukemia

Plasma cell myeloma

Follicular lymphoma

Mantle cell lymphoma

Diffuse large B cell lymphoma

Mediastinal (thymic) large B cell lymphoma

Burkitt lymphoma

B cell proliferations of uncertain malignant potential

T cell neoplasm

Precursor T cell neoplasm

Precursor T lymphoblastic leukemia

Mature T cell and NK cell neuroplasms

Adult T cell leukemia/lymphoma (HTLV-1)

Extranodal NK cell/T cell lymphoma, nasal type

Mycosis fungoides

Peripheral T cell lymphoma, unspecified

Angioimmunoblastic T cell lymphoma

Anaplastic large cell lymphoma (ALCL)

T cell proliferations of uncertain malignant potential

HTLV-1, human T-lymphotropic virus 1; NK, natural killer.
From: World Health Organization (WHO); Swerdlow SH, Campo E, Harris NL, et al. *WHO classification of tumours of haematopoietic and lymphoid tissues,* 4th ed. Lyons: International Agency for Research on Cancer, 2008.

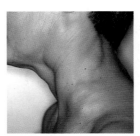

Fig. 8.19 Malignant lymphomas in the neck occur as groups of indolent, partly fixed but often mobile lymph nodes.

can lead to an incorrect diagnosis. The clinical course of the disease progresses in different stages.

Diagnosis. Histological examination is the only way to establish a diagnosis and identify the tumor subgroups by immunohistology.

Staging. The Ann Arbor staging classification is commonly used for the staging of lymphomas. This is the scheme established by the American Joint Committee on Cancer (AJCC) and International Union against Cancer (UICC). Originally developed for Hodgkin disease, this staging scheme was later expanded to include non-Hodgkin lymphoma (**Table 8.6**).

Treatment. Treatment options consist of chemotherapy and radiotherapy. The disease should be treated in a hematology–oncology center.

Lymph-Node Metastases

Apart from primary tumors of the lymphatic tissue (malignant lymphomas), lymph-node metastases represent the largest proportion of malignant cervical lymph-node diseases. Lymph-node metastases in the neck most frequently originate from squamous cell carcinoma of the mucous membranes of the upper respiratory tract and upper alimentary canal. In addition, rare metastases of other histological types can be found, as well as tumors from outside the head and neck area. A special form is cervical metastatic spread from an unknown primary tumor.

Lymphogenic spread of a squamous cell carcinoma requires invasive growth of a primary tumor, with penetration of tumor cells into the lymph vessels. These cells proceed into the next regional lymph node via drainage through afferent lymph vessels. Only a few tumor cells are able to evade the immune system and local influences. These usually

generalized pruritus. Weight loss, night sweats, and fever are of prognostic and therapeutic significance.

In most cases, the disease is initially localized, but then tends to metastasize. At the time of diagnosis, the cervical lymph nodes are affected in 70% (±10%) of patients. In ≈ 10% of patients, there is primary extranodal disease affecting the nasopharynx or oropharynx, gastrointestinal tract, skin, or skeleton. The affected lymph nodes are indolent, firm, usually mobile, and tend to occur in groups (**Fig. 8.19**). Pain is often noticed in these lymph nodes after consumption of alcohol. Spontaneous fluctuation in size is observed fairly commonly and

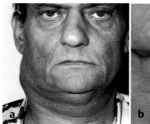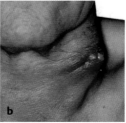

Fig. 8.20a, b   a Lymph-node metastases are solid, indolent, and fixed to the surrounding tissue.
b Exulceration of the metastases produces hemorrhagic secretion and often an inflamed reaction in the surrounding skin.

proliferate in the subcapsular sinus of the lymph node before proceeding to form a micrometastasis (<3 mm), but clinically obvious changes in the lymph node are not yet evident. With continued proliferation, a macrometastasis can develop, with extracapsular and extranodal expansion, as well as further lymphogenic or hematogenic spread (**Fig. 8.20a, b**).

The probability of lymphogenic spread of head and neck cancer correlates with its site and the various underlying densities of the lymph vessel network (**Fig. 8.21a–h**). This is why, for example, cancers of the nasopharynx and tonsils are associated with a higher incidence of metastatic disease than vocal cord and hypopharynx carcinomas (**Table 8.7**). The probability of metastatic spread is also influenced by the size and depth of invasion of the primary tumor, its histological differentiation (grades I–IV), evidence of tumor cells in lymphatic vessels (lymphangiosis carcinomatosa), and tumor invasion into the perineural sheath. Contralateral or bilateral cervical metastatic invasion are observed particularly with midline tumors (e.g., nasopharynx, tongue base, palate, postcricoid region) and in the presence of progressive tumor expansion.

The extent of lymphogenic spread is classified in accordance with the AJCC and UICC systems, using the TNM nomenclature. In addition to the T classification, which describes the extent of the primary tumor, and the M classification, which indicates either the absence or presence of distant metastases, there is also an N classification indicating the presence and extent of lymphogenic spread (**Table 8.8**).

A nomenclature and topography for lymph nodes in the head and neck region has been developed

Table 8.6   Clinical staging of lymphomas (Ann Arbor classification)

Stage	Definition
I	Involvement of a single lymph-node region (I) or of a single extralymphatic organ or site (I_E)
II	Involvement of two or more lymph-node regions on the same side of the diaphragm (II) or localized involvement of extralymphatic organ or site and of one or more lymph-node regions on the same side of the diaphragm (II_E).
III	Involvement of lymph-node regions on both sides of the diaphragm (III), which may also be accompanied by localized involvement of an extralymphatic organ or site (III_E) or by involvement of the spleen (III_S), or both (III_{SE})
IV	Diffuse or disseminated involvement of one or more extralymphatic organs or tissues, with or without associated lymph-node enlargement

Table 8.7   Frequency of metastases from squamous epithelial carcinomas in the head and neck region

Site of primary tumor	Rate of metastasis (%)	Bilateral metastasis (%)	Occult metastasis (%)
Nasopharynx	48–90	25–50	28–50
Mouth floor	30–65	8–12	10–31
Soft palate	30–68	30–32	22–30
Tongue	34–75	10–15	20–36
Tongue base	50–85	20–50	22–38
Tonsils	58–76	7–22	25–32
Piriform sinus	52–87	8–15	30–50
Supraglottic area	31–70	20–32	16–43
Glottic area	0.5–39	7–16	0.5–12

and subsequently modified several times following examinations of the cervicofacial spread of lymph-node metastases in relation to the site of the primary tumor and its surgical management. Six lymph-node regions, or levels, are distinguished in the neck dissection classification presented by Robbins et al. (2002) (**Table 8.9**). Amongst other aspects, this classification does not take into ac-

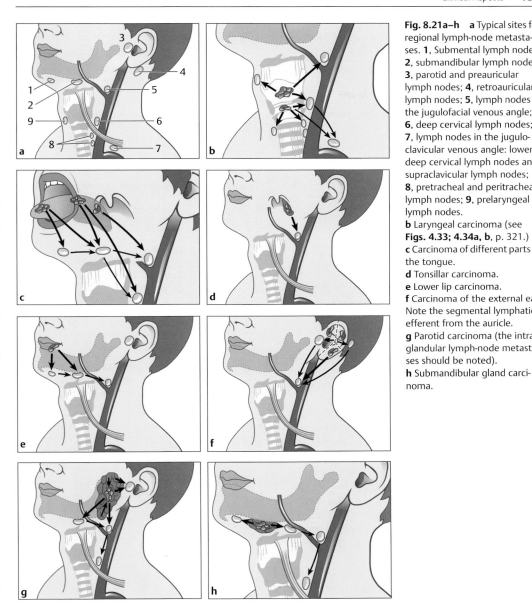

Fig. 8.21a–h **a** Typical sites for regional lymph-node metastases. **1**, Submental lymph nodes; **2**, submandibular lymph nodes; **3**, parotid and preauricular lymph nodes; **4**, retroauricular lymph nodes; **5**, lymph nodes in the jugulofacial venous angle; **6**, deep cervical lymph nodes; **7**, lymph nodes in the jugulo-clavicular venous angle: lower deep cervical lymph nodes and supraclavicular lymph nodes; **8**, pretracheal and peritracheal lymph nodes; **9**, prelaryngeal lymph nodes.
b Laryngeal carcinoma (see **Figs. 4.33; 4.34a, b**, p. 321.)
c Carcinoma of different parts of the tongue.
d Tonsillar carcinoma.
e Lower lip carcinoma.
f Carcinoma of the external ear. Note the segmental lymphatic efferent from the auricle.
g Parotid carcinoma (the intra-glandular lymph-node metastases should be noted).
h Submandibular gland carcinoma.

count retroauricular, preauricular, retropharyngeal, and occipital lymph nodes. The aim of this neck dissection classification is to classify the predominant routes of lymph drainage of the upper aerodigestive tract along relatively constant and predictable paths according to the corresponding topographical lymph-node group, although the drainage pathways may vary in individual cases (**Table 8.10**).

Note: The presence of lymph-node metastases reduces the 5-year survival rate considerably, and the presence of fixed metastases reduces the chance of survival markedly.

Table 8.8 N classification of regional lymph nodes (excluding nasopharynx and thyroid gland) of the head and neck region

NX	Regional lymph nodes cannot be assessed
N0	No regional lymph-node metastasis
N1	Metastasis in a single ipsilateral lymph node, 3 cm or less in largest dimension
N2a	Metastasis in a single ipsilateral lymph node, greater than 3 cm but no more than 6 cm in largest dimension
N2b	Metastases in multiple ipsilateral lymph nodes, none more than 6 cm in largest dimension
N2c	Metastases in bilateral or contralateral lymph nodes, none more than 6 cm in largest dimension
N3	Metastasis in a lymph node more than 6 cm in largest dimension

Table 8.9 Cervical lymph node classification

Level	Site	
IA	Submental LNs	Between the anterior bellies of the digastric muscle and the hyoid bone
IB	Submandibular LNs	Between anterior and posterior bellies of the digastric muscle and the body of the mandible
II	Upper jugular LNs	Between the suprahyoid muscles and posterior border of the sternocleidomastoid, from the skull base to the level of the hyoid bone
IIA		Anterior to CN XI
IIB		Posterior to CN XI
III	Middle jugular LNs	Between the infrahyoid muscles and posterior border of sternocleidomastoid, from the hyoid bone to the level of the cricoid
IV	Lower jugular LN group	Between the infrahyoid muscles and posterior border of sternocleidomastoid, from the level of the cricoid to the clavicle
V	LNs of the posterior triangle	Between posterior border of sternocleidomastoid and anterior border of the trapezius, from the skull base to the clavicle
VA		Superior to the level of the cricoid
VB		Inferior to the level of the cricoid
VI	LNs of the anterior compartment	Between the common carotid arteries, from the hyoid bone to the suprasternal notch

CN, cranial nerve; LN, lymph node.

Virchow's node can be seen or felt in the left supraclavicular fossa at the site of entry of the thoracic duct into the angle between the internal jugular vein and the subclavian vein.

The prescalene lymph nodes are found in the prescalene fat pad, which occupies the space bounded below by the subclavian vein, medially by the internal jugular vein, and laterally by the omohyoid muscle. The floor of the space is formed by the scalenus anticus muscle, with the phrenic nerve. The number of lymph nodes in the prescalene fat pad may vary from three to 30. Metastasis to the supraclavicular prescalene lymph nodes is a contraindication to surgery for abdominal, gynecologic, or thoracic malignancies.

The lymph fluid of the neck usually passes through three lymph node stations before it reaches the venous circulation.

Surgical methods for removing lymph-node metastases play an important part in the treatment of this area.

■ CUP Syndrome

The cancer of unknown primary (CUP) syndrome has a special place in the diagnosis and treatment of malignant diseases associated with cervical lymph-node metastases. It is defined as evidence of one or more histologically confirmed metastases of a malignant tumor, the site of which is uncertain despite intensive diagnostic work-up.

Lymph-node metastases most often manifest in the head and neck area. In 50–70% of cases, the primary tumor is also found in this region. In

Table 8.10 Preferred regional direction of metastatic spread, depending on the site of the primary tumor

Site of primary tumor		Lymphogenous path of metastases
Nasopharynx		II A/B, (III), V A/B, retro-pharyngeal lymph nodes
Oropharynx		II A/B, III, V A/B
Oral cavity		I A/B, II A/B, III
Nasal cavity		I B, II A/B
Lower lip		I A
Hypopharynx		II A/B, III, (IV, VI)
Larynx	Supraglottis	II A/B, III (VI)
	Glottis	II A/B, III(VI)
	Subglottis	III, IV
Parotid glands		II A/B
Submandibular glands		I B,
Thyroid gland		VI

20–30% of cases, a tumor is found outside the ear, nose, and throat area.

Even after intensive clinical examinations and the use of imaging techniques, the primary tumor is not detected in 3–9% of patients with lymph-node metastases in the neck area. Most often, these are cases of unknown squamous cell carcinomas; less often, they involve adenocarcinoma or undifferentiated carcinoma. Occult malignant melanomas are present in fewer than 10% of cases.

One hypothesis regarding the genesis of this condition is that the metastasis may have rapid growth, so that it becomes clinically evident before an undetected small primary tumor. It is also conceivable that there is a recurrence of a primary tumor, influenced by the local immune system. In the CUP syndrome, it appears possible that the lymphogenic or hematogenic stages are bypassed in certain cases, making it difficult to locate the primary tumor.

A diagnosis of CUP syndrome follows an extensive search for the primary tumor, including endoscopic examination of the upper respiratory and digestive tracts under anesthesia, as well as imaging techniques (cervical CT and MRI). Since most primary tumors of metastatic cervical squamous cell carcinoma are detected in the tonsils and on the base of the tongue, as well as on the pharynx and piriform sinus, diagnostic procedures include tonsillectomy, biopsy of the nasopharynx, and deep biopsy of the tongue base and hypopharynx. Depending on the histological findings, particularly in cases of deep cervical lymph-node metastases, the search for primaries should be extended to the area of the infraclavicular organs, and additional imaging techniques (e. g., CT, MRI of the chest and abdomen, PET) should be used if needed. A hidden bronchial carcinoma is detected in up to 30% of cases. Consultation with other medical specialists (pulmonologists, gastroenterologists, gynecologists, urologists, etc.) during the search for the tumor should be carefully considered. Basically, the scope of the diagnostic measures needed in searching for the primary tumor depends on the extent and prognosis of the tumor disease, as well as the patient's general health.

Therapy and prognosis. Treatment depends on the histological results and the site of the lymph-node metastases. If there is a suspicion of an occult squamous cell carcinoma, neck dissection is usually required, combined with radiotherapy. If a primary tumor is confirmed, radical surgery becomes necessary. A modified radical neck dissection is followed by radiotherapy, which includes the lymphatic drainage area of the affected region. The 5-year survival rate after surgery of this type and postoperative radiotherapy is, on average, around 50%, and over 60% when there is an upper cervical location and stage N1 or N2.

The presence of a cervical lymph-node metastasis from an adenocarcinoma always represents an advanced stage of disease, and treatment has to be individually tailored to meet the patient's needs. With upper cervical metastases, a neck dissection and postoperative radiotherapy may be considered. With a deep cervical location, only palliative therapy is usually possible. The 5-year survival rate ranges from 0% to 28%.

Cervical lymph-node metastases from an occult malignant melanoma should be treated with a modified radical neck dissection.

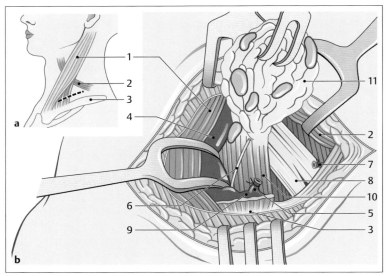

Fig. 8.22a, b Prescalene lymph-node biopsy.
a The incision and limits of dissection: border of the clavicle, omohyoid muscle, and jugulosubclavian venous angle covered by the sternocleidomastoid muscle.
b The intraoperative appearance. **1**, Sternocleidomastoid muscle; **2**, inferior belly of the omohyoid muscle; **3**, clavicle; **4**, internal jugular vein; **5**, subclavian vein; **6**, phrenic nerve ; **7**, transverse cervical artery, divided; **8**, brachial plexus; **9**, jugulosubclavian venous angle; **10**, scalene muscles; **11**, prescalene fat pad with lymph nodes.

■ Principles of Surgery

■ Prescalene Node Biopsy

The lymph nodes lying in the prescalene fatty tissue, anterior to the scalenus anterior muscle and in the omoclavicular triangle, are of considerable clinical and diagnostic importance even if they are not palpable. Because of the central position of these lymph nodes in the lymphatic system as a whole, histological examination of them provides early information about the extent of malignant and inflammatory diseases. Numerically, the highest proportion of positive results, ≈ 80 %, is achieved with biopsy of these lymph nodes in sarcoidosis. Epithelioid cell foci of sarcoid found in the scalene muscles are able to differentiate the lesion from tuberculosis.

Technique (Fig. 8.22a, b). The operation can be performed with the patient under local anesthesia. A horizontal incision, 3–4 cm long, is made above the clavicle. After the platysma has been divided, the posterior border of the sternocleidomastoid muscle is retracted medially, and the inferior belly of the omohyoid muscle is retracted laterally and superiorly. The surgical field is the prescalene omoclavicular triangle, lying between the internal jugular vein, the subclavian vein, and the omohyoid muscle.

The prescalene fat pad is excised, preserving the phrenic nerve and the contents of the carotid sheath, and the eight to 15 lymph nodes are excised. This simplifies histological examination of the nodes.

■ Mediastinoscopy

Mediastinoscopy, especially if combined with prescalene biopsy, is an important complement to modern imaging procedures for diagnosis of lymphadenopathy of the intrathoracic, and especially mediastinal, lymph nodes. The entire upper and paratracheal part of the superior mediastinum can be examined as far as the origin of both superior lobar bronchi. Occasionally, thymomas, teratomas, intrathoracic goiters, pneumoconioses, and even the pericardium lying beyond the bifurcation can be visualized when a search is being made for cysts. Particularly valuable, however, is the ability to take biopsies from the paratracheal, tracheobronchial, and bronchopulmonary lymph nodes.

This procedure is indicated firstly in order to establish a histological diagnosis of metastatic carcinoma, Hodgkin's and non-Hodgkin's lymphoma, or sarcoid and tuberculous lymphadenopathy; and secondly, to assess operability in patients with bronchial and esophageal carcinoma.

Technique (Fig. 8.23). Intubation anesthesia is necessary. A 4-cm horizontal skin incision is made 2 cm above the suprasternal notch. The trachea is exposed as in tracheotomy, with care being taken to identify and divide the pretracheal fascia horizontally.

The mediastinoscope is inserted into a pocket created by finger dissection under the pretracheal fascia and is directed inferiorly along the anterior tracheal wall as far as the carina. Needle aspiration must be performed before a biopsy is taken, in order to avoid serious hemorrhage which may require thoracotomy, although this is uncommon. Further uncommon complications include recurrent nerve paralysis and pneumothorax.

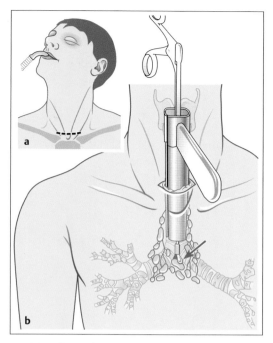

Fig. 8.23a, b   Mediastinoscopy.
a Skin incision.
b Mediastinoscope with biopsy forceps (arrow).

■ **Neck Dissection**

The preferred treatment for an operable tumor with evidence of lymph-node metastases is complete tumor removal, including unilateral or bilateral removal of cervical lymph nodes (neck dissection), followed by radiotherapy. Alternatively, it is possible to treat the patient with radiotherapy alone or with combined and chemoradiotherapy.

Surgical treatment of the cervical lymphatic drainage paths is fundamental in head and neck malignancies. A clinically inconspicuous cervical lymph node, known as N0 neck, is an exception and there is disagreement here with regard to the indication for surgery. When treatment of N0 neck is being planned, tumor-specific parameters (histology, site, and extent) should be considered, as well as patient-specific factors (age, general health, compliance). Further clinical examinations have to be carried out in order to determine whether to use a "wait-and-see" strategy, while following the course of the disease closely, or to perform elective removal of the neck lymph nodes—given the fact that, on average, 30 % of patients have occult metastases.

The principle of neck dissection consists of systematic unilateral or bilateral excision of the fatty and connective tissues containing the lymph nodes between the superficial and deep cervical fascia. It may also be necessary to include further anatomical structures, with the goal of removing occult and solid lymph-node metastases (**Fig. 8.24a, b**).

In order to establish a standard terminology, the Committee for Head and Neck Surgery of the American Academy of Otolaryngology–Head and Neck Surgery (AAO-HNS) published a classification system for neck dissections in 1991 (most recently revised in 2008):

- *Radical neck dissection:* The standard, classic procedure for clearing neck lymph nodes at levels I–V from the base of the skull to the clavicle. For radical results, the following are removed simultaneously: sternocleidomastoid muscle, internal jugular vein, accessory nerve, and submandibular gland.
- *Extended radical neck dissection:* Additional lymph-node groups are removed (e. g., levels VI, occipital lymph nodes) and/or nonlymphatic structures (e. g., carotid artery, hypoglossal and vagus nerves).
- *Modified radical neck dissection:* This form of neck dissection, once described as functional, includes clearing of levels I–V while preserving one or more nonlymphatic structures such as the accessory nerve and internal jugular vein. While bearing in mind the oncological necessity for radical surgery, the preservation of nonlymphatic structures can lead to a substantial reduction in morbidity.

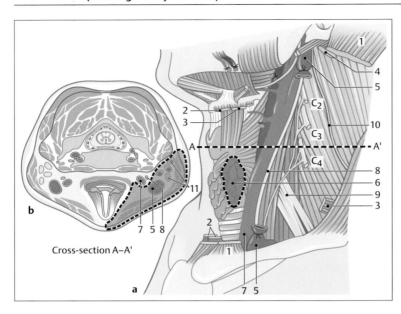

Fig. 8.24a, b The appearance after modified radical neck dissection.
a The situation after removal of: **1**, sternocleidomastoid muscle; **2**, infrahyoid muscles; **3**, omohyoid muscle, divided; **4**, digastric muscle and stylohyoid muscle, divided; **5**, stumps of the internal jugular vein; **6**, partial resection of the thyroid gland. The following are retained: **7**, carotid artery (the *external* carotid artery may need to be resected, depending on the extent of the tumor); **8**, vagus nerve; **9**, brachial plexus; **10**, accessory nerve (this should be preserved if the accessory chain of nodes is not affected).
b The equivalent cross-section through the neck (**A–A'**). The resected area between the deep and superficial cervical fascia is shown in the gray area. **11**, Cervical lymph-node metastases. C2, C3, C4, roots of cervical spinal nerves C2–C4.

- *Selective neck dissection:* One or more levels of the six lymph-node regions and nonlymphatic structures are preserved. When documenting the operation, the removed levels are placed in parenthesis—e. g., "selective neck dissection (II–IV)." This form of neck dissection is practiced especially by advocates of elective neck dissection for N0 neck. Depending on the site of the primary tumor, the appropriate lymph drainage is cleared to include clinically occult metastases and simultaneously reduce surgery-related morbidity.

The classification also mentions that, during all forms of neck dissection, clearing of level I includes removal of the submandibular gland.

Note: A prerequisite for all forms of neck dissection is operability of the primary tumor as well as an absence of distant metastases. Examination of the patient and the clinical history should of course be undertaken, with full consideration of the surgical procedure and the anesthesia required.

Prognosis. Generally, histological evidence of lymph-node metastases leads to a poorer prognosis. In the presence of lymph-node metastases, the prognosis depends on the following:
- The site of the lymph-node metastases: adverse factors for the prognosis are lymph-node metastases in the posterior, supraclavicular, and retropharyngeal and occipital areas.
- The number of lymph-node metastases: more than two lymph-node metastases appear to be adverse for the prognosis.
- The capsule structure of the lymph nodes: the extent of extracapsular carcinoma is one of the most important criteria for prognosis. Extracapsular carcinoma increases the risk of remote metastases by a factor of three (ca. 20 %).

Note: Isolated removal of lymph-node metastases is contraindicated, as this does not deal with the cervical metastatic pathways, and the danger of retrograde, irregular, and contralateral metastases therefore increases.

▪ Thyroid Gland and Otorhinolaryngology

▪ Topographic Anatomy

The normal thyroid gland covers the lower lateral part of the thyroid cartilage on both sides. Its isthmus lies over the cricoid cartilage and the upper tracheal rings. The lobes grasp the upper cervical trachea and the thyroid cartilage to a varying extent (**Fig. 8.25**). Fibrous connections from the gland to the cricoid and thyroid cartilage and to the upper tracheal ring explain the mobility of the thyroid gland, which accompanies all movements of the larynx, particularly on swallowing. A thyroid gland of normal size is not visible externally.

A pyramidal process is often present as a remnant of the thyroglossal duct, leading from the isthmus to the hyoid bone. The terms superior, middle, and inferior in relation to tracheotomy refer to the relationship between the thyroid isthmus and the tracheotomy opening (see **Fig. 6.12a**).

Note: Ear, nose, and throat symptoms caused by thyroid gland disease may or may not be accompanied by a visible enlargement of the gland. Macroscopic findings do not reflect the function of the thyroid gland, although functional disorders often accompany the development of goiter.

The superior thyroid artery arises from the external carotid artery, and arches inferiorly to penetrate the upper pole of the gland. Shortly after its origin from the external carotid artery, the superior thyroid artery lies in fairly close relation at the level of this curve to the external branch of the superior laryngeal nerve (**Fig. 8.26**).

The inferior thyroid arteries arise from the thyrocervical trunk, curve medially at the level of the sixth cervical vertebra, and reach the lower pole of the thyroid gland after dividing into two, and occasionally more, branches. The recurrent laryngeal nerves run on both sides, close to the inferior thyroid artery or its branches in the region of the lower pole of the thyroid gland. More than 25 anatomic variations of the relationship between the nerve and the artery have been described. However, the recurrent nerve runs *anterior to* the artery in 25 % of patients, *posterior to* the artery in 35 %, and *between* the branches of the artery in 35 %.

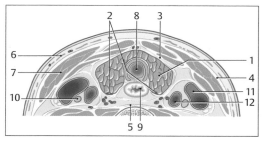

Fig. 8.25 The topography of the thyroid gland, showing a horizontal cross-section at the level of the first cervical thoracic spine. The thyroid gland covers the trachea and borders posteriorly on the neurovascular bundle. There is an internal capsule enclosing the thyroid and parathyroid glands, which is used as a surgical capsule. **1**, Thyroid gland; **2**, parathyroid glands; **3**, thyroid capsule (external capsule); **4**, external cervical fascia (lamina superficialis); **5**, deep cervical fascia (lamina pretrachealis); **6**, platysma; **7**, sternocleidomastoid muscle; **8**, trachea; **9**, esophagus; **10**, vagus nerve; **11**, internal jugular vein; **12**, carotid artery.

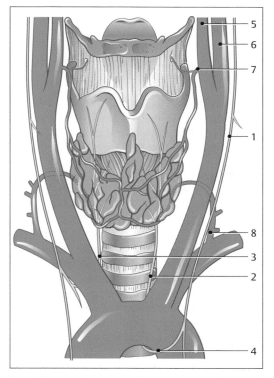

Fig. 8.26 Blood supply and innervation of the thyroid gland. **1**, Vagus nerve; **2**, continuation of the left recurrent laryngeal nerve; **3**, right recurrent laryngeal nerve; **4**, left recurrent laryngeal nerve; **5**, external carotid artery; **6**, internal carotid artery, **7**, superior thyroid artery; **8**, thyrocervical trunk with inferior thyroid artery.

Familiarity with the relative positions of the artery and nerve is absolutely necessary in order to avoid unilateral or bilateral vocal cord paralysis during operations on the thyroid gland.

Function. The thyroid gland produces two hormones—thyroxine, T_4, and triiodothyronine, T_3—in which iodine is bound to the amino acid tyrosine. The hormone is bound mainly in follicular colloid and is stored as thyroglobulin. Hormone reserves are sufficient to last ≈ 2 months. This compensates for changes in iodine intake and changing biological requirements. Hormone secretion is activated by proteolytic enzymes of thyroid-stimulating hormone (TSH) and thyrotropin-releasing hormone (TRH).

The main functions of the thyroid gland are the regulation of metabolism, control of oxygen consumption, and regulation of heat, body growth, and mental development.

■ **Diagnostic Procedures in Thyroid Disorders**

History and general examination. Questioning is directed especially to symptoms of:
- *Thyrotoxicosis* (nervousness, inability to sleep, sweating, loss of weight, and palpitations).
- *Hypothyroidism* (apathy, sensitivity to cold, somnolence, and weight gain).

Physical diagnosis
- Palpation, inspection, measurement of the circumference of the neck, auscultation.
- Laryngoscopy to control recurrent nerve paralysis.
- Tracheobronchoscopy, if tumor or tracheomalacia is suspected.
- CT or MRI.
- Technetium 99 or isotope scans.

Functional diagnosis. The main screening tests are assessment of T_4 and the free T_4 index, T_3, and the TSH response to TRH administration. The TRH test is particularly useful for confirming or excluding a functional disorder. The radioiodine test is still irreplaceable for certain indications, not least to demonstrate ectopic thyroid tissue.

Serologic tests. Antibodies against thyroglobulin or microsomes are useful in cases of thyroiditis.

Histologic or cytologic diagnosis. This is mandatory in cases of cold or hot nodules, or expansive and destructive tissue growth.

■ **Specific Conditions**

Goiter
The term "goiter" has long been associated with the endemic type of thyroid disease that occurs in regions with low-iodine soils. Enlargement of the thyroid gland may be diffuse or nodular. It is due to the increase in tissue caused by an increase of thyrocytes, adenomas, or degenerative changes with cyst formation. Other causes of goiter include malignancy and infection.

Large retrosternal goiters can cause considerable compression and displacement of the trachea or esophagus and can thus affect breathing and swallowing. Pressure on the recurrent laryngeal nerve may affect vocal cord function.

The WHO classification is as follows. In grade I goiter, the gland is palpable but not visible; in grade II, the gland is palpable and visible; in grade III, the gland is clearly visible at a considerable distance with the neck free of clothing. These grades can be subdivided into (a) adenomatous or (b) diffuse.

Ectopic thyroid tissue is most often found in the region of the foramen cecum at the base of the tongue, the lingual thyroid, and rarely in the neck and mediastinum.

During the embryonic period, thyroid tissue may grow into the trachea or larynx and cause dyspnea in the postnatal period or in later life. Dyspnea can occur in women during menstruation, as the result of an endotracheal goiter.

Hypothyroidism
- *Primary hypothyroidism* is spontaneous and is due to loss of the thyroid after total or subtotal resection without subsequent hormonal replacement, congenital hypoplasia or aplasia, ectopic thyroid in children, or disordered synthesis of thyroid hormone.
- *Secondary hypothyroidism* is caused by absent TSH stimulation from the pituitary.

Clinical Features. General symptoms include mental motor inactivity, increased need for sleep, dry scaly skin, and myxedema.

Specific ear, nose, and throat symptoms include a rough voice, hoarseness, a deep, monotonous voice, and slow speech with a nasal twang. Symptoms also include difficulty in swallowing and globus sensation, particularly in the presence of goiter. Deafness and dizziness may occur in prolonged hypothyroidism.

Hypothyroidism is the most common endocrine disorder in children after diabetes mellitus. In addition to aplasia and ectopia, *Pendred syndrome* should be mentioned. The condition includes sensorineural deafness combined with disorders of iodine metabolism leading to the formation of a goiter.

Diagnosis. The literature on nuclear medicine should be consulted. Otologic diagnosis includes pediatric audiology, auditory brainstem response (ABR) testing (see p. **38**), and vestibular tests.

Treatment. This consists of hormone substitution in cooperation with a pediatrician, an endocrinologist, and an expert in nuclear medicine. The management of deafness is described on pages 108–111.

Hyperthyroidism

Generalized symptoms. These include loss of weight, tremor in the fingers, fluttering of the eyelids, tremor of the tongue, attacks of sweating, and sleeplessness. the *Merseburger triad* (goiter, tachycardia, and exophthalmos) consists of classic symptoms of primary thyrotoxicosis. However, thyrotoxicosis demonstrating only one of these symptoms or mild symptoms is more common.

Endocrine orbitopathy with exophthalmos, conjunctivitis, swelling of the lids, chemosis, periocular edema, and oculomotor paralysis can occur on one or both sides and is most often accompanied by thyrotoxicosis. However, exophthalmos also occurs without evidence of abnormal thyroid gland function.

> **Note:** Infections or tumors of the nose and sinuses have to be excluded using special investigations. Orbital abscess or phlegmon, mucopyocele, and malignancy of the base of the skull, for example, may cause proptosis.

Pathogenesis. Endocrine orbitopathy is caused by increased volume in the retrobulbar tissues, probably stimulated by immunologic processes or by abnormal levels of thyrotropic hormone.

Diagnosis. This is based on palpation of a diffuse or nodular goiter, scans, radioiodine studies, serum tests with hormone determination, and a TRH test. Orbitopathy is investigated using computed tomography.

Treatment. Thyroidectomy is performed after medical therapy or radioactive iodine is given. Malignant exophthalmos leads to blindness if untreated. In addition to specific treatment of the thyroid disorder and medical treatment of exophthalmos with cortisone, transnasal endoscopic decompression of the orbit may also be necessary.

Thyroiditis

Definition. The different types of thyroiditis are similar only in relation to the histological findings; the etiology is very different and ranges from infectious to autoimmune causes (**Table 8.11**). Subacute thyroiditis and the acute type in particular are very rare. Subacute disease is found mainly in females.

Etiology. Chronic lymphocytic thyroiditis (Hashimoto thyroiditis) is due to an autoimmune process in which a reaction of lymphocytes and antibodies against thyroid tissue is observed. Lymphocytic and plasma cell infiltrations into thyroid tissue can be detected histologically. The *subacute* type is characterized by a granulomatous inflammation accompanied by giant cells, mainly 10–14 days after a virus infection. The *acute* type is mainly a bacterial inflammation, caused by a purulent infection in the surrounding tissues (e.g., abscess in the tongue base). Other rare causes of thyroiditis are autoimmune inflammatory reactions postpartum, which mostly heal spontaneously. During oncologic therapy with cytokines (tumor necrosis factor-α, interferon, interleukin-1, interleukin-2), a slight thyroiditis may occur, which disappears after the end of treatment.

Clinical Features. In *acute* thyroiditis:
- Acute onset with fever.
- Redness of the skin.
- Tenderness and pain.
- Abscess formation possible.

Table 8.11 Inflammation of the thyroid gland

	Acute thyroiditis	Subacute thyroiditis		Chronic thyroiditis
		Giant cell thyroiditis	Hashimoto thyroiditis (chronic lymphocytic thyroiditis)	Riedel thyroiditis (chronic fibrous thyroiditis)
Symptoms	Swelling, pain, redness of overlying skin, fever	Fever, pain, long-term course	Relatively few symptoms, myxedema after years	Hard, often asymmetrical thyroid swelling; infiltration of surrounding tissue with compression of trachea and esophagus
Pathogenesis	Viral infection (such as influenza), bacterial infection (such as typhus, paratyphoid), or by extension of cervical bacterial infection	Paramyxovirus infection, genetic predisposition (HLA-B35)	Autoimmune disease, familial occurrence indicates genetic factors	Arteritis of the thyroid gland and the periglandular tissue followed by sclerosing and fibrosing processes
Diagnosis	Ultrasound (B-mode), CT scan	Palpation, ultrasound, serology	Immunological evidence of microsomal antibodies	Biopsy shows severe inflammatory infiltrate, especially in the periglandular tissue
Treatment	Antibiotics, steroids, thyroid hormones, incision and drainage if abscess develops	Nonsteroidal anti-inflammatory drugs, corticosteroids in severe cases	Medical treatment with thyroid hormones and steroids; thyroidectomy may be necessary for large goiters	Hemithyroidectomy (to reduce the compression syndrome)

CT, computed tomography.

In *subacute* thyroiditis:
• Prolonged course, with a 14-day delay after virus infection.
• Hard, tough swelling.
• Pain in the thyroid region.
• Odynophagia.
• Fatigue, lack of appetite, loss of weight.
• Nervousness.
• Caloric intolerance.
• Tachycardia.

In *chronic lymphocytic thyroiditis* (Hashimoto thyroiditis), a distinction is made between a classic type with struma and an atrophic type without struma. Hyperthyroidism can occur temporarily. Usually, there are only slight symptoms:
• Struma.
• Pain and tenderness in the thyroid region.
• Symptoms of hypothyroidism may be followed by hyperthyroid symptoms at times.

Riedel struma (Riedel thyroiditis), which is very hard, is probably a rare type of Hashimoto thyroiditis. The inflammation proceeds with fibrotic tissue changes.

Diagnosis. *Laboratory tests:*
• Differential blood tests and C-reactive protein (CRP) show signs of inflammation.
• Thyroid hormone tests show hyperthyroidism at times in patients with chronic thyroiditis. Hashimoto thyroiditis mainly causes hypothyroidism.
• Antibodies against thyroid peroxidases and antibodies against thyroglobulin are raised.

Ultrasound: This is used to assess the volume and echo characteristics. Inflammations show a typical tiger skin–like appearance.

Scintigraphy: There are no specific changes in activity in cases of thyroiditis.

Fine-needle biopsy: This is used to differentiate tumors. Giant cells, lymphocytes and plasma cells are typical cytologic results in thyroiditis.

Treatment. *Acute purulent thyroiditis*: Antibiotics, puncture or drainage of abscess, antirheumatic drugs, local treatment with cooling.

Subacute thyroiditis (De Quervain thyroiditis): In mild cases, only antirheumatic drugs or salicylic acid are necessary; in severe or unclear cases, treatment with steroids can be attempted. The pain should resolve within 5 days. In hyperthyroid phases, β-blockers are helpful as thyrostatic drugs are not effective.

Chronic lymphocytic thyroiditis (Hashimoto thyroiditis): For hypothyroidism, hormone substitution is necessary; in phases of hyperthyroidism, treatment with thyrostatics should be administered.

Thyroid Malignancy

This type of tumor represents 0.5 % of all malignant tumors. Women are affected almost twice as often as men. Cold nodules on radioiodine testing, demonstrated by scanning, are potentially malignant. The term "hot nodule" indicates an autonomous adenoma with a relatively slight tendency to undergo malignant degeneration. Thyroid malignancies are categorized into three types: differentiated, anaplastic carcinomas, and rare types (**Table 8.12**).

- *Differentiated thyroid tumors* include follicular and papillary carcinoma. Follicular thyroid carcinomas tend to rupture the capsule, invade vessels, and produce hematogenous metastases.
  - *Papillary thyroid carcinoma* is the most frequent malignant thyroid tumor. It produces lymphatic metastases in the neck. Regional cervical lymph-node metastases are often the first symptoms of a primary tumor of the thyroid gland, particularly if the tumor is small.
  - In regions in which goiter was formerly endemic, *follicular carcinoma* is the predominant tumor.
- *Anaplastic (undifferentiated) carcinomas* spread rapidly to neighboring organs and metastasize through blood and lymphatic pathways (**Table 8.13**).

Table 8.12 Main types of thyroid carcinoma

Papillary adenocarcinoma
Peak between age 20 and 45 years and after age 60 years
Late development of metastases
Partly cystic, or with shadows on ultrasound

Follicular adenocarcinoma
Solid tumor with fibrotic capsule
Often in goiter-endemic areas
Prognosis good

Anaplastic or non-differentiated thyroid carcinoma
5–10 % of all thyroid carcinomas
High-grade malignancy
Tendency for diffuse growth
Poor prognosis

Medullar thyroid carcinoma (C cell carcinoma)
5–10 % of all thyroid carcinomas
Develops from parafollicular C cells
Early hematogenic and lymphogenic metastases
Tendency for rapid growth

- The *rare types* include medullary carcinoma. This tumor arises from the C cells (the parafollicular cells, which form calcitonin) and not from thyroid cells themselves. The presence of amyloid is one of the histologic characteristics in this type of lesion. Medullary carcinomas usually grow slowly and do not store iodine.

Clinical Features. In contrast to undifferentiated thyroid carcinomas, other malignant tumors of the thyroid glands usually grow slowly. They are often unilateral and present as one or more firm nodules. Occasionally, the primary tumor is too small to be noticed, and the diagnosis is first made on the presence of metastases. Thyroid function, as demonstrated by the peripheral level of hormones, is not affected in the initial stages of the disease. When the thyroid gland has ruptured, its mobility on swallowing is reduced due to infiltration of the surrounding tissues. Globus symptoms, otalgia, or recurrent nerve paralysis may occur.

Table 8.13 N classification of regional lymph nodes in thyroid gland carcinoma

NX	Regional lymph nodes cannot be assessed
N0	No regional lymph-node metastasis
N1	Regional lymph-node metastasis
N1a	Metastasis in level VI (pretracheal and paratracheal, including prelaryngeal and midline prelaryngeal nodes adjacent to the thyroid gland)
N1b	Metastasis in other unilateral, bilateral, or contralateral cervical or upper/superior mediastinal lymph nodes

Pathogenesis. A hereditary disposition appears likely. The medullary carcinoma may be part of an autosomal-dominant syndrome. In carcinomas arising from thyrocytes, there appears to be a correlation with increased TSH stimulation due to iodine deficiency. Thyroid tumors thus often develop from a long-standing goiter. An increased incidence is also observed in recurrent goiter after previous surgery and in advanced Hashimoto disease.

Diagnosis. A needle biopsy or open biopsy is performed if the disease is suspected on the basis of palpation or a scan, particularly if a cold nodule is found. Tumor markers are very important for both diagnosis and follow-up. In medullary carcinoma, there is an increased level of calcitonin, whereas an increased level of serum thyroglobulin is found in both follicular and papillary carcinomas.

Treatment. With the exception of papillary microcarcinomas staged as pT1 N0 M0, the standard therapy for thyroid carcinoma is complete thyroidectomy followed by radioablation and subsequent hormone replacement. Thyroidectomy is performed with preservation of the recurrent nerve and of at least one parathyroid gland. Depending on the primary tumor, unilateral or bilateral selective neck dissection (see p. 405) is indicated particularly for papillary carcinoma. Typical procedural controls include B-mode ultrasound, a full-body scan (with iodine 131), and thyroglobulin detection in serum.

9 Salivary Glands

There are three paired major salivary glands (**Fig. 9.1**):

- Parotid gland.
- Submandibular gland.
- Sublingual gland.

In addition, there are 700–1000 separate minor salivary glands, occurring mainly in the oral and pharyngeal mucosa (**Fig. 9.2**).

Embryology, Structure, and Congenital Anomalies

The major salivary glands arise from solid aggregations of ectodermal cells in the foregut between the fourth and eighth weeks of embryonic development. Thickening of the surrounding mesenchyme encapsulates the developing gland and also includes lymph-node primordia. The ducts become patent in the 22nd week. **Figure 9.3** shows the cellular architecture of the secretory apparatus and drainage system of the salivary glands.

Aplasia of one or more glands may occur, but complete absence of all the major glands is extremely rare.

Diverticula and ectasia of the parotid duct system may predispose to parotitis.

Aberrant salivary gland tissue may be found in the cervical lymph nodes, the middle ear, and the mandible.

Accessory glands are appendages of the major glands, most commonly the parotid; they possess efferent ducts and have functional capabilities.

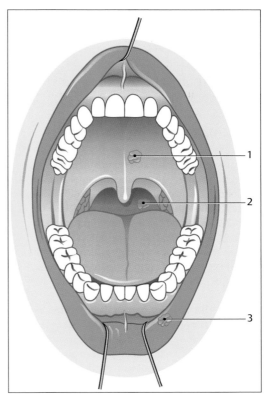

Fig. 9.2 The minor salivary glands. **1**, Palatine glands; **2**, Apharyngeal glands; **3**, labial glands.

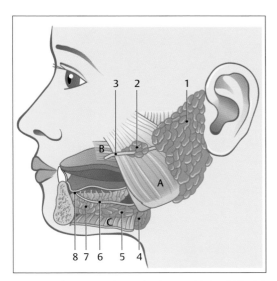

Fig. 9.1 The major salivary glands. Parotid gland (**1**) with small accessory gland (**2**) and Stensen duct (**3**). Submandibular gland (**4**) with uncinate process (**5**) and submandibular (Wharton) duct (**6**). Sublingual gland (**7**) with sublingual caruncle (**8**). **A**, masseter muscle; **B**, buccinator muscle; **C**, mylohyoid muscle.

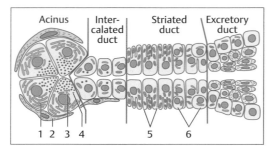

Fig. 9.3 Structure of the salivary glands. **1**, Endoplasmic reticulum; **2**, myoepithelial cell; **3**, Golgi apparatus; **4**, secretory granules; **5**, basal invaginations and mitochondria; **6**, basal cells.

The theory that the parotid gland consists of two lobes located lateral and medial to the facial nerve, connected by an isthmus, has been rejected as incorrect, although the terms "superficial parotidectomy" and "total parotidectomy" are still used (see **Fig. 9.28**).

Anatomy and Physiology of the Major and Minor Salivary Glands

■ Parotid Gland

The largest of the salivary glands lies in the retromandibular fossa, in a subcutaneous pocket surrounded by a capsule of compressed connective tissue. This pseudocapsule is very thick, especially laterally, and is the cause of tension pain in parotid swelling. Inferiorly, there are defects in this connective-tissue mantle through which infections and tumors can penetrate into the pterygopalatine fossa or parapharyngeal space.

Borders. The superior part of the parotid glands is limited anteriorly by the anterior border of the ascending ramus of the mandible, posteriorly by the external acoustic meatus, and above by the zygomatic arch. The inferior portion of the gland is the cervical portion, which lies between the angle of the jaw and mastoid process. The gland is bounded inferiorly by the anterior margin of the sternocleidomastoid muscle and the posterior belly of the digastric muscle.

Clinical significance. Pleomorphic adenomas arising in the cervical part of the gland may form a dumbbell tumor extending into the oropharynx, with only a relatively small external tumor.

The *parotid duct* (Stensen duct) is ≈6 cm long. It leaves the anterior border of the gland, crosses the masseter muscle, and perforates the buccinator muscle and the buccal mucosa. The edges of its orifice are slightly elevated and are red and swollen in inflammation. The orifice lies opposite the second upper molar tooth. The *facial nerve* leaves the base of the skull through the stylomastoid foramen and enters the gland parenchyma as a short trunk 0.7–1.5 cm long. It divides into two or three main branches and then divides again peripherally into the terminal temporal, frontal, zygomatic buccal, and cervical branches. The zygomatic and buccal branches have numerous anastomoses with each other. The forehead branch and the marginal mandibular branch for the lower lip usually have no anastomoses with neighboring branches (see **Fig. 1.114**).

The facial nerve supplies all of the mimetic muscles and the platysma. Medial to the nerve, the pes anserinus major, lie the branches of the external carotid artery—the transverse facial, maxillary, and retroauricular arteries, which supply the parotid gland. Venous drainage is via the internal jugular vein.

> **Note:** The safest point from which to find the facial nerve in conservative parotidectomy—as performed for pleomorphic adenoma, for example—is its trunk (see **Fig. 9.28**).

Lymph drainage. There are several intraglandular and periglandular lymph nodes from which the lymph drains via the submandibular nodes or directly into the upper deep cervical nodes. The first regional lymph-node station for the parotid lies inside the gland—a fact that has major clinical significance in oncology patients.

Autonomic control of salivary secretion. The *preganglionic* fibers originate in the inferior salivatory nucleus. They follow the glossopharyngeal nerve to the jugular foramen, leave that nerve at the inferior ganglion, and then join the tympanic nerve to form the tympanic plexus of the middle ear, from which the lesser superficial petrosal nerve arises. The fibers finally reach the otic ganglion, in which they synapse.

The *postganglionic* parasympathetic fibers run from there with the auriculotemporal nerve to the parotid gland.

The *sympathetic* fibers arise from the carotid plexus and regulate the circulation of the gland by vasoconstriction. They have less effect on salivary production.

■ Submandibular Gland

The submandibular gland is embedded in the submandibular triangle. It is bordered anteriorly by the digastric muscle, posteriorly by the stylomandibular ligament, and superiorly by the mandible.

The main part of the gland lies inferior to the mylohyoid muscle and is covered by the external cervical fascia.

The *submandibular duct* (Wharton duct) is ≈ 5 cm long, runs forward beneath the mucosa of the floor of the mouth, and opens close to the frenulum in the sublingual caruncle *in the floor of the mouth.*

Clinical significance. Infection can spread along the U-shaped body of the gland into the posterior part of the floor of the mouth, causing a phlegmon or abscess in the floor of the mouth.

The duct crosses posterolaterally over the lingual nerve. If the duct is slit over a probe (e. g., for acute obstruction due to a sialolith), the nerve is not in danger. The very thin marginal mandibular branch of the facial nerve running between the upper pole of the gland and the mandible is vulnerable during surgery on the submandibular gland. Injury to the lingual or hypoglossal nerves during removal of the gland for sialolithiasis or benign tumors is avoided by exposing the nerves.

Autonomic supply. The gland receives its autonomic supply from the lingual nerve through preganglionic *parasympathetic fibers* that reach it via the chorda tympani and synapse in the submandibular ganglion to give off postganglionic fibers.

Sympathetic fibers from the superior cervical ganglion control the blood supply.

■ Sublingual Gland

The smallest of the major salivary glands lies beneath the mucosa of the oral floor, its posterior part touching the anterior end of the submandibular gland. Its duct system usually unites with that of

the submandibular gland, and its innervation is the same as that of the submandibular gland.

Clinical significance. A *ranula* is a retention cyst caused by obliteration of one of the smaller openings of the sublingual gland; the principal opening is unaffected. Depending on its size, a ranula can cause difficulty in swallowing and speaking, due to interference with the mobility of the tongue. Treatment consists of surgical removal or epithelial drainage by marsupialization of the ranula.

■ Minor Salivary Glands

These glands are scattered throughout the oropharyngeal, nasal, sinus, laryngeal, and tracheal mucosa. There are also collections on the inner surface of the lip, in the buccal mucosa, and in the palate. The minor salivary glands produce only 5–8 % of the entire volume of saliva, but despite that they ensure satisfactory moistening of the mucosa if one or more of the major salivary glands fails to function. Severe xerostomia may occur if their secretory function is suppressed due to radiotherapy or other causes.

Clinical significance. Tumors of the minor salivary glands are often malignant (adenoid cystic carcinoma, acinar cell tumor). Benign tumors (e. g., pleomorphic adenoma) occur less frequently.

Formation and Function of Saliva

Physical, chemical, and mental factors stimulate the production of saliva. The amount produced in a day ranges from 1000 to 1500 mL, and 99.5 % of it is water. The rest consists of inorganic, organic, and cellular material. The individual salivary glands make a variable contribution to the quantity and quality of the total output (**Table 9.1**).

The secretion is formed in two steps. The primary secretion is formed in the acini and is then partially resorbed and modified during passage through the duct system, in a manner somewhat analogous to urine production by the kidneys.

Physiologic functions of the saliva
- Saliva has a protective effect on the mucosa of the mouth and upper respiratory tract, through mechanical cleansing and an immunologic

Table 9.1 The composition and quality of saliva in unstimulated conditions. The proportion of parotid saliva increases in response to marked stimulation

Gland	Proportion	Quality
Parotid gland	≈ 30 %	Mainly serous
Submandibular gland	55–65 %	Mixed mucous and serous
Sublingual gland	≈ 5 %	Mainly mucous
Minor salivary glands	5–8 %	Mixed, mainly mucous

mechanism based on proteins, lysozymes, and immunoglobulins, especially immunoglobulin A (IgA).
- Saliva has a digestive function; it lubricates the food and initiates the cleavage of starch by amylase.
- Saliva aids in the excretion of autogenous and foreign material, particularly iodine and coagulating factors, alkaloids, viruses including Epstein–Barr virus, poliomyelitis, rubella, coxsackievirus, cytomegalovirus, and hepatitis virus. The excretion of blood group substances in the saliva may be important in forensic medicine.
- Saliva aids in protection of the teeth. The organic and inorganic (e. g., fluoride) content of the saliva is important in the formation and maintenance of the dental enamel. It helps prevent bacterial deposition.
- Saliva helps mediate the sense of taste by lavage of the taste buds.

Composition. The composition of the saliva depends on its flow rate, the circadian rhythm, the season of the year, sex, and nutrition. The wide variability of this parameter needs to be taken into account during analysis, although it should be emphasized that saliva analysis has not become clinically important.

Disturbances of secretion. *Xerostomia* is extremely distressing. It may be caused centrally by lesions of the autonomic nervous supply to the salivary glands, by diseases of the salivary glands, by dehydration due to diarrhea or vomiting, by radiotherapy, or by systemic diseases such as Sjögren syndrome.

Sialorrhea means excessive saliva flow. Predisposing factors are diseases of the oral and lingual mucosa and teeth, as well as psychogenic factors.

Ptyalism is abnormal dribbling of saliva from the mouth in neurologic disease, as may occur in Parkinson disease, epilepsy, and paralysis of the muscles of deglutition.

Saliva production is also influenced by generalized diseases and drugs.

Methods of Investigation

The diagnosis of salivary gland diseases is a difficult and specialized field in otolaryngology, as the findings can be caused either by diseases of the salivary glands themselves or by a systemic disease.

Salivary gland diseases can often be diagnosed on the basis of the history, the patient's age, and the clinical findings (**Table 9.2**). The latter include swelling, consistency, mobility, rapidity of enlargement, pain, and facial nerve function.

Examples of salivary gland dysfunction
- Recurrent attacks of severe pain indicate sialolithiasis or recurrent parotitis.
- Bilateral disease indicates sialadenosis or mumps.
- Sex: myoepithelial sialadenitis, Sjögren disease, occurs almost exclusively in women.
- Malignancy is indicated by pain, facial paralysis, regional lymph-node metastases, and ulceration.

Age-dependent conditions
- Congenital hemangiomas and lymphangiomas occur in neonates.
- Mumps and chronic recurrent parotitis occur in school-age children.
- Adenomas and sialadenosis occur in middle age.
- The proportion of malignancy increases with age.

Normally, only the flat contour of the submandibular gland can be recognized with its soft overlying skin in the submandibular triangle. The parotid gland is not visible unless it is enlarged. Specific findings can be detected by palpation, which should be performed bimanually to allow both sides to be compared and may include both intraoral and extraoral palpation (**Fig. 9.4a, b**).

Table 9.2   Examination of the patient

Clinical history	Swelling: when? How often? After meals?
	Dry mouth: since when? Variable?
	Other (systemic) diseases: rheumatism, wrist pain, dry eye
	Drug use: alcohol; sympatholytic, parasympatholytic or parasympathomimetic drugs; β-blocking drugs; psychotropic drugs; cardiac drugs
Palpation	Check for signs of inflammation (redness, pain, swelling, warmth)
	Swelling: unilateral or bilateral, diffuse, local, painful? Consistency: soft, hard, mobile or immobile?
	Cervical lymph nodes: consistency, mobility, size

Clinical symptoms and interpretation

Swelling	Unilateral: tumor; bilateral: systemic disease, infection
	Whole gland: sialadenosis
	Growth rate: rapid growth suggests a malignant lesion, slow growth a benign lesion or possibly adenoid cystic carcinoma
Pain	Most common in acute or recurrent inflammations, sialadenosis; uncommon with tumors
Saliva	Clear: normal
	Cloudy or milky: sialadenitis
	Fluffy, granular: chronic inflammation
Xerostomia	Decreased salivation due to autonomic nervous system disease, autoimmune disease, dehydration, or drug side effects
Facial palsy	Malignant tumors, Heerfordt syndrome

> **!**
>
> **Note:** Unilateral or bilateral masseteric hypertrophy is often confused with parotid disease. The parotid gland can be distinguished from the masseter muscle by asking the patient to press the teeth together firmly, which causes the muscle to stand out.

The size of the gland in centimeters, its consistency, superficial profile, mobility, tenderness, and reddening of the overlying skin should be noted. Redness and swelling of the ducts and their orifices should also be looked for, and the appearance of the expressed saliva (clear, flocculent, purulent, or bloodstained) should be assessed. Stones in the ducts, particularly the submandibular duct, are often palpable.

■ Diagnostic Imaging

■ Sonography

This is the first imaging study after palpation. Its accuracy depends on the examiner's degree of experience (**Fig. 9.5a–h**). In view of its ease of use, low cost and good diagnostic yield, sonography is the diagnostic method of choice for salivary gland diseases.

■ Computed Tomography, Spiral CT

Contrast administration is helpful (80–150 mL of nonionic iodinated medium). Computed tomography (CT) of the parotid gland, especially when combined with sialography, provides information about the size and extent of parotid tumors, especially lesions involving the deep lobe. CT makes it possible to distinguish tumors arising from the gland itself from tumors that have invaded the gland from other structures, such as metastatic and parapharyngeal tumors. The findings may be equivocal for the diagnosis of small or malignant tumors.

■ Magnetic Resonance Imaging

Magnetic resonance imaging (MRI) provides high-resolution images of soft-tissue structures using T1-weighted and T2-weighted spin-echo sequences. Fluids have a high signal intensity, while solid structures appear hypointense. Contrast medium (gadolinium) is useful for tumor diagnosis.

■ Sialography

Sialography is contrast visualization of the salivary drainage system and portions of the glandular parenchyma. Magnetic resonance sialography is an alternative imaging technique.

Although sialography is not often used today, it is a method that can broaden the practitioner's understanding of salivary gland pathologies.

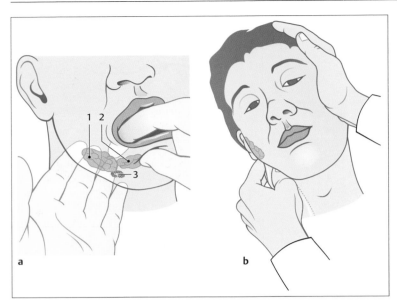

Fig. 9.4a, b   a Bimanual palpation of the submandibular gland (**1**), sublingual gland (**2**), and of a periglandular lymph node or stone (**3**) in the submandibular duct.
b Technique for palpating the retromandibular part of the parotid gland and the lymph nodes below the sternocleidomastoid muscle. The head is bent to relax the cervical fascia.

Technique of sialography. A plastic catheter and a cannula are introduced into the duct of the parotid gland or submandibular gland. Contrast medium is injected slowly in small amounts. Radiographs are taken in two planes or with an image intensifier.

> **Note:** Sialography is contraindicated in patients with an acute infection.

In chronic recurrent sialadenitis, sialographic images show a typical "tree in leaf" pattern, caused by ectasia of the acini and terminal and excretory ducts. Benign tumors frequently appear as a round mass displacing the contrast-filled ducts. Malignant tumors may cause duct tears, sudden changes in duct width, and contrast extravasation. The findings in Sjögren syndrome vary: initially, the picture is that of a "ripe tree" with delicate branching of the ductal system and an indistinct gland periphery. Later cases show a "bare tree" pattern, marked by rarefaction of the ducts and parenchymal atrophy (**Fig. 9.6a–g**).

■ **Positron-Emission Tomography**

Positron-emission tomography (PET) may be useful in special cases such as recurrent tumor or carcinoma with unknown primary (CUP) syndrome.

■ **Plain Radiographs**

Plain radiographs of the oral floor with lateral and tangential views of the submandibular and parotid glands are helpful only if the stone has a high calcium content. Radiolucent stones can often be detected with sialography, which shows a circular filling defect.

■ **Function Studies**

Loss of function (Galen's *functio laesa*) is another clinical manifestation of inflammatory disease, especially in parenchymatous organs. It is therefore important to obtain information about the functional status of the gland.

■ **Methods**

Sialometry. A small catheter is introduced into the papillae of both glands (parotid or submandibular). Saliva is collected for 10 min in a small test tube. It is important to note any difference between the sides and to classify secretory function as normal, increased, or decreased.

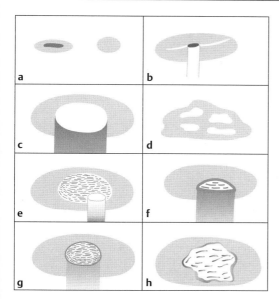

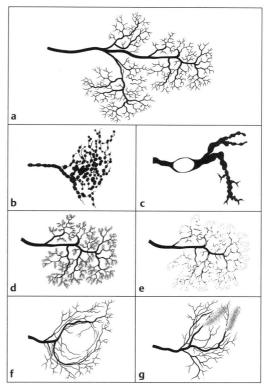

Fig. 9.5a–h Simplified representation of typical sonographic findings (according to Gabriele Behrbohm, MD, Berlin, Germany).
a Intraglandular lymph nodes.
b Salivary stone with distal acoustic shadow (particularly with a dilated duct).
c Cyst with an echo-free interior and distal acoustic enhancement.
d Signs of chronic inflammation: variable gland sizes and nonhomogeneous hyperechoic parenchyma.
e Warthin tumor has smooth, sharply circumscribed margins with solid and cystic components.
f Acute inflammation with an intraglandular abscess: enlarged gland with diffusely hypoechoic parenchyma. The abscess shows a thick wall, internal echoes, and shadowing with distal enhancement.
g Benign tumors such as pleomorphic adenomas are smooth and sharply circumscribed, with a uniformly hypoechoic internal echo pattern and faint distal enhancement.
h A malignant tumor typically has ill-defined, scalloped margins and a nonhomogeneous, hypoechoic parenchyma with evidence of peritumoral infiltration.

Fig. 9.6a–g Typical sialograms.
a A normal submandibular gland.
b Chronic recurrent obstructive parotitis with ectasia of the acini and terminal ducts, showing a "tree in leaf" appearance. The excretory duct shows a "string of beads" pattern.
c A stone in the submandibular duct. There is ectasia due to retention of secretions and extensive parenchymatous atrophy.
d Chronic nonobstructive parotitis, showing an "apple tree in bloom" appearance.
e The "ripe tree," "bare tree," and " frosted tree" patterns seen in different stages of ductal rarefaction and parenchymal atrophy, such as that occurring in Sjögren syndrome.
f Benign tumor of the parotid gland, with basket-shaped displacement around the tumor.
g Malignancy of the parotid gland, with interruption of the ducts and extravasation of contrast medium.

Scintigraphy. This can be used to conduct a functional study of the secretory activity of the gland (**Fig. 9.7**).

■ **Biopsy**

Histological diagnosis is the key to all salivary gland disease. It is the basis on which the decision is made on whether to operate or treat the patient medically, as in patients with sialadenosis or Sjögren disease.

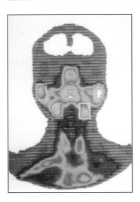

Fig. 9.7 This scintiscan of the salivary glands demonstrates hyposalivation in the right parotid gland and normal salivation in all the other glands.

Table 9.3 Diseases of the salivary glands

Inflammatory

Acute	Viral	Mumps, cytomegalovirus, coxsackievirus, AIDS
	Bacterial	Sialadenitis
Chronic		Chronic sclerosing sialadenitis of sub-mandibular gland (Küttner tumor), non-obstructive or obstructive sialadenitis

Noninflammatory

Cysts	Dysgenetic mucoceles of small glands, salivatory duct cysts, lymphoepithelial cysts
Systemic diseases	Sjögren syndrome, Heerfordt disease, Melkersson–Rosenthal syndrome, sarcoidosis, tuberculosis, syphilis, actinomycosis, AIDS
Sialadenosis	Metabolic (diabetes), endocrinic, neurogenic, side effects (e. g., of psychoactive substances, antihypertensive agents)

Tumors

Benign	Adenomas: pleomorphic; monomorphic: Warthin tumor, cystadenolymphoma, hemangioma, lymphangioma
Malignant	Carcinoma: adenocarcinoma, carcinoma in pleomorphic adenoma, acinus cell carcinoma, adenoid cystic carcinoma
	Malignant lymphoma: MALT type, B cell tumor, metastases

AIDS, acquired immune deficiency syndrome; MALT, mucosa-associated lymphoid tissue.

Fine-needle aspiration biopsy is only beneficial if the findings are positive; if it is inconclusive, the biopsy may need to be repeated. Smaller lesions may need ultrasound guidance during biopsy. The biopsy specimens should be interpreted by an experienced cytologist.

A core needle biopsy, if necessary, should be taken in more than one direction. This is a more useful test, but is difficult in cystic tumors. Care needs to be taken to avoid injury to the facial nerve. It is conceivable that tumor cells might be seeded along the needle track, but this has never been documented. Biopsy of an ulcerated lesion is easy. If the skin is intact, the best site for a parotid gland biopsy is the part of the parotid in the retromandibular fossa, to protect the facial nerve.

If the clinical findings indicate a salivary tumor, superficial parotidectomy or excision of the submandibular gland will provide a large biopsy and is also the correct treatment for a benign tumor. Intraoperative frozen-section biopsy enables the surgeon to decide between carrying out a partial or total parotidectomy, or a more extensive procedure. However, experience has shown that intraoperative diagnosis of a salivary gland tumor is often difficult. Diagnosis is easier with a fixed specimen.

Clinical Aspects

■ Inflammatory Diseases

See **Table 9.3**.

■ Acute Bacterial Infections

Clinical Features. The gland suddenly becomes swollen and tender. Infection of the parotid gland causes a protrusion of the auricle, which is most easily seen from behind the patient.

The overlying skin may be red (**Fig. 9.8**), and fluctuation may be felt if suppuration is present. An infection may rupture spontaneously to the outside or through the Santorini cleft into the external auditory meatus. The duct orifice appears red and swollen. Pus drains spontaneously, or after external massage. Trismus is also present.

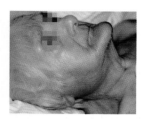

Fig. 9.8   Bacterial parotitis in a 91-year-old woman.

!

Note: If facial paralysis is present, this finding is not consistent with an infectious disease, and a malignant process should be strongly suspected.

Pathogenesis. Reducing salivary flow is an important prerequisite when there is ascending bacterial infection in the duct. Postoperative parotitis, which used to be common particularly after abdominal surgery, has now become much less frequent due to the use of antibiotics, fluid and electrolyte replacement, and postoperative oral hygiene. However, acute purulent infections still occur occasionally in patients with uncontrolled diabetes or renal failure with electrolyte disturbances and dehydration, or in the presence of carious teeth or poor oral hygiene. Nursing-home residents are predisposed to developing acute parotitis.

Diagnosis. The history shows a previous disease or operation. Clinical findings are noted (external appearance, palpable findings, gross characteristics of secretions), and saliva samples can be obtained for microbiological analysis.

Differential diagnosis. The differential diagnosis includes lymphadenitis due to a meatal furuncle, dentogenic abscess of the cheek, unerupted teeth, infected sebaceous cyst, and zygomatic abscess of mastoiditis in children.

Treatment. High-dose parenteral antibiotics are given, particularly agents that are active against Gram-negative organisms. The drug can be changed later if necessary, depending on the results of culture and sensitivity tests. Adequate hydration is provided, the fluid and electrolyte balance is corrected, and sialogogues are given. Fan-shaped external incisions are made for an abscess, with care being taken to avoid the facial nerve (see **Fig. 1.114**).

Antibiotics. Broad-spectrum antimicrobial therapy is indicated to cover all possible aerobic and anaerobic pathogens, including coverage for *Staphylococcus aureus,* hemolytic streptococci, and β-lactamase–producing anaerobic Gram-negative bacilli. A penicillinase-resistant penicillin or first-generation cephalosporin is generally satisfactory. Methicillin-resistant staphylococci may make it necessary to use vancomycin. Clindamycin, cefoxitin, imipenem, a combination of metronidazole and a macrolide, or a penicillin plus a β-lactamase inhibitor, will provide adequate coverage for anaerobic as well as aerobic bacteria.

The same treatment is prescribed for purulent infections of the submandibular gland. The most common cause in this case is obstruction by a stone or dental disease.

■ Viral Infections

Mumps

Clinical Features. Clinical features include swelling of the affected gland, redness and slight swelling of the ductal orifice, and displacement of the auricle. The secretions are not purulent, and 30% of patients are nonfebrile. Both glands are involved in 75% of cases. Swelling on one side may precede swelling on the other by up to 5 days. The submandibular and sublingual glands may also be involved, but they are rarely affected alone without parotid involvement.

An irreversible lesion of the eighth cranial nerve may be caused by this neurotropic virus, leading to unilateral or bilateral complete deafness. The pancreas, testes, ovaries, and central nervous system may also be affected, or any one of these organs may be involved in a synchronous or metachronous fashion.

Pathogenesis. The virus belongs to the Paramyxoviridae family. Local epidemics are known to occur in kindergartens and schools. The incubation period is 20 ± 10 days. An infection usually confers permanent immunity.

Diagnosis. Direct demonstration of the virus is possible only during the early phase of the disease, ranging from a few hours to several days.

The virus can be isolated from saliva, cerebrospinal fluid (CSF), or urine. It is demonstrated by culture in the kidneys of apes or the cells of hens or guinea pigs.

Serologic tests consist of complement-binding reaction or hemagglutination inhibition tests. The initial value is assessed and another reading is taken 2–3 weeks later. A fourfold rise in the antibody titer is evidence of a mumps infection. Increased amylase excretion in the blood and urine reaches its maximum on the third or fourth day of the illness.

> **Note:** Unilateral deafness in children often goes unnoticed by the child and by the parents. Audiologic tests during the course of the illness are therefore important.

Differential diagnosis. The differential diagnosis includes cervical lymphadenitis, purulent parotitis, chronic recurrent parotitis, and sialolithiasis. Dental infections are easy to exclude clinically or by serology.

Mumps is a common misdiagnosis in adults. A tumor is frequently present.

Treatment. It is not possible to treat the cause. Mumps hyperimmunoglobulins are recommended in the early stage. Symptomatic treatment includes analgesics and anti-inflammatory drugs, as required. Ample fluids should be given. A vaccine is available.

Cytomegalovirus

Cytomegalovirus (CMV) infection is mainly a disease of children, which is seen in neonates and infants up to 2 years of age. Congenital infections are mild and have no characteristic symptoms. Severe cases are accompanied by jaundice, petechial eruptions, hepatosplenomegaly, thrombocytopenia, hemolytic anemia, chorioretinitis, and psychomotor and mental retardation.

Acquired cytomegalovirus infection in adults usually does not produce any characteristic signs of infection.

Pathogenesis. The cytomegalovirus is transmitted across the placenta and by droplet inhalation or dirt infection. It preferentially affects the salivary glands, although it is a generalized disease.

Diagnosis. Serology is positive for antibodies. Histology shows owl's-eye cell nuclei and cellular inclusion bodies in the salivary and urinary sediment, or in tissue from the salivary glands.

Treatment. Treatment is symptomatic, as a specific therapy is not yet available.

Course. CMV infections have a high mortality rate in neonates.

Coxsackievirus

Clinical Features. Clinical manifestations include parotid swelling and gingivitis, often beginning with herpangina.

Pathogenesis. Infection is caused by a virus secreted by the pharyngeal and intestinal mucosa.

Diagnosis. The diagnosis is based on epidemiology and serologic testing.

Treatment. Therapy is symptomatic, and local treatment for the mucosa may be given as needed.

■ Chronic Inflammation

Chronic Sclerosing Sialadenitis of the Submandibular Gland (Küttner Tumor)

Clinical Features. Clinical manifestations include induration and enlargement of the gland, which is often difficult to differentiate from a true tumor. Pain is minimal.

Pathogenesis. Histology shows chronic inflammation of the gland, with destruction of the serous acini, lymphocytic infiltration of the interstitial connective tissue, periductal sclerosis, and, in the late stage, "cirrhosis" of the salivary glands due to metaplasia of the glandular parenchyma and connective tissue. The etiologic agents are still unknown, but an autoimmune process may be involved.

Diagnosis and treatment. The gland is removed for differential diagnosis and histology.

Chronic Recurrent Parotitis

Clinical Features. The symptoms tend to be unilateral or alternating, but occasionally there may be a simultaneous bilateral parotid swelling that may be very painful. The disease mainly occurs in children. The saliva is milky, granular, or consists of pure pus and has a salty taste. Trismus is often present. Attacks recur at variable intervals. The patient is asymptomatic between recurrences, but the parotid gland is usually indurated between attacks.

Chronic granulating inflammation of the small salivary glands of the lips: cheilitis granulomatosa (Miescher).

Diagnosis. The syndrome is diagnosed by biopsy of the lip glands at the side of inflammation. Sarcoidosis and Crohn disease need to be excluded.

Treatment. Corticosteroids and clofazimine.

Tuberculosis

Clinical Features. The clinical hallmark is a relatively painless swelling, usually located in the parotid or submandibular area. The periglandular and intraglandular lymph nodes are almost always the primary site of infection. Caseation, infiltration of the salivary parenchyma and surrounding tissues, external fistulas, and cutaneous tuberculosis have become less common.

Pathogenesis. Primary lymph-node infection is unusual today. The most common form at present results from postprimary hematogenous spread to the lymph nodes of the salivary glands.

Diagnosis. Intraglandular or periglandular lymph-node involvement is very difficult to distinguish by palpation from a salivary gland tumor. Radiography may show calcification, which requires differentiation from sialoliths or extravasated material. Tuberculosis of other organs, especially the lung, has to be excluded. Microscopy and culture for tuberculosis organisms are important investigations, in addition to histology. The disease is notifiable.

Treatment. Antituberculous drugs are given.

> **Note:** Serious errors, such as a failure to diagnose malignancy, can be avoided only by biopsy.

Radiation Sialadenitis

Clinical Features. The initial reaction is a reduction in salivary flow, followed later by a sicca syndrome that is often combined with hypogeusia or ageusia. The end stage may be characterized by an extremely distressing xerostomia, depending on the size of the field and the radiation dose.

Pathogenesis. Membrane damage to the nuclei and intra-cytoplasmic cell organelles occurs in the major and minor salivary glands during radiotherapy for malignant head and neck tumors above a dose of 10–15 Gy. This leads to interstitial fibrosis of the secretory elements. Permanent damage is likely to occur above a dose of 40–50 Gy.

Diagnosis. The diagnosis is based on a history of radiation exposure.

Treatment. Treatment is symptomatic. An attempt can be made to stimulate salivary secretion by one of the following: 1 % pilocarpine hydrochloride, 10 drops three times a day on a piece of sugar; artificial saliva; or having the patient take frequent sips of water or milk.

Course. In some cases, the production of saliva and the sense of taste may return to some extent after a period of months or years.

■ Sialolithiasis

Clinical Features. Clinical manifestations are related to eating or to psychological gustatory stimulation, which produce a severe, often painful swelling of the affected salivary gland (salivary colic). In many cases, swelling of the salivary gland due to retained secretions persists for variable periods of time.

Pathogenesis. Sialolithiasis is the end stage of a disease known as *electrolyte sialadenitis*. It is probably due to a primary dyschylic disturbance of salivary electrolyte secretion. The increased viscosity of the saliva leads to mucus obstruction, which subsequently aggravates the primary secretion disorder. Lumps of secretion form, consisting of an organic mucoprotein complex matrix. Inorganic material is deposited in onion-ring formations around this center. Factors that promote mineralization include mechanical causes such as dilation of the ducts, stenoses, localized attacks of inflammation, and neurohumoral dysfunction.

The scale deposited around the organic center consists of calcium phosphate and calcium carbonate with an apatite structure. The stones may be single, but are more often multiple and vary in size from a pinhead to the size of a cherry stone. Sialolithiasis is more common in men (2 : 1) and occurs mainly in adults. In most cases, only one gland is affected at any one time. The stone is located in the submandibular gland in 85 % of cases and in the parotid gland in

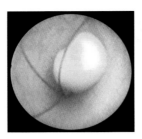

Fig. 9.13 Sialoendoscopic extraction of an intraductal salivary stone with a wire basket (with permission by F. Marchal).

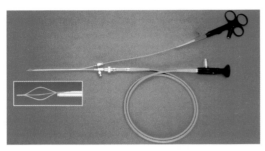

Fig. 9.14 Karl Storz instrumentation for sialoendoscopy (designed by F. Marchal).

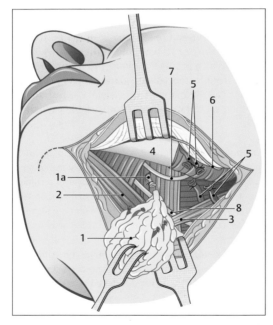

Fig. 9.15 Removal of the submandibular gland. **1**, Submandibular gland; **1a**, ligated submandibular duct; **2**, anterior belly of the digastric muscle; **3**, stylohyoid muscle, covered by the posterior belly of the digastric muscle; **4**, **horizontal ramus of the mandible; 5**, facial artery and vein ligated; **6**, marginal mandibular branch of the facial nerve (must be preserved, as it innervates the muscles of the lower lip); **7**, lingual nerve; **8**, hypoglossal nerve.

15 %. This ratio is explained by differences in flow. Submandibular saliva flows upward against gravity and is more viscous due to its greater mucin content.

Diagnosis. The stone is often palpable in the floor of the mouth or the cheek. A grating sensation is noted when a probe is inserted into the duct. The initial imaging study is ultrasound. If the calcium content is high enough, the stones may be visible on plain radiographs. Radiolucent stones can be detected indirectly by the presence of a filling defect on the sialogram (see **Fig. 9.6c**).

Differential diagnosis. Differentiation is required from a facial phlebolith, calcified tuberculous lymph node, and intraglandular tumor.

Treatment. Conservative treatment consists of sialogogues and glandular massage to stimulate spontaneous expulsion of the stone. Antibiotics are given if there is concomitant inflammation of the gland.

Surgical treatment. Papillotomy is indicated in patients with palpable prepapillary or extraglandular stones. The stone is removed by splitting the duct over a probe, providing immediate relief of pain.

- *Lithotripsy*: Extracorporeal (with piezoelectric and electromagnetic systems) or intracorporeal (laser lithotripsy).
- *Sialoendoscopy*: This procedure allows extensive exploration of the duct system (the main duct plus secondary and tertiary branches) and makes it possible to extract intraductal and intraglandular stones (**Figs. 9.13, 9.14**).

If it is not possible to avoid repeated attacks of stone formation and ductal obstruction, leading to chronic inflammatory parenchymal damage, the diseased gland should be removed (**Fig. 9.15**; see also **Fig. 9.30**).

■ Cysts

It is important to differentiate between cystic tumors and cysts of the salivary glands. There are four different types of cyst:

Dysgenetic cysts. An example of this type is the ranula ("frog tumor"), located below the mucosa of the oral floor. It may be divided into multiple compartments. As the cyst penetrates to the oral mucosa, it takes on an hourglass shape.

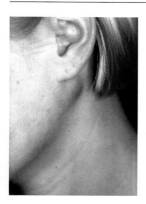

Fig. 9.16 A young woman with a lymphatic epithelial cyst of the parotid gland.

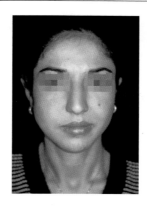

Fig. 9.17 Sialadenosis. A young woman with facial asymmetry caused by diffuse enlargement of the parotid gland.

Mucoceles of the small salivary glands. The mucoceles may appear as extravascular protrusions, frequently occurring in the lower lip of an adolescent patient. Retention mucoceles in patients over the age of 60 are caused by obstruction of the salivary ducts.

Salivary duct cysts. These are 2–3 cm in size and are common in older patients. The pathogenic mechanism is the same as with retention cysts.

Lymphatic epithelial cysts (Fig. 9.16). The cyst epithelium is surrounded by lymphatic stroma with lymphatic inclusions. The pathogenesis is probably related to lymph-node inclusions with an inflammatory reaction. Multifocal lymphoepithelial cysts of the parotid gland appear in 5% of patients with human immunodeficiency virus (HIV) infection as an early sign of general lymphatic hyperplasia and pathology.

■ Sialadenosis

Clinical Features. The symptoms include recurrent, or more often persistent, bilateral *painless* swelling, mainly of the parotid gland (**Fig. 9.17**). *Painful* sialadenosis may occur during treatment with antihypertensive drugs such as clonidine.

Pathogenesis. Salivary gland disorders with acinar swelling, degenerative lesions of the myoepithelium, and hydropic swelling of the axoplasm of autonomic nerve fibers may occur in endocrine and metabolic disorders such as diabetes, pregnancy, puberty, menopause, adrenal dysfunction, avitaminosis, protein deficiency, starvation dystrophy,

alcoholism, and central neurogenic and autonomic dysfunction. They may also develop in response to treatment with antihypertensive agents and other drugs such as clozapine (**Fig. 9.18**).

Diagnosis. The endocrine and metabolic systems are evaluated. Sialography initially is unimpressive, but later shows narrowing of the ducts and a "bare tree" pattern. Histology and electron microscopy demonstrate the specific lesions in the autonomic nervous system and glandular parenchyma.

Treatment. Metabolic or endocrine disorders are treated, and the antihypertensive agents are discontinued or changed. Corticosteroids are helpful in reducing tension in the parotid capsule and the volume of the parotid gland.

■ Trauma

■ Injury to the Nerves or Ducts and Salivary Fistulas

Nerve damage. Injury to the facial nerve in the parotid area or to the lingual or hypoglossal nerve in the sublingual area should be treated without delay (see pp. 112–114).

Injuries to the ducts. Only injuries to major ducts need to be repaired. A fine plastic catheter is introduced, and the two parts of the duct are reanastomosed using microsurgical technique. If part of the duct is lost, an attempt can be made to reconstruct it or to implant the shortened duct into the buccal mucosa, creating a new orifice.

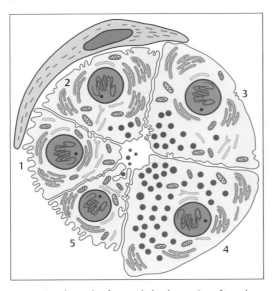

Fig. 9.18   The cycle of parotid gland secretion after adrenergic stimulation. Model of sialadenosis (Seifert and Donath). **1**, Start of synthesis and formation of endoplasmic reticulum; **2**, **3**, proliferation and maturation of secretory granules; **4**, extended storage of secretory granules and expansion of acinar volume with decreased protein synthesis; **5**, end of adrenergic stimulation.

Table 9.4   Distribution of tumors in specific salivary glands

Parotid tumors	80 % of all salivary tumors, of which 30 % are malignant
Submandibular tumors	10 % of all salivary tumors, of which 50 % are malignant
Tumors of the minor salivary glands	10 % of all salivary tumors, of which 50 % are malignant
Sublingual tumors	1 % of all salivary tumors, of which 80 % are malignant

Salivary fistulas.   Provided the main duct system is intact, treatment of parenchymatous fistulas usually causes no difficulty. In most cases, a fistula in the external parenchyma will heal spontaneously, but it may take several weeks. Occasionally, it may be necessary to suppress secretions temporarily with atropine, botulinum toxin injection, or radiotherapy. If this does not succeed in closing the salivary fistula, it should be excised and the soft tissues, particularly the capsule, closed in layers.

Auriculotemporal Syndrome or Frey Syndrome (Gustatory Sweating)

Clinical Features.   The patient reports sweating and reddening of the skin in the preauricular area before, during, and after eating. Pain is uncommon. Mild forms that can be diagnosed with the starch–iodine test are more common than the fully developed form with excessive sweating, which is very distressful for the patient. The symptoms develop slowly and often do not appear until several months after the primary traumatic or inflammatory cause.

Pathogenesis.   This disease is usually due to trauma or surgery and only rarely to parotitis. There is aberrant regeneration and anastomosis of postganglionic parasympathetic nerves supplying the gland, with sympathetic autonomic fibers running in the auriculotemporal nerve supplying the skin. This results in hypersensitivity of the cutaneous sweat glands to cholinergic impulses.

Treatment.   Botulinum toxin (cumulative dose of 6–10 IU SC) after mapping the involved area. An ointment containing 1 % glycopyrronium bromide can be applied to the affected skin area, the tympanic plexus can be divided in the middle ear, or lyophilized dura or a sheet of fascia can be implanted subdermally in the affected area.

■ Salivary Tumors

Ninety percent of all salivary tumors are epithelial in origin. The remainder are nonepithelial tumors such as hemangioma, lymphangioma, malignant lymphoma, and periglandular tumors.

■ Benign Tumors

Adenoma

The distribution and histology of this tumor are summarized in **Tables 9.4 and 9.5**.

Different adenomas have a very similar clinical presentation. A long history, slow growth, absence of metastases, skin infiltration and ulceration, and the preservation of facial nerve function suggest a benign salivary tumor. The definitive diagnosis is made by histologic examination of the surgical specimen. All adenomas should be treated surgically. The details are discussed below.

Table 9.5 Classification of benign epithelial salivary tumors

Pleomorphic adenoma (formerly known as "mixed tumor")	85 %
Monomorphic adenoma	
Cystadenolymphoma, Warthin tumor	15 %
Adenomas of other types	

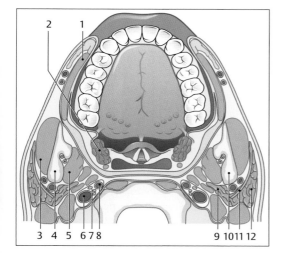

Fig. 9.19 Topographic relations of the parotid gland, neck, and pharyngeal structures. **1**, Buccinator muscle; **2**, palatine tonsil; **3**, masseter muscle; **4 & 10**, mandibular ramus; **5**, pterygoid muscle; **6**, internal jugular vein; **7**, cranial nerves IX, X, and XII; **8**, internal carotid artery; **9**, retromandibular lobe of parotid gland; **11**, facial nerve; **12** superficial lobe of parotid gland.

Pleomorphic Adenoma

Clinical Features. The site of predilection is the parotid gland, where 80 % of these tumors arise. They are almost always unilateral. Pleomorphic adenomas grow slowly over many years. The average history is 5–7 years, but a history of 20 years may be elicited in some patients. Women are affected more frequently than men. The tumor is firm, often nodular, and nonpainful. Facial nerve function is preserved even with very large tumors, provided they remain benign. Difficulty in swallowing due to tumor size may be caused by extension of the tumor into the pharynx or by adenomas of the minor salivary glands of the palate or pharynx (**Fig. 9.19**).

Iceberg tumors are large pleomorphic adenomas that extend into the tonsillar region (**Fig. 9.20a–c**).

Pathogenesis. The epithelial origin of pleomorphic adenoma has been proved. Approximately two-thirds arise in the superficial lobe of the parotid gland (**Fig. 9.21**). The histologic appearance is highly variable. Increasing experience has identified subtypes with scant stroma, which have a clinical propensity to malignant degeneration.

Approximately 50 % of adenomas have a capsule. Otherwise there is an indistinct boundary between the tumor and the gland. A truly multilocular tumor is uncommon. Recurrent "multicentric" pleomorphic adenomas are usually the result of using faulty surgical technique for tumor enucleation.

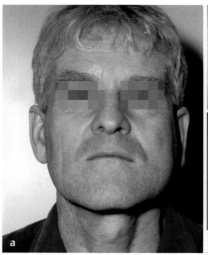

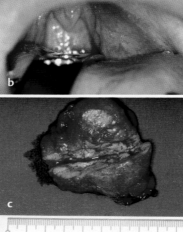

Fig. 9.20a–c Iceberg tumor of the parotid gland in a 47-year-old patient.
a The tumor is located in the retromandibular fossa.
b The tumor is palpable and visible in the tonsillar fossa.
c The tumor after dissection.

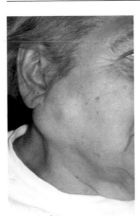

Fig. 9.21 Typical appearance of pleomorphic adenoma, with a smooth, bulging surface.

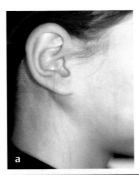

Fig. 9.22a, b **a** Warthin tumor in a 15-year-old girl. **b** T2-weighted magnetic resonance image.

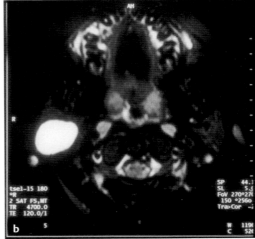

Diagnosis. Palpation and sonography. Sialography (see **Fig. 9.6f**) and fine-needle biopsy provide a preoperative diagnosis only in tumors of indeterminate nature. Intraoperative diagnosis may be made by frozen section, but the definitive diagnosis is made by histologic examination of the surgical specimen.

Treatment. Parotid tumors are treated with superficial parotidectomy or total parotidectomy in deep lobe tumors, with preservation of the facial nerve. For submandibular gland tumors, treatment is excision of the gland along with the tumor and surrounding tissue. Tumors of the minor glands are treated using excision with a margin of healthy tissue (see **Figs. 9.15, 9.28**).

Prognosis. The outlook is very good. Malignant transformation occurs in 3–5% of pleomorphic adenomas. The frequency of malignant degeneration is higher in recurrent tumors, inadequately resected lesions, and in patients with a long history.

Cystadenolymphoma (Warthin Tumor)

Clinical Features. This tumor is usually unilateral, but 10% are bilateral. It presents as a firm, elastic, mobile, nontender mass. Most cases occur in elderly men.

Pathogenesis. This soft cystic tumor usually develops in the inferior part of the parotid gland (**Fig. 9.22a**). It probably arises from segments of the salivary ducts that have been included in intraglandular or extraglandular lymph nodes during embryonic development. The histology therefore shows a rich lymphoreticular stroma, with lymph follicles between the epithelial glandular segments—giving rise to the term "papillary cystadenoma lymphomatosum."

Diagnosis. This is aided by careful palpation and sonography. Salivary scintiscans show uptake of technetium Tc 99 m. Aspiration or needle biopsy is less helpful in this cystic tumor. Definitive diagnosis rests on histologic examination of the surgical specimen.

Treatment. Depending on the site of the lesion, treatment consists of partial excision of the parotid gland (preserving the facial nerve) or excision of the submandibular gland.

Prognosis. The outlook is very good and malignant degeneration is uncommon.

Hemangioma

Clinical Features. Two types are distinguished—cavernous and capillary hemangiomas. Hemangiomas are a common childhood lesion in the parotid and submandibular glands (**Fig. 9.23**). The affected gland is enlarged, and the chin is pale red or blue. The tumor is soft and compressible.

Diagnosis. The diagnosis relies on ultrasound, MRI, and angiography to distinguish between high-flow and low-flow lesions.

Treatment. The growth tendency of the lesion is assessed using ultrasound or MRI. Surgical treatment is difficult, and rigorous selection criteria should be applied. Preoperative embolization is indicated for high-flow lesions. Other options are magnesium wire implantation and laser obliteration.

Lymphangioma (Cystic Hygroma)

Clinical Features. This tumor is manifested by partial or complete facial asymmetry (**Figs. 9.24, 9.25**). It grows diffusely into all glandular spaces and surrounding tissues.

Diagnosis. Lymphangioma appears as a soft, cystic mass that slowly fills and enlarges when the head is bent forward. MRI should also be performed.

Treatment. All portions of the tumor should be completely excised in carefully selected patients. The procedure should only be carried out by highly experienced surgeons.

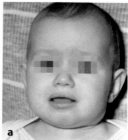
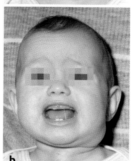

Fig. 9.23a, b
a Hemangioma of the parotid region in a young boy.
b It protrudes when the boy is crying.

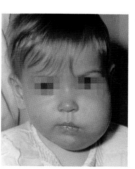

Fig. 9.24 A girl with a large lymphangioma of the left side of the face.

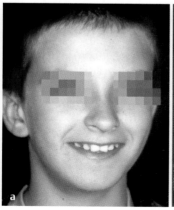
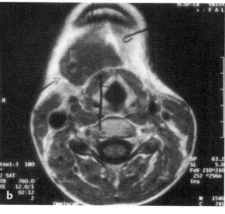

Fig. 9.25a, b **a** Lymphangioma of the oral floor in a 12-year-old boy.
b T1-weighted magnetic resonance image of the region.

Table 9.6 Histologic classification of salivary gland tumors

Adenomas

Pleomorphic adenoma

Myoepithelioma (myoepithelial adenoma)

Basal cell adenoma

Warthin tumor (adenolymphoma)

Oncocytoma (oncocytic adenoma)

Canalicular adenoma

Sebaceous adenoma

Ductal papilloma

- Inverted ductal papilloma
- Intraductal papilloma
- Sialadenoma papilliferum

Cystadenoma

- Papillary cystadenoma
- Mucinous cystadenoma

Carcinomas

Acinic cell adenocarcinoma

Mucoepidermoid carcinoma

Adenoid cystic carcinoma

Polymorphous low-grade adenocarcinoma

Epithelial–myoepithelial carcinoma

Basal cell adenocarcinoma

Sebaceous carcinoma

Papillary cystadenocarcinoma

Mucinous adenocarcinoma

Oncocytic carcinoma

Salivary duct carcinoma

Adenocarcinoma

Malignant myoepithelioma (myoepithelial carcinoma)

Carcinoma in pleomorphic adenoma (malignant mixed tumor)

Squamous cell carcinoma

Small cell carcinoma

Undifferentiated carcinoma

Other carcinomas

■ Malignant Tumors

Some 25–30 % of salivary gland tumors are malignant (**Table 9.6**). The following signs are suggestive of malignancy:

- Rapid growth or periods of rapid growth (except for adenoid cystic carcinoma, which grows very slowly).
- Pain.
- Firm infiltration, occasional ulceration of the skin or mucosa, poor mobility of the tumor.
- Cervical lymph-node metastases.
- Facial paralysis with parotid tumors (**Table 9.7**).

Note: Survival is reduced in patients with facial paralysis or regional lymph-node metastases. As a rule, the smaller the gland of origin, the greater the clinical likelihood of malignant growth in firm salivary gland tumors.

The classification of epithelial malignancies is shown in **Table 9.6**; the TNM classification is shown in **Table 9.8**.

Acinar Cell Tumors

Clinical Features. These are caused by local growth of the tumor.

Diagnosis. The diagnosis is based on histologic examination. The tumor cells resemble acinar cells.

Treatment. Total parotidectomy is performed, as the recurrence rate after less extensive surgery is very high. The decision on whether to remove or preserve the facial nerve or individual branches with the help of neuromonitoring is based on the clinical presentation and intraoperative findings. Neck dissection is advised.

Course and prognosis. These tumors are malignant, but their prognosis is better than that of carcinoma. Regional or distant metastases are uncommon and occasionally occur late in the course. The peak incidence is between 30 and 60 years of age. The 5-year and 15-year survival rates are 75 % and 55 %, respectively.

Mucoepidermoid Tumors

Clinical Features. When these tumors are of low-grade malignancy they grow slowly, whereas high-grade tumors grow very rapidly and cause pa

facial paralysis, and regional lymph-node metastases in 40–50 % of cases. Distant blood-borne metastases are also more common in the latter group.

Pathogenesis. Well-differentiated tumors (low-grade, ≈ 75 %) have to be distinguished from undifferentiated tumors (high-grade, ≈ 25 %).

The grade of malignancy is determined by the ratio between epidermoid and mucous cells. Tumors with predominantly mucous cells have a better prognosis. The most common sites of occurrence are the parotid gland and the minor salivary glands of the palate. The peak age incidence is between 40 and 50 years, but the tumor may also occur in children.

Diagnosis. The diagnosis is based on histologic examination.

Treatment. Parotidectomy is performed for parotid lesions, regardless of the grade of malignancy. A neck dissection is also indicated for high-grade tumors. The need for facial nerve excision and reconstruction has to be determined on a case-by-case basis.

Prognosis. Five-year survival rates of ≈ 90 % are achieved with low-grade mucoepidermoid tumors, but this rate declines considerably with high-grade tumors.

Adenoid Cystic Carcinoma (Cylindroma)

Clinical Features. Growth is usually slow, but fulminating growth may occasionally occur. Pain or paresthesia are typical complaints. Facial paralysis occurs in ≈ 25 % of patients. Cranial nerve deficits are common, especially with tumors extending to the skull base, and typically involve cranial nerves V, VII, IX, and XII. Regional lymph-node metastases are present in ≈ 15 % of patients at the initial diagnosis. Blood-borne distant metastases to the lung and skeleton are common, occurring in up to 20 % of patients (**Fig. 9.26**).

Pathogenesis. Histologically, this tumor consists of primitive duct epithelium and myoepithelial cells, which form glandular-cystic, cribriform cell nests and also solid trabecular structures. The older term "cylindroma" for this tumor led to underestimation of its seriousness, and for this reason it is no longer used. In fact, the tumor should be considered particularly malignant, as its growth pattern involves extensive local diffuse perivascular and perineural infiltration. It

Table 9.7 Frequency of facial paralysis in parotid malignancy at the time of presentation

Adenoid cystic carcinoma	25 %
Undifferentiated carcinoma	25 %
Carcinoma in pleomorphic adenoma	15 %
Adenocarcinoma	10 %
Mucoepidermoid carcinoma	10 %

Table 9.8 TNM classification for carcinoma of the major salivary glands

TX	Primary tumor cannot be assessed
T0	No evidence of primary tumor
T1	Tumor ≤ 2 cm or less in greatest dimension, without extraparenchymal extension
T2	Tumor > 2 cm to 4 cm in greatest dimension, without extraparenchymal extension
T3	Tumor > 4 cm and/or tumor with extraparenchymal extension
T4-a	Tumor invades skin, mandible, ear canal, and/or facial nerve
T4-b	Tumor invades base of skull and/or pterygoid plates and/or encases carotid artery

For N and M staging, see **Table 3.10**, p. 283
From: F.L. Greene et al., *AJCC Cancer Staging Manual*, 6th ed. (New York: Springer, 2002) and UICC, *TNM Classification of Malignant Tumours*, 6th ed. (New York: Wiley-Liss, 2002).

can metastasize to the chest, and late recurrence is common.

Adenoid cystic carcinomas are also relatively common in the minor salivary glands, especially those in the palate, followed by the sublingual, submandibular, and parotid glands. The average age of the patient is 55 ± 10 years.

Diagnosis. MRI scans show the size and location of the tumor, as well as perineural spread. Histology (e.g., fine-needle aspiration biopsy) confirms the diagnosis.

Treatment. Hematogenous metastases to the lung and skeleton need to be excluded before surgery. The only chance of cure is with a radical primary

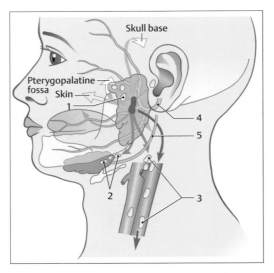

Fig. 9.26 Routes of spread of parotid tumors. Light orange arrow: contiguous extension; medium orange arrow: lymphatic metastasis; red arrow: hematogenous metastasis. **1**, Intraparotid and periparotid spread; **2**, submandibular spread; **3**, jugular lymph-node metastases; **4**, facial nerve; **5**, hypoglossal nerve.

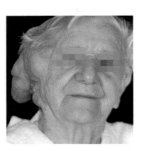

Fig. 9.27 Carcinoma in pleomorphic adenoma.

operation dictated by the site of the tumor. The facial nerve must be resected for an adenoid cystic carcinoma of the parotid gland, and it should then be reconstructed with a free graft. Primary radiotherapy for adenoid cystic carcinoma is of less value than radical surgery. Radiotherapy, usually neutron radiotherapy, is indicated for nonresectable or recurrent tumors. Postoperatively, all patients should be treated with radiotherapy or chemoradiotherapy. In patients with completely resected T1 or T2 N0 tumors and low-grade histology, postoperative radiotherapy can be dispensed with.

Prognosis and course (Fig. 9.26). Locoregional infiltration, early regional and systemic metastases to the lungs, brain and skeleton, and lack of response to radiotherapy and chemotherapy result in a poor prognosis. A prolonged course over 10 years or more, even in the presence of distant metastases, is not exceptional. The standard calculation of the 5-year survival rate is not relevant with the particular characteristics of adenoid cystic carcinoma; the outcome is almost invariably fatal.

Adenocarcinoma
Papillary and mucus-secreting carcinomas arise from the salivary duct system and infiltrate and destroy local tissues. Both sexes are equally affected. Pain, facial paralysis, and cervical lymphnode metastases are common.

Squamous Cell Carcinoma
This infiltrating, rapidly growing tumor mainly attacks the parotid gland, accounting for 5–10 % of all parotid tumors. Regional lymph-node metastases are found in approximately one-third of the patients.

> **Note:** Before accepting the diagnosis of a primary squamous cell carcinoma of the salivary gland, the physician should consider the possibility of metastases from other head and neck carcinomas to the salivary lymph nodes.

Carcinoma in Pleomorphic Adenoma
Clinical Features. The history is often characteristic. In most cases, the tumor has been present for years, causing nothing more than a cosmetically unacceptable parotid swelling. This is followed by abrupt enlargement of the mass (**Fig. 9.27**), often with pain radiating to the ear, total facial paralysis, or paralysis of individual nerve branches. In 25 % of patients, regional lymph-node metastases develop, with infiltration of the tumor into the skin and external ulceration.

Pathogenesis. It is very unusual for pleomorphic adenoma to develop as a primary malignancy. It is now thought more likely that malignant transformation occurs after a long latent period, particularly in the subtype of pleomorphic adenoma that has scant stroma. Approximately 3–5 % of pleomorphic adenomas undergo malignant transformation, and this percentage rises with the length of the history. As a result, these patients are a decade older on average than patients with benign pleomorphic adenoma.

Diagnosis. The diagnosis is based on the history, the clinical findings of facial paralysis and regional lymph-node metastases, intraoperative frozen section, and definitive histologic examination.

Treatment. Radical parotidectomy, which requires complete excision of the tumor with good margins, is performed with en bloc neck dissection.

Prognosis. These tumors have a guarded prognosis.

■ **Basic Principles in the Treatment of Salivary Tumors**

The following treatment recommendations can be made on the basis of the specific biology of salivary gland tumors and clinical experience. For both benign and malignant tumors, the initial operation almost always determines the success of the treatment (pleomorphic adenoma) or the prospects for patient survival (adenoid cystic carcinoma). Radiotherapy for benign epithelial tumors is not justified by radiation biology. The results of irradiation alone for malignant epithelial salivary tumors are inferior to those of surgery. However, radiotherapy be appropriate for inoperable tumors, carcinomas that cannot be removed completely, and especially for malignant lymphomas.

The extent of the operation is determined by the location and extent of the tumor and especially by the condition of neighboring structures such as the facial nerve, hypoglossal and lingual nerves, pharynx, contents of the carotid sheath, external auditory meatus, skull base, facial skeleton, lymph nodes, and overlying skin.

Techniques for preserving or reconstructing the facial nerve using autologous nerve grafting represent a substantial advance in parotid surgery (see also pp. 112–114).

Note: Lymph-node metastases from primary tumors of the eye, such as melanoma, or from other tributary areas in the head may simulate primary tumors of the major salivary glands, especially the parotid, and particularly if the primary tumor (such as squamous carcinoma of the skin) has previously been treated with surgery or radiation and the surgical scar or radiation dermatitis is hidden by hair.

Table 9.9 House–Brackman facial paralysis scale

Grade		Facial movement
I	Normal	Normal facial function at all times
II	Mild dysfunction	Forehead: moderate to good function, eye: complete closure, mouth: slight asymmetry
III	Moderate dysfunction	Forehead: slight to moderate movement, eye: complete closure with effort, mouth: slightly weak with maximum effort
IV	Moderately severe dysfunction	Forehead: none, eye: incomplete closure, mouth: asymmetric with maximum effort
V	Severe dysfunction	Forehead: none, eye: incomplete closure, mouth: slight movement
VI	Total paralysis	No movement

Neck dissection is indicated for adenoid cystic carcinomas, carcinomas, high-grade mucoepidermoid tumors, carcinoma in pleomorphic adenomas, and metastases to the parotid lymph nodes from the skin of the face and scalp.

The first stations for lymph-node metastases are the intraglandular and periglandular parotid or submandibular nodes, followed by the deep cervical nodes. Distant hematogenous metastases are a relatively common finding, especially in adenoid cystic carcinoma.

Note: Contiguous tumor spread, especially of adenoid cystic carcinoma along nerves and vessels, is so extensive that the prognosis remains poor even after an extensive resection.

Medicolegal issues. Before any parotid surgery is performed, the patient should be warned about the possibility of injury to the facial nerve and its consequences (**Table 9.9**). It is also useful to warn patients about the possibility of a salivary fistula and Frey syndrome.

Histologic Diagnosis, Staging, Follow-up

The histologic diagnosis defines the biological malignancy of a tumor and has a decisive influence on the prognosis. Experience has shown that examination of intraoperative frozen sections of salivary gland tissue is difficult for the pathologist.

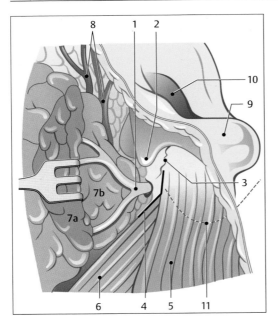

Fig. 9.28 Conservative parotidectomy. Sites for exposing the main trunk of the facial nerve (**1**): apex of the cartilaginous meatus ("pointer"), (**2**); the tympanomastoid fissure (**3**); angle (**4**) between the anterior border of the sternocleidomastoid muscle (**5**) and the posterior belly of the digastric muscle (**6**). Superficial lobe of the parotid gland (**7a**), deep lobe of the parotid gland (**7b**), superficial temporal artery and vein (**8**), retracted lobe of the auricle (**9**), meatal introitus (**10**), mastoid apex (**11**).

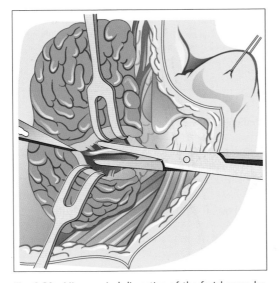

Fig. 9.29 Microsurgical dissection of the facial nerve between the superficial and deep lobes of the parotid gland.

The size of a malignant tumor and lymph-node staging are assessed using CT and/or MRI (depending on the anatomic region) before treatment is initiated. Lymph-node staging is based on CT sections 3–5 mm thick, from the base of the skull to the superior thoracic aperture. Use of contrast medium is mandatory.

Chest radiography in two planes should be performed during the course of primary staging and at follow-up. Much better information is provided by thoracic CT before treatment is begun and at annual follow-up examinations. An abdominal CT is recommended before treatment is started, but if the findings are normal, annual sonographic monitoring is sufficient.

Radioisotope scanning for tumor staging serves to rule out or prove the presence of distant metastases in the skeletal system. Use of PET-CT may be indicated in special cases, such as CUP syndrome with metastasis.

Follow-up: The first review MRI and/or CT studies of the neck are performed 3 months after the operation or at the conclusion of chemotherapy or radiotherapy, and annually thereafter.

Basic Surgical Procedures

Superficial Parotidectomy with Preservation of the Facial Nerve for Benign Tumors (Figs. 9.28, 9.29)

An S-shaped or Y-shaped skin incision is made in front of or behind the auricle and extended down to the sternocleidomastoid muscle. The main trunk of the facial nerve is identified ≈ 5 mm below the triangular apex of the cartilaginous meatus. The trunk is followed to the branches. The trunk can also be located by starting at the tympanomastoid fissure and dissecting 6–8 mm in the medial direction. An even better method is to expose the anterior borders of the sternocleidomastoid muscle and the posterior belly of the digastric; a line bisecting the angle formed by their borders points to the facial nerve trunk. The facial nerve branches are dissected peripherally using a binocular loupe or operating microscope. The nerve stimulator is very helpful for identifying the facial nerve branches during surgery.

The extent of this operation is determined by the size and location of the tumor. It may be necessary to carry out either a superficial or total parotidectomy with preservation of the facial nerve.

Radical Parotidectomy for Malignant Tumors

The extent of the operation is determined by the size and location of the tumor. Thus, it may be necessary to perform a mandibulectomy, petrosectomy, resection of the supraglandular or periglandular skin, and a neck dissection. Resection of the facial nerve is absolutely indicated in patients with partial or complete facial paralysis. Since the malignant cells penetrate the nerve sheath, especially in adenoid cystic carcinoma, removal of the nerve is almost always indicated even if there is no clinical evidence of paralysis.

Facial paralysis after operations for malignancy can be treated using free nerve grafting or the placement of fascial slings (**Figs. 9.30, 9.31**).

Removal of the Submandibular Gland
(see Fig. 9.15)

The skin incision is made 2 cm below and parallel to the horizontal ramus of the mandible. The dissection is carried down to the gland, starting posteriorly. To preserve the nerve supply to the lower lip, the marginal mandibular branch is protected by elevating the facial artery and vein after they have been ligated. Another way of protecting the nerve is to dissect the platysma carefully away from the submandibular fascia, keeping deep to the pla-

tysma, and to look for the nerve. The hypoglossal and lingual nerves are preserved by precise dissection on the capsule of the gland and, if necessary, by exposing the nerves. The duct is ligated anteriorly after the gland has been freed.

The principles described for radical parotidectomy also apply to malignant tumors of the submandibular gland.

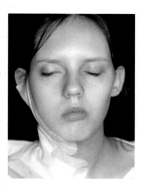

Fig. 9.30 Adenoid cystic carcinoma of the right parotid gland in a 21-year-old woman, 1 day after total parotidectomy, modified radical neck dissection, and facial nerve reconstruction with a free graft from the great auricular nerve. Eyelid closure has already been restored.

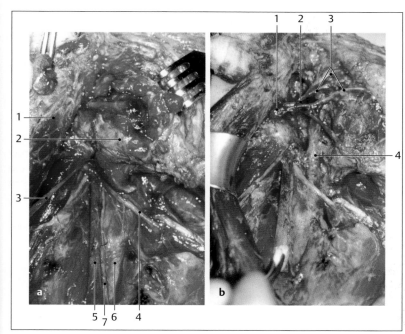

Fig. 9.31a, b The same patient as in **Fig. 9.30**.
a The intraoperative appearance following complete resection. **1**, sternocleidomastoid muscle; **2**, total parotidectomy; **3**, accessory nerve (XI); **4**, hypoglossal nerve (XII); **5**, jugular vein; **6**, common carotid artery; **7**, vagus nerve (X).
b Facial nerve reconstruction. **1**, Facial nerve trunk (VII); **2**, anastomosis; **3**, free transplants; **4**, external carotid artery.

Appendix

Emergencies in ENT and First Aid Procedures

Acute bleeding

Bleeding from the ear   see p. 84
Bleeding from the nose (epistaxis)   see p. 191
Bleeding from the mouth, larynx,
     trachea and esophagus   see pp. 245, 269,
         278, 282 ff.

Acute dyspnea

Differential diagnoses   see pp. 301–303, 305,
         345, 282, 257
Emergency bronchoscopy   see p. 347
Tracheotomy   see pp. 345, 351 355
Intubation   see pp. 310, 311, 355
Laryngotomy   see p. 353

Foreign bodies

In the hypopharynx and esophagus   see pp. 278,
         364, 367, 368
In the larynx, trachea, and bronchi   see pp. 313, 357
In the nose   see p. 152
In the ear   see p. 55

Trauma

To the nose   see p. 201
To the midface   see p. 203
Frontobasal injury   see p. 207

Corrosions and burns

In the mouth   see p. 277
In the pharynx   see p. 277
In the esophagus   see p. 365

Sudden-onset hearing loss

Causes in the external ear canal and
     middle ear   see pp. 55, 58, 62, 84, 87
Causes due to disturbances of the inner
     ear and brain stem   see pp. 86, 88, 101

Acute vertigo   see pp. 62, 85, 86, 95, 97 ff.

Facial palsy   see pp. 62, 75, 84, 111, 112

Complications of sinus infections   see pp. 186 ff.

Complications after tonsillectomy see pp. 268, 272
Secondary tonsillar hemorrhage   see pp. 269, 273

Essential Information for Infection Control

Andrew C. Swift

Introduction

Before the discovery and introduction of antibiotics, infections in the head and neck were an important cause of serious morbidity and often resulted in major complications and death. However, antibiotics transformed this situation, and previous infections that were once life-threatening became controllable and treatable.

As antibiotics were used more and more frequently, the bacteria responded by developing resistance. Recognition of this change led to the development of more varieties of antibiotics that would maintain activity against the bacteria, but the organisms still seemed able to adapt and become antibiotic-resistant.

With the passage of time, the situation became more serious, as patients started to acquire severe infections that often led to significant morbidity or death whilst in hospital. The two bacterial infections that have plagued hospitals in recent years have been methicillin-resistant *Staphylococcus aureus* (MRSA) and *Clostridium difficile*. There have been considerable numbers of deaths during outbreaks of the latter.

These infections are no longer restricted to specific parts of the hospital, but can affect any patient or clinical area. Otolaryngologists therefore need to have a working knowledge and understanding of these diseases, especially if performing head and neck surgical procedures. In addition to the potentially serious clinical consequences of the infections, there are now legal implications that could affect the individual doctor. A basic working knowledge of these issues is therefore essential.

It became imperative for further measures to be introduced rapidly to control and attempt to eradicate these infections. The response varies amongst different countries, but the following describes the changes instigated in the United Kingdom as an example of the way in which the threat is being addressed.

Infection Control Response in the UK

As a consequence of the increased incidence of these infections, together with public awareness of the issue and a demand for safer hospital environments, various changes were instigated by the UK government through the Department of Health. A new Health Act was introduced in 2006 that made it a statutory requirement for hospital trusts to introduce an infection policy. A Health Care Commission was set up that oversees these policies, ensures that they are strictly adhered to and receives proof of action through regular audit data. Individual staff at all levels have to comply with the hospital infection policy, and failure to comply is now a breach of contract that leads to formal disciplinary action. If a patient were to die from an MRSA infection that was subsequently found to have resulted from a breach of policy, a case of corporate manslaughter could be brought against the hospital trust concerned. In addition to this, if an individual is found to be responsible, criminal charges can be instigated, with the ultimate threat of imprisonment. It has also been noted that solicitors would actively pursue such claims. The situation has therefore taken on a new level of importance, in addition to the normal desire to prevent and treat these infections vigorously if they occur.

Many hospitals have therefore introduced a concept of "zero tolerance" for breaches of infection policy. They have also set up systems to administer infection policy, including infection control teams, and have appointed leading clinicians to be responsible for infection control within their own specialty group.

The thrust of these changes is to minimize the use of antibiotics and restrict their use to only those patients in whom they are deemed essential. There is also a restriction on the types of antibiotic used, with an emphasis on avoiding those that predispose to the development of *C. difficile* infection. Antibiotic prophylaxis is still encouraged when there is evidence to show that it is effective, but strict guidelines on the prescription and duration of administration have to be followed. For example, in the Head and Neck Unit at Aintree University Hospital in Liverpool, patients undergoing open head and neck surgery with breach of the pharyngeal mucosa were, until recently, prescribed cefuroxime and metronidazole, commencing with induction and followed by three 8-hourly doses. However, to combat rising *C. difficile* infection numbers cefuroxime has been replaced by a single dose of tazocin.

There has also been a huge emphasis on hygiene and cleanliness. Frequent and proper handwashing is encouraged, and alcohol gel is placed strategically in dispensers throughout all clinical areas—although it is recognized that this type of gel will not be active against *C. difficile* spores.

A more contentious area with medical staff is the introduction of a specific dress code. In particular, medical staff are required to comply with having arms bare below the elbows and to avoid wearing a watch or jewellery around the wrist when in clinical areas. In practical terms, this does facilitate proper handwashing between contacts with patients. However, there is a lack of an evidence base for other aspects of dress code such as wearing ties, although such aspects are nevertheless still being encouraged and enforced. The wearing of white coats is no longer acceptable in many UK hospitals.

New hospital medical staff are required to undergo a proper induction course before starting clinical work so that they are informed about local policies and can familiarize themselves with the local hospital rules.

C. difficile Infection

Infection with *C. difficile* is now a significant threat in the hospital environment and has led to prolonged hospital stays for many patients, as well as some deaths.

Pathogenesis. *C. difficile* is carried in 2–3% of adults as a commensal, but in 10–20% of elderly people. It is transmitted directly by hands and from contaminated surfaces. The bacterium is an anaerobic spore-forming Gram-positive bacillus. The spores are very resilient and are resistant to many disinfectants, including alcohol gel, but they are killed by chlorine-releasing disinfectants.

The sequence of events is that a hospitalized patient is exposed to a toxigenic strain of *C. difficile* that colonizes the gut. Infection results when the patient is prescribed an antibiotic that disrupts the normal gut flora and facilitates transformation of spores and proliferation of the clostridial bacterial load. Pathogenic strains produce an enterotoxin (toxin A) and a cytotoxin (toxin B) that bind onto intestinal mucosal cells.

Complications of infection are dehydration, electrolyte imbalance, pseudomembranous colitis, colonic perforation, toxic megacolon, and death.

Risk factors. Certain antibiotics are much more likely to induce this process of events—particularly broad-spectrum antibiotics and clindamycin. This has led to preferred antibiotics being recommended by the local hospital microbiologists and some being available only in exceptional circumstances.

It is not uncommon for patients to be taking protein-pump inhibitors for gastroesophageal reflux before hospital admission. These drugs promote the growth of *C. difficile* and are a significant risk factor for developing infection. Other risk factors are age over 65, a course of antibiotics within 3 months before admission, previous hospitalization, inflammatory bowel disease, and cytotoxic medication.

Clinical features. The diagnostic criteria for infection are liquid feces or toxic megacolon and a positive enzyme immunoassay for *C. difficile* toxin. In mild cases, the patients may only have liquid feces, but the features of a more significant moderate infection include pyrexia, severe abdominal pain, lower gastrointestinal bleeding, and neutrophilia. With severe infection, these features become much worse. Diarrhea is profuse, serum albumin falls, serum lactate rises, and renal dysfunction ensues.

Management. Early diagnosis and treatment is imperative. *C. difficile* infection should be suspected in any in-patient with diarrhea, especially those with more than three liquid bowel movements in 24 h. Such patients should be isolated to a side room within 4 h, and isolation procedures such as handwashing after every contact and use of gloves and aprons should be adopted. The vacated area should be disinfected with hypochlorite solution. Two fecal samples should be sent for culture and detection of the enterotoxin within 4 h, and the infection control team should be contacted.

Treatment should include intravenous hydration. Metronidazole or possibly vancomycin should be administered orally for 10 days. In severe infection, the antibiotics of choice are oral vancomycin or intravenous metronidazole. All patients suspected of having a severe infection should have an urgent abdominal radiograph and intervention from a senior gastroenterologist, surgeon, and microbiologist.

Protein-pump inhibitors and other antibiotics should be stopped after discussion with a microbiologist.

MRSA Infection

MRSA is a significant public health problem in many countries, and the incidence has increased in the UK over the last decade. It has been mandatory to report MRSA bacteremia in the UK since 2001, and rates are now declining. In 2008, all UK hospitals were set a target to reduce their infection rates by 50 %.

Epidemiology. Infection associated with health care is an international problem, and hospital-acquired infection rates range from 5 % to 10 %. However, the reported rates of S. aureus bloodstream infections that represent MRSA vary between different European countries. In 2002, the range of this reported rate was 0.7 % in Sweden and 45 % in Greece (data from the European Antimicrobial Resistance Surveillance System, EARSS).

Public attention has been captured by media reports that have described MRSA as a lethal superbug that resists antibiotics. In reality, MRSA is no more pathogenic than methicillin-sensitive S. aureus (MSSA). Patients have died from bacteremia, but the death rates quoted in the media are often crude estimates that refer to all hospital-acquired infections. In the UK, figures from the Office for National Statistics for 2005 show that MRSA was recorded as contributing to death in 1629 patients and was attributed as the main cause of death in

467 patients. This compares with 7233 patients with MRSA bacteremia during the same period (Health Protection Agency figures).

Risk factors. Infection follows contact from contaminated hands and poor aseptic technique. Otoscopes, marker pens, stethoscopes, and tourniquets have been recognized as potential fomites in the hospital setting. Most affected patients will have colonization rather than infection, but once they are affected, there is a significant potential for spread by contact that may lead to bacteremia in a susceptible patient.

A "Confidential Study of Deaths" following MRSA infection showed that most occurred in elderly patients with significant underlying chronic medical conditions, such as diabetes, renal failure, or immunosuppression. The most frequently identified cause of MRSA bacteremia was via invasive devices such as an intravenous cannula and/or a urinary catheter.

Prevention. The main focus with MRSA has been on prevention; all hospitals will have their own individual policies on how best to approach this. A high standard of hand hygiene is essential. Hospital staff are encouraged to wash their hands between contacts with patients and to use alcohol gel frequently. Aseptic technique protocols must be followed for all procedures, and devices such as cannulas or urinary catheters should be labeled and documented correctly according to the local hospital protocol.

All patients should be screened at preoperative clinics or on hospital admission if they are in high-risk groups. Screening sites include the nose, tracheostomy sites, groin, wounds or sores, stoma sites, intravenous cannula sites, and sputum if expectorating.

Treatment. Patients who have MRSA colonization should bathe or shower with triclosan (Aquasept) or octenidine (Octenisan) for 10 days. Nasal colonization is eradicated by applying mupirocin ointment to the anterior nares three times daily for 5 days. Three sets of negative weekly screens are then required to ensure that colonization is fully controlled.

MRSA bacteremia is treated with intravenous vancomycin or teicoplanin. However, some vancomycin-resistant strains of MRSA are now emerging, and local microbiological advice should be sought.

References and Further Reading

American Joint Committee on Cancer. Greene FL, Page DL, Fleming ID, et al., eds. AJCC Cancer Staging Manual. 6th ed. New York: Springer; 2002

American Joint Committee on Cancer. Greene FL, Page DL, Fleming ID, et al., eds. AJCC Cancer Staging Manual. 6th ed. New York: Springer; 2002

Behrbohm H, Kaschke O, Nawka T. Endoskopische Diagnostik und Therapie in der HNO. Stuttgart: Gustav Fischer;1997.

Behrbohm H, Tardy ME. Essentials of septorhinoplasty. Stuttgart–New York: Thieme; 2004.

Bachert C. Pharmakologische Therapie der Polyposis nasi. Allergologie 2004;27:484–494

Bailey BJ, Johnson JT, Newlands SD. Head and Neck Surgery: Otolaryngology. 4th ed. Philadelphia: Lippincott Williams & Wilkins; 2006

Bohnstedt RM. Krankheitssymptome an der Haut in Beziehung zu Störungen anderer Organe. Stuttgart: Thieme; 1965

Bull T, Almeyda J. Color atlas of ENT Diagnosis. 5th ed. New York: Thieme; 2009

Chandler JR, Langenbrunner DJ, Stevens ER. The pathogenesis of orbital complications in acute sinusitis. Laryngoscope 1970;80(9):1414–14285470225

Committee for Head and Neck Surgery and Oncology, American Academy of Otolaryngology–Head and Neck Surgery. Neck Dissection Classification Committee, American Head and Neck Society. Pocket guide to TNM staging of head and neck cancer and neck dissection classification. Alexandria, VA: American Academy of Otolaryngology–Head and Neck Surgery Foundation, Inc.; 2008. Available from: http://www.entnet.org/EducationAndResearch/NeckDissection.cfm.

Draf W. Endonasal micro-endoscopic frontal sinus surgery: The Fulda concept. Oper Tech Otolaryngol–Head Neck Surg 1991;2:234–240

Fisch U, May JS, Linder T, Porcellini B. Tympanoplasty, Mastoidectomy, and Stapes surgery. 2nd ed. New York: Thieme; 2008

Fokkens W, Lund V, Mullol J; European Position Paper on Rhinosinusitis and Nasal Polyps group. European position paper on rhinosinusitis and nasal polyps 2007. Rhinol Suppl 2007;20(20):1–13617844873

Gleeson MJ, Browning GG, Burton MJ, et al, eds. Scott-Brown's Otorhinolaryngology, Head and Neck Surgery. 7th ed. London: Hodder Arnold; 2008. 3 vols

Gwaltney JM Jr, Jones JG, Kennedy DW; The International Conference on Sinus Disease. Medical management of sinusitis: educational goals and management guidelines. The International Conference on sinus Disease. Ann Otol Rhinol Laryngol Suppl 1995;167: 22–307574266

Harnsberger R, Hudgins P, Wiggins R, Davidson C. Diagnostic Imaging: Head and Neck. Salt Lake City: Amirsys; 2004

Hirano M, Sato K. Histological Color Atlas of the Human Larynx. San Diego: Singular; 1993

Jackler RK, Driscoll CLW. Tumors of the Ear and Temporal Bone. Philadelphia: Lippincott Williams & Wilkins; 2000

Johnson AF, Jacobson BH. Medical Speech-language Pathology: A Practitioner's Guide. New York: Thieme; 2007

Kennedy DW. International Conference on Sinus Disease: Terminology, Staging, Therapy. Ann Otol Rhinol Laryngol 1995; 104(10, Suppl 167)

Kennedy DW, Bolger WE, Zinnreich SF. Diseases of the sinuses – diagnosis and management. Hamilton; BC Decker; 2001.

Lee KJ. Essential Otolaryngology: Head and Neck Surgery. 9th ed. New York: McGraw-Hill; 2008

Luxon LM, Furman JM, Martini A, Stephens D, eds. Textbook of Audiological Medicine: Clinical Aspects of Hearing and Balance. London: Dunitz; 2003

Mafee MF, Valvassori GE, Becker M. Imaging of the Head and Neck. 2nd ed. New York: Thieme; 2005

Messerklinger W. Die Rolle der lateralen Nasenwand in der Pathogenese, Diagnose und Therapie der rezidivierenden und chronischen Rhinosinusitis. Laryngol Rhinol Otol (Stuttg) 1987;66:293–299

Myers EN. Operative Otolaryngology, Head and Neck Surgery. 2nd ed. Philadelphia: Saunders; 2008

Naumann HH, Tardy ME, Kastenbauer ER, eds. Head and Neck Surgery. New York: Thieme; 1995–1998. 3 vols

Papel ID. Facial Plastic and Reconstructive Surgery. 3 rd ed. New York: Thieme; 2009

Probst R, Grevers G, Iro H. Basic Otorhinolaryngology: A Step-by-step Learning Guide. New York: Thieme; 2006

Remacle M, Eckel HE, Antonelli A, . Endoscopic cordectomy. A proposal for a classification by the Working Committee, European Laryngological Society. Eur Arch Otorhinolaryngol 2000;257(4):227–23110867840

Remacle M, Van Haverbeke C, Eckel H, . Proposal for revision of the European Laryngological Society classification of endoscopic cordectomies. Eur Arch Otorhinolaryngol 2007;264(5):499–50417377801

Robbins KT. Classification of neck dissection: current concepts and future considerations. Otolaryngol Clin North Am 1998;31(4):639–6559687326

Robbins KT, Medina JE, Wolfe GT, Levine PA, Sessions RB, Pruet CW. Standardizing neck dissection terminology. Official report of the Academy's Committee for Head and Neck Surgery and Oncology. Arch Otolaryngol Head Neck Surg 1991;117(6):601–6052036180

Robbins KT, Clayman G, Levine PA, ; American Head and Neck Society; American Academy of Otolaryngology—Head and Neck Surgery. Neck dissection classification update: revisions proposed by the American Head and Neck Society and the American Academy of Otolaryngology-Head and Neck Surgery. Arch Otolaryngol Head Neck Surg 2002;128(7):751–75812117328

Royal College of Surgeons of England, Clinical Effectiveness Unit. National Prospective Tonsillectomy Audit: final report of an audit carried out in England and Northern Ireland between July 2003 and September 2004. London: Royal College of Surgeons of England; 2005. Available at: http://www.rcseng.ac.uk/publications/docs/national_prospective.html/attachment_download/pdffile.

Sanna M. The Temporal Bone: A Manual for Dissection and Surgical Approaches. New York: Thieme; 2006

Sataloff RT. Professional Voice: The Science and Art of Clinical Care. 3 rd ed. San Diego: Plural; 2005

Schuenke M, Schulte E, Schumacher U, Ross LM, Lamperti ED. Thieme Atlas of Anatomy: Neck and Internal Organs [DVD]. New York: Thieme; 2007

Schuenke M, Schulte E, Schumacher U, Ross LM, Lamperti ED. Thieme Atlas of Anatomy: Head and Neuroanatomy [DVD]. New York: Thieme; 2008

Seiden AM, Tami TA, Pensak ML, Cotton RT, Gluckman JL. Otolaryngology: The Essentials. New York: Thieme; 2002

Shah JP. Head and Neck Surgery and Oncology. 3 rd ed. Philadelphia: Mosby; 2003

Simmen D, Jones NS. Manual of Endoscopic Sinus Surgery and its Extended Applications. New York: Thieme; 2005

Stammberger H. Endoscopic endonasal surgery: concepts in treatment of recurring rhinosinusitis, part I: anatomic and pathologic considerations. Otolaryngol Head Neck Surg 1986;94:143–146

Stammberger H. Endoscopic endonasal surgery: concepts in treatment of recurring rhinosinusitis, part II: surgical technique. Otolaryngol Head Neck Surg 1986;94:147–156

Stammberger H. Functional endoscopic sinus surgery. Philadephia: BC Decker; 1991.

Stammberger H, Posawetz W. Functional endoscopic sinus surgery. Concept, indications and results of Messerklinger technique. Eur Arch Otorhinolaryngol 1989;247:63–76

UICC/International Union Against Cancer. Sobin LH, Wittekind C, eds. TNM Classification of Malignant Tumours. 6th ed. New York: Wiley-Liss; 2002

von Lanz T, Wachsmuth W. Praktische Anatomie. Eine Lehr- und Hilfsbuch der Anatomischen Grundlagen ärztlichen Handelns. 2nd ed. Berlin: Springer; 1950

Weerda H. Surgery of the Auricle: Tumors—Traum—Defects—Abnormalities. New York: Thieme; 2007

Wigand M. Endoscopic Surgery of the Paranasal Sinuses and Anterior Skull Base. 2nd ed. New York: Thieme 2008

Bousquet J, Van Cauwenberge P, Khaltaev N; Aria Workshop Group; World Health Organization. Allergic rhinitis and its impact on asthma. J Allergy Clin Immunol 2001; 108(5, Suppl)S147–S33411707753

World Health Organization (WHO). Allergic rhinitis and its impact on asthma. Geneva: World Health Organization; 2008. Available at: http://www.guidelines.gov/.

World Health Organization (WHO). Swerdlow SH, Campo E, Harris NL, et al. WHO Classification of Tumours of Haematopoietic and Lymphoid Tissues. 4th ed. Lyons: International Agency for Research on Cancer; 2008. (WHO classification of tumours, vol. 2)

Wormald PJ. Endoscopic Sinus Surgery: Anatomy, Three-dimensional Reconstruction, and Surgical Technique. 2nd ed. Stuttgart, New York: Thieme Publishers; 2008

Subject Index

Page numbers in *italics* denote figures and those in **bold** denote tables

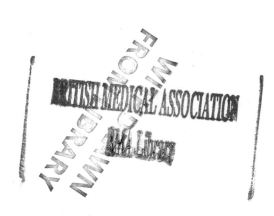